CLINICAL NEUROANATOMY FOR MEDICAL STUDENTS

By the Same Author:

Atlas of Clinical Anatomy
Gross Anatomy Dissector
Clinical Anatomy: A Review with Questions and Explanations
Clinical and Functional Histology for Medical Students
Clinical Anatomy for Medical Students, Sixth Edition
Clinical Neuroanatomy: A Review with Questions and Explanations, Third Edition

Translation:

Clinical Neuroanatomy for Medical Students, Spanish Edition 1999
Editorial Medica Pan Americana S.A.

CLINICAL NEUROANATOMY FOR MEDICAL STUDENTS

FIFTH EDITION

Richard S. Snell, M.D., Ph.D.
Emeritus Professor of Anatomy
George Washington University
School of Medicine and Health Sciences
Washington, D.C.

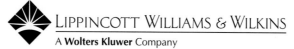
LIPPINCOTT WILLIAMS & WILKINS
A **Wolters Kluwer** Company
Philadelphia • Baltimore • New York • London
Buenos Aires • Hong Kong • Sydney • Tokyo

Editor: Rob Anthony
Managing Editor: Ulita Lushnycky
Marketing Manager: Aimee Sirmon
Production Manager: Susan Rockwell

Library of Congress Cataloging-in-Publication Data

Snell, Richard S.
  Clinical neuroanatomy for medical students / Richard S. Snell.—5th ed.
    p. ; cm.
  Includes bibliographical references and index.
  ISBN 0–7817–2831–2
    1. Neuroanatomy. I. Title
  [DNLM: 1. Nervous System—anatomy & histology. WL 101 S671c 2001]
  QM451 .S64 2001
  616.8—dc21

                                                          00–047789

01 02 03
1 2 3 4 5 6 7 8 9 10

To My Students——Past, Present, and Future

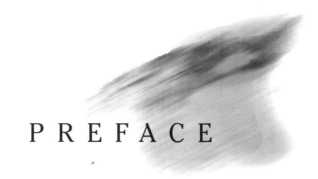

PREFACE

This book provides the basic neuroanatomical facts necessary for the practice of medicine. It is designed for first and second year medical students, dental students, and allied health students. Neurological residents have found the book to be of great help during their rotations.

The information provides students with an understanding of the functional organization of the nervous system and clearly indicates how injury and disease can result in neurological deficits. The book prepares the student to interpret the many symptoms and signs presented by a neurological patient so that he or she may confidently make a diagnosis, and, where possible, institute appropriate treatment. **The amount of factual information has been strictly limited to that which is clinically important.** This is not a book for the Basic Neuroscientist in training.

As we enter the second millenium, with the explosion of knowledge of the normal and pathophysiological structure of the nervous system, faculty and students should pause and seriously consider what information is strictly necessary for the diagnosis and treatment of patients. Gone are the days when students were presented with masses of detail involving complicated neural connections, which not only confused the student but prevented them from recalling the essential features at the bedside.

The fifth edition has been substantially reorganized. Many of the topics have been grouped together to avoid repetition and many duplicated figures have been eliminated. The content of each chapter has been updated, obsolete material discarded and new material added.

As in the previous edition, the design of each chapter allows the reader easy access and fast retrieval of information. Each chapter is divided into the following categories:

1. **Clinical Example.** A short case report that serves to dramatize the relevance of neuroanatomy introduces each chapter.
2. **Chapter Outline.** A list of selected headings with page numbers is provided so that immediate access is possible. This information is supplied in addition to the detailed index at the end of the book.
3. **Chapter Objectives.** This section details the material that is most important to learn and understand in each chapter. It emphasizes the basic information in the area being studied. This section also points out information on which examiners have repeatedly asked questions in national examinations.
4. **Basic Neuroanatomy.** This section provides basic information on neuroanatomical structures that are of clinical importance. Numerous examples of normal radiographs, CT scans, MRIs, and PET scans are also provided. Many cross-sectional diagrams have been included to stimulate students to think in terms of three-dimensional anatomy, which is so important in the interpretation of CT scans and MR images.
5. **Clinical Notes.** This section provides the practical application of neuroanatomical facts that are essential in clinical practice. It emphasizes the structures that the physician will encounter when making a diagnosis and treating a patient. It also provides the information necessary to understand many procedures and techniques and notes the anatomical "pitfalls" commonly encountered.
6. **Clinical Problem Solving.** This section provides the student with many examples of clinical situations in which a knowledge of neuroanatomy is necessary to solve clinical problems and to institute treatment; solutions to the problems are provided at the end of the chapter.

7. **Review Questions.** The purpose of the questions is threefold: to focus attention on areas of importance, to enable students to assess their areas of weakness, and to provide a form of self-evaluation when questions are answered under examination conditions. Some of the questions are centered around a clinical problem that requires a neuroanatomical answer. Solutions to the problem are provided at the end of each chapter.

The book is extensively illustrated. The majority of the figures have been kept simple; color has been used throughout this book. The number of tables in this edition has been increased. References to neuroanatomical literature are included should readers wish to acquire a deeper knowledge of an area of interest.

R.S.S.

ACKNOWLEDGMENTS

I am greatly indebted to the following colleagues who provided me with photographic examples of neuroanatomical material: Dr. N. Cauna, Emeritus Professor of Anatomy, University of Pittsburgh School of Medicine; Dr. F. M. J. Fitzgerald, Professor of Anatomy, University College, Galway, Ireland; and Dr. A. Peters, Professor of Anatomy, Boston University School of Medicine.

I am also grateful to members of the Department of Radiology at the George Washington University School of Medicine and Health Sciences for the loan of radiographs and CT scans that have been reproduced in different sections of this book. I am most grateful to Dr. G. Size of the Department of Radiology at Yale University Medical Center for examples of CT scans and MR images of the brain. I also thank Dr. H. Dey, Director of the Pet Scan Unit of the Department of Radiology, Veterans Affairs Medical Center, West Haven, CT, for several examples of Pet scans of the brain. I thank the Medical Photographers of the Department of Radiology at Yale for their excellent work in reproducing the radiographs.

As in the past, I express my sincere thanks to Mya Feldman and Ira Grunther, AMI, for the preparation of the very fine artwork.

Finally, to the staff of Lippincott Williams and Wilkins, I express my deep appreciation for their continued enthusiasm and support throughout the preparation of this book.

CONTENTS

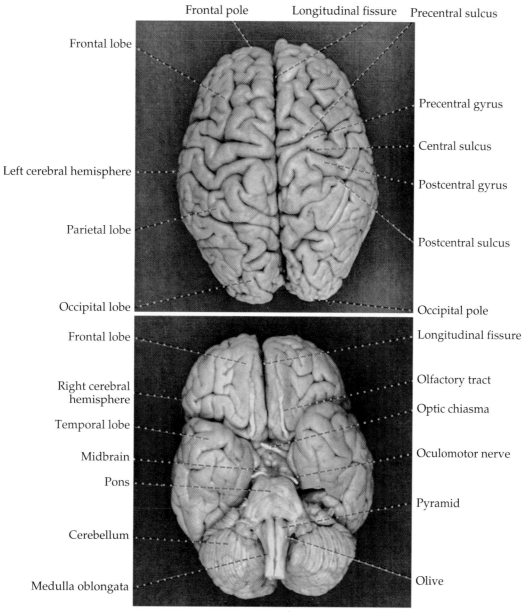

Fig. P–1. **Top**. Superior view of the brain. **Bottom**. Inferior view of the brain.

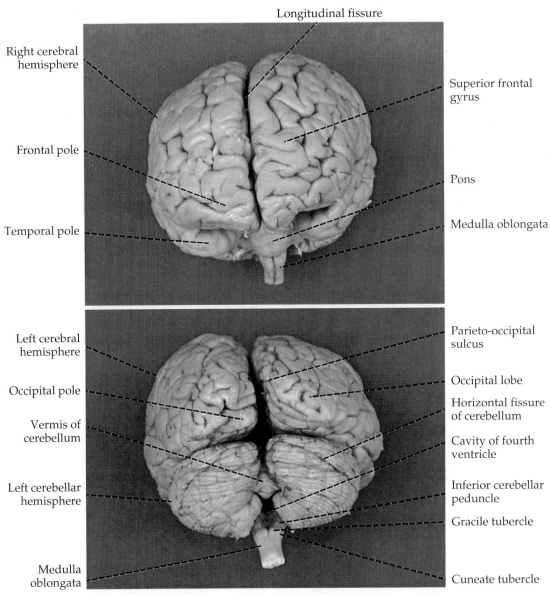

Longitudinal fissure

Right cerebral hemisphere

Superior frontal gyrus

Frontal pole

Pons

Temporal pole

Medulla oblongata

Left cerebral hemisphere

Parieto-occipital sulcus

Occipital pole

Occipital lobe

Vermis of cerebellum

Horizontal fissure of cerebellum

Cavity of fourth ventricle

Left cerebellar hemisphere

Inferior cerebellar peduncle

Gracile tubercle

Medulla oblongata

Cuneate tubercle

Fig. P–2. **Top**. Anterior view of the brain. **Bottom**. Posterior view of the brain.

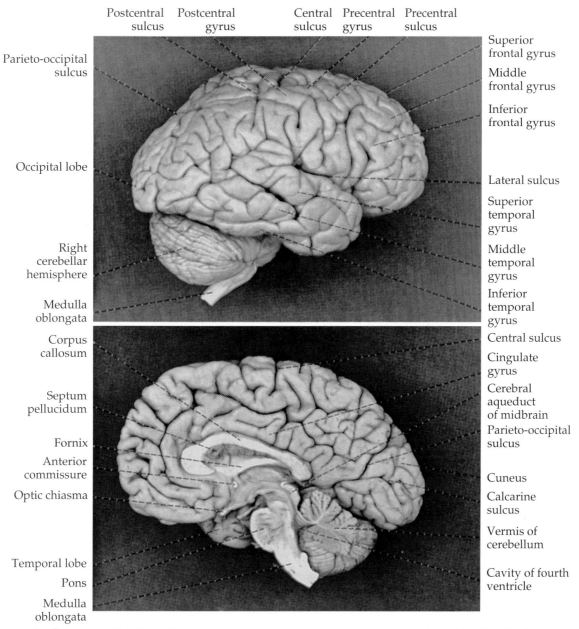

Postcentral sulcus   Postcentral gyrus   Central sulcus   Precentral gyrus   Precentral sulcus

Parieto-occipital sulcus

Occipital lobe

Right cerebellar hemisphere

Medulla oblongata

Corpus callosum

Septum pellucidum

Fornix

Anterior commissure

Optic chiasma

Temporal lobe

Pons

Medulla oblongata

Superior frontal gyrus

Middle frontal gyrus

Inferior frontal gyrus

Lateral sulcus

Superior temporal gyrus

Middle temporal gyrus

Inferior temporal gyrus

Central sulcus

Cingulate gyrus

Cerebral aqueduct of midbrain

Parieto-occipital sulcus

Cuneus

Calcarine sulcus

Vermis of cerebellum

Cavity of fourth ventricle

Fig. P–3. **Top**. Right lateral view of the brain. **Bottom**. Medial view of the right side of the brain following median sagittal section.

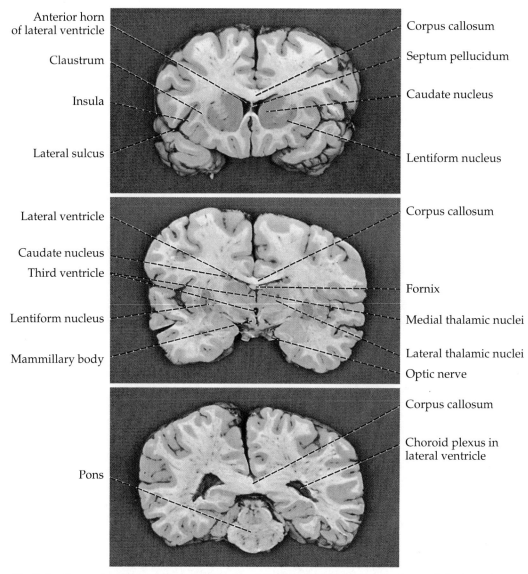

Fig. P–4. Coronal sections of the brain passing through (**Top**) the anterior horn of the lateral ventricle, (**Middle**) the mammillary bodies, and (**Bottom**) the pons.

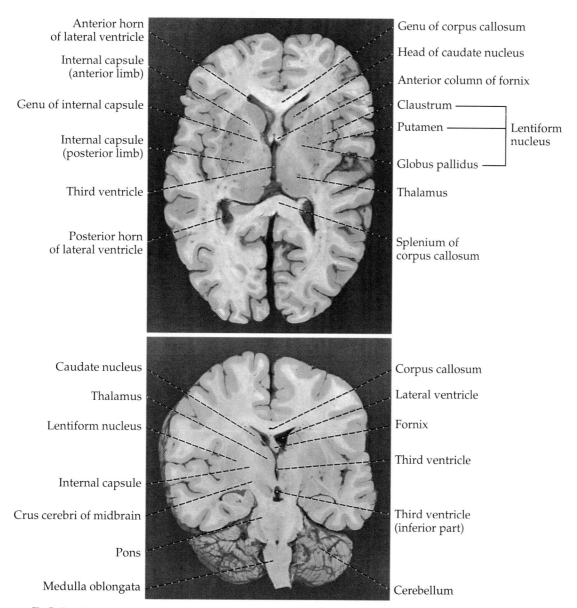

Anterior horn of lateral ventricle

Internal capsule (anterior limb)

Genu of internal capsule

Internal capsule (posterior limb)

Third ventricle

Posterior horn of lateral ventricle

Genu of corpus callosum

Head of caudate nucleus

Anterior column of fornix

Claustrum

Putamen

Globus pallidus

Lentiform nucleus

Thalamus

Splenium of corpus callosum

Caudate nucleus

Thalamus

Lentiform nucleus

Internal capsule

Crus cerebri of midbrain

Pons

Medulla oblongata

Corpus callosum

Lateral ventricle

Fornix

Third ventricle

Third ventricle (inferior part)

Cerebellum

Fig P–5. **Top**. Horizontal section of the cerebrum showing the lentiform nucleus, the caudate nucleus, the thalamus, and the internal capsule. **Bottom**. Oblique coronal section of the brain.

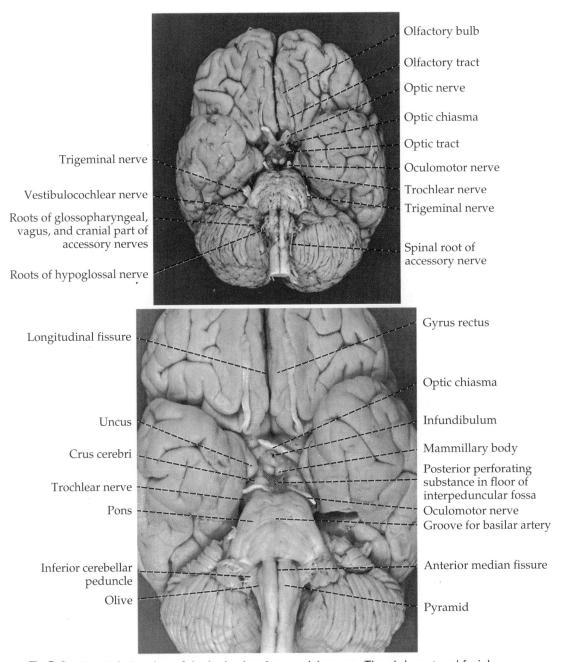

Olfactory bulb

Olfactory tract

Optic nerve

Optic chiasma

Optic tract

Oculomotor nerve

Trochlear nerve

Trigeminal nerve

Spinal root of
accessory nerve

Trigeminal nerve

Vestibulocochlear nerve

Roots of glossopharyngeal,
vagus, and cranial part of
accessory nerves

Roots of hypoglossal nerve

Longitudinal fissure

Gyrus rectus

Optic chiasma

Uncus

Infundibulum

Crus cerebri

Mammillary body

Trochlear nerve

Posterior perforating
substance in floor of
interpeduncular fossa

Pons

Oculomotor nerve

Groove for basilar artery

Inferior cerebellar
peduncle

Anterior median fissure

Olive

Pyramid

Fig. P–6. **Top**. Inferior view of the brain showing cranial nerves. The abducent and facial nerves cannot be seen. **Bottom**. Enlarged inferior view of the central part of the brain.

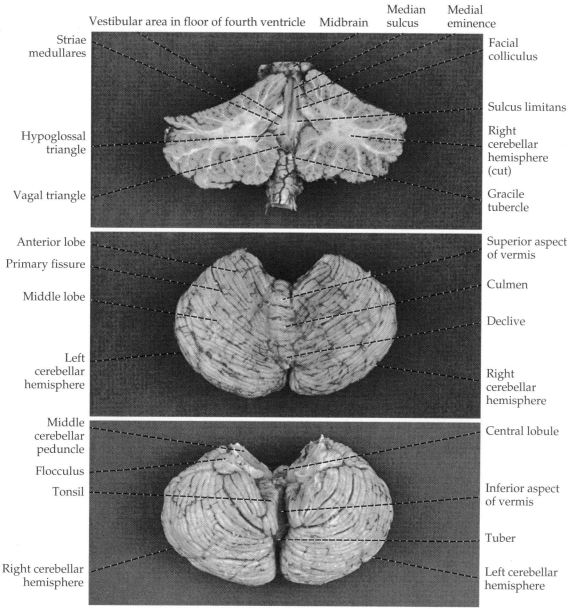

Fig. P–7. **Top**. Posterior view of the brainstem. The greater part of the cerebellum had been removed to expose the floor of the fourth ventricle. **Middle**. Superior view of the cerebellum showing the vermis and right and left cerebellar hemispheres. **Bottom**. Inferior view of the cerebellum showing the vermis and right and left cerebellar hemispheres.

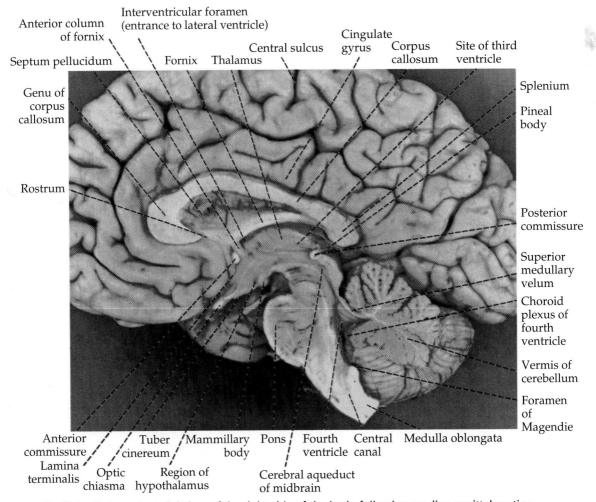

Anterior column of fornix

Interventricular foramen (entrance to lateral ventricle)

Septum pellucidum

Fornix

Thalamus

Central sulcus

Cingulate gyrus

Corpus callosum

Site of third ventricle

Genu of corpus callosum

Rostrum

Splenium

Pineal body

Posterior commissure

Superior medullary velum

Choroid plexus of fourth ventricle

Vermis of cerebellum

Foramen of Magendie

Anterior commissure

Lamina terminalis

Optic chiasma

Tuber cinereum

Region of hypothalamus

Mammillary body

Pons

Fourth ventricle

Central canal

Medulla oblongata

Cerebral aqueduct of midbrain

Fig. P–8. Enlarged medial view of the right side of the brain following median sagittal section, showing the continuity of the central canal, fourth ventricle, cerebral aqueduct, and the third ventricle and entrance into the lateral ventricle through the interventricular foramen.

CHAPTER 1

Introduction and Organization of the Nervous System

A 23-year-old student was driving home from a party and crashed his car head-on into a tree. On examination in the emergency department of the local hospital, he had a fracture dislocation of the seventh thoracic vertebra, with signs and symptoms of severe damage to the spinal cord. Later, he was found to have paralysis of the left leg. Testing of cutaneous sensibility revealed a band of cutaneous hyperesthesia (increased sensitivity) extending around the abdominal wall on the left side at the level of the umbilicus. Just below this, he had a narrow band of anesthesia and analgesia. On the right side, he had total analgesia, thermoanesthesia, and partial loss of the sensation of touch of the skin of the abdominal wall below the level of the umbilicus and involving the whole of the right leg.

With his or her knowledge of anatomy, a physician knows that a fracture dislocation of the seventh thoracic vertebra would result in severe damage to the tenth thoracic segment of the spinal cord. Because of the small size of the vertebral foramen in the thoracic region, such an injury inevitably results in damage to the spinal cord. Knowledge of the vertebral levels of the various segments of the spinal cord enables the physician to determine the likely neurologic deficits. The unequal sensory and motor losses on the two sides indicate a left hemisection of the cord. The band of anesthesia and analgesia was caused by the destruction of the cord on the left side at the level of the tenth thoracic segment; all afferent nerve fibers entering the cord at that point were interrupted. The loss of pain and thermal sensibilities and the loss of light touch below the level of the umbilicus on the right side were caused by the interruption of the lateral and anterior spinothalamic tracts on the left side of the cord.

To comprehend what has happened to this patient, a knowledge of the relationship between the spinal cord and its surrounding vertebral column must be understood. The various neurologic deficits will become easier to understand after the reader has learned how the nervous pathways pass up and down the spinal cord. This information will be discussed in Chapter 4.

C H A P T E R   O U T L I N E

C H A P T E R   O B J E C T I V E S

It is essential that students, at the very outset of their studies of neuroanatomy, understand the basic organization of the main structures that form the nervous system. A three-dimensional appreciation of the parts of the brain and their relative positions to one another is a must before one considers the maze of neuronal circuitries that must be understood to localize and diagnose neurologic problems. Geographically, one would not contemplate starting a journey unless one first studied a map. This is the objective of Chapter 1.

INTRODUCTION

The nervous system and the endocrine system control the functions of the body. The nervous system is composed basically of specialized cells, whose function is to receive sensory stimuli and to transmit them to effector organs, whether muscular or glandular (Fig. 1-1). The sensory stimuli that arise either outside or inside the body are correlated within the nervous system, and the efferent impulses are coordinated so that the effector organs work harmoniously together for the well-being of the individual. In addition, the nervous system of higher species has the ability to store sensory information received during past experiences; and this information, when appropriate, is integrated with other nervous impulses and channeled into the common efferent pathway.

CENTRAL AND PERIPHERAL NERVOUS SYSTEMS

The nervous system is divided into two main parts, for purposes of description: the **central nervous system** (Fig. 1-2A), which consists of the brain and spinal cord, and the **peripheral nervous system** (Fig. 1-2B), which consists of the cranial and spinal nerves and their associated ganglia (Box 1-1).

In the central nervous system, the brain and spinal cord are the main centers where correlation and integration of nervous information occur. Both the brain and spinal cord are covered with membranes, the **meninges,** and are suspended in the **cerebrospinal fluid;** they are further protected by the bones of the skull and the vertebral column (Fig. 1-3).

The central nervous system is composed of large numbers of excitable nerve cells and their processes, called **neurons,** which are supported by specialized tissue called **neuroglia** (Fig. 1-4). The long processes of a nerve cell are called **axons** or **nerve fibers.**

The interior of the central nervous system is organized into gray and white matter. **Gray matter** consists of nerve cells embedded in neuroglia; it has a gray color. **White matter** consists of nerve fibers embedded in neuroglia; it has a white color due to the presence of lipid material in the myelin sheaths of many of the nerve fibers.

In the peripheral nervous system, the cranial and spinal nerves, which consist of bundles of nerve fibers or axons, conduct information to and from the central nervous sys-

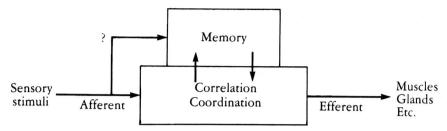

Figure 1–1 The relationship of afferent sensory stimuli to memory bank, correlation and coordinating centers, and common efferent pathway.

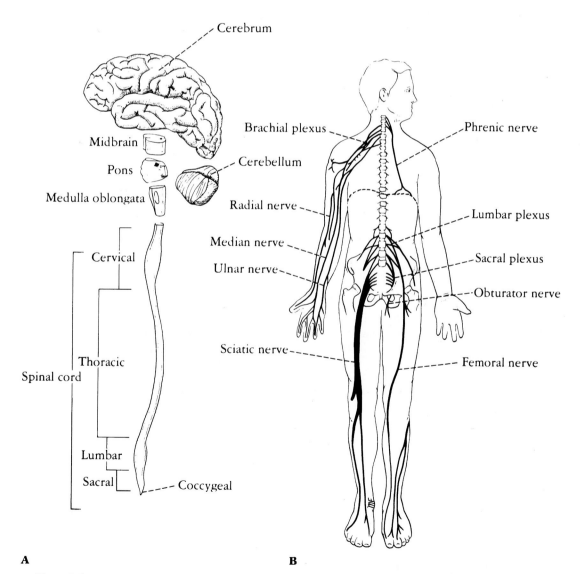

A   **B**

Figure 1–2 **A.** The main divisions of the central nervous system. **B.** The parts of the peripheral nervous system (the cranial nerves have been omitted).

Box 1–1   Major Divisions of the Central and Peripheral Nervous Systems

Central Nervous System

Brain
  Forebrain
    Cerebrum
    Diencephalon (between brain)
  Midbrain
  Hindbrain
    Medulla oblongata
    Pons
    Cerebellum
Spinal cord
  Cervical segments
  Thoracic segments
  Lumbar segments
  Sacral segments
  Coccygeal segments

Peripheral Nervous System

Cranial nerves and their ganglia—12 pairs that exit the skull through the foramina
Spinal nerves and their ganglia—31 pairs that exit the vertebral column through the intervertebral foramina
  8 Cervical
  12 Thoracic
  5 Lumbar
  5 Sacral
  1 Coccygeal

tem. Although surrounded by fibrous sheaths as they run to different parts of the body, they are relatively unprotected and are commonly damaged by trauma.

Autonomic Nervous System

The autonomic nervous system is the part of the nervous system concerned with the innervation of involuntary structures, such as the heart, smooth muscle, and glands within the body. It is distributed throughout the central and peripheral nervous systems. The autonomic system may be divided into two parts, the **sympathetic** and the **parasympathetic,** and in both parts there are afferent and efferent nerve fibers. The activities of the sympathetic part of the autonomic system prepare the body for an emergency. The activities of the parasympathetic part of the autonomic system are aimed at conserving and restoring energy.

MAJOR DIVISIONS OF THE CENTRAL NERVOUS SYSTEM

Before proceeding to a detailed description of the spinal cord and brain, it is essential to understand the main features of these structures and their general relationship to one another.

Spinal Cord

The spinal cord is situated within the **vertebral canal** of the vertebral column and is surrounded by three meninges (Figs. 1-3A and 1-6): the **dura mater,** the **arachnoid mater,** and the **pia mater.** Further protection is provided by the **cerebrospinal fluid,** which surrounds the spinal cord in the **subarachnoid space.**

The spinal cord is roughly cylindrical (Fig. 1-6) and begins superiorly at the foramen magnum in the skull, where it is continuous with the **medulla oblongata** of the brain (Figs. 1-5 and 1-6). It terminates inferiorly in the lumbar region. Below, the spinal cord tapers off into the **conus medullaris,** from the apex of which a prolongation of the pia mater, the **filum terminale,** descends to attach to the back of the coccyx (Fig. 1-5B).

Along the entire length of the spinal cord are attached 31 pairs of spinal nerves by the **anterior** or **motor roots** and the **posterior** or **sensory roots** (Figs. 1-6 and 1-7). Each root is attached to the cord by a series of rootlets, which extend the whole length of the corresponding segment of the cord. Each posterior nerve root possesses a **posterior root ganglion,** the cells of which give rise to peripheral and central nerve fibers.

STRUCTURE OF THE SPINAL CORD

The spinal cord is composed of an inner core of **gray matter,** which is surrounded by an outer covering of **white matter** (Fig. 1-7). The gray matter is seen on cross section as an H-shaped pillar with **anterior** and **posterior gray columns,** or **horns,** united by a thin **gray commissure** containing the small **central canal.** The white matter, for purposes of description, may be divided into **anterior, lateral,** and **posterior white columns** (Fig. 1-7).

Brain

The brain lies in the cranial cavity and is continuous with the spinal cord through the foramen magnum (Fig. 1-6A). It is surrounded by three meninges (Fig. 1-3): the **dura mater,** the **arachnoid mater,** and the **pia mater,** and these are continuous with the corresponding meninges of the spinal cord. The cerebrospinal fluid surrounds the brain in the subarachnoid space.

The brain is conventionally divided into three major divisions. These are, in ascending order from the spinal cord, the **hindbrain,** the **midbrain,** and the **forebrain.** The hindbrain may be subdivided into the **medulla oblongata,** the **pons,** and the **cerebellum.** The forebrain may also be subdivided into the **diencephalon** (between brain), which is the central part of the forebrain, and the **cerebrum.** The **brainstem** (a collective term for the medulla oblongata, pons, and midbrain) is that part of the brain that remains after the cerebral hemispheres and cerebellum are removed.

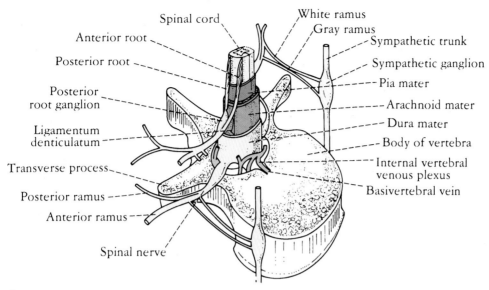

Spinal cord
White ramus
Gray ramus
Anterior root
Posterior root
Sympathetic trunk
Sympathetic ganglion
Pia mater
Posterior root ganglion
Arachnoid mater
Dura mater
Ligamentum denticulatum
Body of vertebra
Transverse process
Internal vertebral venous plexus
Posterior ramus
Basivertebral vein
Anterior ramus
Spinal nerve

A

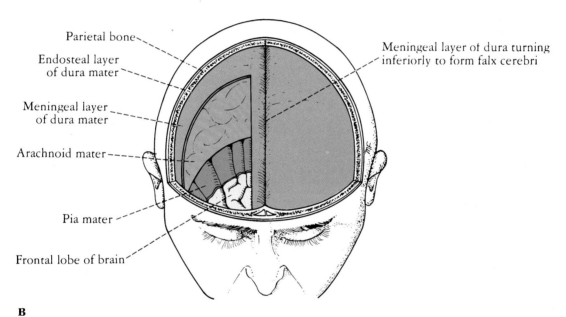

Parietal bone
Endosteal layer of dura mater
Meningeal layer of dura turning inferiorly to form falx cerebri
Meningeal layer of dura mater
Arachnoid mater
Pia mater
Frontal lobe of brain

B

Figure 1–3 **A.** Protective coverings of the spinal cord. **B.** Protective coverings of the brain.

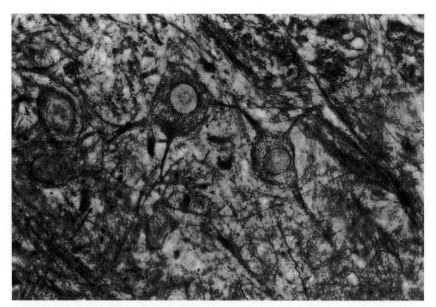

Figure 1–4 Photomicrograph of several large nerve cells with surrounding neuroglia.

HINDBRAIN
Medulla Oblongata

The medulla oblongata is conical in shape and connects the pons superiorly to the spinal cord inferiorly (Fig.1-9). It contains many collections of neurons, called **nuclei,** and serves as a conduit for ascending and descending nerve fibers.

Pons

The pons is situated on the anterior surface of the cerebellum, inferior to the midbrain and superior to the medulla oblongata (Figs. 1-9 and 1-10). The pons, or bridge, derives its name from the large number of transverse fibers on its anterior aspect connecting the two cerebellar hemispheres. It also contains many nuclei and ascending and descending nerve fibers.

Cerebellum

The cerebellum lies within the posterior cranial fossa (Figs.1-8,1-9, and 1-10), posterior to the pons and the medulla oblongata. It consists of two hemispheres connected by a median portion, the **vermis.** The cerebellum is connected to the midbrain by the **superior cerebellar peduncles,** to the pons by the **middle cerebellar peduncles,** and to the medulla by the **inferior cerebellar peduncles** (see Fig. 6-9). The peduncles are composed of large bundles of nerve fibers connecting the cerebellum to the remainder of the nervous system.

The surface layer of each cerebellar hemisphere is called the **cortex** and is composed of gray matter (Fig. 1-12). The cerebellar cortex is thrown into folds, or folia, separated by closely set transverse fissures. Certain masses of gray matter are found in the interior of the cerebellum, embedded in the white matter; the largest of these is known as the **dentate nucleus** (see Fig.6-7).

The medulla oblongata, the pons, and the cerebellum surround a cavity filled with cerebrospinal fluid, called the **fourth ventricle.** This is connected superiorly to the third ventricle by the **cerebral aqueduct,** and inferiorly it is continuous with the central canal of the spinal cord (Figs.1-11 and 1-12). It communicates with the subarachnoid space through three openings in the inferior part of the roof. It is through these openings that the cerebrospinal fluid within the central nervous system can enter the subarachnoid space.

MIDBRAIN

The midbrain is the narrow part of the brain that connects the forebrain to the hindbrain (Figs. 1-2A and 1-11). The narrow cavity of the midbrain is the **cerebral aqueduct,** which connects the third and fourth ventricles (Fig. 1-11). The midbrain contains many nuclei and bundles of ascending and descending nerve fibers.

DIENCEPHALON

The diencephalon is almost completely hidden from the surface of the brain. It consists of a dorsal **thalamus** and a ventral **hypothalamus** (Fig. 1-11). The thalamus is a large egg-shaped mass of gray matter that lies on either side of the third ventricle. The anterior end of the thalamus forms the posterior boundary of the **interventricular foramen,** the opening between the third and lateral ventricles (Fig. 1-11). The hypothalamus forms the lower part of the lateral wall and floor of the third ventricle (Fig. 1-11).

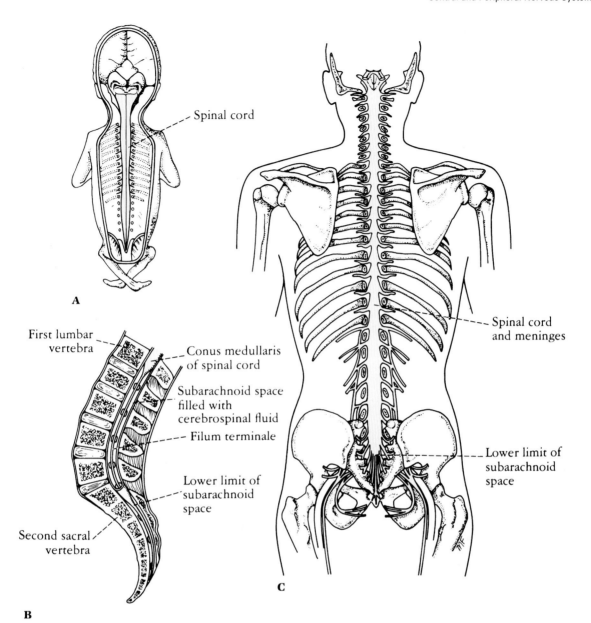

Spinal cord

A

First lumbar vertebra

Conus medullaris of spinal cord

Subarachnoid space filled with cerebrospinal fluid

Filum terminale

Lower limit of subarachnoid space

Second sacral vertebra

B

Spinal cord and meninges

Lower limit of subarachnoid space

C

Figure 1–5   A. Fetus with the brain and spinal cord exposed on the posterior surface. Note that the spinal cord extends the full length of the vertebral column. **B.** Sagittal section of the vertebral column in an adult, showing the spinal cord terminating inferiorly at the level of the lower border of the first lumbar vertebra. **C.** Adult spinal cord and covering meninges, showing the relationship to surrounding structures.

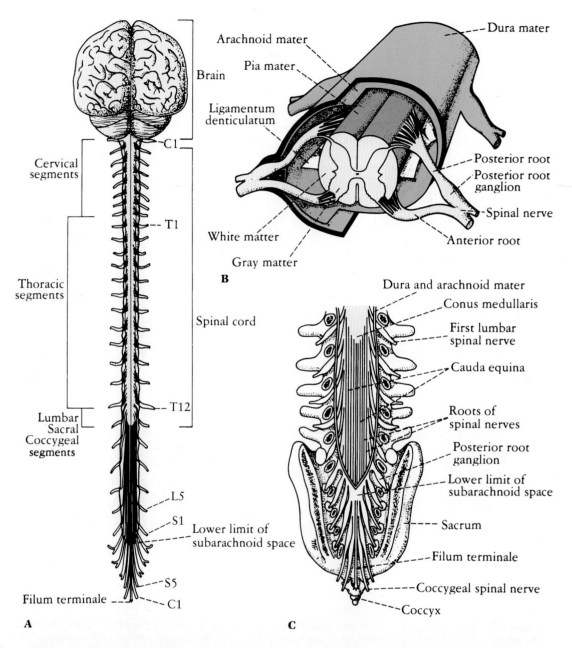

Figure 1–6 A. Brain, spinal cord, spinal nerve roots, and spinal nerves as seen on their posterior aspect. **B.** Transverse section through the thoracic region of the spinal cord, showing the anterior and posterior roots of a spinal nerve and the meninges. **C.** Posterior view of the lower end of the spinal cord and cauda equina, showing their relationship with the lumbar vertebrae, sacrum, and coccyx.

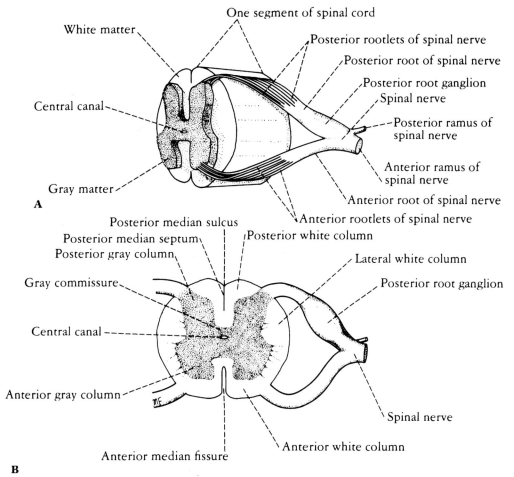

Figure 1–7 **A.** Transverse section through the lumbar part of the spinal cord, oblique view. **B.** Transverse section through the lumbar part of the spinal cord, face view, showing the anterior and posterior roots of a spinal nerve.

CEREBRUM

The cerebrum, the largest part of the brain, consists of two cerebral hemispheres, which are connected by a mass of white matter called the **corpus callosum** (Figs. 1-10, and 1-11). Each hemisphere extends from the frontal to the occipital bones, superior to the anterior and middle cranial fossae; posteriorly, the cerebrum lies above the tentorium cerebelli (See Fig. 15-3). The hemispheres are separated by a deep cleft, the **longitudinal fissure,** into which projects the **falx cerebri** (See Fig. 15-1).

The surface layer of each hemisphere, the **cortex,** is composed of gray matter. The cerebral cortex is thrown into folds, or **gyri,** separated by fissures, or **sulci** (Fig.1-10). The surface area of the cortex is greatly increased by this means. A number of the large sulci are conveniently used to subdivide the surface of each hemisphere into **lobes.** The lobes are named from the bones of the cranium under which they lie.

Within the hemisphere is a central core of white matter, containing several large masses of gray matter, the **basal nuclei** or **ganglia.** A fan-shaped collection of nerve fibers, termed the **corona radiata** (Fig.1-13), passes in the white matter to and from the cerebral cortex to the brainstem. The corona radiata converges on the basal nuclei and passes between them as the **internal capsule.** The tailed nucleus situated on the medial side of the internal capsule is referred to as the **caudate nucleus** (Fig.1-14) and the lens-shaped nucleus on the lateral side of the internal capsule is called the **lentiform nucleus.**

The cavity present within each cerebral hemisphere is called the **lateral ventricle** (See Fig. 16-2 and 16-3). The lateral ventricles communicate with the third ventricle through the **interventricular foramina.**

During the process of development, the cerebrum becomes enormously enlarged and overhangs the diencephalon, the midbrain, and the hindbrain.

Text continued on p. 13

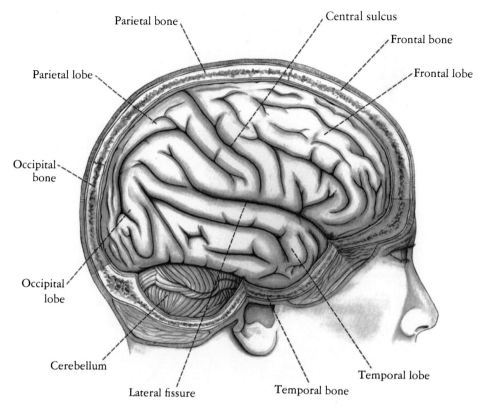

Parietal bone

Central sulcus

Frontal bone

Frontal lobe

Parietal lobe

Occipital bone

Occipital lobe

Cerebellum

Lateral fissure

Temporal bone

Temporal lobe

Figure 1–8   Lateral view of the brain within the skull.

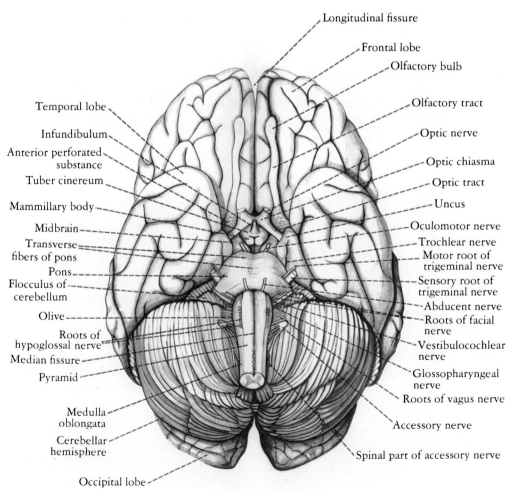

Longitudinal fissure

Frontal lobe

Olfactory bulb

Olfactory tract

Temporal lobe

Infundibulum

Anterior perforated substance

Tuber cinereum

Mammillary body

Midbrain

Transverse fibers of pons

Pons

Flocculus of cerebellum

Olive

Roots of hypoglossal nerve

Median fissure

Pyramid

Medulla oblongata

Cerebellar hemisphere

Occipital lobe

Optic nerve

Optic chiasma

Optic tract

Uncus

Oculomotor nerve

Trochlear nerve

Motor root of trigeminal nerve

Sensory root of trigeminal nerve

Abducent nerve

Roots of facial nerve

Vestibulocochlear nerve

Glossopharyngeal nerve

Roots of vagus nerve

Accessory nerve

Spinal part of accessory nerve

Figure 1–9   Inferior view of the brain.

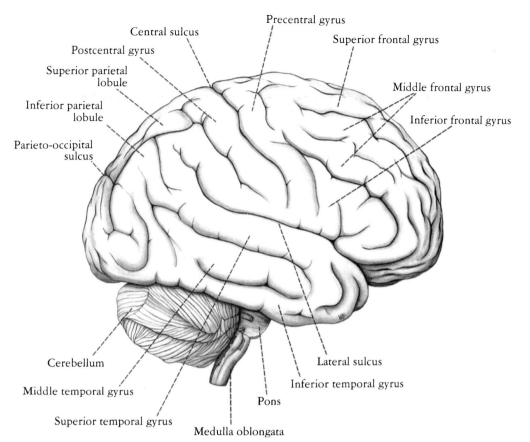

Figure 1–10 Brain viewed from its right lateral aspect.

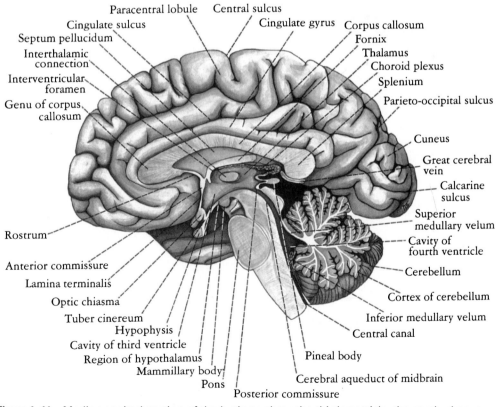

Figure 1–11 Median sagittal section of the brain to show the third ventricle, the cerebral aqueduct, and the fourth ventricle.

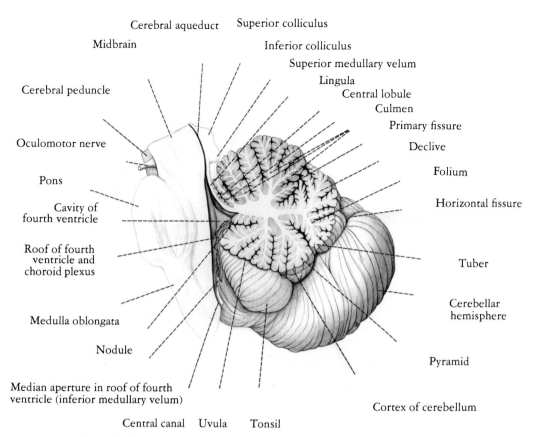

Cerebral aqueduct Superior colliculus
Midbrain Inferior colliculus
Superior medullary velum
Lingula
Central lobule
Cerebral peduncle Culmen
Primary fissure
Oculomotor nerve Declive
Folium
Pons
Horizontal fissure
Cavity of
fourth ventricle
Roof of fourth
ventricle and
choroid plexus Tuber
Cerebellar
hemisphere
Medulla oblongata
Nodule Pyramid
Median aperture in roof of fourth
ventricle (inferior medullary velum)
Cortex of cerebellum
Central canal Uvula Tonsil

Figure 1–12 Sagittal section through the brainstem and the cerebellum.

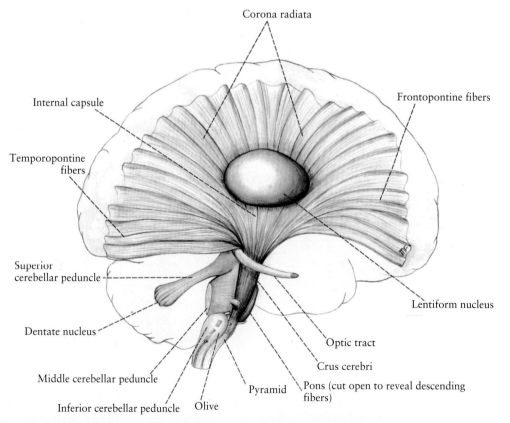

Corona radiata

Internal capsule Frontopontine fibers

Temporopontine
fibers

Superior
cerebellar peduncle

Lentiform nucleus

Dentate nucleus

Optic tract

Crus cerebri

Middle cerebellar peduncle Pons (cut open to reveal descending
fibers)
Pyramid
Inferior cerebellar peduncle Olive

Figure 1–13 Right lateral view showing continuity of the corona radiata, the internal capsule, and the crus cerebri of the cerebral peduncles. Note the position of the lentiform nucleus lateral to the internal capsule.

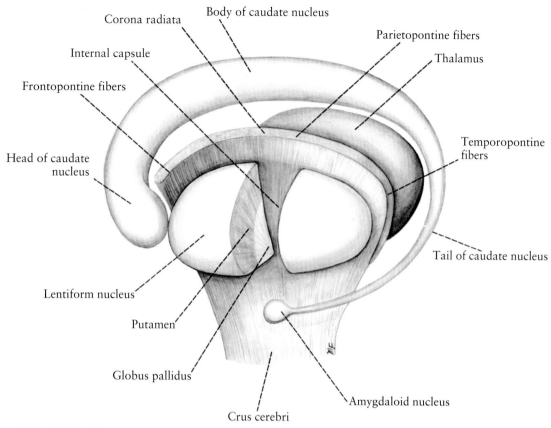

Figure 1–14 Diagram showing the relationship between the lentiform nucleus, the caudate nucleus, the thalamus, and the internal capsule, as seen from the left lateral side.

STRUCTURE OF THE BRAIN

Unlike the spinal cord, the brain is composed of an inner core of white matter, which is surrounded by an outer covering of gray matter. However, as already mentioned, certain important masses of gray matter are situated deeply within the white matter. For example, within the cerebellum, there are the gray cerebellar nuclei and within the cerebrum, the gray thalamic, caudate, and lentiform nuclei.

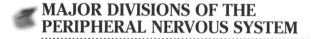

MAJOR DIVISIONS OF THE PERIPHERAL NERVOUS SYSTEM

The peripheral nervous system consists of the cranial and spinal nerves and their associated ganglia.

Cranial And Spinal Nerves

The cranial and spinal nerves are made up of bundles of nerve fibers supported by connective tissue.

There are 12 pairs of **cranial nerves** (Fig.1-9), which leave the brain and pass through foramina in the skull. There are 31 pairs of **spinal nerves** (Fig.1-6), which leave the spinal cord and pass through intervertebral foramina in the vertebral column. The spinal nerves are named accord-

ing to the regions of the vertebral column with which they are associated: 8 **cervical,** 12 **thoracic,** 5 **lumbar,** 5 **sacral,** and 1 **coccygeal.** Note that there are 8 cervical nerves and only 7 cervical vertebrae and that there is 1 coccygeal nerve and there are 4 coccygeal vertebrae.

Each spinal nerve is connected to the spinal cord by two roots: the **anterior root** and the **posterior root** (Fig. 1-6b). The anterior root consists of bundles of nerve fibers carrying nerve impulses away from the central nervous system. Such nerve fibers are called **efferent fibers.** Those efferent fibers that go to skeletal muscles and cause them to contract are called **motor fibers.** Their cells of origin lie in the anterior gray horn of the spinal cord.

The posterior root consists of bundles of nerve fibers, called **afferent fibers**, that carry nervous impulses to the central nervous system. Because these fibers are concerned with conveying information about sensations of touch, pain, temperature, and vibration, they are called **sensory**

Many neuroscientists refer to the anterior and posterior nerve roots as ventral and dorsal nerve roots, respectively, even though in the upright human, the roots are anterior and posterior. This is probably due to the fact that the early basic research was performed on animals. In any event, the student must get used to hearing both sets of terms.

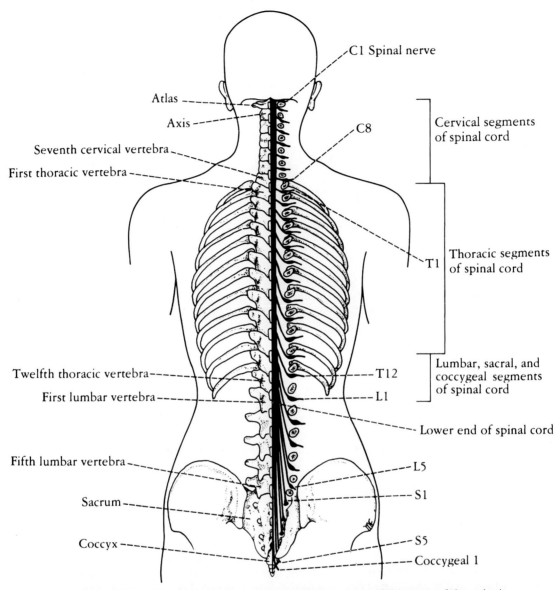

Figure 1–15 Posterior view of the spinal cord, showing the origins of the roots of the spinal nerves and their relationship to the different vertebrae. On the right, the laminae have been removed to expose the right half of the spinal cord and the nerve roots.

fibers. The cell bodies of these nerve fibers are situated in a swelling on the posterior root called the **posterior root ganglion** (Fig. 1-6).

The spinal nerve roots pass from the spinal cord to the level of their respective intervertebral foramina, where they unite to form a **spinal nerve** (Fig. 1-15). Here the motor and sensory fibers become mixed together, so that a spinal nerve is made up of a mixture of motor and sensory fibers.

Because of the disproportionate growth in length of the vertebral column during development, compared with that of the spinal cord, the length of the roots increases progressively from above downward (Fig. 1-15). In the upper cervical region the spinal nerve roots are short and run almost horizontally, but the roots of the lumbar and sacral nerves below

the level of the termination of the cord (lower border of the first lumbar vertebra in the adult) form a vertical leash of nerves around the **filum terminale** (Fig. 1-16). Together these lower nerve roots are called the **cauda equina.**

After emerging from the intervertebral foramen, each spinal nerve immediately divides into a large **anterior ramus** and a smaller **posterior ramus,** each containing both motor and sensory fibers. The posterior ramus passes posteriorly around the vertebral column to supply the muscles and skin of the back. The anterior ramus continues anteriorly to supply the muscles and skin over the anterolateral body wall, and all the muscles and skin of the limbs.

The anterior rami join one another at the root of the limbs to form complicated **nerve plexuses** (Fig.1-2B). The

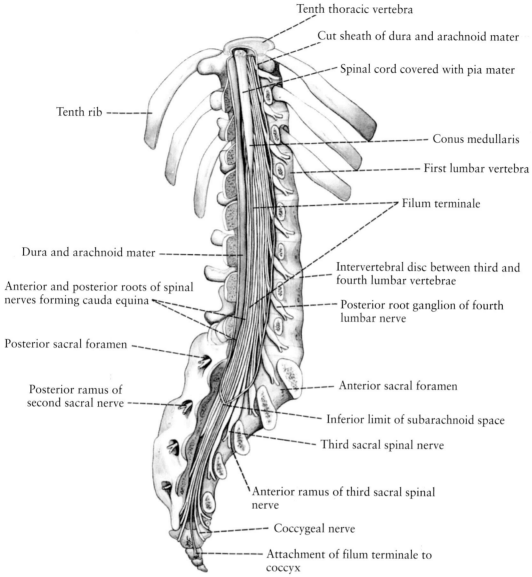

Tenth thoracic vertebra

Cut sheath of dura and arachnoid mater

Spinal cord covered with pia mater

Tenth rib

Conus medullaris

First lumbar vertebra

Filum terminale

Dura and arachnoid mater

Intervertebral disc between third and fourth lumbar vertebrae

Anterior and posterior roots of spinal nerves forming cauda equina

Posterior root ganglion of fourth lumbar nerve

Posterior sacral foramen

Anterior sacral foramen

Posterior ramus of second sacral nerve

Inferior limit of subarachnoid space

Third sacral spinal nerve

Anterior ramus of third sacral spinal nerve

Coccygeal nerve

Attachment of filum terminale to coccyx

Figure 1–16 Oblique posterior view of the lower end of the spinal cord and the cauda equina. On the right, the laminae have been removed to expose the right half of the spinal cord and the nerve roots.

cervical and brachial plexuses are found at the root of the upper limbs and the **lumbar and sacral plexuses** are found at the root of the lower limbs.

Ganglia

Ganglia may be divided into sensory ganglia of spinal nerves (posterior root ganglia) and cranial nerves, and autonomic ganglia.

SENSORY GANGLIA

Sensory ganglia are fusiform swellings (see Fig. 1-6) situated on the posterior root of each spinal nerve just proximal to the root's junction with a corresponding anterior root. They are referred to as **posterior root ganglia.** Similar ganglia that are also found along the course of cranial nerves V, VII, VIII, IX, and X are called **sensory ganglia** of these nerves.

AUTONOMIC GANGLIA

Autonomic ganglia, which are often irregular in shape, are situated along the course of efferent nerve fibers of the autonomic nervous system. They are found in the paravertebral sympathetic chains (See Figs. 14-1 and 14-2) around the roots of the great visceral arteries in the abdomen and close to, or embedded within, the walls of various viscera.

CLINICAL NOTES

RELATIONSHIP OF SPINAL CORD SEGMENTS TO VERTEBRAL NUMBERS

Because the spinal cord is shorter than the vertebral column, the spinal cord segments do not correspond numerically with the vertebrae that lie at the same level (Fig.1-15). The following table will help a physician determine which spinal segment is related to a given vertebral body.

On examination of a patient's back, one can see that the spinous processes lie approximately at the same level as the vertebral bodies. In the lower thoracic region, however, because of the length and extreme obliquity of the spinous processes, the tips of the spines lie at the level of the vertebral body below.

Vertebrae	Spinal Segment
Cervical vertebrae	Add 1
Upper thoracic vertebrae	Add 2
Lower thoracic vertebrae (7–9)	Add 3
Tenth thoracic vertebra	L1 and 2 cord segments
Eleventh thoracic vertebra	L3 and 4 cord segments
Twelfth thoracic vertebra	L5 cord segment
First lumbar vertebra	Sacral and coccygeal cord segments

INJURIES TO THE SPINAL CORD AND BRAIN

The spinal cord and brain are well protected. Both are suspended in fluid, the **cerebrospinal fluid,** and are surrounded by the bones of the vertebral column and skull. Unfortunately, if the forces of violence are sufficiently great, these protective structures can be overcome, with consequent damage to the delicate underlying nervous tissue. Moreover, the cranial and spinal nerves and blood vessels are also likely to be injured.

Spinal Cord Injuries

The degree of spinal cord injury at different vertebral levels is governed largely by anatomical factors. In the cervical region, dislocation or fracture dislocation is common, but the large size of the vertebral canal often prevents severe injury to the spinal cord. However, when there is considerable displacement of the bones or bone fragments, the cord is sectioned. Respiration ceases if the lesion occurs above the segmental origin of the phrenic nerves (C3, 4, and 5), since the intercostal muscles and the diaphragm are paralyzed, and death occurs.

In fracture dislocations of the thoracic region, displacement is often considerable and because of the small size of the vertebral canal, severe injury to this region of the spinal cord results.

In fracture dislocations of the lumbar region, two anatomical facts aid the patient. First, the spinal cord in the adult extends down only as far as the level of the lower border of the first lumbar vertebra (Fig.1-16). Second, the large size of the vertebral foramen in this region gives the roots of the cauda equina ample room. Nerve injury may therefore be minimal in this region.

Injury to the spinal cord may produce partial or complete loss of function at the level of the lesion, and partial or complete loss of function of afferent and efferent nerve tracts below the level of the lesion. The symptoms and signs of such injuries are considered after the detailed structure of the spinal cord is discussed, and the ascending and descending tracts are considered in Chapter 4.

Spinal Nerve Injuries

DISEASE AND THE INTERVERTEBRAL FORAMINA

The intervertebral foramina (Fig. 1-17) transmit the spinal nerves and the small segmental arteries and veins, all of which are embedded in areolar tissue. Each foramen is bounded superiorly and inferiorly by the pedicles of adjacent vertebrae, anteriorly by the lower part of the vertebral body and by the intervertebral disc, and posteriorly by the articular processes and the joint between them. In this situation, the spinal nerve is very vulnerable and may be pressed on or irritated by disease of the surrounding structures. Herniation of the intervertebral disc, fractures of the vertebral bodies, and osteoarthritis involving the joints of the articular processes or the joints between the vertebral bodies may all result in pressure, stretching, or edema of the emerging spinal nerve. Such pressure would give rise to dermatomal pain, muscle weakness, and diminished or absent reflexes.

HERNIATED INTERVERTEBRAL DISCS

Herniation of the intervertebral discs occurs most commonly in those areas of the vertebral column where a mobile part joins a relatively immobile part, for example, the cervicothoracic junction and the lumbosacral junction. In these areas the posterior part of the anulus fibrosus of the disc ruptures, and the central nucleus pulposus is forced posteriorly like toothpaste out of a tube. This herniation of the nucleus pulposus may result either in a central protrusion in the midline under the posterior longitudinal ligament of the vertebrae or in a lateral protrusion at the side of the posterior ligament close to the intervertebral foramen (Fig.1-18).

Cervical disc herniations are less common than in the lumbar region. The discs most susceptible to this condition are those between the fifth and sixth and the sixth and seventh cervical vertebrae. Lateral protrusions cause pressure on a spinal nerve or its roots. Each spinal nerve emerges above the corresponding vertebra; thus, the protrusion of the disc between the fifth and sixth cervical vertebrae may compress the C6 spinal nerve or its roots. Pain is felt near the lower part of the back of the neck and shoulder and along the area in the distribution of the spinal nerve involved. Central protrusions may press on the spinal

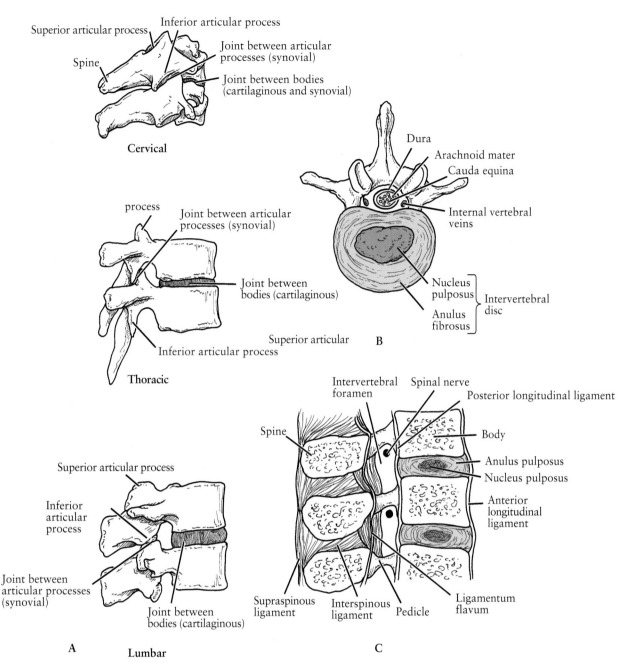

Figure 1–17 **A.** Joints in the cervical, thoracic, and lumbar regions of the vertebral column. **B.** Third lumbar vertebra seen from above, showing the relationship between the intervertebral disc and the cauda equina. **C.** Sagittal section through three lumbar vertebrae, showing the ligaments and the intervertebral discs. Note the relationship between the emerging spinal nerve in an intervertebral foramen and the intervertebral disc.

cord and the anterior spinal artery and involve the various spinal tracts.

Lumbar disc herniations are more common than cervical disc herniations (Fig. 1-18). The discs usually affected are those between the fourth and fifth lumbar vertebrae and between the fifth lumbar vertebra and the sacrum. In the lumbar region, the roots of the cauda equina run pos-

teriorly over a number of intervertebral discs (Fig. 1-18). A lateral herniation may press on one or two roots and often involves the nerve root going to the intervertebral foramen just below. The nucleus pulposus occasionally herniates directly backward and, if it is a large herniation, the whole cauda equina may be compressed, producing paraplegia.

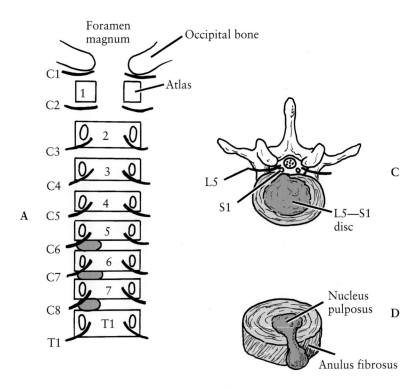

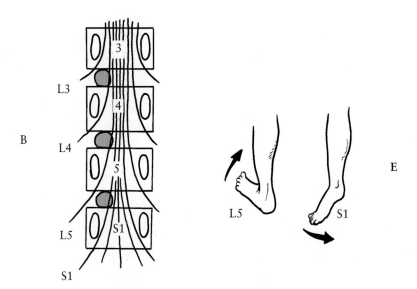

Figure 1–18 **A** and **B.** Posterior views of the vertebral bodies in the cervical and lumbar regions, showing the relationship that might exist between a herniated nucleus pulposus and spinal nerve roots. Note there are 8 cervical spinal nerves and only 7 cervical vertebrae. In the lumbar region, for example, the emerging L4 nerve roots pass out laterally close to the pedicle of the fourth lumbar vertebra and are not related to the intervertebral disc between the fourth and fifth lumbar vertebrae. **C.** Posterolateral herniation of the nucleus pulposus of the intervertebral disc between the fifth lumbar vertebra and the first sacral vertebra, showing pressure on the S1 nerve root. **D.** An intervertebral disc that has herniated its nucleus pulposus posteriorly. **E.** Pressure on the L5 motor nerve root produces weakness of dorsiflexion of the ankle; pressure on the S1 motor nerve root produces weakness of plantar flexion of the ankle joint.

In lumbar disc herniations, pain is referred down the leg and foot in the distribution of the affected nerve. Because the sensory posterior roots most commonly pressed upon are the fifth lumbar and first sacral, pain is usually felt down the back and lateral side of the leg, radiating to the sole of the foot. This condition is often called **sciatica.** In severe cases, paresthesia or actual sensory loss may occur.

Pressure on the anterior motor roots causes muscle weakness. Involvement of the fifth lumbar motor root weakens dorsiflexion of the ankle, whereas pressure on the first sacral motor root causes weakness of plantar flexion. The ankle jerk reflex may be diminished or absent (Fig.1-18).

A large, centrally placed protrusion may give rise to bilateral pain and muscle weakness in both legs. Acute retention of urine may also occur.

SPINAL TAP (LUMBAR PUNCTURE)

Spinal tap may be performed to withdraw a sample of cerebrospinal fluid for microscopic or bacteriological examination, or to inject drugs to combat infection or induce anesthesia. Fortunately, the spinal cord terminates inferiorly at the level of the lower border of the first lumbar vertebra in the adult. (In the infant it may reach inferiorly to

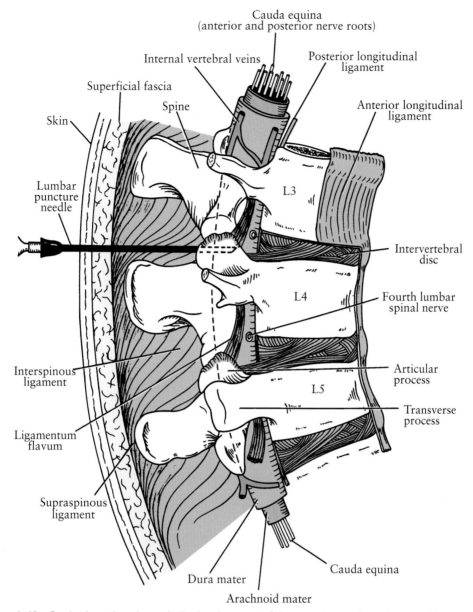

Figure 1–19   Sagittal section through the lumbar part of the vertebral column in a position of flexion. Note that the spines and laminae are well separated in this position, allowing introduction of the lumbar puncture needle into the subarachnoid space.

the third lumbar vertebra.) The subarachnoid space extends inferiorly as far as the lower border of the second sacral vertebra. The lower lumbar part of the vertebral canal is thus occupied by the subarachnoid space, which contains the lumbar and sacral nerve roots and the filum terminale (the cauda equina). A needle introduced into the subarachnoid space in this region usually pushes the nerve roots to one side without causing damage.

With the patient lying on his or her side or in the upright sitting position, with the vertebral column well flexed, the space between adjoining laminae in the lumbar region is opened to a maximum (Fig.1-19). An imaginary line joining the highest points on the iliac crests passes over the fourth lumbar spine. Using a careful aseptic technique and local

anesthesia, the physician passes the lumbar puncture needle, fitted with a stylet, into the vertebral canal above or below the fourth lumbar spine. The needle will pass through the following anatomical structures before it enters the subarachnoid space: (1) skin, (2) superficial fascia, (3) supraspinous ligament, (4) interspinous ligament, (5) ligamentum flavum, (6) areolar tissue containing the internal vertebral venous plexus, (7) dura mater, and (8) arachnoid mater. The depth to which the needle will have to pass will vary from 1 inch (2.5 cm) or less in a child to as much as 4 inches (10 cm) in an obese adult.

As the stylet is withdrawn, a few drops of blood commonly escape. This usually indicates that the point of the needle is situated in one of the veins of the internal verte-

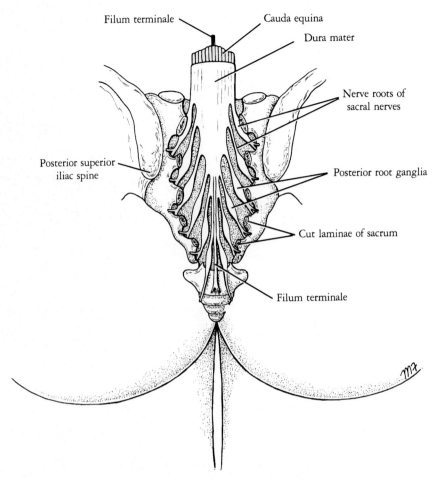

Filum terminale
Cauda equina
Dura mater
Nerve roots of
sacral nerves
Posterior superior
iliac spine
Posterior root ganglia
Cut laminae of sacrum
Filum terminale

Figure 1–20 Posterior view of the sacrum. Laminae have been removed to show the sacral nerve roots lying within the sacral canal.

bral plexus and has not yet reached the subarachnoid space. If the entering needle should stimulate one of the nerve roots of the cauda equina, the patient will experience a fleeting discomfort in one of the dermatomes or a muscle will twitch, depending on whether a sensory or a motor root was impaled.

The cerebrospinal fluid pressure may be measured by attaching a manometer to the needle. When the patient is in the recumbent position, the **normal pressure is about 60 to 150 mm of water.** The pressure shows oscillations corresponding to the movements of respiration and the arterial pulse.

A block of the subarachnoid space in the vertebral canal, which may be caused by a tumor of the spinal cord or the meninges, may be detected by compressing the internal jugular veins in the neck. This raises the cerebral venous pressure and inhibits the absorption of cerebrospinal fluid in the arachnoid granulations, thus producing an increase in the manometer reading of the cerebrospinal fluid pressure. If this rise fails to occur, the subarachnoid space is blocked and the patient is said to exhibit a positive **Queckenstedt's sign.**

CAUDAL ANESTHESIA

Anesthetic solutions may be injected into the sacral canal through the sacral hiatus. The solutions pass upward in the loose connective tissue and bathe the spinal nerves as they emerge from the dural sheath (Fig. 1-20). Obstetricians use this method of nerve block to relieve the pains of the first and second stages of labor. The advantage is that when administered by this method, the anesthetic does not affect the infant. Caudal anesthesia may also be used in operations in the sacral region, including anorectal surgery.

HEAD INJURIES

A blow to the head may cause the scalp to be merely bruised; severe blows may cause the scalp to be torn or split. Even if the head is protected by a crash helmet, the brain may be severely damaged without clinical evidence of scalp injury.

Fractures Of The Skull

Severe blows to the head often result in the skull's changing shape at the point of impact. Small objects may penetrate the skull and produce local laceration of the brain. Larger

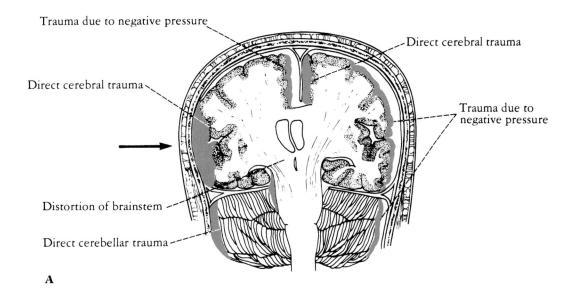

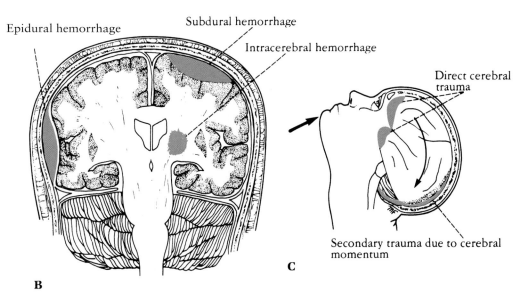

Figure 1–21 **A.** Mechanisms of acute cerebral injury when a blow is applied to the lateral side of the head. **B.** Varieties of intracranial hemorrhage. **C.** Mechanism of cerebral trauma following a blow on the chin. The movement of the brain within the skull can also tear the cerebral veins.

objects applied with great force may shatter the skull, and fragments of bone are driven into the brain at the site of impact.

In the adult, fractures of the skull are common, but in the young child less so. In the infant, the skull bones are more resilient than in the adult, and they are separated by fibrous sutural ligaments. In the adult, the inner table of the skull is particularly brittle. Moreover, the sutural ligaments begin to ossify during middle age.

The type of fracture that occurs in the skull will depend on the age of the patient, the severity of the blow, and the area of the skull receiving the trauma. The **adult skull** may be likened to an eggshell because it possesses a certain limited resilience, beyond which it splinters. A severe, localized blow will produce a local indentation, often accompanied

by splintering of the bone. Blows to the vault often result in a series of linear fractures, which radiate out through the thin areas of the bone. The petrous parts of the temporal bones and the occipital crests strongly reinforce the base of the skull and tend to deflect linear fractures.

The **young child's skull** may be likened to a table tennis ball because a localized blow produces a depression without splintering. This common type of circumscribed lesion is referred to as a "pond" fracture.

Brain Injuries

Brain injuries are produced by displacement and distortion of the neuronal tissues at the moment of impact (Fig. 1-21). The brain, which is incompressible, may be likened to a water-soaked log floating submerged in water. The brain is floating in the cerebrospinal fluid in the subarachnoid space and is capable of a certain amount of anteroposterior and lateral gliding movement. The anteroposterior movement is limited by the attachment of the superior cerebral veins to the superior sagittal sinus. Lateral displacement of the brain is limited by the falx cerebri. The tentorium cerebelli and the falx cerebelli also restrict displacement of the brain.

It follows from these anatomical facts that blows on the front or back of the head lead to displacement of the brain, which may produce severe cerebral damage, stretching and distortion of the brainstem, and stretching and even tearing of the commissures of the brain. Blows to the side of the head produce less cerebral displacement, and the injuries to the brain consequently tend to be less severe. It should be noted, however, that the falx cerebri is a tough structure and may cause considerable damage to the softer brain tissue in cases where there has been a severe blow to the side of the head (Fig.1-21). Furthermore, it is important to remember that glancing blows to the head may cause considerable rotation of the brain, with shearing strains and distortion of the brain, particularly in areas where further rotation is prevented by bony prominences in the anterior and middle cranial fossae. Brain lacerations are very likely to occur when the brain is forcibly thrown against the sharp edges of bone within the skull—the lesser wings of the sphenoid, for example.

When the brain is suddenly given momentum within the skull, the part of the brain that moves away from the skull wall is subjected to diminished pressure, because the cerebrospinal fluid has not had time to accommodate to the brain movement. This results in a suction effect on the brain surface, with rupture of surface blood vessels.

A sudden severe blow to the head, as in an automobile accident, may result in damage to the brain at two sites: (1) at the point of impact, and (2) at the pole of the brain opposite the point of impact, where the brain is thrown against the skull wall. This is referred to as **contrecoup injury.**

The movement of the brain within the skull at the time of head injuries not only is likely to cause avulsion of cranial nerves but commonly leads to rupture of tethering blood vessels. Fortunately, the large arteries found at the base of the brain are tortuous and this, coupled with their strength, explains why they are rarely torn. The thin-walled cortical veins, which drain into the large dural venous sinuses, are very vulnerable and can produce severe subdural or subarachnoid hemorrhage (Fig.1-21).

Intracranial Hemorrhage

Although the brain is cushioned by the surrounding cerebrospinal fluid in the subarachnoid space, any severe hemorrhage within the relatively rigid skull will ultimately exert pressure on the brain.

Intracranial hemorrhage may result from trauma or cerebral vascular lesions (Fig.1-21). Four varieties are considered here: (1) epidural, (2) subdural, (3) subarachnoid, and (4) cerebral.

Epidural (extradural) **hemorrhage** results from injuries to the meningeal arteries or veins. The anterior division of the middle meningeal artery is the common artery to be damaged. A comparatively minor blow to the side of the head, resulting in fracture of the skull in the region of the anterior inferior portion of the parietal bone, may sever the artery (see Fig. 1-21). Arterial or venous injury is especially likely to occur if the vessels enter a bony canal in this region. Bleeding occurs and strips the meningeal layer of dura from the internal surface of the skull. The intracranial pressure rises, and the enlarging blood clot exerts local pressure on the underlying precentral gyrus (motor area). Blood may also pass laterally through the fracture line to form a soft swelling on the side of the head. To stop the hemorrhage, the torn artery must be ligated or plugged. The burr hole through the skull wall should be placed about 1 1/2 inches (4 cm) above the midpoint of the zygomatic arch.

Subdural hemorrhage results from tearing of the superior cerebral veins where they enter the superior sagittal sinus (See Fig. 15-1). The cause is usually a blow on the front or back of the head, resulting in excessive anteroposterior displacement of the brain within the skull. This condition, which is much more common than middle meningeal hemorrhage, can be produced by a sudden minor blow. Once the vein is torn, blood under low pressure begins to accumulate in the potential space between the dura and the arachnoid. In a few patients the condition is bilateral.

Acute and chronic forms of the clinical condition occur, depending on the speed of accumulation of fluid in the subdural space. For example, if the patient starts to vomit, the venous pressure will rise as the result of a rise in the intrathoracic pressure. Under these circumstances the subdural blood clot will rapidly increase in size and produce acute symptoms. In the chronic form, over a course of several months, the small blood clot will attract fluid by osmosis, so that a hemorrhagic cyst forms and gradually expands and produces pressure symptoms. In both forms the blood clot must be removed through burr holes in the skull.

Subarachnoid hemorrhage results from nontraumatic leakage or rupture of a congenital aneurysm on the cerebral arterial circle or, less commonly, from an arteriovenous malformation. The symptoms, which are sudden in onset, will include severe headache, stiffness of the neck, and loss of consciousness. The diagnosis is established by performing computed tomography (CT) or magnetic resonance imaging (MRI) or by withdrawing heavily blood-stained cerebrospinal fluid through a lumbar puncture.

Cerebral hemorrhage. Spontaneous **intracerebral hemorrhage** (Fig. 1-21) is most common in patients with hypertension. It is generally due to rupture of the thin-walled **lenticulostriate artery** (Fig. 17-11), a branch of the middle cerebral artery (Fig. 17-4). The hemorrhage involves important descending nerve fibers in the internal capsule and produces hemiplegia on the opposite side of the body. The patient immediately loses consciousness, and the paralysis is evident when consciousness is regained. The diagnosis is established by performing brain CT or MRI.

THE SHAKEN-BABY SYNDROME

Inflicted head injury is the most common cause of traumatic death in infancy. It is believed that the sudden decel-

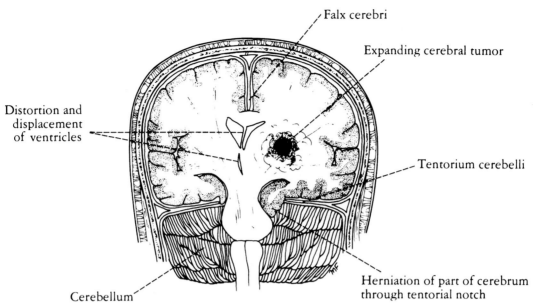

Falx cerebri

Expanding cerebral tumor

Distortion and displacement of ventricles

Tentorium cerebelli

Herniation of part of cerebrum through tentorial notch

Cerebellum

Figure 1–22 Sudden displacement of the cerebral hemispheres through the tentorial notch into the posterior cranial fossa following a lumbar puncture; the cerebral tumor is situated in the right cerebral hemisphere. Computed tomography (CT) or magnetic resonance imaging (MRI) should be used rather than a lumbar puncture when investigating a cerebral tumor.

eration that occurs when an infant is held by the arms or trunk and shaken or the head is forcefully struck against a surface is responsible for the brain injuries. Biomechanical studies have shown that the rotation of the floating brain about its center of gravity causes diffuse brain injuries, including diffuse axonal injury and subdural hematoma. In shaken-baby syndrome major rotational forces have to occur which clearly exceed those encountered in normal child play activities.

The majority of cases take place during the first year and they are usually restricted to infants under 3 years of age. Common symptoms include lethargy, irritability, seizures, altered muscle tone, and symptoms indicating raised intracranial pressure, such as, impaired consciousness, vomiting, breathing abnormalities, and apnea. In severe cases the baby may be unresponsive, the fontanelles are bulging, and the child may have retinal hemorrhages. Spinal tap may reveal blood in the cerebrospinal fluid. Subdural or subarachnoid hemorrhages can be readily detected on CT or MRI scans. Autopsy findings commonly include localized subdural hemorrhage in the parietal-occipital region and subarachnoid blood, associated with massive cerebral swelling and widespread neuronal loss.

SPACE-OCCUPYING LESIONS WITHIN THE SKULL

Space-occupying or expanding lesions within the skull include tumor, hematoma, and abscess. Since the skull is a rigid container of fixed volume, these lesions will add to the normal bulk of the intracranial contents.

An expanding lesion is first accommodated by the expulsion of cerebrospinal fluid from the cranial cavity. Later the

veins become compressed, interference with the circulation of blood and cerebrospinal fluid begins, and the intracranial pressure starts to rise. The venous congestion results in increased production and diminished absorption of cerebrospinal fluid, the volume of the cerebrospinal fluid begins to rise, and so a vicious circle is established.

The position of the tumor within the brain may have a dramatic effect on the signs and symptoms. For example, a tumor that obstructs the outflow of cerebrospinal fluid or directly presses upon the great veins will cause a rapid increase in intracranial pressure. The signs and symptoms that enable the physician to localize the lesion will depend on the interference with the brain function and the degree of destruction of the nervous tissue produced by the lesion. Severe headache, possibly due to the stretching of the dura mater, and vomiting, due to pressure on the brainstem, are common complaints.

A spinal tap should not be performed in patients with suspected intracranial tumor. The withdrawal of cerebrospinal fluid may lead to a sudden displacement of the cerebral hemisphere through the notch in the tentorium cerebelli into the posterior cranial fossa (Fig.1-22) or herniation of the medulla oblongata and cerebellum through the foramen magnum. CT scans or MRIs are used in making the diagnosis.

COMPUTED TOMOGRAPHY (CT)

CT is used for the detection of intracranial lesions. The procedure is quick, safe, and accurate. The total dose of irradiation is no greater than for a conventional skull radiograph.

CT relies on the same physics as conventional x-rays, in that structures are distinguished from one another by their

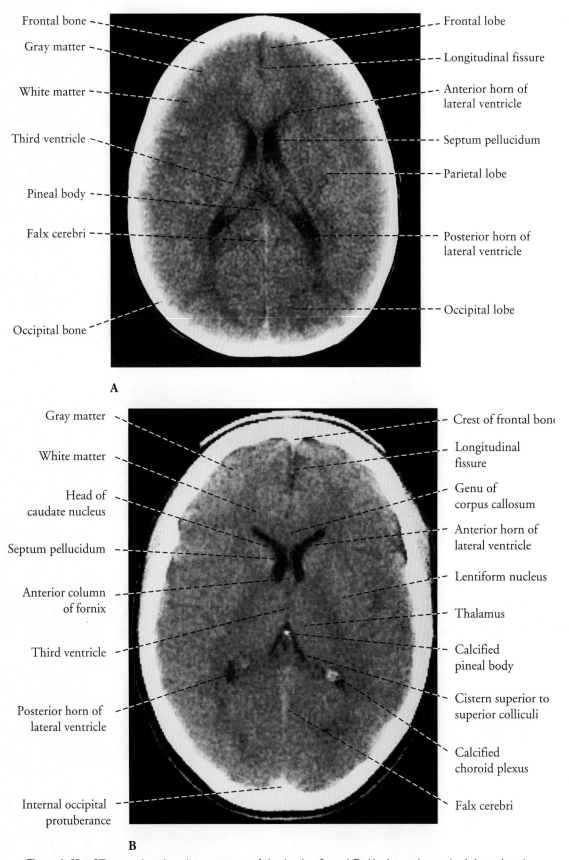

Frontal bone

Gray matter

White matter

Third ventricle

Pineal body

Falx cerebri

Occipital bone

Frontal lobe

Longitudinal fissure

Anterior horn of lateral ventricle

Septum pellucidum

Parietal lobe

Posterior horn of lateral ventricle

Occipital lobe

A

Gray matter

White matter

Head of caudate nucleus

Septum pellucidum

Anterior column of fornix

Third ventricle

Posterior horn of lateral ventricle

Internal occipital protuberance

Crest of frontal bone

Longitudinal fissure

Genu of corpus callosum

Anterior horn of lateral ventricle

Lentiform nucleus

Thalamus

Calcified pineal body

Cistern superior to superior colliculi

Calcified choroid plexus

Falx cerebri

B

Figure 1–23 CT scan showing the structure of the brain. **A** and **B.** Horizontal cuts (axial sections).

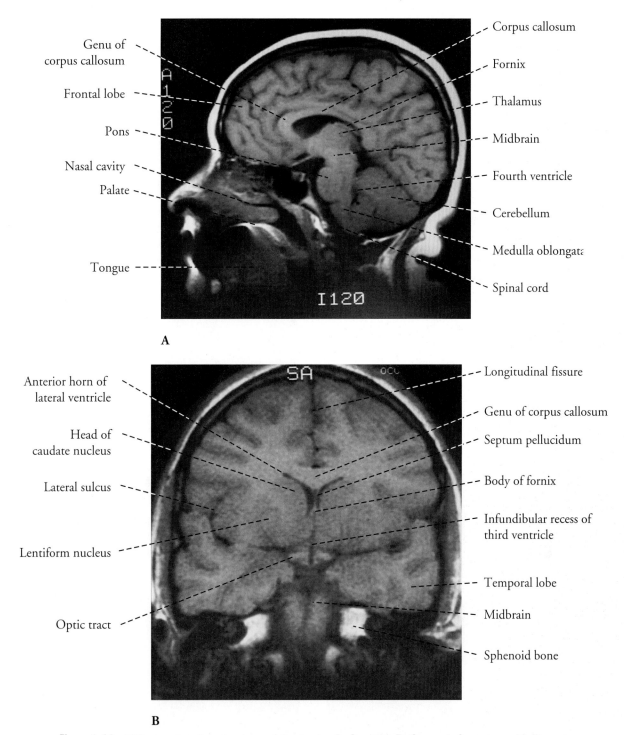

Genu of corpus callosum

Frontal lobe

Pons

Nasal cavity

Palate

Tongue

Corpus callosum

Fornix

Thalamus

Midbrain

Fourth ventricle

Cerebellum

Medulla oblongata

Spinal cord

A

Anterior horn of lateral ventricle

Head of caudate nucleus

Lateral sulcus

Lentiform nucleus

Optic tract

Longitudinal fissure

Genu of corpus callosum

Septum pellucidum

Body of fornix

Infundibular recess of third ventricle

Temporal lobe

Midbrain

Sphenoid bone

B

Figure 1–24 MRI showing the structure of the brain. **A.** Sagittal. **B.** Coronal. Compare with Figure 1-23. Note the better differentiation between gray and white matter.

ability to absorb energy from x-rays. The x-ray tube emits a narrow beam of radiation as it passes in a series of scanning movements through an arc of 180 degrees around the patient's head. The x-rays having passed through the head are collected by a special x-ray detector. The information is fed to a computer that processes the information, which is then displayed as a reconstructed picture on a television-like screen. Essentially, the observer sees an image of a thin slice through the head, which may then be photographed for later examination (Fig. 1-23).

The sensitivity is such that small differences in x-ray absorption can be easily displayed. The gray matter of the cerebral cortex, white matter, internal capsule, corpus callosum, ventricles, and subarachnoid spaces can all be recognized. An iodine-containing medium can be injected intravascularly, which enhances greatly the contrast between tissues having a different blood flow.

MAGNETIC RESONANCE IMAGING (MRI)

The technique of MRI uses the magnetic properties of the hydrogen nucleus excited by radiofrequency radiation transmitted by a coil surrounding the head. The excited hydrogen nuclei emit a signal that is detected as induced electric currents in a receiver coil. MRI is absolutely safe to the patient and, because it provides better differentiation between gray and white matter, MRI can be more revealing than a CT scan. The reason for this is that gray matter contains more hydrogen in the form of water than does white matter and the hydrogen atoms are less bound in fat (Fig. 1-24).

POSITRON EMISSION TOMOGRAPHY (PET)

This technique uses radioactive isotopes that decay with the emission of positively charged electrons (positrons) to map the biochemical, physiological, and pharmacological processes taking place in the brain.

The appropriate isotope is incorporated into molecules of known biochemical behavior in the brain and then is injected into the patient. The metabolic activity of the compound can then be studied by making cross-sectional tomo-

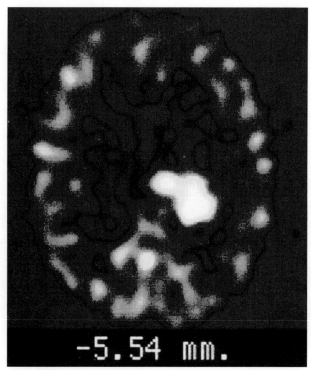

Figure 1–26 Axial (horizontal) PET scan of a 62-year-old male patient with a malignant glioma in the left parietal lobe, following the injection of 18-fluorodeoxyglucose. A high concentration of the compound (circular yellow area) is seen in the region of the tumor. (Courtesy Dr. Holley Dey.)

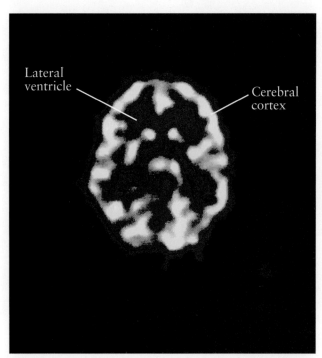

Figure 1–25 Axial (horizontal) positron emission tomography (PET) scan of a normal brain following the injection of 18-fluorodeoxyglucose. Regions of active metabolism (yellow areas) are seen in the cerebral cortex. The lateral ventricles are also demonstrated. (Courtesy Dr. Holley Dey.)

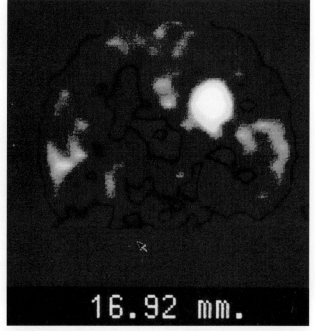

Figure 1–27 Coronal PET scan of a 62-year-old male patient with a malignant glioma in the left parietal lobe, following the injection of 18-fluorodeoxyglucose (same patient as in Fig. 1-26). A high concentration of the compound (circular yellow area) is seen in the region of the tumor. (Courtesy Dr. Holley Dey.)

graphic images of the brain using the same principles as in CT (Fig. 1-25). By making a series of time lapse images at different anatomical sites, it is possible to study the variations in brain metabolism at these sites. This technique has been used to study the distribution and activity of neurotrans-

mitters, the variations in oxygen utilization, and cerebral blood flow.

PET has been successfully used in the evaluation of patients with brain tumors (Figs. 1-26 and 1-27), movement disorders, seizures, and schizophrenia.

Clinical Problem Solving

1. A 45-year-old woman was examined by her physician and found to have carcinoma of the thyroid gland. Apart from the swelling in the neck, the patient also complained of back pain in the lower thoracic region, with a burning soreness radiating around the right side of her thorax over the tenth intercostal space. Although the back pain was often relieved by changing posture, it was worsened by coughing and sneezing. A lateral radiograph of the thoracic part of the vertebral column revealed a secondary carcinomatous deposit in the tenth thoracic vertebral body. Further physical examination revealed muscular weakness of both legs. Using your knowledge of neuroanatomy, explain the following: (a) the pain in the back, (b) the soreness over the right tenth intercostal space, (c) the muscular weakness of both legs, and (d) which segments of the spinal cord lie at the level of the tenth thoracic vertebral body.

2. A 35-year-old coal miner was crouching down at the mine face to inspect a drilling machine. A large rock suddenly became dislodged from the roof of the mine shaft and struck the miner on the upper part of his back. Examination by a physician showed an obvious forward displacement of the upper thoracic spines on the eighth thoracic spine. What anatomical factors in the thoracic region determine the degree of injury that may occur to the spinal cord?

3. A 20-year-old man with a long history of tuberculosis of the lungs was examined by an orthopedic surgeon because of the sudden development of a humpback (kyphosis). He also had symptoms of a stabbing pain radiating around both sides of his thorax intensified by coughing or sneezing. A diagnosis of tuberculous osteitis of the fifth thoracic vertebra was made, with the collapse of the vertebral body responsible for the kyphosis. Using your knowledge of neuroanatomy, explain why the collapse of the fifth thoracic vertebral body should produce pain in the distribution of the fifth thoracic segmental nerve on both sides.

4. A 50-year-old man woke up one morning with a severe pain near the lower part of the back of the neck and left shoulder. The pain was also referred along the outer side of the left upper arm. Movement of the neck caused an increase in the intensity of the pain, which was also accentuated by coughing. A lateral radiograph of the neck showed a slight narrowing of the space between the fifth and sixth cervical vertebral bodies. An MRI showed disruption of the intervertebral disc between the fifth and sixth cervical vertebrae. State which nerve root was involved, using your knowledge of anatomy. Also state the nature of the disease.

5. A medical student offered to help a fellow student straighten out the bumper of his foreign sports car. He had just finished his course in neuroanatomy and was in poor physical shape. Undaunted, he attempted to lift the end of the bumper while his friend stood on the other end. Suddenly he felt an acute pain in the back that extended down the back and outer side of his right leg. Later he was examined by an orthopedic surgeon, who found that the pain was accentuated by coughing. A lateral radiograph of the lumbar vertebral column revealed nothing abnormal. An MRI, taken in the sagittal plane, showed a small posterior prolapse of the nucleus pulposus in the disc between the fifth lumbar and the first sacral vertebrae. A diagnosis of herniation of the intervertebral disc between the fifth lumbar and first sacral vertebrae was made. Explain the symptoms of this disease, using your knowledge of neuroanatomy. Which spinal nerve roots were pressed upon?

6. A 5-year-old child was seen in the emergency department and a diagnosis of acute meningitis was made. The resident decided to perform a lumbar puncture in order to confirm the diagnosis. Using your knowledge of neuroanatomy, where would you perform a lumbar puncture? Name, in order, the structures pierced when a lumbar puncture needle is introduced into the subarachnoid space.

7. A pregnant young woman told her friends that she hated the idea of going through the pain of childbirth but she equally detested the thought of having a general anesthetic. Is there a specialized local analgesic technique that will provide painless labor?

8. While crossing the road, a pedestrian was struck on the right side of his head by a passing car. He fell to the ground but did not lose consciousness. After resting for an hour and then getting up, he appeared to be confused and irritable. Later, he staggered and fell to the floor. On questioning, he was seen to be drowsy, and twitching of the lower left half of his face and left arm was noted. A diagnosis of epidural hemorrhage was made. Which artery is likely to have been damaged? What is responsible for the drowsiness and muscle twitching?

9. A 45-year-old woman was examined by a neurologist and found to have an intracranial tumor. She complained of severe headaches, which occurred during the night and early morning. She described the pain as

"bursting" in nature, and although at first, 6 months ago, they were intermittent, they were now more or less continuous. Coughing, stooping, and straining at stool made the pain worse. The pain was accompanied by vomiting on three recent occasions. What is the sequence of events that occurs within the skull as the intracranial pressure rises? Would you perform a routine lumbar puncture on every patient you suspected of having an intracranial tumor?

10. While examining an unconscious 18-year-old man admitted to the emergency room following a motorcycle accident, the neurosurgeon asked the attending medical student what happens to the brain in an accident in which it is suddenly decelerated within the skull. What is the value of wearing a crash helmet?

Answers to Clinical Problem Solving

1. Carcinoma of the thyroid, breast, kidney, lung, and prostate commonly gives rise to metastases in bone. (a) The pain in the back was caused by the carcinoma invading and destroying the tenth thoracic vertebral body. (b) Compression of the posterior nerve root of the tenth thoracic spinal nerve by the carcinoma of the vertebral column produced the hyperesthesia and hyperalgesia over the right tenth intercostal space. (c) Muscular weakness of the legs was caused by pressure on the descending motor nerve fibers in the spinal cord by the carcinoma's invasion of the vertebral canal. (d) Although there is disproportionate growth in length of the vertebral column during development compared with that of the spinal cord, the upper cervical segments of the spinal cord still lie posterior to the vertebral bodies of the same number; however, the spinal cord in the adult terminates inferiorly at the level of the lower border of the first lumbar vertebra and, therefore, the first and second lumbar segments of the spinal cord lie at the level of the tenth thoracic vertebral body.

2. This patient had a severe fracture dislocation between the seventh and eighth thoracic vertebrae. The vertical arrangement of the articular processes and the low mobility of this region because of the thoracic cage mean that a dislocation can occur in this region only if the articular processes are fractured by a great force. The small circular vertebral canal leaves little space around the spinal cord, so that severe cord injuries are certain.

3. Each spinal nerve is formed by the union of a posterior sensory root and an anterior motor root and leaves the vertebral canal by traveling through an intervertebral foramen. Each foramen is bounded superiorly and inferiorly by the pedicles of adjacent vertebrae, anteriorly by the lower part of the vertebral body and by the intervertebral disc, and posteriorly by the articular processes and the joint between them. In this patient the fifth thoracic vertebral body had collapsed and the intervertebral foramina on both sides had been considerably reduced in size, causing compression of the posterior sensory roots and the spinal nerves. The consequent irritation of the sensory fibers was responsible for the pain.

4. This patient had symptoms suggestive of irritation of the left sixth cervical posterior nerve root. The radiograph revealed narrowing of the space between the fifth and sixth cervical vertebral bodies, suggesting a herniation of the nucleus pulposus of the intervertebral disc at this level. The MRI showed the nucleus pulposus extending posteriorly beyond the anulus fibrosus, thus confirming the diagnosis.

5. The herniation occurred on the right side and was relatively small. The pain occurred in the distribution of the fifth lumbar and first sacral segments of the spinal cord, and the posterior sensory roots of these segments of the cord were pressed upon on the right side.

6. In a 5-year-old child, the spinal cord terminates inferiorly at about the level of the second lumbar vertebra (certainly no lower than the third lumbar vertebra). With the child lying on his side and comforted by a nurse, and with the operator using an aseptic technique, the skin is anesthetized in the midline just below the fourth lumbar spine. The fourth lumbar spine lies on an imaginary line joining the highest points on the iliac crests. The lumbar puncture needle, fitted with a stylet, is then passed carefully into the vertebral canal. The needle will pass through the following anatomical structures before it enters the subarachnoid space: (a) skin, (b) superficial fascia, (c) supraspinous ligament, (d) interspinous ligament, (e) ligamentum flavum, (f) areolar tissue containing the internal vertebral venous plexus, (g) dura mater, and (h) arachnoid mater.

7. Caudal analgesia (anesthesia) is very effective in producing a painless labor if it is performed skillfully. The anesthetic solutions are introduced into the sacral canal through the sacral hiatus. Sufficient solution is given so that the nerve roots up as far as T11 and 12 and L1 are blocked. This will make the uterine contractions painless during the first stage of labor. If the nerve fibers of S2, 3, and 4 are also blocked, the perineum will be anesthetized.

8. A blow on the side of the head may easily fracture the thin anterior part of the parietal bone. The anterior branch of the middle meningeal artery commonly enters a bony canal in this region and is sectioned at the time of the fracture. The resulting hemorrhage causes gradual accumulation of blood under high pressure out-

side the meningeal layer of the dura mater. The pressure is exerted on the underlying brain as the blood clot enlarges, and the symptoms of confusion and irritability become apparent. This is followed later by drowsiness. Pressure on the lower end of the motor area of the cerebral cortex (the right precentral gyrus) causes twitching of the facial muscles and, later, twitching of the left arm muscles. As the blood clot progressively enlarges, the intracranial pressure rises and the patient's condition deteriorates.

9. A detailed account of the various changes that occur in the skull in patients with an intracranial tumor is given on page 23. A patient suspected of having an intracranial tumor should **not** undergo a spinal tap. The withdrawal of cerebrospinal fluid may lead to a sudden displacement of the cerebral hemisphere through the opening in the tentorium cerebelli into the posterior cranial fossa, or herniation of the medulla oblongata and cerebellum through the foramen magnum. CT scans or MRIs are now used in making the diagnosis.

10. The brain is floating in the cerebrospinal fluid within the skull, so that a blow to the head or sudden deceleration leads to displacement of the brain. This may produce severe cerebral damage, stretching or distortion of the brainstem, avulsion of cranial nerves, and, commonly, rupture of tethering cerebral veins. (For further details, see p 22.) A crash helmet helps to protect the brain by cushioning the blow and thus slowing up the brain's rate of deceleration.

Review Questions

Directions: Each of the incomplete statements in this section is followed by completions of the statement. Select the ONE lettered completion that is BEST in each case.

1. The spinal cord has
   (a) an outer covering of gray matter and an inner core of white matter
   (b) an enlargement below that forms the conus medullaris
   (c) anterior and posterior roots of a single spinal nerve attached to a single segment
   (d) cells in the posterior gray horn that give rise to efferent fibers that supply skeletal muscles
   (e) a central canal that is situated in the white commissure

2. The medulla oblongata has
   (a) a tubular shape
   (b) the fourth ventricle lying posterior to its lower part
   (c) the midbrain directly continuous with its upper border
   (d) no central canal in its lower part
   (e) the spinal cord directly continuous with its lower end in the foramen magnum

3. The midbrain has
   (a) a cavity called the cerebral aqueduct
   (b) a large size
   (c) no cerebrospinal fluid around it
   (d) a cavity that opens above into the lateral ventricle
   (e) a location in the middle cranial fossa of the skull

Directions: Each of the numbered items in this section is followed by answers that are positively phrased. Select the ONE lettered answer that is an EXCEPTION.

4. The following statements concerning the cerebellum are correct **except:**
   (a) It lies within the posterior cranial fossa.
   (b) The cerebellar cortex is composed of gray matter.
   (c) The vermis is the name given to that part joining the cerebellar hemispheres together.
   (d) The cerebellum lies anterior to the fourth ventricle.
   (e) The dentate nucleus is a mass of gray matter found in each cerebellar hemisphere.

5. The following statements concerning the cerebrum are correct **except:**
   (a) The cerebral hemispheres are separated by a deep cleft called the longitudinal fissure.
   (b) The lobes are named for the skull bones under which they lie.
   (c) The corpus callosum is a mass of gray matter lying within each cerebral hemisphere.
   (d) The internal capsule is an important collection of nerve fibers having the caudate nucleus and the thalamus on its medial side and the lentiform nucleus on its lateral side.
   (e) The cavity present within each cerebral hemisphere is called the lateral ventricle.

6. The following statements concerning the peripheral nervous system are correct **except:**
   (a) There are 12 pairs of cranial nerves.
   (b) There are 8 pairs of cervical spinal nerves.
   (c) The posterior root of a spinal nerve contains many efferent motor nerve fibers.
   (d) A spinal nerve is formed by the union of an anterior and a posterior root in an intervertebral foramen.
   (e) A posterior root ganglion contains the cell bodies of sensory nerve fibers entering the spinal cord.

7. The following statements concerning the central nervous system are correct **except:**
   (a) A CT brain scan can distinguish between white matter and gray matter.

(b) The lateral ventricles are in direct communication with the fourth ventricle.

(c) An MRI of the brain uses the magnetic properties of the hydrogen nucleus excited by radiofrequency radiation transmitted by a coil surrounding the patient's head.

(d) Following trauma and sudden movement of the brain within the skull, the large arteries at the base of the brain are rarely torn.

(e) The movement of the brain at the time of head injuries may damage the small sixth cranial nerve.

8. The following statements concerning the cerebrospinal fluid are correct **except:**

(a) The cerebrospinal fluid in the central canal of the spinal cord is unable to enter the fourth ventricle.

(b) With the patient in the recumbent position, the normal pressure is about 60 to 150 mm of water.

(c) It protects the brain and spinal cord from traumatic injury.

(d) Compression of the internal jugular veins in the neck raises the cerebrospinal fluid pressure.

(e) The subarachnoid space is filled with cerebrospinal fluid.

9. The following statements concerning the vertebral levels and the spinal cord segmental levels are correct **except**:

(a) The first lumbar vertebra lies opposite the sacral and coccygeal segments of the cord.

(b) The third thoracic vertebra lies opposite the fifth thoracic spinal cord segment.

(c) The fifth cervical vertebra lies opposite the seventh cervical spinal cord segment.

(d) The eighth thoracic vertebra lies opposite the eleventh thoracic spinal cord segment.

(e) The third cervical vertebra lies opposite the fourth cervical spinal cord segment.

Directions: Read the case histories then answer the questions.

You will be required to select ONE BEST lettered answer.

A 23-year-old woman was unconscious when admitted to the emergency department. While crossing the road, she had been hit on the side of the head by a bus. Within an hour, she was found to have a large doughlike swelling over the right temporal region. She also had signs of muscular paralysis on the left side of the body. A lateral radiograph of the skull showed a fracture line running downward and forward across the anterior inferior angle of the right parietal bone. Her coma deepened and she died 5 hours after the accident.

10. Select the most likely cause of the swelling over the right temporal region in this patient?

(a) Superficial bruising of the skin

(b) Hemorrhage from a blood vessel in the temporalis muscle

(c) Rupture of the right middle meningeal vessels

(d) Edema of the skin

(e) Hemorrhage from a blood vessel in the superficial fascia

11. Select the most likely cause of the muscular paralysis of the left side of the body in this patient?

(a) Laceration of the right side of the cerebral hemisphere

(b) Right-sided epidural hemorrhage

(c) Left-sided epidural hemorrhage

(d) Injury to the cerebral cortex on the left side of the brain

(e) Injury to the right cerebellar hemisphere

A 69-year-old man was admitted to the neurology unit complaining of severe discomfort of the lower back. Radiological examination of the lumbar region of the vertebral column revealed significant narrowing of the spinal canal caused by advanced osteoarthritis.

12. Explain the discomfort in the lower back experienced by this patient?

(a) Muscle fatigue

(b) Prolapsed intervertebral disc

(c) Torn ligament in the joints of the lumbar region of the spine

(d) Compression of the cauda equina

(e) Bad posture

Later, in this same patient, the back pain became more severe and now radiated down the back of the left leg; the patient was also experiencing difficulty walking. Examination of the patient revealed weakness and some wasting of the muscles of the left leg. Radiological examination showed that the osteoarthritic changes had spread to involve the boundaries of many of the lumbar intervertebral foramina.

13. Explain the change in the symptoms and signs found in this patient.

(a) The sciatic nerve was compressed in the pelvis by a spreading rectal cancer.

(b) The patient had developed advanced atherosclerosis of the arteries of the right lower limb.

(c) The osteoarthritic process had produced osteophytes that encroached on the intervertebral foramina, compressing the segmental spinal nerve roots.

(d) Neuritis had developed in the sciatic nerve trunk.

(e) The patient was experiencing psychiatric problems.

Answers to Review Questions

1. C
2. E
3. A
4. D
5. C
6. C
7. B
8. A
9. C
10. C. The swelling over the right temporal region and the radiological finding of a linear fracture over the anterior inferior angle of the right parietal bone would strongly suggest that the right middle meningeal artery had been damaged and an epidural (extradural) hemorrhage had occurred. Blood had spread through the fracture line into the overlying temporalis muscle and soft tissue.

11. B. The left-sided paralysis (left hemiplegia) was due to pressure exerted by the right-sided epidural hemorrhage on the precentral gyrus of the right cerebral hemisphere.
12. D. In persons in whom the spinal canal was originally small, significant narrowing of the canal in the lumbar region can lead to neurological compression of the cauda equina with pain radiating to the back, as in this patient.
13. C. One of the complications of osteoarthritis of the vertebral column is the growth of osteophytes, which commonly encroach on the intervertebral foramina, causing pain along the distribution of the segmental nerve. In this patient the segmental nerves L4 and 5 and S1, 2, and 3, which form the important sciatic nerve, were involved. This would explain the pain radiating down the left leg and the atrophy of the leg muscles.

ADDITIONAL READING

American Academy of Neurology Therapeutics Subcommittee. Positron emission tomography. *Neurology* 41:163, 1991.

Becker, D. P., and Gudeman, S. K. *Textbook of Head Injury.* Philadelphia: Saunders, 1989.

Brooks, D. J. PET: Its clinical role in neurology. *J. Neurol. Neurosurg. Psychiatry* 54:1, 1991.

Duhaime, A.C., Christian,C.W., Rorke, L.B., and Zimmerman, R.A. Nonaccidental Head Injury in Infants-The "Shaken-Baby Syndrome." *N. Engl. J. Med.* 338:1822-1829,1998.

Prichard, J.W., and Brass, L.M. New anatomical and functional imaging methods. *Ann. Neurol.* 32:395, 1992.

Snell, R.S. *Clinical Anatomy for Medical Students* (6th ed.). Philadelphia. Lippincott Williams & Wilkins, 2000.

Williams, P. L.,et al (eds.), *Gray's Anatomy* (38th Brit. ed.). Churchill Livingstone, New York, 1995.

CHAPTER 2

The Neurobiology of the Neuron and the Neuroglia

A 38-year-old man with a history of involuntary movements, personality changes, and mental deterioration was referred to a neurologist. The symptoms started insidiously 8 years ago and have gotten progressively worse. The first symptoms were involuntary, abrupt, and purposeless movements of the upper limbs associated with clumsiness and dropping of objects. At presentation the patient had difficulty walking, speaking, and swallowing. Associated with these movement defects were an impairment of memory and loss of intellectual capacity. Impulsive behavior and bouts of depression also occurred. Close questioning of the patient and his wife revealed that the patient's father and his older brother had had similar symptoms before they died. A diagnosis of Huntington's disease was made.

Huntington's disease is an autosomal dominant disorder with the defect localized to the short arm of chromosome 4. Histologically, the caudate nucleus and the putamen show extensive degeneration, mainly involving the acetylcholine and gamma-aminobutyric acid (GABA)-producing neurons; the dopamine neurons are unaffected. There is also secondary degeneration of the cerebral cortex. This case is an example of a hereditary disorder that mainly involves a particular group of neurons.

CHAPTER OUTLINE

CHAPTER OBJECTIVES

The neuron is defined and its processes are named. The varieties of neurons are described and examples found in the different parts of the nervous system are given. The cell biology of a neuron is reviewed so that the reader can understand the function of a nerve cell and its processes. Emphasis is placed on the structure of the plasma membrane as it is related to its physiology. The transport of materials from the cell body to the axon terminals is described and the structure and function of synapses and neurotransmitters are discussed in detail.

The supporting function of the neuroglial cells for nerve cells is emphasized and the possible role that they play in neuronal metabolism, function, and neuronal death is described.

The purpose of this chapter is to prepare the student to understand how the basic excitable cell, the neuron, communicates with other neurons. It also considers certain injuries to the neuron and the effects of drugs on the mechanism by which neurons communicate with one another.

 DEFINITION OF A NEURON

Neuron is the name given to the nerve cell and all its processes (Fig. 2-1). Neurons are excitable cells that are specialized for the reception of stimuli and the conduction of the nerve impulse. They vary considerably in size and shape, but each possesses a **cell body** from whose surface project one or more processes called **neurites** (Fig. 2-2). Those neurites responsible for receiving information and conducting it toward the cell body are called **dendrites.** The single long tubular neurite that conducts impulses away from the cell body is called the **axon.** The dendrites and axons are often referred to as **nerve fibers.**

Neurons are found in the brain and spinal cord and in ganglia. Unlike most other cells in the body, normal neurons in the mature individual do not undergo division and replication.

VARIETIES OF NEURONS

Although the cell body of a neuron may be as small as 5 μm or as large as 135 μm in diameter, the processes or neurites may extend over a distance of more than 1 meter. The number, length, and mode of branching of the neurites provide a morphological method for classifying neurons.

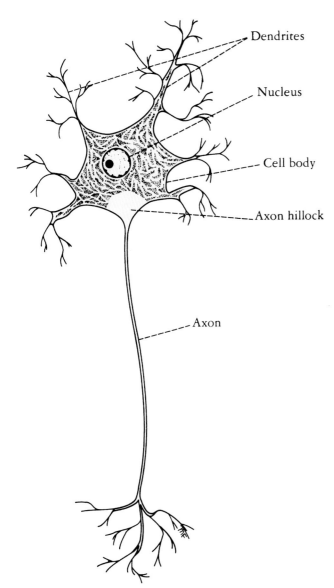

Figure 2–1   A neuron.

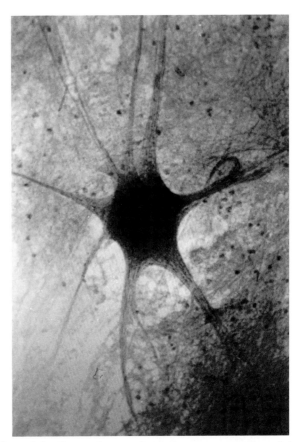

Figure 2–2   Photomicrograph of a smear preparation of the spinal cord showing a neuron with its cell body and its processes or neurites.

Unipolar neurons are those in which the cell body has a single neurite that divides a short distance from the cell body into two branches, one proceeding to some peripheral structure and the other entering the central nervous system (Fig. 2-3). The branches of this single neurite have the structural and functional characteristics of an axon. In this type of neuron the fine terminal branches found at the peripheral end of the axon at the receptor site are often referred to as the dendrites. Examples of this form of neuron are found in the posterior root ganglion.

Bipolar neurons possess an elongated cell body, from each end of which a single neurite emerges (Fig. 2-3). Examples of this type of neuron are found in the retinal bipolar cells and the cells of the sensory cochlear and vestibular ganglia.

Multipolar neurons have a number of neurites arising from the cell body (Fig. 2-3). With the exception of the long process, the axon, the remainder of the neurites are dendrites. Most neurons of the brain and spinal cord are of this type.

Neurons may also be classified according to size:

Golgi type I neurons have a long axon that may be 1 meter or more in length in extreme cases (Figs. 2-4, 2-5, and 2-6). The axons of these neurons form the long fiber tracts of the brain and spinal cord and the nerve fibers of peripheral nerves. The pyramidal cells of the cerebral cortex, the Purkinje cells of the cerebellar cortex, and the motor cells of the spinal cord are good examples.

Golgi type II neurons have a short axon that terminates in the neighborhood of the cell body or is entirely absent (Figs. 2-5 and 2-6). They greatly outnumber the Golgi type I neurons. The short dendrites that arise from these neurons give them a star-shaped appearance. These neurons are very numerous in the cerebral and cerebellar cortex and are often inhibitory in function. Table 2-1 summarizes the classification of neurons.

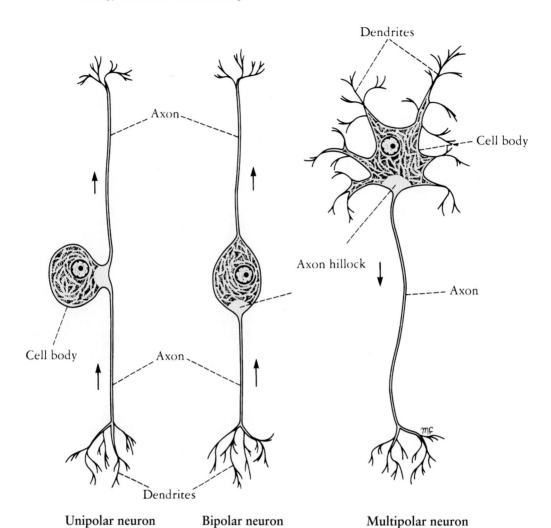

Unipolar neuron   **Bipolar neuron**   **Multipolar neuron**

Figure 2–3   The classification of neurons according to the number, length, and mode of branching of the neurites.

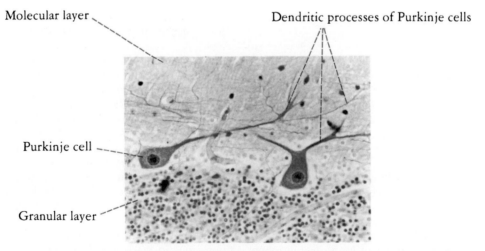

Figure 2–4   Photomicrograph of a silver-stained section of the cerebellar cortex showing two Purkinje cells. These are examples of Golgi type I neurons.

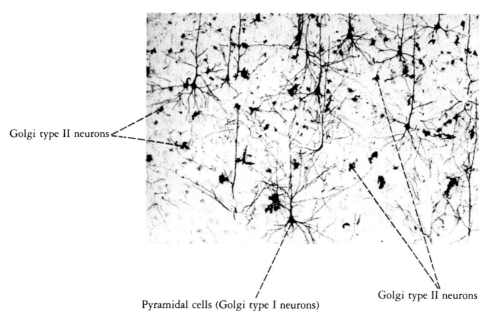

Golgi type II neurons

Golgi type II neurons

Pyramidal cells (Golgi type I neurons)

Figure 2–5 Photomicrograph of a silver-stained section of the cerebral cortex. Note the presence of large pyramidal cells, which are examples of Golgi type I neurons, and numerous Golgi type II neurons.

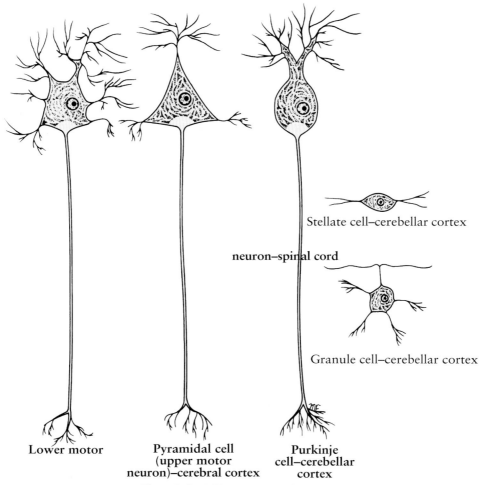

Stellate cell–cerebellar cortex

neuron–spinal cord

Granule cell–cerebellar cortex

Lower motor

Pyramidal cell (upper motor neuron)–cerebral cortex

Purkinje cell–cerebellar cortex

Figure 2–6 Different types of neurons.

Table 2–1	Classification of Neurons	
Morphological Classification	Arrangement of Neurites	Location
Number, Length, Mode of Branching of Neurites		
Unipolar	Single neurite divides a short distance from cell body	Posterior root ganglion
Bipolar	Single neurite emerges from either end of cell body	Retina, sensory cochlea, and vestibular ganglia
Multipolar	Many dendrites and one long axon	Fiber tracts of brain and spinal cord, peripheral nerves, and motor cells of spinal cord
Size of Neuron		
Golgi type I	Single long axon	Fiber tracts of brain and spinal cord, peripheral nerves, and motor cells of spinal cord
Golgi type II	Short axon that with dendrites resembles a star	Cerebral and cerebellar cortex

STRUCTURE OF THE NEURON

Nerve Cell Body

The nerve cell body, like that of other cells, consists essentially of a mass of cytoplasm in which a nucleus is embedded (Figs. 2-7 and 2-8); it is bounded externally by a plasma membrane. It is interesting to note that the volume of cytoplasm within the nerve cell body is often far less than the total volume of cytoplasm in the neurites. The cell bodies of the small granular cells of the cerebellar cortex measure about 5 μm in diameter, whereas those of the large anterior horn cells may measure as much as 135 μm in diameter.

NUCLEUS*

The nucleus, which stores the genes, is commonly centrally located within the cell body and is typically large and rounded. In mature neurons the chromosomes no longer duplicate themselves and function only in gene expression. The chromosomes are therefore not arranged as compact structures but exist in an uncoiled state. The nucleus is thus

---

*The term *nucleus* used in cytology must not be confused with the term *nucleus* in neuroanatomy, which refers to a discrete group of nerve cell bodies in the central nervous system.

pale and the fine chromatin granules are widely dispersed (Figs. 2-6 and 2-7). There is usually a single prominent nucleolus, which is concerned with ribosomal ribonucleic acid (rRNA) synthesis and ribosome subunit assembly. The large size of the nucleolus probably is due to the high rate of protein synthesis, which is necessary to maintain the protein level in the large cytoplasmic volume that is present in the long neurites as well as in the cell body.

In the female one of the two X chromosomes is compact and is known as the **Barr body.** It is composed of sex chromatin and is situated at the inner surface of the nuclear envelope.

The **nuclear envelope** (Figs. 2-8 and 2-9) can be regarded as a special portion of the rough endoplasmic reticulum of the cytoplasm and is continuous with the endoplasmic reticulum of the cytoplasm. The envelope is double-layered and possesses fine **nuclear pores**, through which materials can diffuse into and out of the nucleus (Fig. 2-8). The nucleoplasm and the cytoplasm can be considered as functionally continuous. Newly formed ribosomal subunits can be passed into the cytoplasm through the nuclear pores.

CYTOPLASM

The cytoplasm is rich in granular and agranular endoplasmic reticulum (Figs. 2-9 and 2-10) and contains the following organelles and inclusions: (1) Nissl substance; (2) the Golgi complex; (3) mitochondria; (4) microfilaments; (5) microtubules; (6) lysosomes; (7) centrioles; and (8) lipofuscin, melanin, glycogen, and lipid.

Nissl substance consists of granules that are distributed throughout the cytoplasm of the cell body, except for the region close to the axon, called the **axon hillock** (Fig. 2-11). The granular material also extends into the proximal parts of the dendrites; it is not present in the axon.

Electron micrographs show that the Nissl substance is composed of rough-surfaced endoplasmic reticulum (Fig. 2-12) arranged in the form of broad cisternae stacked one on top of the other. Although many of the ribosomes are attached to the surface of the endoplasmic reticulum, many more lie free in the intervals between the cisternae. Since the ribosomes contain RNA, the Nissl substance is basophilic and can be well demonstrated by staining with toluidine blue or other basic aniline dyes (Fig. 2-11) and using the light microscope.

The Nissl substance is responsible for synthesizing protein, which flows along the dendrites and the axon and replaces the proteins that are broken down during cellular activity. Fatigue or neuronal damage causes the Nissl substance to move and become concentrated at the periphery of the cytoplasm. This phenomenon, which gives the impression that the Nissl substance has disappeared, is known as **chromatolysis.**

The **Golgi Complex,** when seen with the light microscope after staining with a silver-osmium method, appears as a network of irregular wavy threads around the nucleus. In electron micrographs it appears as clusters of flattened cisternae and small vesicles made up of smooth-surfaced endoplasmic reticulum (Figs. 2-8 and 2-9).

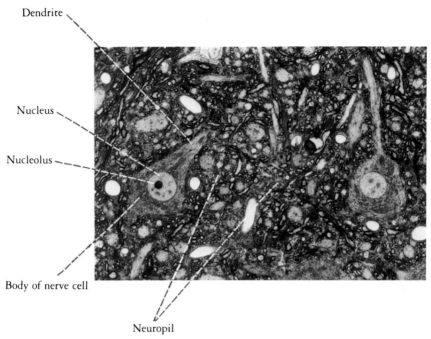

Dendrite

Nucleus

Nucleolus

Body of nerve cell

Neuropil

Figure 2–7 Photomicrograph of a section of the anterior gray column of the spinal cord showing two large motor nerve cells with nuclei. Note the prominent nucleolus in one of the nuclei.

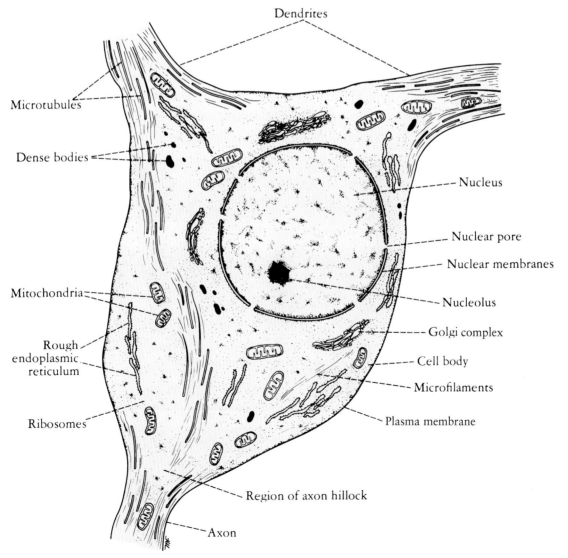

Dendrites

Microtubules

Dense bodies

Nucleus

Nuclear pore

Nuclear membranes

Mitochondria

Nucleolus

Golgi complex

Rough endoplasmic reticulum

Cell body

Microfilaments

Ribosomes

Plasma membrane

Region of axon hillock

Axon

Figure 2–8 Diagrammatic representation of the fine structure of a neuron.

Fine chromatin granules in nucleus

Nucleolus   Nuclear membranes   Golgi complex

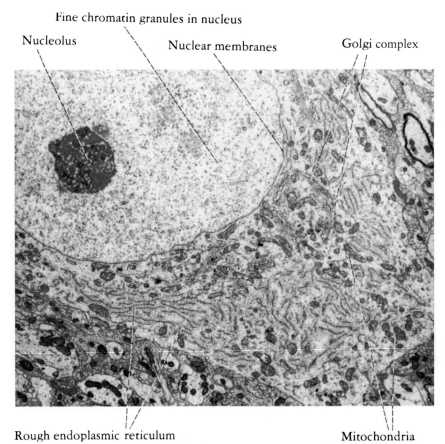

Rough endoplasmic reticulum   Mitochondria

Figure 2–9 Electron micrograph of a neuron showing the structure of the nucleus and a number of cytoplasmic organelles. (Courtesy Dr. J. M. Kerns.)

Cytoplasm of neuron

Nucleus   Plasma membrane

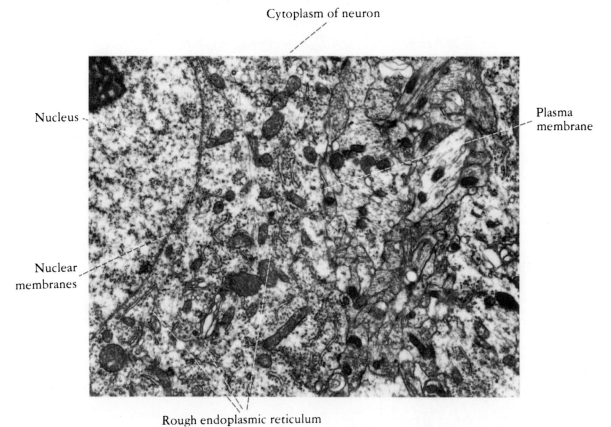

Nuclear membranes

Rough endoplasmic reticulum

Figure 2–10 Electron micrograph of a neuron showing nuclear and plasma membranes and cytoplasmic organelles. (Courtesy Dr. J. M. Kerns.)

Nissl substance

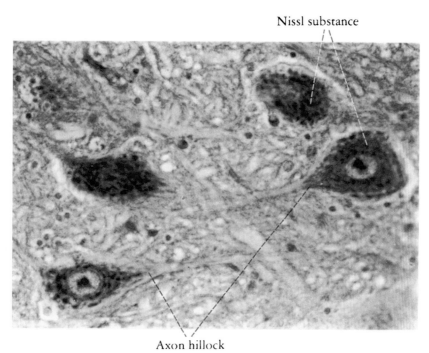

Axon hillock

Figure 2–11 Photomicrograph of a section of the anterior gray column of the spinal cord stained with toluidine blue. Note the presence of dark-staining Nissl substance in the cytoplasm of four neurons.

Nissl substance

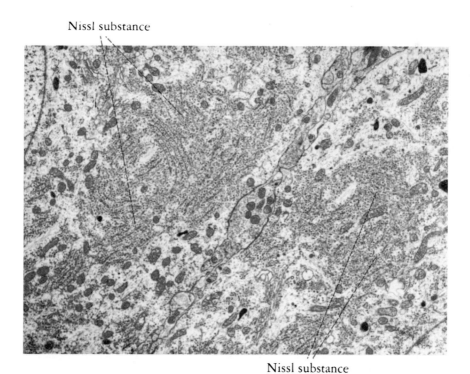

Nissl substance

Figure 2–12 Electron micrograph of the cytoplasm of two neurons showing the structure of Nissl bodies (substance). (Courtesy Dr. J. M. Kerns.)

The protein produced by the Nissl substance is transferred to the cis side of the Golgi complex in transport vesicles, where it is temporarily stored and where carbohydrate may be added to the protein. The proteins are believed to travel from one cisterna to another via transport vesicles. Each cisterna of the Golgi complex is specialized for different types of enzymatic reaction. At the trans side of the complex the macromolecules are packaged in vesicles for transport to the nerve terminals. The Golgi complex is also thought to be active in lysosome production and in the synthesis of cell membranes. The latter function is particularly important in the formation of synaptic vessels at the axon terminals.

Mitochondria are found scattered throughout the cell body, dendrites, and axons (Figs. 2-8 and 2-9). They are spherical or rod-shaped. In electron micrographs the walls show a characteristic double membrane (see Fig. 2-8). The inner membrane is thrown into folds or cristae that project into the center of the mitochondrion. Mitochondria possess many enzymes, which are localized chiefly on the inner mitochondrial membrane. These enzymes take part in the tricarboxylic acid cycle and the cytochrome chains of respiration. Mitochondria are therefore important in nerve cells, as in other cells, in the production of energy.

Neurofibrils, as seen with the light microscope after staining with silver, are numerous and run parallel to each other through the cell body into the neurites (Fig. 2-13). With the electron microscope, the neurofibrils may be resolved into bundles of **neurofilaments,** each filament measuring about 10 nm in diameter (Fig. 2-14). The neurofilaments form the main component of the cytoskeleton. Chemically neurofilaments are very stable and belong to the cytokeratin family.

Microfilaments measure about 3-5nm in diameter and are formed of actin. Microfilaments are concentrated at the periphery of the cytoplasm just beneath the plasma membrane where they form a dense network. Together with microtubules, microfilaments play a key role in the formation of new cell processes and the retraction of old ones. They also assist the microtubules in axon transport.

Microtubules are revealed with the electron microscope and are similar to those seen in other types of cells. They measure about 25 nm in diameter and are found interspersed among the neurofilaments (Fig. 2-14). They extend throughout the cell body and its processes. In the axon, all the microtubules are arranged in parallel with one end pointing to the cell body and the other end pointing distally away from the cell body.

The microtubules and the microfilaments provide a stationary track which permits specific organelles to move by molecular motors. The stop and start movement is caused by the periodic dissociation of the organelles from the track or the collision with other structures.

Cell transport involves the movement of membrane organelles, secretory material, synaptic precursor membranes, large dense core vesicles, mitochondria, and smooth endoplasmic reticulum.

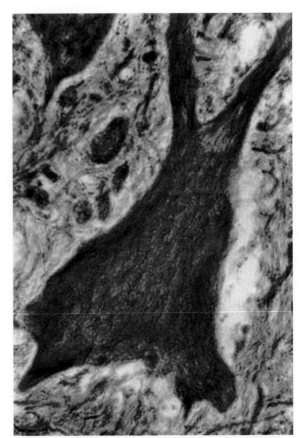

Figure 2–13 Photomicrograph of a silver-stained section of a neuron, showing the presence of large numbers of neurofibrils in the cytoplasm of the cell body and the neurites.

Cell transport can take place in both directions in the cell body and its processes. It is of two kinds: rapid (100-400 mm per day) and slow (0.1 to 3 mm per day).

Rapid transport is brought about by two motor proteins associated with the microtubule adenosine triphosphate (ATP)-ase sites; these are kinesin for anterograde (away from the cell) movement and dynein for retrograde movement. It is believed that in anterograde movement, kinesin coated organelles are moved toward one end of the tubule and in retrograde movement that dynein coated organelles are moved toward the other end of the tubule. The direction and speed of the movement of an organelle can be brought about by the activation of one or other or both of the motor proteins simultaneously.

Slow transport involves the bulk movement of the cytoplasm and includes the movement of mitochondria and other organelles. Slow axonal transport occurs only in the anterograde direction. The molecular motor has not been identified but is probably one of the kinesin family.

Lysosomes are membrane-bound vesicles measuring about 8 nm in diameter. They serve the cell by acting as intracellular scavengers and contain hydrolytic enzymes.

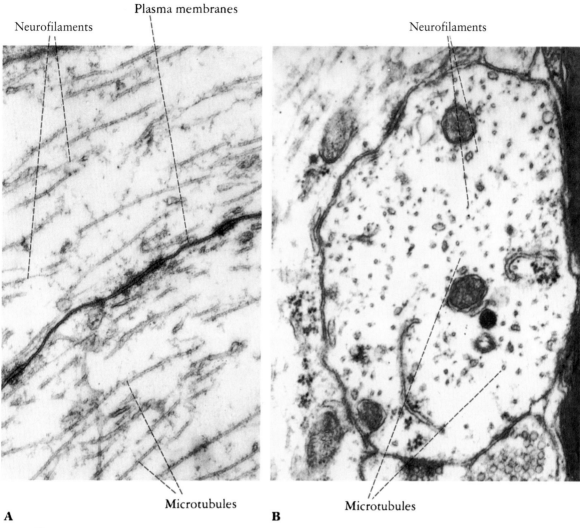

Neurofilaments

Plasma membranes

Neurofilaments

Microtubules

Microtubules

A   **B**

Figure 2–14   Electron micrograph of dendrites showing the presence of neurofilaments and micro-tubules within their cytoplasm. (Courtesy Dr. J. M. Kerns.) **A.** Longitudinal section of two adjacent dendrites. **B.** Transverse section of a dendrite.

They are formed by the budding off of the Golgi apparatus. Lysosomes exist in three forms: (1) **primary lysosomes,** which have just been formed; (2) **secondary lysosomes,** which contain partially digested material (myelin figures); and (3) **residual bodies,** in which the enzymes are inactive and which have evolved from digestible materials such as pigment and lipid.

Centrioles are small, paired structures found in immature dividing nerve cells. Each centriole is a hollow cylinder whose wall is made up of bundles of microtubules. They are associated with the formation of the spindle during cell division and in the formation of microtubules. Centrioles are also found in mature nerve cells, where they are believed to be involved in the maintenance of microtubules.

Lipofuscin (pigment material) occurs as yellowish-brown granules within the cytoplasm (Fig. 2-15). It is believed to be formed as the result of lysosomal activity and

it represents a harmless metabolic by-product. Lipofuscin accumulates with age.

Melanin granules are found in the cytoplasm of cells in certain parts of the brain (e.g., the substantia nigra of the midbrain). Their presence may be related to the catecholamine-synthesizing ability of these neurons whose neurotransmitter is dopamine.

The main structures present in a nerve cell body are summarized in Table 2-2.

Plasma Membrane

The plasma membrane forms the continuous external boundary of the cell body and its processes and in the neuron it is the site for the initiation and conduction of the nerve impulse (Figs. 2-10 and 2-14). The membrane is about 8 nm thick, too thin to be seen with the light microscope.

Lipofuscin granules

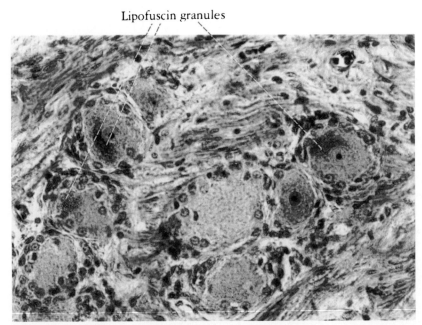

Figure 2–15 Photomicrograph of a longitudinal section of a posterior root ganglion showing the presence of lipofuscin granules within the cytoplasm of sensory neurons.

When viewed under the electron microscope, the plasma membrane appears as two dark lines with a light line between them.

The plasma membrane is composed of an inner and an outer layer of very loosely arranged protein molecules, each layer being about 2.5 nm thick, separated by a middle layer of lipid about 3 nm thick. The lipid layer is made up of two rows of phospholipid molecules arranged so that their hydrophobic ends are in contact with each other and their polar ends are in contact with the protein layers. Certain protein molecules lie within the phospholipid layer and span the entire width of the lipid layer. These molecules provide the membrane with hydrophilic channels through which inorganic ions may enter and leave the cell. Carbohydrate molecules are attached to the outside of the plasma membrane and are linked to the proteins or the lipids, forming what is known as the **cell coat,** or **glycocalyx.**

The plasma membrane and the cell coat together form a semipermeable membrane that allows diffusion of certain ions through it, but restricts others. In the resting state (unstimulated state) the K^+ ions diffuse through the plasma membrane from the cell cytoplasm to the tissue fluid (Fig. 2-16). The permeability of the membrane to K^+ ions is much greater than that to the Na^+ ions, so that the passive efflux of K^+ is much greater than the influx of Na^+. This results in a steady potential difference of about -80 mV, which can be measured across the plasma membrane since the inside of the membrane is negative with respect to the outside. This potential is known as the **resting potential.**

EXCITATION OF THE PLASMA MEMBRANE OF THE NERVE CELL BODY

When the nerve cell is excited (stimulated) by electrical, mechanical, or chemical means, a rapid change in membrane permeability to Na^+ ions takes place and Na^+ ions diffuse through the plasma membrane into the cell cytoplasm from the tissue fluid (Fig. 2-16). This results in the membrane's becoming progressively depolarized. The sudden influx of Na^+ ions followed by the altered polarity produces the so-called **action potential,** which is approximately $+40$ mV. This potential is very brief, lasting about 5 msec. The increased membrane permeability for Na^+ ions quickly ceases and that for K^+ ions increases, so that the K^+ ions start to flow from the cell cytoplasm and return the localized area of the cell to the resting state.

Once generated, the action potential spreads over the plasma membrane, away from the site of initiation, and is conducted along neurites as the **nerve impulse.** This impulse is self-propagated and its size and frequency do not alter (Fig. 2-16). Once the nerve impulse has spread over a given region of plasma membrane, another action potential cannot be elicited immediately. The duration of this nonexcitable state is referred to as the **refractory period.**

The greater the strength of the initial stimulus, the larger will be the initial depolarization and the greater the spread into the surrounding areas of the plasma membrane. Should multiple excitatory stimuli be applied to the surface of a neuron, then the effect can be **summated.** For example, subthreshold stimuli may pass over the surface of the cell

Table 2–2   The Main Structures in a Nerve Cell Body

Structure	Shape	Appearance	Location	Function
Nucleus	Large, rounded	Pale, chromatin widely scattered; single prominent nucleolus; Barr body present in female	Centrally placed; displaced to periphery in cell injury	Controls cell activity
Cytoplasmic organelles				
Nissl substance	Granules of rough endoplasmic reticulum	Broad cisternae; ribosomes are basophilic	Throughout cytoplasm and proximal part of dendrites; absent from axon hillock and axon; fatigue and injury result in concentration at periphery	Synthesizes protein
Golgi complex	Wavy threads; clusters of flattened cisternae and small vesicles	Smooth endoplasmic recticulum	Close to the nucleus	Adds carbohydrate to protein molecule, packages products for transport to nerve terminals; forms cell membranes
Mitochondria	Spherical, rod-shaped	Double membrane with cristae	Scattered	Form chemical energy
Neurofibrils	Linear fibrils	Run parallel to each other; composed of bundles of microfilaments, each 10 nm in diameter	Run from dendrites through cell body to axon	Determines the shape of the neuron
Microfilaments	Linear fine fibrils	Form a dense network beneath the plasma membrane, 3–5 mm in diameter	Role in formation and retraction of cell processes and in cell transport	
Microtubules	Linear tubes	Run between neurofibrils, 25 nm in diameter	Run from dendrites through cell body to axon	Cell transport
Lysosomes	Vesicles	8 nm in diameter; three forms: primary, secondary, and residual bodies	Throughout cell	Cell scavengers
Centrioles	Paired hollow cylinders	Wall made up of bundles of microtubules	Confined to cytoplasm of cell body	Take part in cell division; maintain microtubules
Lipofuscin	Granules	Yellowish-brown	Scattered through cytoplasm	Metabolic by-product
Melanin	Granules	Yellowish-brown	Substantia nigra of midbrain	Related to formation of dopa

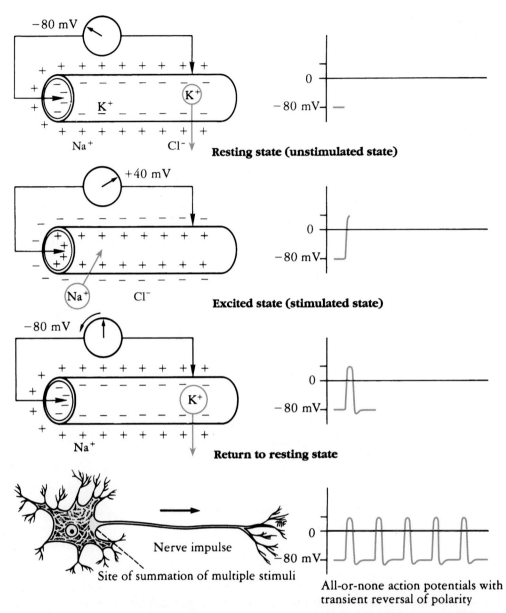

Figure 2–16   Ionic and electrical changes that occur in a neuron when it is stimulated.

body and be summated at the root of the axon and so initiate an action potential.

Inhibitory stimuli are believed to produce their effect by causing an influx of Cl⁻ ions through the plasma membrane into the neuron, thus producing hyperpolarization and reducing the excitatory state of the cell (Fig. 2-17).

SODIUM AND POTASSIUM CHANNELS

The sodium and potassium channels, through which the sodium and potassium ions diffuse through the plasma membrane, are formed of the protein molecules that extend through the full thickness of the plasma membrane (Fig. 2-18). Why a particular channel permits the passage of

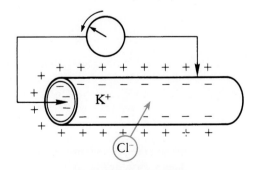

Hyperpolarization

Figure 2–17   Ionic and electrical changes that occur in a neuron during hyperpolarization.

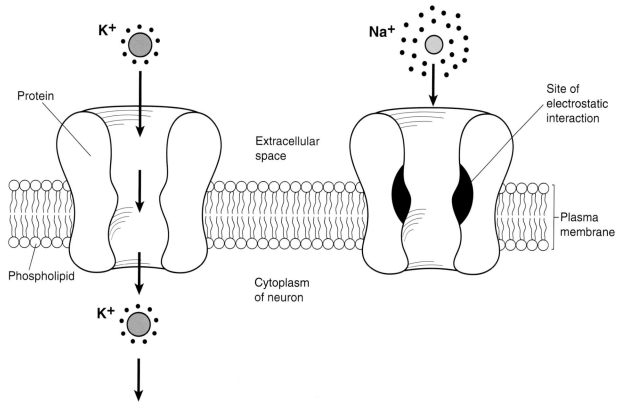

Figure 2–18 Ionic permeability of the plasma membrane. Diagram shows the interactions of the ions with water, the membrane lipid bilayer, and the ion channels.

K ions while excluding Na ions is difficult to explain. The selectivity cannot be due to the diameter of the ions, since the K ion is larger than the Na ion. However, the movement of ions in solution depends not only on the size of the ion but also on the size of the shell of water surrounding it. K ions have weaker electric fields than Na ions and thus K ions attract less water than Na ions. Thus K ions behave as if they are smaller than Na ions. This physico-chemical explanation does not entirely account for why a channel is selective. It is possible that the channels have narrow regions along their length that act as sieves or molecular filters. The ions may also participate in electrostatic interactions with the amino acid residues lining the walls of the channel.

The ion channel proteins are relatively stable but they exist in at least two conformational states which represent an open functional state and a closed functional state. The mechanism responsible for the opening and closing of a channel is not understood but may be likened to a gate that is opened and closed. **Gating** may involve the twisting and distortion of the channel thus creating a wider or narrower lumen. Gating appears to occur in response to such stimuli as voltage change, the presence of a ligand, or stretch or pressure.

In the nonstimulated state, the gates of the potassium channels are open wider than those of the sodium chan-

nels, which are nearly closed. This permits the potassium ions to diffuse out of the cell cytoplasm more readily than the sodium ions can diffuse in. In the stimulated state, the gates of the sodium channels are at first wide open; then the gates of the potassium channels are opened and the gates of the sodium channels are nearly closed again. It is the opening and closing of the sodium and potassium channels that is thought to produce the depolarization and repolarization of the plasma membrane.

The absolute refractory period, which occurs at the onset of the action potential when a second stimulus is unable to produce a further electrical change, is thought to be due to the inability to get the sodium channels open. During the relative refractory period, when a very strong stimulus can produce an action potential, presumably the sodium channels are opened.

The Nerve Cell Processes

The processes of a nerve cell, often called neurites, may be divided into dendrites and an axon.

The **dendrites** are the short processes of the cell body (Fig. 2-19). Their diameter tapers as they extend from the cell body and they often branch profusely. In many neurons the finer branches bear large numbers of small projections called **dendritic spines**. The cytoplasm of the dendrites

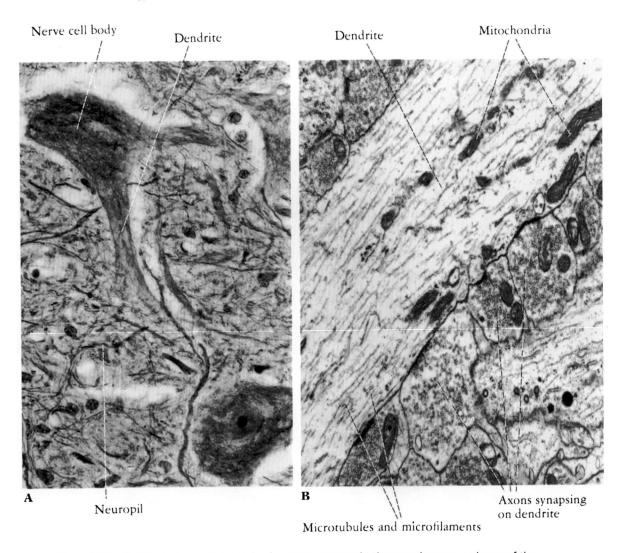

Nerve cell body   Dendrite   Dendrite   Mitochondria

A   Neuropil

B   Microtubules and microfilaments   Axons synapsing on dendrite

Figure 2–19   A. Light photomicrograph of a motor neuron in the anterior gray column of the spinal cord, showing the nerve cell body, two dendrites, and the surrounding neuropil. **B.** Electron micrograph of a dendrite showing axodendritic synapses. (Courtesy Dr. J. M. Kerns.)

closely resembles that of the cell body and contains Nissl granules, mitochondria, microtubules, microfilaments, ribosomes, and agranular endoplasmic reticulum. Dendrites should be regarded merely as extensions of the cell body to increase the surface area for the reception of axons from other neurons. Essentially they conduct the nerve impulse toward the cell body.

Axon is the name given to the longest process of the cell body. It arises from a small conical elevation on the cell body, devoid of Nissl's granules, called the **axon hillock** (Figs. 2-8 and 2-20). Occasionally, an axon arises from the proximal part of a dendrite. An axon is tubular and is uniform in diameter; it tends to have a smooth surface.

Axons usually do not branch close to the cell body; collateral branches may occur along their length. Shortly before their termination, axons commonly branch profuse-

ly. The distal ends of the terminal branches of the axons are often enlarged; they are called **terminals** Fig. 2-21). Some axons (especially those of autonomic nerves) near their termination show a series of swellings resembling a string of beads; these swellings are called **varicosities.**

Axons may be very short (0.1 mm), as seen in many neurons of the central nervous system, or extremely long (3 m), as seen when they extend from a peripheral receptor in the skin of the toe to the spinal cord and thence to the brain.

The diameter of axons varies considerably with different neurons. Those of larger diameter conduct impulses rapidly and those of smaller diameter conduct impulses very slowly.

The plasma membrane bounding the axon is called the **axolemma.** The cytoplasm of the axon is termed the **axoplasm.** Axoplasm differs from the cytoplasm of the cell

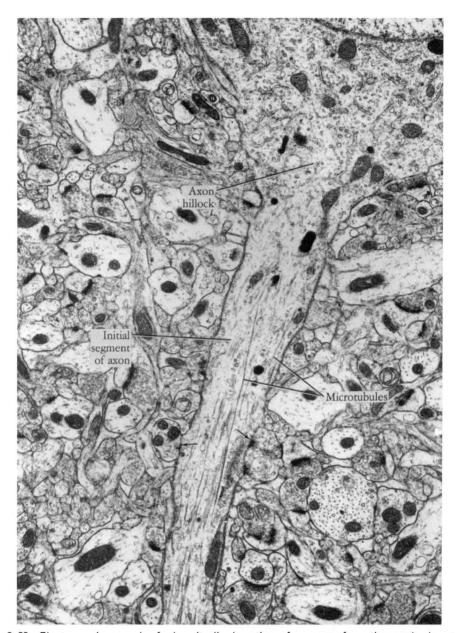

Figure 2–20   Electron micrograph of a longitudinal section of a neuron from the cerebral cortex, showing the detailed structure of the region of the axon hillock and the initial segment of the axon. Note the absence of Nissl substance (rough endoplasmic reticulum) in the axon hillock and the presence of numerous microtubules in the axoplasm. Note also the axon terminals (arrows) forming axoaxonal synapses with the initial segment of the axon. (Courtesy Dr. A. Peters.)

body in possessing no Nissl granules or Golgi complex. The sites for the production of protein, namely RNA and ribosomes, are absent. Thus, axonal survival depends on the transport of substances from the cell bodies.

The **initial segment** of the axon is the first 50 to 100 μm after it leaves the axon hillock of the nerve cell body (Fig. 2-20). This is the most excitable part of the axon and is the site

at which an action potential originates. It is important to remember that under normal conditions an action potential does not originate on the plasma membrane of the cell body, but always at the initial segment.

It is usual to state that an axon always conducts impulses away from the cell body. The axons of sensory posterior root ganglion cells are an exception; here the long neurite,

Axon containing large numbers of presynaptic vesicles

Terminal expansion of axon (bouton terminal)

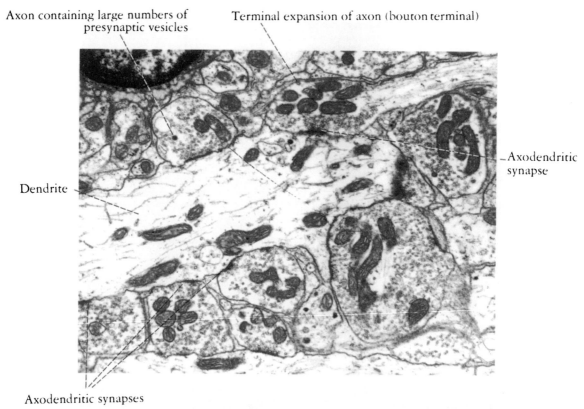

Axodendritic synapse

Dendrite

Axodendritic synapses

Figure 2–21 Electron micrograph showing multiple axodendritic synapses. Note the presence of large numbers of presynaptic vesicles within the axons. (Courtesy Dr. J. M. Kerns.)

which is indistinguishable from an axon, carries the impulse toward the cell body. (See unipolar neurons, p. 36.)

AXON TRANSPORT

Materials are transported from the cell body to the axon terminals (**anterograde transport**) and to a lesser extent in the opposite direction (**retrograde transport**).

Fast anterograde transport of 100 to 400 mm per day refers to the transport of proteins and transmitter substances or their precursors. **Slow anterograde transport** of 0.1 to 3 mm per day refers to the transport of axoplasm and includes the microfilaments and microtubules.

Retrograde transport explains how the cell bodies of nerve cells respond to changes in the distal end of the axons. For example, activated growth factor receptors can be carried along the axon to their site of action in the nucleus. Pinocytotic vesicles arising at the axon terminals can be quickly returned to the cell body. Worn-out organelles can be returned to the cell body for breakdown by the lysosomes.

Axon transport is brought about by microtubules assisted by the microfilaments.

Synapses

The nervous system consists of a large number of neurons that are linked together to form functional conducting path-

ways. Where two neurons come into close proximity and functional interneuronal communication occurs, the site of such communication is referred to as a **synapse*** (Fig. 2-22). Most neurons may make synaptic connections to a 1000 or more other neurons and may receive up to 10,000 connections from other neurons. Communication at a synapse, under physiological conditions, takes place in one direction only. Synapses occur in a number of forms (Fig. 2-22). The most common type is that which occurs between an axon of one neuron and the dendrite or cell body of the second neuron. As the axon approaches the synapse it may have a terminal expansion (bouton terminal) or it may have a series of expansions (bouton de passage), each of which makes synaptic contact. In other types of synapses the axon synapses on the initial segment of another axon, that is, proximal to where the myelin sheath begins, or there may be synapses between terminal expansions from different neurons. Depending on the site of the synapse, they are often referred to as **axodendritic, axosomatic,** or **axoaxonic** (Fig. 2-22).

The manner in which an axon terminates varies considerably in different parts of the nervous system. For example,

---

*The definition has come to include the site at which a neuron comes into close proximity with a skeletal muscle cell and functional communication occurs.

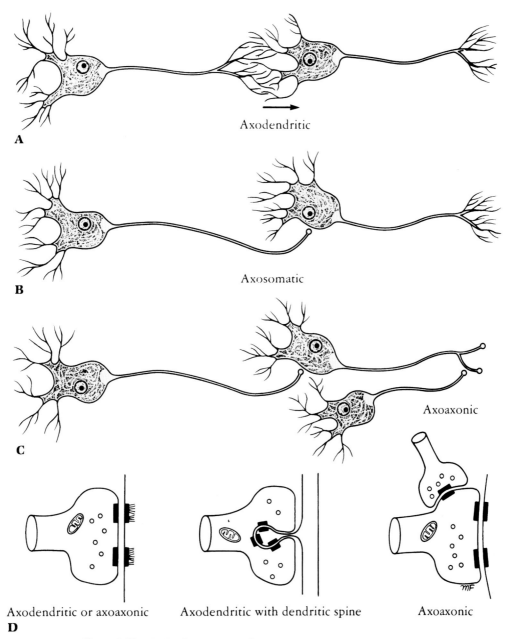

A

Axodendritic

B

Axosomatic

C

Axoaxonic

Axodendritic or axoaxonic

D

Axodendritic with dendritic spine

Axoaxonic

Figure 2–22 **A, B, C,** and **D.** Different types of chemical synapses.

a single axon may terminate on a single neuron, as in the case of a climbing fiber in the cerebellar cortex ending on a single Purkinje cell; or a single axon may synapse with multiple neurons, as in the case of the parallel fibers of the cerebellar cortex synapsing with multiple Purkinje cells. In the same way, a single neuron may have synaptic junctions with axons of many different neurons. The arrangement of these synapses will determine the means by which a neuron can be stimulated or inhibited. **Synaptic spines,** extensions of the surface of a neuron, form receptive sites for synaptic contact with afferent boutons (Fig. 2-22).

Synapses are of two types: chemical and electrical. Most synapses are chemical, in which a chemical substance, the **neurotransmitter,** passes across the narrow space between the cells and becomes attached to a protein molecule in the postsynaptic membrane called the **receptor.**

In most chemical synapses, several neurotransmitters may be present. One neurotransmitter is usually the principal activator and acts directly on the postsynaptic membrane, while the other transmitters function as modulators and modify the activity of the principal transmitter.

Axons near termination   Presynaptic vesicles   Terminal expansion
of axon

Dendrite

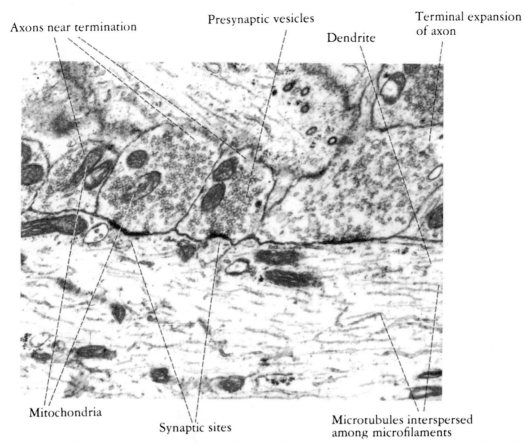

Mitochondria

Synaptic sites

Microtubules interspersed
among microfilaments

Figure 2–23   High-power electron micrograph of axodendritic synapses showing the thickening of the cell membranes at the synaptic sites, presynaptic vesicles, and the presence of mitochondria within the axons near their termination. (Courtesy Dr. J. M. Kerns.)

CHEMICAL SYNAPSES

Ultrastructure of Chemical Synapses

On examination with the electron microscope, synapses are seen to be areas of structural specialization (Figs. 2-21 and 2-23). The apposed surfaces of the terminal axonal expansion and the neuron are called the **presynaptic** and **postsynaptic membranes,** respectively, and they are separated by a **synaptic cleft** measuring about 20-30 nm wide. The presynaptic and postsynaptic membranes are thickened and the adjacent underlying cytoplasm shows increased density. On the presynaptic side, the dense cytoplasm is broken up into groups and on the postsynaptic side the density often extends into a **subsynaptic web. Presynaptic vesicles,** mitochondria, and occasional lysosomes are present in the cytoplasm close to the presynaptic membrane (Fig. 2-23). On the postsynaptic side, the cytoplasm often contains parallel cisternae. The synaptic cleft contains polysaccharides.

The presynaptic terminal contains many small presynaptic vesicles that contain the molecules of the neurotransmitter(s). The vesicles fuse with the presynaptic membrane and discharge the neurotransmitter(s) into the synaptic cleft by a process of exocytosis (Fig. 2-24).

When synapses are first formed in the embryo, they are recognized as small zones of density separated by a synaptic cleft. Later they mature into well-differentiated structures. The presence of simple, undifferentiated synapses in the postnatal nervous system has led to the suggestion that synapses can be developed as required and possibly undergo atrophy when redundant. This plasticity of synapses may be of great importance in the process of learning and in the development and maintenance of memory.

Neurotransmitters at Chemical Synapses

The presynaptic vesicles and the mitochondria play a key role in the release of neurotransmitter substances at synapses. The vesicles contain the neurotransmitter substance that is released into the synaptic cleft; the mitochondria provide adenosine triphosphate (ATP) for the synthesis of new transmitter substance.

The majority of neurons produce and release only one principal transmitter at all their nerve endings. For example, acetylcholine is widely used as a transmitter by different neurons in the central and peripheral parts of the nervous

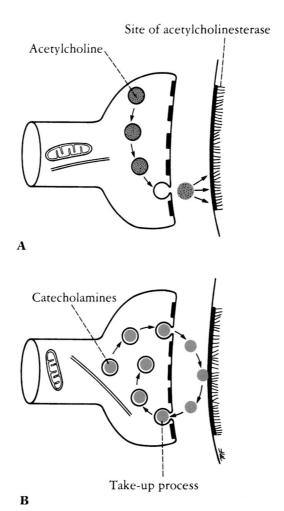

Figure 2–24 Release of neurotransmitters. **A.** Acetylcholine. **B.** Catecholamines.

Table 2–3 Examples of Principal (Classic) Neurotransmitters and Neuromodulators at Synapses				
Neuromediators*	Function	Receptor Mechanism	Ionic Mechanism	Location
Principal neurotransmitters				
Acetylcholine (nicotinic), L-glutamate	Rapid excitation	Ion channel receptors	Opens cation channel (fast EPSP)	Main sensory and motor systems
GABA	Rapid inhibition		Opens anion channel for Cl⁻ (fast IPSP)	
Neuromodulators				
Acetylcholine (muscarinic), serotonin, histamine, adenosine	Modulation and modification of activity	G-protein–coupled receptors	Opens or closes K⁺ or Ca²⁺ channels (slow IPSP and slow EPSP)	Systems that control homeostasis

EPSP = excitatory postsynaptic potential; IPSP = inhibitory postsynaptic potential.
*Note that these are only a few examples of an ever-increasing number of known neuromediators.

system, whereas dopamine is released by neurons in the substantia nigra. Glycine, another transmitter, is found principally in synapses in the spinal cord.

The following are chemical substances known to act as neurotransmitters and there are probably many more yet to be discovered: acetylcholine (ACh), norepinephrine, epinephrine, dopamine, glycine, serotonin, gamma-aminobutyric acid (GABA), enkephalins, substance P, and glutamic acid.

Action of Neurotransmitters

All neurotransmitters are released from their nerve endings by the arrival of the nerve impulse (action potential). This results in an influx of calcium ions, which causes the synaptic vesicles to fuse with the presynaptic membrane. The neurotransmitters are then ejected into the synaptic cleft. Once in the cleft they achieve their objective by raising or lowering the resting potential of the postsynaptic membrane for a brief period of time.

The receptor proteins on the postsynaptic membrane bind the transmitter substance and undergo an immediate conformational change that opens the ion channel, generating an immediate but brief excitatory postsynaptic potential (EPSP) or an inhibitory postsynaptic potential (IPSP). The rapid excitation is seen with acetylcholine (nicotinic) and L-glutamate, or the inhibition is seen with GABA (Table 2-3). Other receptor proteins bind the transmitter substance and activate a second messenger system, usually through a molecular transducer, a G-protein. These receptors have a longer latent period and the duration of the response may last several minutes or longer. Acetylcholine (muscarinic), serotonin, histamine, neuropeptides, and adenosine are good examples of this type of transmitter, which is often referred to as a neuromodulator (see next section).

The excitatory and the inhibitory effects on the postsynaptic membrane of the neuron will depend on the summation of the postsynaptic responses at the different synapses. If the overall effect is one of depolarization, the neuron will be excited and an action potential will be initiated at the initial segment of the axon and a nerve impulse will travel along the axon. If, on the other hand, the overall effect is one of hyperpolarization, the neuron will be inhibited and no nerve impulse will arise.

Distribution and Fate of Neurotransmitters

The distribution of the neurotransmitters varies in different parts of the nervous system. **Acetylcholine,** for example, is found at the neuromuscular junction, in autonomic ganglia, and at parasympathetic nerve endings. In the central nervous system, the motor neuron collaterals to the **Renshaw cells** are cholinergic. In the hippocampus, the ascending reticular pathways, and the afferent fibers for the visual and auditory systems, the neurotransmitters are also cholinergic.

Norepinephrine is found at sympathetic nerve endings. In the central nervous system, it is found in high concentration in the hypothalamus. **Dopamine** is found in high concentration in different parts of the central nervous system, for example, in the basal nuclei (ganglia).

The effect produced by a neurotransmitter is limited by its destruction or reabsorption. For example, in the case of acetylcholine, the effect is limited by the destruction of the transmitter in the synaptic cleft by the enzyme **acetylcholinesterase** (AChE) (Fig. 2-24). However, with the **catecholamines** the effect is limited by the return of the transmitter to the presynaptic nerve ending (Fig. 2-24).

Neuromodulators at Chemical Synapses

It is interesting to note that in many synapses certain substances other than the principal neurotransmitters are ejected from the presynaptic membrane into the synaptic cleft. These are capable of modulating and modifying the activity of the postsynaptic neuron and are called **neuromodulators.**

Action of Neuromodulators

Neuromodulators can coexist with the principal neurotransmitter at a single synapse. Usually, but not always, the neuromodulators are in separate presynaptic vesicles. Whereas on release into the synaptic cleft the principal neurotransmitters have a rapid, brief effect on the postsynaptic membrane, the neuromodulators on release into the cleft do not have a direct effect on the postsynaptic membrane. Rather they enhance, prolong, inhibit, or limit the effect of the principal neurotransmitter on the postsynaptic membrane. The neuromodulators act through a second messenger system, usually through a molecular transducer, a G-protein, and alter the response of the receptor to the neurotransmitter. In a given area of the nervous system, many different afferent neurons can release several different neuromodulators that are picked up by the postsynaptic neuron. Such an arrangement can lead to a wide variety of responses, depending on the input from the afferent neurons.

ELECTRICAL SYNAPSES

Electrical synapses are gap junctions containing channels that extend from the cytoplasm of the presynaptic neuron to that of the postsynaptic neuron. The neurons communicate electrically; there is no chemical transmitter. The bridging channels permit ionic current flow to take place from one cell to the other with the minimum of delay. In electrical synapses the rapid spread of activity from one neuron to another ensures that a group of neurons performing an identical function act together. Electrical synapses also have the advantage that they are bidirectional; chemical synapses are not.

DEFINITION OF NEUROGLIA

The neurons of the central nervous system are supported by several varieties of nonexcitable cells, which together are called **neuroglia** (Fig. 2-25). Neuroglial cells are generally smaller than neurons and outnumber them 5 to 10 times; they comprise about half the total volume of the brain and spinal cord.

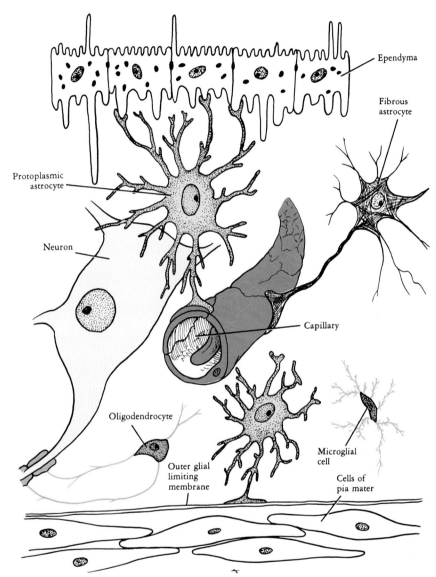

Figure 2–25   Diagrammatic representation of the arrangement of different types of neuroglial cells.

Table 2–4   The Structural Features, Location, and Functions of the Different Neuroglial Cells

Neuroglial Cell	Structure	Location	Function
Astrocytes			
Fibrous	Small cell bodies, long slender processes, cytoplasmic filaments, perivascular feet	White matter	Provide supporting framework, are electrical insulators, limit spread of neurotransmitters, take up K$^+$ ions, store glycogen, have a phagocytic function, take place of dead neurons, are a conduit for metabolites or raw materials, produce trophic substances
Protoplasmic	Small cell bodies, short thick processes, many branches, few cytoplasmic filaments, perivascular feet	Gray matter	
Oligodendrocytes	Small cell bodies, few delicate processes, no cytoplasmic filaments	In rows along myelinated nerves, surrounding neuron cell bodies	Form myelin in CNS, influence biochemistry of neurons
Microglia	Smallest of neuroglial cells, wavy branches with spines	Scattered throughout CNS	Are inactive in normal CNS, proliferate in disease and phagocytose, joined by blood monocytes
Ependyma			
Ependymocytes	Cuboidal or columnar in shape with cilia and microvilli, gap junctions	Line ventricles, central canal	Circulate CSF, absorb CSF
Tanycytes	Long basal processes with end feet on capillaries	Line floor of third ventricle	Transport substances from CSF to hypophyseal-portal system
Choroidal epithelial cells	Sides and bases thrown into folds, tight junctions	Cover surfaces of choroid plexuses	Produce and secrete CSF

CNS = central nervous system; CSF = cerebrospinal fluid.

There are four types of neuroglial cells: (1) astrocytes, (2) oligodendrocytes, (3) microglia, and (4) ependyma (Fig. 2-25). A summary of the structural features, location, and functions of the different neuroglial cells is provided in Table 2-4.

ASTROCYTES

Astrocytes have small cell bodies with branching processes that extend in all directions. There are two types of astrocytes: fibrous and protoplasmic.

Fibrous astrocytes are found mainly in the white matter, where their processes pass between the nerve fibers (Fig. 2-26). Each process is long, slender, smooth, and not much branched. The cell bodies and processes contain many filaments in their cytoplasm.

Protoplasmic astrocytes are found mainly in the gray matter, where their processes pass between the nerve cell bodies (Figs. 2-27 and 2-28). The processes are shorter, thicker, and more branched than those of the fibrous astrocyte. The cytoplasm of these cells contains fewer filaments than that of the fibrous astrocyte.

Many of the processes of astrocytes end in expansions on blood vessels (perivascular feet), where they form an almost complete covering on the external surface of capillaries. Large numbers of astrocytic processes are interwoven at the outer and inner surfaces of the central nervous system, where they form the **outer** and **inner glial limiting membranes**. Thus the outer glial limiting membrane is found beneath the pia mater and the inner glial limiting membrane is situated beneath the ependyma lining the ventricles of the brain and the central canal of the spinal cord.

Astrocytic processes are also found in large numbers around the initial segment of most axons and in the bare segments of axons at the nodes of Ranvier. Axon terminals at many sites are separated from other nerve cells and their processes by an envelope of astrocytic processes.

Functions of Astrocytes

Astrocytes with their branching processes form a supporting framework for the nerve cells and nerve fibers. In the embryo they serve as a scaffolding for the migration of immature neurons. By covering the synaptic contacts between neurons, they may serve as electrical insulators preventing axon terminals from influencing neighboring and unrelated neurons. They may even form barriers for the spread of neurotransmitter substances released at synapses. Astrocytes have been shown to absorb gamma-aminobutyric acid (GABA) and glutamic acid secreted by the nerve terminals, thereby limiting the influence of these neurotransmitters. Astrocytes appear to be able to take up excess K$^+$ ions from the extracellular space so that they may have an important function during repetitive firing of a neuron. They store glycogen within their cytoplasm. The glycogen can be broken down into glucose and released to surrounding neurons in response to norepinephrine.

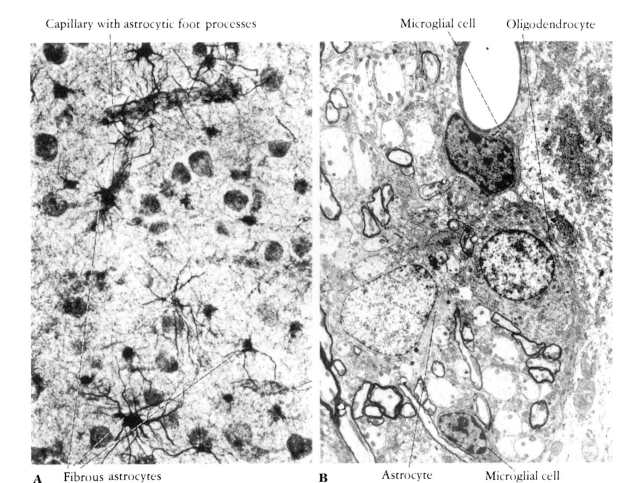

Capillary with astrocytic foot processes   Microglial cell   Oligodendrocyte

A   Fibrous astrocytes   B   Astrocyte   Microglial cell

Figure 2–26   **A.** Photomicrograph of a section of the gray matter of the spinal cord showing fibrous astrocytes. **B.** Electron micrograph showing an astrocyte. (Courtesy Dr. J. M. Kerns.)

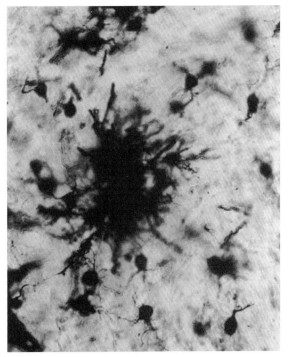

Figure 2–27   Photomicrograph of a protoplasmic astrocyte in the cerebral cortex.

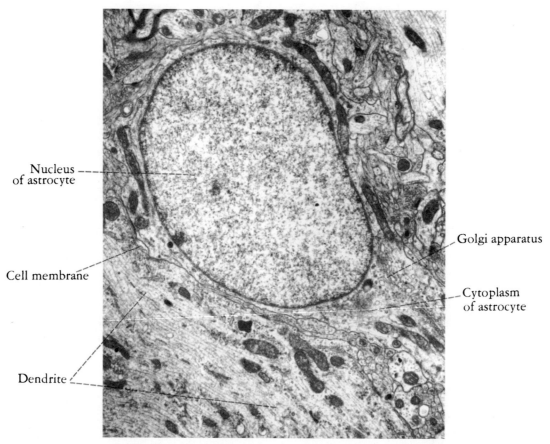

Nucleus of astrocyte

Cell membrane

Dendrite

Golgi apparatus

Cytoplasm of astrocyte

Figure 2–28 Electron micrograph of a protoplasmic astrocyte in the cerebral cortex. (Courtesy Dr. A. Peters.)

Astrocytes may serve as phagocytes by taking up degenerating synaptic axon terminals. Following the death of neurons due to disease, they proliferate and fill in the spaces previously occupied by the neurons, a process called **replacement gliosis.** It is possible that astrocytes can serve as a conduit for the passage of metabolites or raw materials from blood capillaries to the neurons through their perivascular feet. The fact that astrocytes are linked together by gap junctions would enable ions to pass from one cell to another without entering the extracellular space. Astrocytes may produce substances that have a trophic influence on neighboring neurons.

OLIGODENDROCYTES

Oligodendrocytes have small cell bodies and a few delicate processes; there are no filaments in their cytoplasm. Oligodendrocytes are frequently found in rows along myelinated nerve fibers and surround nerve cell bodies (Fig. 2-29). Electron micrographs show the processes of a single oligodendrocyte joining the myelin sheaths of several nerve

fibers (Fig. 2-30). However, only one process joins the myelin between two adjacent nodes of Ranvier.

Functions of Oligodendrocytes

Oligodendrocytes are responsible for the formation of the myelin sheath of nerve fibers in the central nervous system, much as the myelin of peripheral nerves is formed from Schwann cells. Because oligodendrocytes have several processes, unlike Schwann cells, they can each form several internodal segments of myelin on the same or different axons. A single oligodendrocyte can form as many as 60 internodal segments. It should also be noted that unlike Schwann cells in the peripheral nervous system, oligodendrocytes and their associated axons are **not** surrounded by a basement membrane. Myelination begins at about the sixteenth week of intrauterine life and continues postnatally until practically all the major nerve fibers are myelinated by the time the child is walking.

Oligodendrocytes also surround nerve cell bodies (satellite oligodendrocytes) and probably have a similar function

Oligodendrocytes

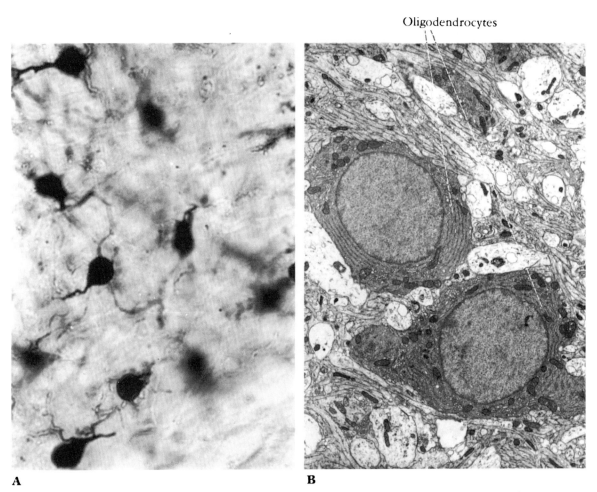

A   **B**

Figure 2–29 **A.** Photomicrograph of a group of oligodendrocytes. **B.** Electron micrograph of two oligodendrocytes. (Courtesy Dr. J. M. Kerns.)

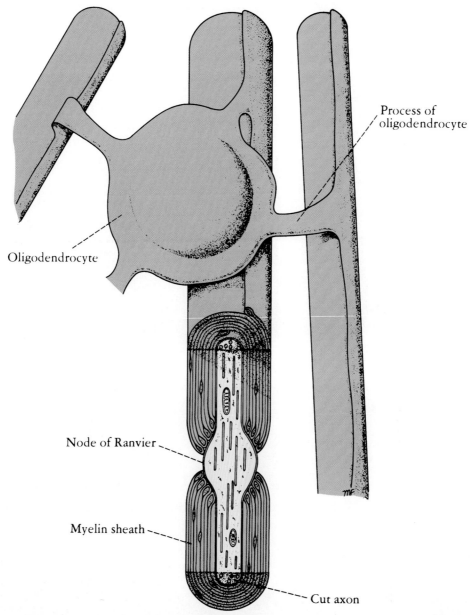

Figure 2–30 A single oligodendrocyte whose processes are continuous with the myelin sheaths of four nerve fibers within the central nervous system.

to the satellite or capsular cells of peripheral sensory ganglia. They are thought to influence the biochemical environment of neurons.

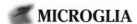
MICROGLIA

The microglial cells are embryologically unrelated to the other neuroglial cells and are derived from macrophages outside the nervous system. They are the smallest of the neuroglial cells and are found scattered throughout the central nervous system (Fig. 2-31). From their small cell bodies arise wavy branching processes that give off numer-

ous spinelike projections. They closely resemble connective tissue macrophages. They migrate into the nervous system during fetal life. Microglial cells increase in number in the presence of damaged nervous tissue and many of these new cells are monocytes that have migrated from the blood.

Function of Microglial Cells

Microglial cells in the normal brain and spinal cord appear to be inactive and are sometimes called **resting microglial cells.** In inflammatory and degenerative lesions of the central nervous system, they retract their processes and migrate

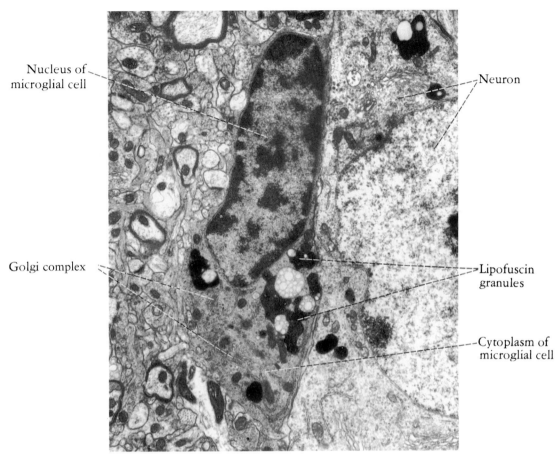

Nucleus of microglial cell

Neuron

Golgi complex

Lipofuscin granules

Cytoplasm of microglial cell

Figure 2–31   Electron micrograph of a microglial cell in the cerebral cortex. (Courtesy Dr. A. Peters.)

to the site of the lesion. Here they proliferate and are actively phagocytic; their cytoplasm becomes filled with lipids and cell remnants. The microglial cells are joined by monocytes from neighboring blood vessels.

 EPENDYMA

Ependymal cells line the cavities of the brain and the central canal of the spinal cord. They form a single layer of cells that are cuboidal or columnar in shape and possess microvilli and cilia (Fig. 2-32). The cilia are often motile and their movements contribute to the flow of the cerebrospinal fluid. The bases of the ependymal cells lie on the internal glial limiting membrane.

Ependymal cells may be divided into three groups:

1. **Ependymocytes,** which line the ventricles of the brain and the central canal of the spinal cord and are in contact with the cerebrospinal fluid. Their adjacent surfaces have gap junctions, but the cerebrospinal fluid is in free communication with the intercellular spaces of the central nervous system.
2. **Tanycytes,** which line the floor of the third ventricle overlying the median eminence of the hypothalamus.

These cells have long basal processes that pass between the cells of the median eminence and place end feet on blood capillaries.

3. **Choroidal epithelial cells,** which cover the surfaces of the choroid plexuses. The sides and bases of these cells are thrown into folds and near their luminal surfaces the cells are held together by tight junctions that encircle the cells. The presence of tight junctions prevents the leakage of cerebrospinal fluid into the underlying tissues.

Functions of Ependymal Cells

Ependymocytes assist in the circulation of the cerebrospinal fluid within the cavities of the brain and the central canal of the spinal cord by the movements of the cilia. The microvilli on the free surfaces of the ependymocytes would indicate that they also have an absorptive function. Tanycytes are thought to transport chemical substances from the cerebrospinal fluid to the hypophyseal portal system. In this manner they may play a part in the control of the hormone production by the anterior lobe of the pituitary. Choroidal epithelial cells are involved in the production and secretion of cerebrospinal fluid from the choroid plexuses.

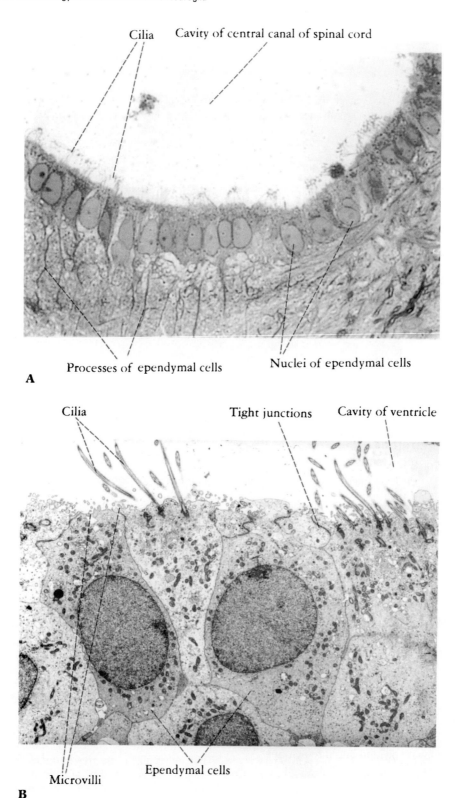

Figure 2–32 **A.** Photomicrograph of ependymal cells lining the central canal of the spinal cord. **B.** Electron micrograph of ependymal cells lining the cavity of the third ventricle. (Courtesy Dr. J. M. Kerns.)

EXTRACELLULAR SPACE

When nervous tissue is examined under an electron microscope, a very narrow gap separates the neurons and the neuroglial cells. These gaps are linked together and filled with tissue fluid; they are called the **extracellular space**. The extracellular space is in almost direct continuity with the cerebrospinal fluid in the subarachnoid space externally and with the cerebrospinal fluid in the ventricles of the brain and the central canal of the spinal cord internally. The

extracellular space also surrounds the blood capillaries in the brain and spinal cord. (There are no lymphatic capillaries in the central nervous system.)

The extracellular space thus provides a pathway for the exchange of ions and molecules between the blood and the neurons and glial cells. The plasma membrane of the endothelial cells of most capillaries is impermeable to many chemicals, and this forms the blood-brain barrier.

CLINICAL NOTES

GENERAL CONSIDERATIONS

The neuron is the basic functional unit of the nervous system. In the mature human if it is destroyed by trauma or disease, it is not replaced. It is incapable of undergoing cell division.

The neuron consists of the cell body and its processes, the axons, and the dendrites. All three parts are concerned with the process of conduction. The cell body is necessary for the normal metabolism of all its processes. Should these processes become separated from the cell body, as the result of disease or simple trauma, they will quickly degenerate. This would explain the necessity for the transport of macromolecules down the axon from the cell body and also emphasizes the dependence of the axon on the cell body. The rate of axoplasmic transport is insufficient to satisfy the release of transmitter substances at the nerve terminals. This problem is overcome in two ways. First, enzymes are present within the nerve terminals in order to synthesize the transmitters from amino acids derived from the extracellular fluid, and, second, at some terminals the transmitter is reabsorbed back into the terminal following its release. Clinically, it is possible, by the use of drugs, to influence this reuptake mechanism.

Neuroglial cells, in contrast to neurons, are nonexcitable and do not have axons, nor do axon terminals synapse upon them. They are smaller than neurons and yet outnumber them 5 to 10 times. They comprise about one-half the total volume of the central nervous system.

REACTION OF A NEURON TO INJURY

The first reaction of a nerve cell to injury is loss of function. Whether the cell recovers or dies will depend on the severity and duration of the damaging agent. If death occurs quickly, say in a few minutes from lack of oxygen, no morphological changes will be immediately apparent. Morphological evidence of cell injury requires a minimum of 6 to 12 hours of survival. The nerve cell becomes swollen and rounded off, the nucleus swells and is displaced toward the periphery of the cell, and the Nissl granules become dispersed toward the periphery of the cytoplasm. At this stage

the neuron could recover. If the kind of neuronal injury were not so severe as to cause death, the reparative changes would start to appear. The cell would resume its former size and shape, the nucleus would return to the center of the cell body, and the Nissl granules would take up their normal position.

When cell death is imminent or has just occurred, the cell cytoplasm stains dark with basic dyes (hyperchromatism) and the nuclear structure becomes unclear. The final stage occurs after cell death. The cytoplasm becomes vacuolated and the nucleus and cytoplasmic organelles disintegrate. The neuron now is dissolved and removed by the activity of the phagocytes. In the central nervous system this function is performed by the microglial cells and in the peripheral nervous system by local members of the reticuloendothelial system.

In chronic forms of injury, the size of the cell body is reduced, the nucleus and cytoplasm show hyperchromatism, and the nuclear membranes and those of the cytoplasmic organelles show irregularity.

Axonal Reaction And Axonal Degeneration

Axonal reaction and axonal degeneration are the changes that take place in a nerve cell when its axon is cut or injured. The changes start to appear within 24 to 48 hours after injury; the degree of change will depend on the severity of the injury to the axon, and will be greater if the injury occurred close to the cell body. The nerve cell becomes rounded off and swollen, the nucleus swells and becomes eccentrically placed, and the Nissl granules become dispersed toward the periphery of the cytoplasm. These changes reach their maximum in about 12 days.

In the peripheral nervous system, section of an axon is followed by attempts at regeneration and reparative changes take place in the cell body.

In the central nervous system degeneration is not followed by regeneration. If the corticospinal tracts, for example, are destroyed by disease, the nerve cells that give rise to these axons degenerate and disappear completely.

There is an important exception to the axonal reaction of nerve cells described above. This occurs in the nerve cells of the posterior root ganglia of the spinal nerves. If the peripheral axons are sectioned, the nerve cells show degenerative changes; if, however, the central axons are sectioned or destroyed by disease, such as tabes dorsalis, the nerve cells show no degenerative changes.

AXONAL TRANSPORT AND THE SPREAD OF DISEASE

Rabies, which is an acute viral disease of the central nervous system, is transmitted by the bite of an infected animal. The virus is present in the saliva of the infected animal and following a bite, travels to the central nervous system by way of axonal transport in both sensory and motor nerves. The incubation period is related to the length of the peripheral nerve involved: The longer the nerve, the longer the duration of the incubation period. **Herpes simplex and herpes zoster** are viral diseases that also involve axonal transport to spread to different parts of the body. Axonal transport is also believed to play a role in the spread of the **poliomyelitis** virus from the gastrointestinal tract to the motor cells of the anterior gray horns of the spinal cord and the brainstem.

TUMORS OF NEURONS

When considering tumors of the nervous system, one must not forget that the nervous system is made up of many different types of tissues. In the central nervous system there are neurons, neuroglia, blood vessels, and meninges and in the peripheral nervous system there are neurons, Schwann cells, connective tissue, and blood vessels. Tumors of neurons in the central nervous system are rare but tumors of peripheral neurons are not uncommon .

The **neuroblastoma** occurs in association with the suprarenal gland; it is highly malignant and occurs in infants and children. The **ganglioneuroma** occurs in the suprarenal medulla or sympathetic ganglia; it is benign and occurs in children and adults. The **pheochromocytoma** occurs in the suprarenal medulla; it is usually benign and gives rise to hypertension, since it secretes norepinephrine and epinephrine.

SYNAPTIC BLOCKING AGENTS

Transmission of a nervous impulse across a synapse is accomplished by the release of neurotransmitters into the synaptic cleft. Transmission occurs in one direction and subthreshold stimulation of many synapses leads to summation. The released transmitter then exerts its effect on the postsynaptic membrane, by increasing the permeability of the postsynaptic membrane to sodium and causing excitation or by increasing the permeability of the postsynaptic membrane to chloride and causing inhibition.

The synapse is a region in which transmission is easily blocked. As a general rule, long chains of neurons with multiple synapses are more easily blocked than are shorter, simpler chains of neurons. General anesthetic agents are effective because they have the ability to block synaptic transmission.

At autonomic ganglia, preganglionic fibers enter the ganglia and synapse with the postganglionic sympathetic or parasympathetic neurons. The nerve impulse, on reaching the termination of the preganglionic nerve, brings about the release of **acetylcholine,** which excites a nervous impulse in the postganglionic neuron.

Ganglionic blocking agents may be divided into three groups, depending on their mechanism of action. The first group of agents, which include the **hexamethonium** and **tetraethylammonium salts,** resemble acetylcholine at the postsynaptic membrane; they thus inhibit transmission across a synapse. The second group of agents, which include **nicotine,** have the same action as acetylcholine on the postsynaptic membrane but they are not destroyed by the cholinesterase. This results in a prolonged depolarization of the postsynaptic membrane, so that it is insensitive to further stimulation by acetylcholine. Unfortunately, this depolarization block is associated with initial stimulation and therefore these drugs are not suitable for clinical use. The third group of agents, which include **procaine,** inhibit the release of acetylcholine from the preganglionic fibers.

In the central nervous system, it is much more difficult to demonstrate the release of a particular transmitter substance at specific synapses, due to inaccessibility. For example, it is impossible to perfuse specific localized brain areas through their vascular system and it is very difficult to stimulate an isolated neuronal pathway within the brain or spinal cord. The motor neuron collaterals to the Renshaw cells have been shown to liberate acetylcholine at their endings. Many synapses in the central nervous system are also cholinergic. The development of monoclonal antibody techniques has opened a whole new approach to the identification and localization of chemical mediators in the central nervous system. Substance P, somatostatin, and cholecystokinin are a few examples of the neuropeptides that have been located in the central nervous system.

The nonuniform concentrations of norepinephrine in the central nervous system have led many investigators to believe that it might function as a central neurotransmitter. The concentrations are greater in gray matter than in white matter and the highest concentrations are found in the hypothalamus. Dopamine is found in high concentrations in the central nervous system and is secreted by neurons that originate in the substantia nigra.

Many of the cholinergic blocking agents used in the peripheral nervous system have little or no effect on the cholinergic synapses of the central nervous system because they are unable to cross the blood-brain barrier in significant concentrations. **Atropine, scopolamine,** and **diisopropylphosphorofluoridate** (DPF) can effectively cross the barrier and their effects on human behavior have been extensively studied. Similarly, it is believed that many psychotropic drugs bring about changes in the activities of the central nervous system by influencing the release of catecholamines at synaptic sites. The **phenothiazines,** for example, are thought to block dopamine receptors on postsynaptic neurons.

TREATMENT OF CERTAIN NEUROLOGICAL DISEASES BY THE MANIPULATION OF NEUROTRANSMITTERS

The increasing numbers of neurotransmitters being discovered in the central nervous system and the location of their site of action are raising the possibility that certain diseases can be modified by the administration of specific drugs. In Huntington's chorea, for example, there is a loss of neurons that use GABA and acetylcholine as transmitters. GABA is unable to cross the blood-brain barrier, but physostigmine, a cholinesterase inhibitor, can cross the barrier and its use has brought about some improvement. The use of L-dopa in the treatment of parkinsonism has been most successful; in this disease it replaces the deficiency of dopamine, which is normally released to the basal ganglia by the neurons of the substantia nigra.

REACTIONS OF NEUROGLIA TO INJURY

The reaction of neuroglial cells to injury, whether caused by physical trauma or by vascular occlusion, is characterized by the hyperplasia and hypertrophy of the astrocytes, which become fibrous irrespective of their antecedent morphology. The proliferation of the astrocytes is referred to as **astrocytosis** or **gliosis.** The loss of neuronal tissue is not compensated for in volume by the glial hypertrophy. The cytoplasm of the enlarged astrocytes contains large numbers of fibrils and glycogen granules. The dense feltwork of astrocytic processes that occurs in the areas of neuronal degeneration produces the so-called **gliotic scar.** The degree of gliosis is much greater in the presence of residual damaged neuronal tissue as compared with a clean surgical excision in which no traumatized brain remains. This is why, in patients with focal epilepsy due to a large gliotic scar, the scar is excised surgically, leaving a minimal glial reaction.

Oligodendrocytes respond to injury by expanding and showing vacuolation of their cytoplasm; the nuclei also tend to become pyknotic. Severe damage to oligodendrocytes would result in demyelination.

Microglial cells in inflammatory and degenerative lesions of the central nervous system retract their processes and migrate to the site of the lesion. Here they proliferate and are actively phagocytic and their cytoplasm becomes filled with lipids and cell remnants. They are joined in their scavenger activity by monocytes that migrate from the neighboring blood vessels.

Microglial cells are active in a number of diseases including multiple sclerosis, dementia in AIDS, Parkinson's disease and Alzheimer's disease.

NEOPLASMS OF NEUROGLIA

Tumors of neuroglia account for 40 to 50 percent of intracranial tumors. Such tumors are referred to as **gliomas.** Tumors of astrocytes are those most commonly encountered and include **astrocytomas** and **glioblastomas.** Apart from the ependymomas, tumors of the neuroglia are highly invasive. This explains the difficulty in achieving complete surgical removal and the great possibility of recurrence after surgery. Another feature is that as these tumors infiltrate, they often do so without interfering with the function of neighboring neurons. As a result, the tumor is often very much larger than the symptoms and physical signs would indicate.

MULTIPLE SCLEROSIS

Multiple sclerosis (MS) is one of the most common central nervous system diseases and affects about 250,000 Americans. It is characterized by the appearance of patches of demyelination in the white matter of the central nervous system, generally starting in the optic nerve, spinal cord, or cerebellum. The myelin sheaths degenerate and the myelin is removed by microglial cells. Astrocytes proliferate leading to the formation of a gliotic scar. As demyelination occurs, the conduction of the nerve impulses in the axons is impeded. Because raising the temperature shortens the duration of the action potential, one of the early signs of multiple sclerosis is that the symptoms and signs can be improved by cooling and made worse by heating by a hot bath. Most cases occur between the ages of 20 and 40. The cause of the disease is unknown, although an interplay between a viral infection and a host immune response may be responsible. For further discussion of this disease see Chapter 4.

CEREBRAL EDEMA

Cerebral edema is a very common clinical condition that can follow head injuries, cerebral infections, or tumors. The resultant swelling of the brain may lead to flattening of the cerebral gyri, herniation of the brain through the tentorial notch or the foramen magnum, and even death.

Cerebral edema may be defined as an abnormal increase in the water content of the tissues of the central nervous system. There are three forms: (1) vasogenic, (2) cytotoxic, and (3) interstitial. **Vasogenic edema** is the most common type and is due to the accumulation of tissue fluid in the extracellular space following damage to the vascular capillary walls or the presence of new capillaries without fully formed blood-brain barriers. It can result from infections, trauma, and tumors. **Cytotoxic edema** is due to the accumulation of fluid within the cells of nervous tissue (neurons and glial), resulting in cellular swelling. The cause may be toxic or metabolic and produces a failure in the plasma membrane ATP sodium pump mechanism. **Interstitial edema** occurs in obstructive hydrocephalus when the rise in cerebrospinal fluid pressure forces the fluid out of the ventricular system into the extracellular space.

Two anatomical factors must always be remembered in cerebral edema: (1) The brain volume is restricted by the surrounding skull and (2) the tissue fluid is drained primarily into the venous sinuses via cerebral veins, there being no lymphatic drainage.

Clinical Problem Solving

1. During an operation for the repair of a sectioned radial nerve in the arm, the neurosurgeon understood that he was operating on a large bundle of nerve fibers supported by connective tissue. He realized that the nerve fibers were either axons or dendrites, or the nerve was made up of a mixture of axons and dendrites. What is your understanding of the composition of the radial nerve?

2. A well-known textbook of neurosurgery makes these statements regarding the prognosis following peripheral nerve repair: (a) The younger the patient, the better the return of function. (b) The more distal the injury to a nerve, the more effective regeneration will be. (c) The closer a lesion is to the nerve cell body, the more profound will be the effect on this trophic center. (d) Sensory nerve cells are affected more by this retrograde phenomenon than are motor nerve cells. Comment on these statements.

3. An 18-year-old male patient was examined by a neurosurgeon 12 months after injury to the right forearm in which the median nerve was severed. At the initial operation, shortly after the injury had occurred, debridement was performed and the separated nerve ends were tagged with radiopaque sutures. Unfortunately, the wound was infected and surgical repair of the nerve was deferred. Is it practical to consider repairing a peripheral nerve after a delay of 12 months?

4. While examining a pathology specimen of nervous tissue under a microscope, the pathologist was able to determine the sex of the individual from whom the tissue had been removed. How would you be able to do this?

5. Axoplasmic flow is involved in the transport of certain viruses in the nervous system. What structures present in the cytoplasm of the neuron take part in this process?

6. About 1 percent of all deaths are due to intracranial tumors. Many different tissues are present within the skull in addition to the nervous system. Moreover, the nervous system itself is composed of many different types of tissues. In fact, tumors that arise as neoplasms of nerve cells and fibers are rare. Name the different types of tissues that are found in the central nervous system and in the peripheral nervous system.

7. When a nerve cell is stimulated, the permeability of the plasma membrane changes, permitting certain ionic movements to take place across the membrane. (a) What is the structure of the plasma membrane? (b) Is the permeability of the plasma membrane increased or decreased when the nerve cell is stimulated? (c) What is the action of local analgesics on the cell membrane?

8. The synapse is a region where nervous transmission is easily blocked. Clinically, the ganglion-blocking drugs used act by competing with acetylcholine released from the nerve endings in the ganglia. Name two groups

of drugs that have been used for this purpose and indicate the site at which they act.

9. A 2-year-old boy was taken to a pediatrician because his mother had noticed that his right eye was protruding (proptosis). When questioned, the mother stated that she had first noticed this protrusion 1 month previously and that it had progressively worsened since that time. The child was otherwise perfectly fit. On physical examination, the child was observed to be healthy in every respect except for the marked proptosis of the right eye. A careful palpation of the abdomen, however, revealed a large, soft mass in the upper part of the abdomen that extended across the midline. X-ray examination, including a CT body scan, revealed a large, soft tissue mass that displaced the right kidney downward. A diagnosis of malignant tumor of the suprarenal or neighboring sympathetic nervous tissue, with metastases in the right orbital cavity, was made, the latter being responsible for the right-side proptosis. Name a tumor of the suprarenal gland or sympathetic nervous tissue that occurs commonly in children and may metastasize in the bones of the orbit.

10. At an autopsy a third-year medical student was handed a slice of the cerebrum and was asked what proportion of central nervous tissue is made up by neuroglia. How would you have answered that question? Which cells are present in the largest numbers, neurons or neuroglial cells?

11. A 23-year-old man, while in the army in Vietnam, received a penetrating gunshot wound to the left side of his head. At the operation the neurosurgeon was able to remove the bullet from the left frontal lobe of his brain. Apart from a slight weakness of his right leg, the patient made an uneventful recovery. Eighteen months later the patient started to have severe generalized attacks of convulsions, during which he lost consciousness. Since this time the attacks have occurred irregularly at about monthly intervals. Each attack is preceded by a feeling of mental irritability, and twitching of the right leg occurs. A diagnosis of epilepsy was made by the examining neurologist. Is it possible that this patient's attacks of epilepsy are related to his gunshot wound in Vietnam? Is traumatic epilepsy a common condition? What treatment would you recommend?

12. A 42-year-old woman visited her physician because she was suffering from very severe headaches. Until 6 months ago she experienced only an occasional mild headache. Since that time her headaches gradually have become more severe and their duration has increased. They now last 3 to 4 hours and are so intense that she has to lie down. She has felt sick on two occasions but she has vomited on only one occasion. The headaches are generalized in nature and are made worse by coughing or straining. A physical examination revealed swelling of both optic discs with congestion of

the retinal veins and the presence of multiple retinal hemorrhages. Weakness of the lateral rectus muscle of the right eye also was detected. Anteroposterior radiographs of the skull showed displacement of the calcified pineal gland to the left side. Anteroposterior and lateral radiographs of the skull showed some degree of calcification in a localized area in the right cerebral hemisphere. These findings, together with those obtained from CT scans of the brain and MRIs, made the diagnosis of a right-sided cerebral tumor certain. Surgical exploration confirmed the presence of a large infiltrating tumor of the right parietal lobe. What is the most common type of tumor found in such a site in a middle-aged patient? How would you treat such a patient?

Answers to Clinical Problem Solving

1. The radial nerve is made up of nerve fibers derived from motor, sensory, and autonomic neurons. By definition the nerve fibers, or nerve cell processes, are referred to as neurites. The short neurites are called dendrites and the long neurites are called axons. It is customary to refer to those neurites that conduct the nervous impulse toward the cell body as the dendrites and to those that conduct the impulses away from the cell body as the axons. However, in the case of the unipolar sensory neurons found in the posterior root ganglia, the neurite carrying nervous information toward the cell body has all the structural characteristics of an axon and is referred to as an axon. Thus the radial nerve, which is composed of sensory and motor fibers, is made up of axons.

2. (a) It is a general rule that all reparative phenomena throughout the body occur more readily in the young than in the old. (b) As the distal end of a peripheral nerve is approached, fewer branches remain and thus there are fewer structures yet to innervate; consequently, there are fewer possibilities of nerve fibers innervating the wrong structure during the process of regeneration. Moreover, the more distal the injury, the less the metabolism of the proximal nerve cell body is affected by the injury. (c) This is a physiological fact. A very severe nerve injury close to its nerve cell body may result in the death of the entire neuron. (d) The physiology of sensory neurons is more susceptible to change by retrograde phenomena than that of motor neurons.

3. If the wound is not infected, the best time to perform a nerve suture is about 3 weeks after the injury. Satisfactory results have been obtained after a delay of as much as 14 months, provided that paralyzed muscles have not been overstretched and joint adhesions have been avoided by passive movements of the joints. In other words, the neuron still retains the ability to regenerate its processes even after 14 months, but the degree of recovery of function will depend a great deal on the care that the denervated structures receive in the intervening time.

4. In 1949, Barr and Bertram noticed the presence of a small, stainable body of chromatin (Barr body) situated at the inner surface of the nuclear envelope in the female that could not be seen in the cells of the male. It is one of the two X chromosomes present in the female. The presence or absence of the Barr body enables one to readily determine the sex of the individual from whom the tissue was removed.

5. With the electron microscope it is possible to resolve within the cytoplasm of a neuron small tubules that measure about 25 nm in diameter; there are also microfilaments measuring about 3-5 nm in diameter. The possible role that these structures play in cell transport is discussed on page 42.

6. The central nervous system is made up of the following tissues: (a) neurons, (b) neuroglia, (c) blood vessels, and (d) meninges. The peripheral nervous system is composed of the following tissues: (a) neurons, (b) Schwann cells, (c) connective tissue, and (d) blood vessels.

7. (a) The structure of the plasma membrane is described on page 43. (b) When a neuron is excited, the permeability of the plasma membrane to Na^+ ions is increased and these diffuse from the tissue fluid into the neuron cytoplasm. (c) Local analgesics act as membrane stabilizers and inhibit the increase in permeability to Na^+ ions in response to stimulation. It is not understood how this stabilization is brought about. One theory is that the analgesic agent becomes attached to receptor sites on the protein layer of the plasma membrane, reducing the permeability to Na^+ ions and preventing depolarization from taking place. Small-diameter nerve fibers are more readily blocked than are large fibers, and nonmyelinated fibers are more readily blocked than are myelinated ones. For these reasons, nerve fibers that conduct pain and temperature are most easily blocked and the large motor fibers are the least easily blocked. The small autonomic nerve fibers are blocked early and account for the rapid appearance of vasodilatation.

8. Tetraethylammonium salts and hexamethonium salts are the two groups of drugs. These salts closely resemble acetylcholine in structure and compete with acetylcholine at the postsynaptic membrane. By this means they successfully block a ganglion, although the amount of acetylcholine released is unaffected.

9. The neuroblastoma is a tumor of primitive neuroblasts and arises either in the suprarenal medulla or in the upper abdominal sympathetic ganglia. It is very malignant and is confined to children. The tumor metastasizes early and the metastasis may be the reason why the child receives medical attention, as in this case. The bones of the orbit are a common site for metastasis of a neuroblastoma.

10. Neuroglia comprises about one-half the total volume of the central nervous system. Neuroglial cells outnumber neurons by 5 to 10 times.
11. The reaction of tissue of the central nervous system to injury is characterized by the hyperplasia and hypertrophy of the astrocytes. The proliferation of the astrocytes is often referred to to as *astrocytosis* or *gliosis*. The degree of gliosis is much greater in the presence of residual damaged brain tissue than with a clean surgical incision. The resulting scar tissue, so-called *gliotic scar*, in the case of a penetrating gunshot wound, may be extensive and may give rise to focal or generalized epileptic attacks. The majority of such patients who become epileptic do so within 2 years. After careful examination of these patients, including the performance of radiography, CT brain scans, MRIs, and electroencephalography, the trauma site should be explored with a view to removing the gliotic scar. Such a scar will be replaced by a much smaller surgical scar. This operative intervention cures many of these patients.

12. A history of severe headaches and nausea and the finding of a choked optic disc (swelling of the optic disc, congestion of the retinal veins, and retinal hemorrhages) are not always diagnostic of a brain tumor. However, the finding of weakness of the lateral rectus muscle of the right eye owing to compression of the right sixth cranial nerve against the floor of the skull, together with the positive results on radiological and other laboratory tests, made the diagnosis certain. The glioma (tumor of neuroglia) is the most common type of tumor found in such a patient. Unfortunately, gliomas tend to infiltrate the brain tissue and cannot be completely removed surgically. Biopsy is performed to establish the diagnosis, as much of the tumor is removed as is clinically feasible, and the area is treated by deep x-ray therapy postoperatively. Survival time may also be increased by the use of chemotherapy.

Review Questions

Directions: Each of the numbered items in this section is followed by answers that are positively phrased. Select the ONE lettered answer that is an EXCEPTION.

1. The following statements concerning the cytology of a neuron are correct **except:**
   (a) A unipolar neuron is one that gives rise to a single neurite that remains unbranched until it reaches its destination and synapses with a second neuron.
   (b) A bipolar neuron is one that gives rise to a neurite that emerges from each end of the cell body. The sensory ganglia of the vestibulocochlear nerve (eighth cranial nerve) possess bipolar neurons.
   (c) Nissl substance is not found in the axon of a neuron.
   (d) The Golgi complex is important in the synthesis of cell membranes.
   (e) Melanin granules are found in the neurons of the substantia nigra, and it is these neurons that are responsible for the neurotransmitter dopamine.
2. The following statements concerning the cytology of a neuron are correct **except:**
   (a) The protein molecules projecting from the surface of the microtubules take part in rapid transport in axoplasm.
   (b) The protein molecules that extend through the full thickness of the plasma membrane of a neuron serve as sodium and potassium channels.
   (c) There is strong experimental evidence to suggest that the gates of the sodium and potassium channels are formed by actin molecules.
   (d) The large size of the nucleolus in a neuron is related to the very large volume of cytoplasm possessed by certain neurons.

   (e) A synapse is the site where two neurons come into close proximity and where functional interneuronal communication occurs.
3. The following statements concerning the axon are true **except:**
   (a) The initial segment of the axon is the first 50 to 100 μm after it leaves the axon hillock.
   (b) The nerve impulse generated by a neuron does not originate at the initial segment of an axon but on the dendrite.
   (c) The action potential is produced by the sudden influx of Na^+ ions into the cytoplasm.
   (d) Following the influx of Na^+ ions in the production of the action potential, the permeability for Na^+ ions ceases and that for K^+ ions increases, so that K^+ ions start to flow from the cell cytoplasm.
   (e) The spread of the action potential along the plasma membrane of the axon constitutes the nerve impulse.
4. The following statements concerning a nerve impulse are true **except:**
   (a) The refractory period is the duration of the nonexcitable state of the plasma membrane following the passage of a wave of depolarization.
   (b) Subthreshold stimuli when applied to the surface of a neuron can be summated.
   (c) Inhibitory stimuli are believed to produce their effect by causing an influx of K^+ ions through the plasma membrane of the neuron.
   (d) Hyperpolarization can be produced by causing an influx of Cl^- ions through the plasma membrane.
   (e) The axolemma is the site of nerve conduction.

5. The following statements concerning the structure of a synapse are true **except:**
   (a) Synapses may be axodendritic, axosomatic, or axoaxonic.
   (b) The synaptic cleft is the space between the presynaptic and postsynaptic membranes and measures about 20 nm.
   (c) The subsynaptic web lies beneath the postsynaptic membrane.
   (d) Presynaptic vesicles may contain the neurotransmitter substance.
   (e) Most neurons produce and release many different types of principal transmitter substances at all their nerve endings.
6. The following statements concerning a neuron are correct **except:**
   (a) Nerve fibers are the dendrites and axons of a neuron.
   (b) The volume of cytoplasm within the nerve cell body always far exceeds that found in the neurites.
   (c) Golgi type I neurons have very long axons.
   (d) Golgi type II neurons have very short axons.
   (e) Golgi type I neurons form the Purkinje cells of the cerebellar cortex.
7. The following statements concerning the neuron organelles and inclusions are correct **except:**
   (a) Centrioles are found in mature nerve cells as well as in immature dividing nerve cells.
   (b) Lipofuscin granules tend to accumulate with age.
   (c) The Nissl substance fills the axon hillock but is absent from other areas of the cytoplasm.
   (d) Microfilaments contain actin and probably assist in cell transport.
   (e) Mitochondria are found in the dendrites and axons.
8. The following statements concerning a dendrite are correct **except:**
   (a) A dendrite conveys a nerve impulse toward the nerve cell body.
   (b) Dendritic spines are small projections of the plasma membrane that increase the receptor surface area of the dendrite.
   (c) The cytoplasm of dendrites contains Nissl granules, microtubules, microfilaments, ribosomes, and agranular endoplasmic reticulum.
   (d) Most dendrites expand in width as they extend from the nerve cell body.
   (e) Dendrites often branch profusely.
9. The following statements concerning neuromodulators are correct **except:**
   (a) Neuromodulators may coexist with the principal (classic) transmitter at a single synapse.
   (b) They often enhance and prolong the effect of the principal transmitter.
   (c) They act through a second messenger.
   (d) They have a brief effect on the postsynaptic membrane.

(e) Acetylcholine (muscarinic) is a good example of a neuromodulator.
10. The following statements concerning the neurobiology of neuron structures are correct **except:**
    (a) A lysosome is a membrane bound vesicle.
    (b) A terminal bouton is the presynaptic part of an axon.
    (c) A receptor is a protein molecule on the postsynaptic membrane.
    (d) Nissl substance is formed of the smooth surfaced endoplasmic reticulum.
    (e) Microtubules provide a stationary track which allows specific organelles to move by molecular motors.
11. The following statements concerning neuroglia are correct **except:**
    (a) Fibrous astrocytes are located mainly in the white matter of the central nervous system.
    (b) Replacement gliosis follows the death of neurons in the central nervous system and is due to the proliferation of oligodendrocytes.
    (c) Astrocytes are involved in the absorption of gamma-aminobutyric acid (GABA) secreted by the nerve terminals.
    (d) Oligodendrocytes are responsible for the formation of the myelin of nerve fibers in the central nervous system.
    (e) Unlike Schwann cells in the peripheral nervous system, a single oligodendrocyte can form by means of its many processes several internodal segments of myelin on the same or different axons.
12. The following statements concerning the microglial cells are correct **except:**
    (a) Microglial cells resemble connective tissue macrophages.
    (b) Microglial cells are smaller than astrocytes or oligodendrocytes.
    (c) Microglial cells migrate into the central nervous system during fetal life.
    (d) In the presence of damaged neurons microglial cells increase in number.
    (e) In degenerative lesions of the central nervous system, the circulating blood contributes no cells to the population of microglial cells.
13. The following statements concerning the ependymal cells are correct **except:**
    (a) The ependymal cells form a single layer and many possess microvilli and cilia.
    (b) The ependymocytes line the ventricular system but permit the cerebrospinal fluid to enter the extracellular spaces of the nervous tissue.
    (c) Tanycytes have long, branching basal processes, many of which have end feet placed on the capillaries of the median eminence.
    (d) Choroidal epithelial cells secrete cerebrospinal fluid.

(e) Ependymal cells are incapable of absorbing substances from the cerebrospinal fluid.

14. The following statements concerning the extracellular space are true **except:**
    (a) The space is formed by the gaps between the neurons and the neuroglial cells.
    (b) The space surrounds the lymphatic capillaries present in the brain and spinal cord.
    (c) The space is in almost direct continuity with the subarachnoid space.
    (d) The space is filled with tissue fluid.
    (e) The space is continuous with the synaptic cleft between two neurons.

15. The following statements concerning tumors of neuroglia are correct **except:**
    (a) They form about 40 to 50 percent of all intracranial tumors.
    (b) Apart from the ependymomas, tumors of neuroglia are highly invasive.
    (c) They commonly infiltrate between neurons, causing initially the minimum disturbance of function.
    (d) They are nonmalignant and easily removed surgically.
    (e) As they expand, they raise the intracranial pressure.

16. The following statements concerning neuroglial cells are correct **except:**
    (a) They tend to be larger than nerve cell bodies.
    (b) Heat reduces the action potential in an axon and accentuates the signs and symptoms in multiple sclerosis.
    (c) Oligodendrocytes are found close to nerve cell bodies and their neurites.
    (d) Multiple sclerosis is a disease involving the oligodendrocyte.
    (e) Unlike Schwann cells, oligodendrocytes are not surrounded by a basement membrane.

17. The following general statements concerning the neuroglial cells are correct **except:**
    (a) The microglial cells have wavy processes with spinelike projections.
    (b) The astrocytes form a scaffold for developing neurons.
    (c) Oligodendrocyte processes are continuous with the myelin sheaths.
    (d) The ependymal cells have cilia on their free borders.
    (e) Macroglia is the term used to distinguish the larger oligodendrocytes from the smaller astrocyte.

Directions: Read the case histories then answer the questions. You will be required to select ONE BEST lettered answer.

An 8-year-old boy and a 12-year-old girl were taking a walk in the country when a sick-looking raccoon suddenly crossed their path. They both attempted to stroke the animal, which promptly bit them. The boy was bitten on the leg and the girl on the cheek. Later it was found that the animal was rabid.

18. Which of the following statements concerning this case is **incorrect?**
    (a) The rabies virus is present in the saliva of the infected animal.
    (b) The virus eventually spreads to the central nervous system.
    (c) The incubation period for rabies in the girl was much longer than that in the boy.
    (d) The virus reaches the central nervous system by traveling along peripheral nerves.
    (e) The virus is carried along the nerve by means of axonal transportation.

A 13-year-old girl fell off her horse and was unconscious when admitted to the emergency department of a local hospital. On questioning, her parents stated that when she fell, she hit her head on a log. She was wearing a riding helmet at the time. Neurological examination revealed that although unconscious, she responded to pain stimuli and there was no evidence of a focal lesion. Several hours later, she had a generalized seizure and examination of her retina showed bilateral papilledema; she was now in a state of coma.

The neurologist was concerned about the increasing intracranial pressure and the occurrence of cerebral edema.

19. Assuming that the patient was developing cerebral edema, which of the following statements is **incorrect?**
    (a) The trauma to the head was probably responsible for the development of the vasogenic form of cerebral edema.
    (b) The extracellular space contained more fluid than normal.
    (c) There was increased capillary permeability.
    (d) The tissue fluid was increased around both neurons and neuroglial cells.
    (e) The cerebral edema could be improved by the administration of intravenous 5% glucose solution.

20. Which of the following statements concerning cerebral edema is **incorrect?**
    (a) The rise in intracranial pressure may cause herniation of the cerebral cortex through the tentorial notch.
    (b) There is increased drainage of tissue fluid through the lymphatic vessels.
    (c) The skull bones limit the expansion of the brain.
    (d) Plasma proteins escape from the damaged endothelial cells of the capillaries into the extracellular space.
    (e) Cerebral edema can cause focal or generalized signs of brain dysfunction.

Answers to Review Questions

1. A
2. C
3. B
4. C
5. E
6. B
7. C
8. D
9. D
10. D
11. B
12. E
13. E
14. B
15. D
16. A
17. E

18. C. In this clinical problem, the rabies virus spread to the central nervous system in the boy along the axoplasm of the nerve fibers contained in the sciatic nerve of the leg. In the girl, the virus entered the axoplasm of the nerve fibers of the trigeminal nerve. Clearly, the virus had a much shorter distance to travel to the central nervous system in the girl and consequently the duration of the incubation period for the onset of symptoms in the girl was very much shorter than that in the boy.

19. E. Intravenous infusion of 5% glucose solution would result in a further significant increase in intracranial pressure because hypo-osmolality increases the outpouring of fluid from the capillaries into the extracellular space. If intravenous fluids are necessary in patients with head injuries, normal saline solution or 5% glucose and saline solution should be used.

20. B. The central nervous system does not have lymphatic drainage.

ADDITIONAL READING

Adams, J. H., and Duchen, L. W. (eds.), *Greenfield's Neuropathology* (5th ed.). New York: Oxford University Press, 1992.

Alberts, B., Bray, D., Lewis, J., Raff, M,. Roberts, K., Watson, JD. *Molecular Biology of the Cell, 3rd* ed. New York: Garland, 1994.

Andersen, OS., Koeppe, RE.11. Molecular Determinants of Channel Function. *Physiol Rev. 72:S89-S158, 1992.*

Armstrong, CM. Voltage-Dependent Ion Channels and Their Gating, *Physiol Rev 72:S5-13, 1992*

Armstrong, CM., Hille, B. Voltage-Gated Ion Channels and Electrical Excitability. *Neuron, 20:371-378, 1998.*

Bannister, R. Brain's Clinical Neurology *(6th ed.). New York: Oxford University Press, 1985.*

Barr, M. L. The significance of the sex chromatin. *Int. Rev. Cytol. 19:35, 1966.*

Bernstein, J. J., and Bernstein, E. M. Axonal regeneration and formation of synapses proximal to the site of lesion following hemisection of the rat spinal cord. *Exp. Neurol. 30:336, 1971.*

Berry, M. Regeneration of Axons in the Central Nervous System. In V. Navaratnam and R. J. Harrison (eds.), *Progress in Anatomy. Vol. 3.* New York: Cambridge University Press, 1983. P. 213.

Berry, M. Neurogenesis and gliogenesis in the human brain. *Food Chem. Toxicol.* 24:79, 1986.

Catterall, W. A., Structure and Function of Voltage-Gated Ion Channels. *Trends Neurosci.* 16:500-506, 1993.

Cooper, JR., Bloom, FE., Roth, RH. *The Biochemical Basis of Neuropharmacology,* 7th ed. New York: Oxford Univ. Press, 1996.

Hayes, G. M., Woodroofe, M. N., and Cuzner, M. L. Characterization of microglia isolated from adult human brain. *J. Neuroimmunol.* 19:177, 1988.

Henn, F. A., and Henn, S. W. The psychopharmacology of astroglial cells. *Prog. Neurobiol.* 15:1, 1983.

Hertz, L. Functional Interactions between Astrocytes and Neurons. In *Glial and Neuronal Cell Biology.* New York: Liss, 1981. P. 45.

Hille, B. *Ionic Channels of Excitable Membranes,* 2nd ed. Sunderland, MA: Sinauer. 1992.

Hille, B. Modulation of Ion-Channel Function by G-Protein-Coupled Receptors. *Trends Neurosci* 17:531-536, 1994.

Imamoto, V. Origin of Microglia: Cell Transformation from Blood Monocytes into Macrophagic Ameboid Cells and Microglia. In *Glial and Neuronal Cell Biology.* New York: Liss, 1981. P. 125.

Jessell, TM., Kandel, ER. Synaptic Transmission: A Bidirectional and Self-Modifiable Form of Cell-Cell Communication. *Cell* 72:1-30, 1993.

Kelly, RB. Storage and Release of Neurotransmitters. *Cell* 72:43-53, 1993.

Koester, J. Passive Membrane Properties of the Neuron. In E. R. Kandel, J. H. Schwartz, and T. M. Jessell (eds.). *Principles of Neural Science* (3rd ed.). New York: Elsevier, 1991. P. 95.

Koester, J. Voltage-Gated Ion Channels and the Generation of the Action Potential. In E. R. Kandel, J. H. Schwartz, and T. M. Jessell (eds.), *Principles of Neural Science* (3rd ed.). New York: Elsevier, 1991. P. 104.

Kukuljan, M., Labarca, P., Latorre, R. Molecular Determination of Ion Conduction and Inactivation in K+ Channels. *Am. J. Physiol.* 268:C535-C556.

Kupfermann, I. Modulatory actions of neurotransmitters. *Ann. Rev. Neurosci.* 2:447, 1979.

Lemke, G. The Molecular Genetics of Myelination: an Update. *Glia* 7:263-271, 1993.

Matthews, G. Synaptic Exocytosis and Endocytosis: Capacitance Measurements. *Curr. Opin. Neurobiol.* 6(3): 358-364, 1996.

McCormick, D. A. Membrane Properties and Neurotransmitter Actions. In G. M. Shepherd (ed.), *The Synaptic Organization of the Brain* (3rd ed.). New York: Oxford University Press, 1990. P. 32.

McEwen, B. S., and Grafstein, B. Fast and slow components in axonal transport of protein. *J. Cell Biol.* 38:494, 1968.

Nicholls, JG., Martin, AR., Wallace, BG. *From Neuron to Brain: A Cellular and Molecular Approach to the Function of the Nervous System,* 3rd ed. Sunderland, MA: Sinauer, 1992.

Perry, VH. Microglia in the Developing and Mature Central Nervous System. In: KR Jessen, WD Richardson (eds). *Glial Cell Development: Basic Principles and Clinical Relevance, pp. 123-140.* Oxford: Bios. 1996.

Peters, A., Palay, SL., Webster, HdeF. *The Fine Structure of the Nervous System: Neurons and Their Supporting Cells,* 3rd ed. New York: Oxford Univ. Press, 1991.

Siegel, GJ., Agranoff, BW., Albers, RW., Molinoff, PB. (eds). *Basic Neurochemistry: Molecular, Cellular, and Medical Aspects,* 6th ed. Philadelphia: Lippincott-Raven, 1999.

Sudarsky, L. *Pathophysiology of the Nervous System.* Boston: Little, Brown, 1990.

Von Gersdorff, H., Matthews, G. Dynamics of Synaptic Fusion and Membrane Retrieval in Synaptic Terminals. *Nature* 367:735-739, 1994.

Waxman, S.G. Demyelinating Diseases-New Pathological Insights, New Therapeutic Targets. *N. Engl. J. Med.* 338:323-325, 1998.

CHAPTER 3

Nerve Fibers, Peripheral Nerves, Receptor and Effector Endings, Dermatomes, and Muscle Activity

A 45-year-old man was recovering from a mild upper respiratory tract infection when he suddenly noticed weakness in both legs while walking up stairs. He also developed a numb sensation over the lower part of both legs and the feet. Two days later, while shaving, he noticed a weakness of the muscles on the right side of his face.

On physical examination the patient did not appear to be ill. He had no pyrexia. Examination of his leg muscles showed obvious signs of muscle weakness involving both legs, especially below the knees. Both ankle reflexes were absent and the right knee jerk was diminished. He had sensory deficits for touch and pain sensations in the distribution of the stocking area of both feet and lower legs, and a mild form of facial nerve palsy involving the right side of the face. There was no neurological evidence of loss of function of the brain or spinal cord.

The patient was suspected of having Guillain-Barré syndrome and was admitted to the hospital for observation. The cause of this disease is unknown, although it is believed to be viral and involve the immune system. Histologically, the peripheral nerves show focal scattered areas of demyelination with an accumulation of lymphocytes and macrophages. As the myelin is lost, the axons are left naked and the Schwann cell bodies remain intact. In the majority of patients, recovery occurs in 2 to 4 weeks as remyelination occurs. Hospitalization is necessary in the early stages because the disease can spread rapidly to involve the intercostal and phrenic nerves, resulting in paralysis of the intercostal muscles and diaphragm. For the same reason, the coughing and swallowing reflexes should be carefully watched. A physician would find this disease impossible to understand without a knowledge of the structure of peripheral nerves.

CHAPTER OUTLINE

First, the basic structure and function of nerve fibers are considered. The process of nerve degeneration and regeneration is described in detail, because nerve lesions are very common in clinical practice and can be caused by a wide variety of diseases, including trauma, neoplasms, infection, metabolic dysfunction (diabetes), and chemical toxins such as lead. The process of nerve degeneration is fast and can take place in nerves in the central and peripheral nervous systems. The regeneration of nerves is slow and confined to the peripheral nervous system. Because so much research today is being devoted to investigating why regeneration in the central nervous system ceases within 2 weeks, the histological changes that occur must be learned.

Special organs that lie at the ends of sensory and motor nerves are also considered. A brief overview of the physical examination of the different sensory modalities is provided. Terms used in assessing skin sensory loss and abnormal muscle activity are also described. The material in this chapter commonly forms the basis for examination questions.

NERVE FIBERS

A nerve fiber is the name given to an axon (or a dendrite) of a nerve cell. The structure of axons and dendrites is described on page 47. Bundles of nerve fibers found in the central nervous system are often referred to as **nerve tracts** (Fig. 3-1); bundles of nerve fibers found in the peripheral nervous system are called **peripheral nerves** (Fig. 3-2).

Two types of nerve fibers are present in the central and peripheral parts of the nervous system, namely, myelinated and nonmyelinated fibers.

Myelinated Nerve Fibers

A myelinated nerve fiber is one that is surrounded by a myelin sheath. The myelin sheath is not part of the neuron but is formed by a supporting cell (Fig. 3-2 and Fig. 3-3). In the central nervous system the supporting cell is called the **oligodendrocyte**; in the peripheral nervous system it is called the **Schwann cell**.

The myelin sheath is a segmented, discontinuous layer interrupted at regular intervals by the **nodes of Ranvier** (Figs. 3-4 and 3-6). Each segment of the myelin sheath measures approximately 0.5 to 1.0 mm in length. In the central nervous system each oligodendrocyte may form and maintain myelin sheaths for as many as 60 nerve fibers (axons). In the peripheral nervous system there is only one Schwann cell for each segment of one nerve fiber.

FORMATION OF MYELIN

Myelin sheaths begin to form before birth and during the first year postnatally. The process has been studied with the electron microscope.

In the **peripheral nervous system**, the nerve fiber or axon first indents the side of a Schwann cell (Fig. 3-4). Later, as the axon sinks farther into the Schwann cell, the external plasma membrane of the Schwann cell forms a **mesaxon**, which suspends the axon within the Schwann cell. Subsequently, it is thought, the Schwann cell rotates on the axon so that the plasma membrane becomes wrapped around and around the axon in a spiral. The direction of the spiral is clockwise in some segments and counterclockwise in others. To begin with, the wrappings are loose, but gradually the cytoplasm between the layers of the cell membrane disappears, leaving cytoplasm near the surface and in the region of the nucleus. The wrappings become tight with maturation of the nerve fiber. The thickness of the myelin depends on the number of spirals of Schwann cell membrane. Some nerve fibers are surrounded by only a few turns of the membrane while others have as many as 50 turns. In electron micrographs of cross sections of mature myelinated nerve fibers, the myelin is seen to be laminated (Fig. 3-5). Each lamella measures 13 to 18 nm thick. The dark **major dense line**, about 2.5 nm thick, consists of two inner protein layers of the plasma membrane that are fused together. The lighter **minor dense line**, about 10 nm thick, is formed by the approximation of the outer surfaces of adjacent plasma membranes and is made up of lipid. The fused outer protein layers of the plasma membranes are very thin and form a thin intraperiod line situated in the center of the lighter lipid layer (Figs. 3-4 and 3-5). At the node of Ranvier, two adjacent Schwann cells terminate and the myelin sheaths become thinner by the turning off of the lamellae (Fig. 3-6). At these regions the plasma membrane of the axon, the axolemma, is exposed.

The **incisures of Schmidt-Lanterman** are seen on longitudinal sections of myelinated nerve fibers. They represent areas where the dark major dense line is not formed as a result of the localized persistence of Schwann cell cytoplasm (Fig. 3-7). This persistence of cytoplasm involves all the layers of the myelin and thus there is a continuous spiral of cytoplasm from the outermost region of the Schwann cell to the region of the axon. This spiral of cytoplasm may provide a pathway for the conduction of metabolites from the surface region of the Schwann cell to the axon.

In the **central nervous system**, oligodendrocytes are responsible for the formation of the myelin sheaths. The plasma membrane of the oligodendrocyte becomes wrapped around the axon and the number of layers will determine the thickness of the myelin sheath (Fig. 3-3). The **nodes of Ranvier** are situated in the intervals between adjacent oligodendrocytes. A single oligodendrocyte may be connected to the myelin sheaths of as many as 60 nerve fibers. For this reason, the process of myelination in the central nervous system cannot take place by rotation of the

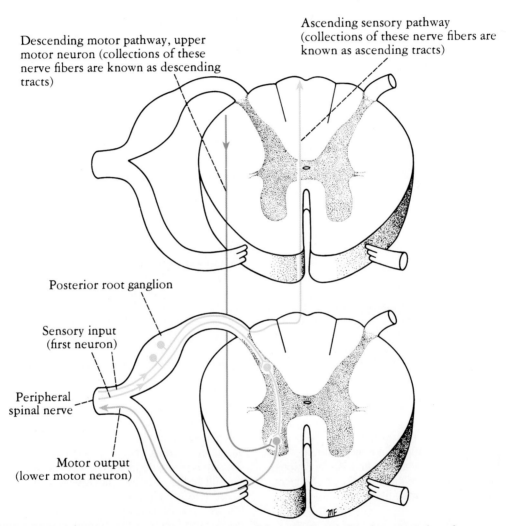

Descending motor pathway, upper motor neuron (collections of these nerve fibers are known as descending tracts)

Ascending sensory pathway (collections of these nerve fibers are known as ascending tracts)

Posterior root ganglion

Sensory input (first neuron)

Peripheral spinal nerve

Motor output (lower motor neuron)

Figure 3–1 Sections through the thoracic region of the spinal cord showing examples of nerve fibers entering or leaving the central nervous system; ascending and descending nerve fibers (tracts or pathways) are also shown.

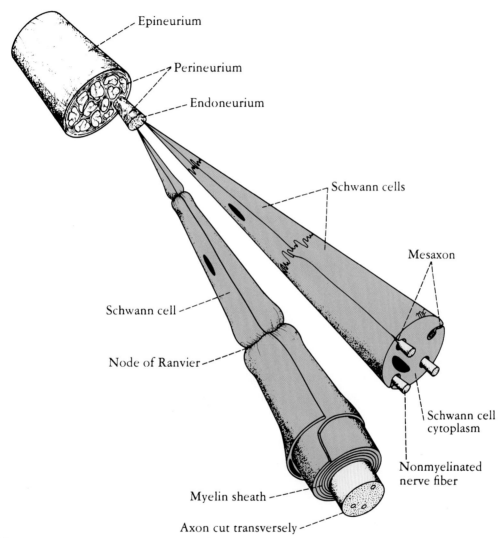

Figure 3–2 Exploded view of a peripheral nerve, showing the connective tissue sheaths and the structure of myelinated and nonmyelinated nerve fibers.

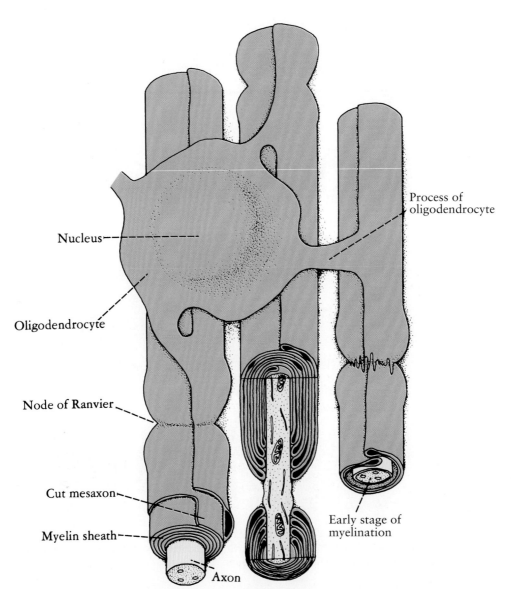

Figure 3–3   The relationship between an oligodendrocyte and myelinated nerve fibers in the central nervous system. Note the absence of a basement membrane.

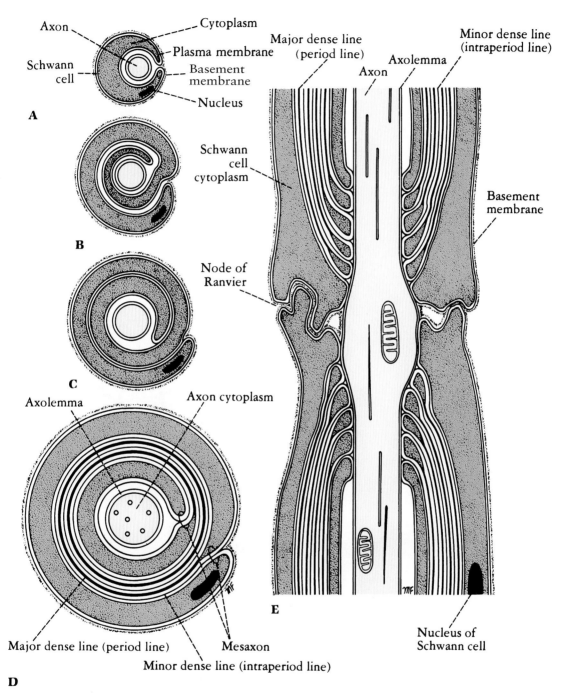

Figure 3–4 A myelinated nerve fiber in the peripheral nervous system. A, B, C, and D. Cross sections showing the stages in the formation of the myelin sheath. E. A longitudinal section of a mature myelinated nerve fiber showing a node of Ranvier. Note the presence of a basement membrane.

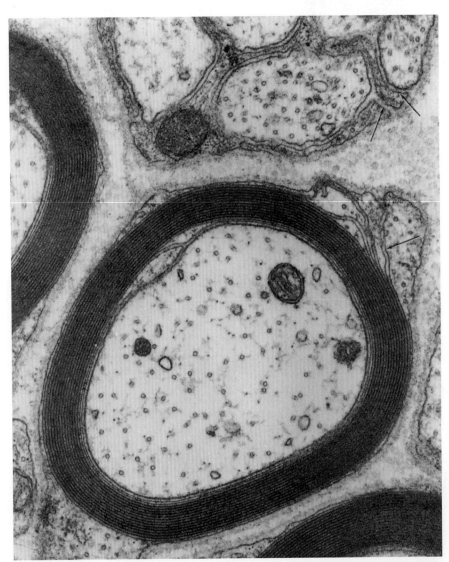

Figure 3–5   Electron micrograph of a transverse section of a peripheral nerve, showing a myeli-nated axon with spiral myelin lamellae (center). Note the mesaxon (arrow). Parts of two other myelinated fibers are also shown. A number of nonmyelinated axons are enclosed in the periph-eral cytoplasm of a Schwann cell (top). The mesaxons are indicated by arrows. (× 28,000.) (Courtesy Dr. H. de F. Webster.)

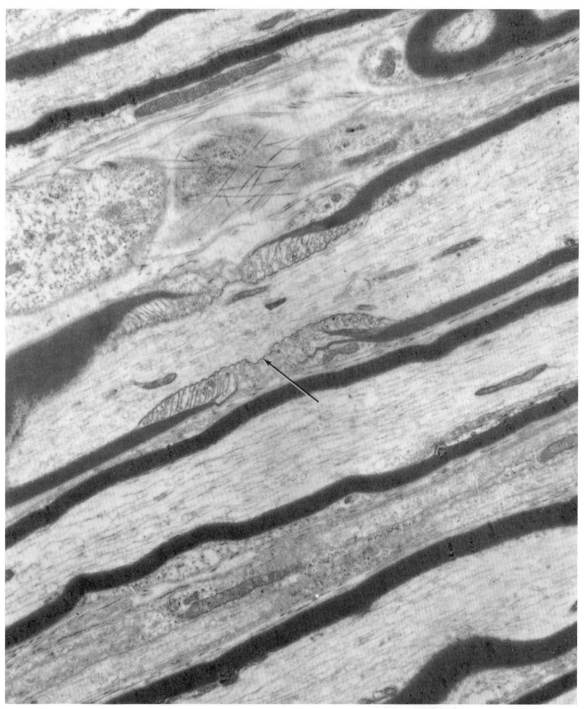

Figure 3–6 Electron micrograph of a longitudinal section of several myelinated axons, showing the structure of a node of Ranvier (arrow). At the node, two adjacent Schwann cells terminate and the myelin sheaths become thinner by the turning off of the lamellae. Note the many microtubules and microfilaments within the axons. (× 12,220.) (Courtesy Dr. H. de F. Webster.)

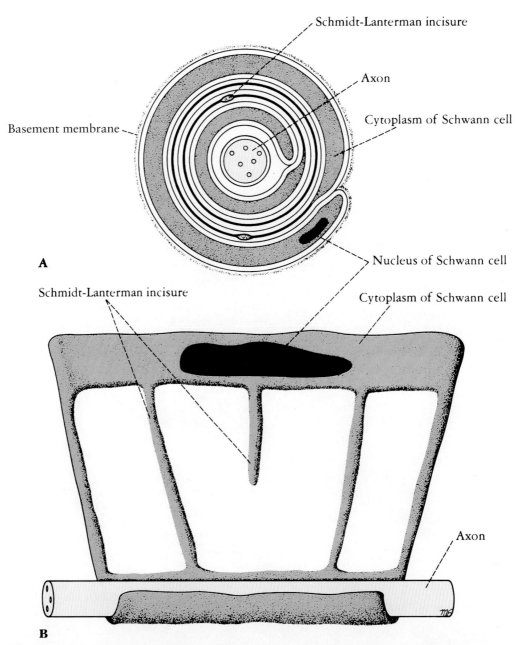

Figure 3–7   Schmidt-Lanterman incisures in the myelin sheath of a peripheral nerve. **A.** Transverse section of a myelinated nerve fiber. **B.** Schematic diagram of a myelinated nerve fiber in which the myelin sheath has been unrolled.

oligodendrocyte on the axon, as did the Schwann cell in the peripheral nervous system. It is possible that myelination in the central nervous system occurs by the growth in length of the process of the oligodendrocyte, the process wrapping itself around the axon. There are incisures of Schmidt-Lanterman in nerve fibers of the central nervous system. Table 3-1 provides a summary of facts concerning myelination in the central and peripheral nervous systems.

Nonmyelinated Nerve Fibers

The smaller axons of the central nervous system, the postganglionic axons of the autonomic part of the nervous system, and some fine sensory axons associated with the reception of pain are nonmyelinated.

In the **peripheral nervous system** each axon, which is usually less than 1 μm in diameter, indents the surface of the Schwann cell so that it lies within a trough (Fig. 3-2). As

| | | Number of | | Schmidt- | |
Location	Cell Responsible	Nerve Fibers Served by Cell	Nodes of Ranvier	Lanterman Incisures	Mesaxon
Peripheral nerve	Schwann cell	1	Present	Present	Present
CNS tract	Oligodendrocyte	Up to 60	Present	Present	Absent

Table 3–1   Myelination in the Peripheral and Central Nervous System

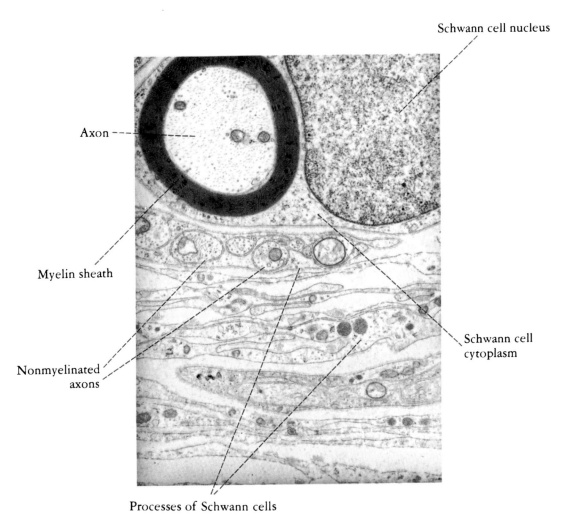

Figure 3–8   Electron micrograph of a transverse section of a myelinated nerve fiber and several nonmyelinated nerve fibers. (Courtesy Dr. J. M. Kerns.)

many as 15 or more axons may share a single Schwann cell, each lying within its own trough or sometimes sharing a trough. In some situations the troughs are deep and the axons are embedded deep in the Schwann cells, forming a **mesaxon** from the Schwann cell plasma membrane (Figs. 3-5 and 3-8). The Schwann cells lie close to one another along the length of the axons and there are no nodes of Ranvier.

In areas where there are synapses or where motor transmission occurs, the axon emerges from the trough of the

Schwann cell for a short distance, thus exposing the active region of the axon (Fig. 3-9).

In the **central nervous system** nonmyelinated nerve fibers run in small groups and are not particularly related to the oligodendrocytes.

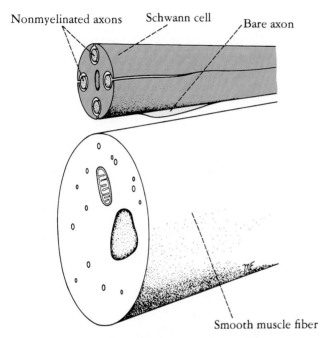

Figure 3–9 Autonomic neuromuscular junction between a nonmyelinated axon and a smooth muscle fiber.

 PERIPHERAL NERVES

The peripheral nerves are the cranial and spinal nerves. Each peripheral nerve consists of parallel bundles of nerve fibers, which may be efferent or afferent axons, and may be myelinated or nonmyelinated, and are surrounded by connective tissue sheaths (Figs. 3-10 and 3-11).

The nerve trunk is surrounded by a dense connective tissue sheath called the **epineurium** (Fig. 3-12). Within the sheath are bundles of nerve fibers, each of which is surrounded by a connective tissue sheath called the **perineurium**. Between the individual nerve fibers is a loose, delicate connective tissue referred to as the **endoneurium**. The connective tissue sheaths serve to support the nerve fibers and their associated blood vessels and lymph vessels. Peripheral nerve fibers can be classified according to their speed of conduction and size (Table 3-2).

Spinal Nerves and Spinal Nerve Roots

There are 31 pairs of spinal nerves, which leave the spinal cord and pass through intervertebral foramina in the vertebral column. (For details, see p. 14.) Each spinal nerve is connected to the spinal cord by **two roots**: the **anterior root** and the **posterior root** (Fig. 3-13). The anterior root consists of bundles of nerve fibers carrying nerve impulses away from the central nervous system; these nerve fibers are called **efferent fibers**. The **posterior root** consists of bundles of nerve fibers carrying nerve impulses to the central nervous system; these nerve fibers are called **afferent fibers**. Because these fibers are concerned with conveying information to the central nervous system, they are called **sensory fibers**. The cell bodies of these nerve fibers are situated in a swelling on the posterior root called the **posterior root ganglion**.

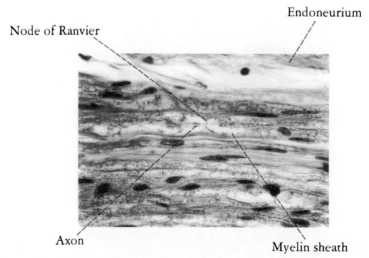

Figure 3–10 Photomicrograph of a longitudinal section of a peripheral nerve stained with hematoxylin and eosin. (× 400.)

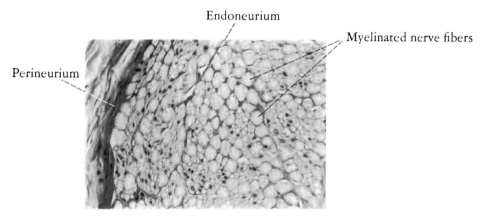

Figure 3–11 Photomicrograph of a transverse section of a peripheral nerve stained with hematoxylin and eosin. (× 275.)

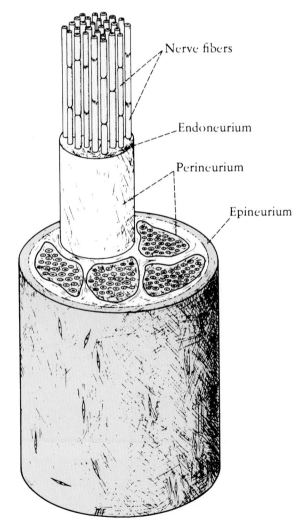

Figure 3–12 Structure of a peripheral nerve.

Table 3–2   Classification of Nerve Fibers by Speed of Conduction and Size

Fiber Type	Conduction Velocity (meters per second)	Fiber Diameter (μm)	Functions	Myelin	Sensitivity to Local Anesthetics
A Fibers					
Alpha	70–120	12–20	Motor, skeletal muscle	Yes	Least
Beta	40–70	5–12	Sensory, touch, pressure, vibration	Yes	
Gamma	10–50	3–6	Muscle spindle	Yes	
Delta	6–30	2–5	Pain (sharp, localized), temperature, touch	Yes	
B Fibers	3–15	<3	Preganglionic autonomic	Yes	
C Fibers	0.5–2.0	0.4–1.2	Pain (diffuse, deep), temperature, postganglionic autonomic	No	Most

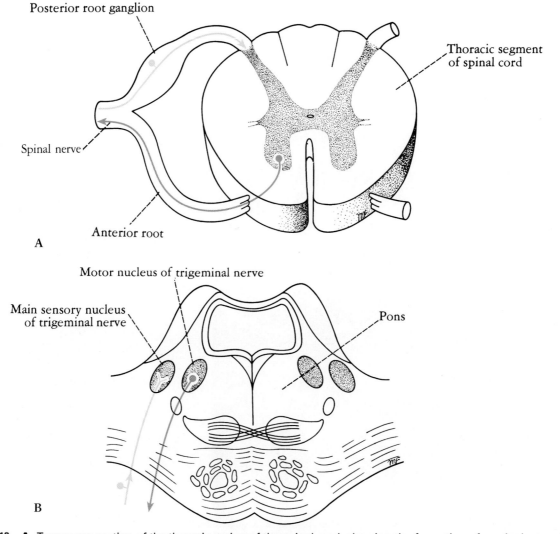

Figure 3–13   A. Transverse section of the thoracic region of the spinal cord, showing the formation of a spinal nerve from the union of an anterior and a posterior nerve root. **B.** Transverse section of the pons showing the sensory and motor roots of the trigeminal nerve.

Cranial Nerves

There are 12 pairs of cranial nerves (Fig. 3-13), which leave the brain and pass through foramina in the skull. Some of these nerves are composed entirely of afferent nerve fibers bringing sensations to the brain (olfactory, optic, vestibulocochlear), others are composed entirely of efferent fibers (oculomotor, trochlear, abducent, accessory, hypoglossal), while the remainder possess both afferent and efferent fibers (trigeminal, facial, glossopharyngeal, and vagus). The cranial nerves are described in detail in Chapter 11.

Sensory Ganglia

The sensory ganglia of the posterior spinal nerve roots and of the trunks of the trigeminal, facial, glossopharyngeal, and vagal cranial nerves have the same structure. Each ganglion is surrounded by a layer of connective tissue that is continuous with the epineurium and perineurium of the peripheral nerve. The neurons are unipolar, possessing cell bodies that are rounded or oval in shape (Fig. 3-14). The cell bodies tend to be aggregated and separated by bundles of nerve fibers. A single nonmyelinated process leaves each cell body and after a convoluted course bifurcates at a T junction into peripheral and central branches. The former axon terminates in a series of dendrites in a peripheral sensory ending, and the latter axon enters the central nervous system. The nerve impulse, on reaching the T junction, passes directly from the peripheral axon to the central axon, thus bypassing the nerve cell body.

Each nerve cell body is closely surrounded by a layer of flattened cells called **capsular cells** or **satellite cells** (see Fig. 3-14). The capsular cells are similar in structure to Schwann cells and are continuous with these cells as they envelop the peripheral and central processes of each neuron.

Autonomic Ganglia

The autonomic ganglia (sympathetic and parasympathetic ganglia) are situated at a distance from the brain and spinal cord. They are found in the sympathetic trunks, in prevertebral autonomic plexuses—for example, in the cardiac, celiac, and mesenteric plexuses—and as ganglia in or close to viscera. Each ganglion is surrounded by a layer of connective tissue that is continuous with the epineurium and perineurium of the peripheral nerve. The neurons are multipolar and possess cell bodies that are irregular in shape (Fig. 3-15). The dendrites of the neurons make synaptic connections with the myelinated axons of preganglionic neurons. The axons of the neurons are of small diameter (C fibers) and unmyelinated, and they pass to viscera, blood vessels, and sweat glands.

Each nerve cell body is closely surrounded by a layer of flattened cells called **capsular cells** or **satellite cells**. The capsular cells, like those of sensory ganglia, are similar in structure to Schwann cells and are continuous with them as they envelop the peripheral and central processes of each neuron.

Peripheral Nerve Plexuses

Peripheral nerves are composed of bundles of nerve fibers. In their course, peripheral nerves sometimes divide into branches that join neighboring peripheral nerves. If this should occur frequently, a network of nerves, called a **nerve plexus,** is formed. It should be emphasized that the formation of a nerve plexus allows individual nerve fibers to pass from one peripheral nerve to another and **in most instances branching of nerve fibers does not take place**. A plexus thus permits a redistribution of the nerve fibers within the different peripheral nerves.

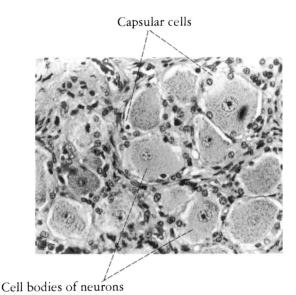

Capsular cells

Cell bodies of neurons

Figure 3–14 Photomicrograph of a longitudinal section of a posterior root ganglion of a spinal nerve stained with hematoxylin and eosin. (x 400.)

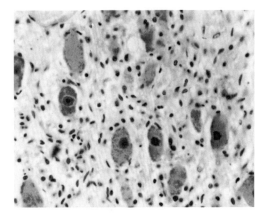

Figure 3–15 Photomicrograph of a longitudinal section of a ganglion of the sympathetic trunk stained with hematoxylin and eosin. (x 300.)

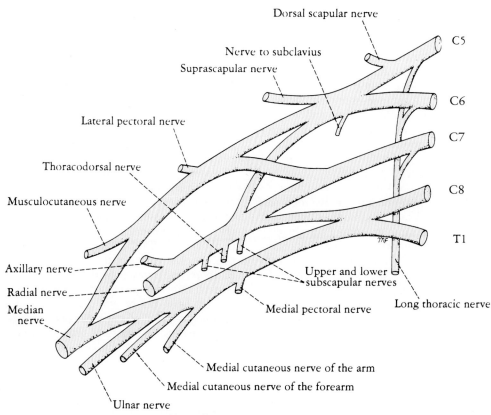

Figure 3–16 Brachial plexus.

At the root of the limbs the anterior rami of the spinal nerves form complicated plexuses. The cervical and brachial plexuses are at the root of the upper limbs (Fig. 3-16), and the lumbar and sacral plexuses are at the root of the lower limbs. This allows the nerve fibers derived from different segments of the spinal cord to be arranged and distributed efficiently in different nerve trunks to the various parts of the upper and lower limbs.

Cutaneous nerves, as they approach their final destination, commonly form fine plexuses that again permit a rearrangement of nerve fibers before they reach their terminal sensory endings.

The autonomic nervous system also possesses numerous nerve plexuses that consist of preganglionic and postganglionic nerve fibers and ganglia.

CONDUCTION IN PERIPHERAL NERVES

In the resting unstimulated state a nerve fiber is polarized so that the interior is negative to the exterior; the potential difference across the axolemma is about −80 mV and is called the **resting membrane potential** (Fig. 3-17). As has been explained previously (See page 44), this so-called resting potential is produced by the diffusion of sodium and potas-

sium ions through the channels of the plasma membrane and is maintained by the sodium-potassium pump. The pump involves active transport across the membrane and requires adenosine triphosphate (ATP) to provide the energy.

A nerve impulse (action potential) starts at the initial segment of the axon and is a self-propagating wave of electrical negativity that passes along the surface of the plasma membrane (axolemma). The wave of electrical negativity is initiated by an adequate stimulus being applied to the surface of the neuron. Under normal circumstances this occurs at the initial segment of the axon, which is the most sensitive part of the neuron. The stimulus alters the permeability of the membrane to Na^+ ions at the point of stimulation. Now Na^+ ions rapidly enter the axon (see Fig. 3-17). The positive ions outside the axolemma quickly decrease to zero. The membrane potential therefore is reduced to zero and is said to be depolarized. A typical resting potential is −80 mV, with the outside of the membrane positive to the inside; the action potential is about +40 mV, with the outside of the membrane negative to the inside.

The negatively charged point on the outside of the axolemma now acts as a stimulus to the adjacent positively charged axolemma and in less than 1 msec the polarity of the adjacent resting potential is reversed (see Fig. 3-17). The action potential now has moved along the axolemma from the point originally stimulated to the adjacent point on the

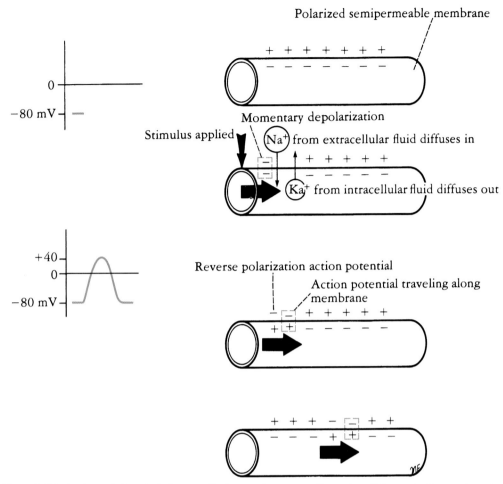

Figure 3–17 Ionic and electrical changes that occur in a nerve fiber when it is conducting an impulse.

membrane. It is in this manner that the action potential travels along the full length of a nerve fiber.

As the action potential moves along the nerve fiber, the entry of the Na$^+$ ions into the axon ceases and the permeability of the axolemma to K$^+$ ions increases. Now K$^+$ ions rapidly diffuse outside the axon (since the concentration is much higher within the axon than outside), so that the original resting membrane potential is restored. The permeability of the axolemma now decreases and the status quo is restored by the active transport of the Na$^+$ ions out of the axon and the K$^+$ ions into the axon. The outer surface of the axolemma is again electrically positive compared to the inner surface.

For a short time after the passage of a nerve impulse along a nerve fiber, while the axolemma is still depolarized, a second stimulus, however strong, is unable to excite the nerve. This period of time is called the **absolute refractory period**. This period is followed by a further short interval during which the excitability of the nerve gradually returns to normal. This latter period is called the **relative refractory period**. It is clear from this that the refractory period makes a continuous excitatory state of the nerve impossible and it limits the frequency of the impulses.

The **conduction velocity** of a nerve fiber is proportional to the cross-sectional area of the axon, the thicker fibers conducting more rapidly than those of smaller diameter. In the large motor fibers (alpha fibers), the rate may be as high as 70 to 120 meters per second; the smaller sensory fibers have slower conduction rates (see Table 3-2).

In nonmyelinated fibers, the action potential passes continuously along the axolemma, progressively exciting neighboring areas of membrane (Fig. 3-18). In myelinated fibers, the presence of a myelin sheath serves as an insulator. Consequently, a myelinated nerve fiber can be stimulated only at the nodes of Ranvier, where the axon is naked and the ions can pass freely through the plasma membrane between the extracellular fluid and the axoplasm. In these fibers the action potential jumps from one node to the next (Fig. 3-18). The action potential at one node sets up a current in the surrounding tissue fluid, which quickly produces depolarization at the next node. This leaping of the action potential from one node to the next is referred to as **saltatory conduction** (Fig. 3-18). This is a more rapid mechanism than is found in nonmyelinated fibers (120 meters per second in a large myelinated fiber compared with 0.5 meter per second in a very small unmyelinated fiber).

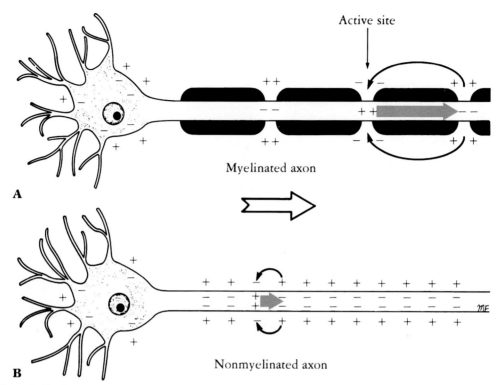

Figure 3–18   Electrical changes that occur in: **A.** Stimulated myelinated axon (saltatory conduction). **B.** Stimulated nonmyelinated axon.

 RECEPTOR ENDINGS

An individual receives impressions from the outside world and from within the body by special sensory nerve endings or receptors.

Sensory receptors can be classified into five basic functional types:

Mechanoreceptors. These respond to mechanical deformation.

Thermoreceptors. These respond to changes in temperature; some receptors respond to cold and others to heat.

Nociceptors. These respond to any stimuli that bring about damage to the tissue.

Electromagnetic receptors. The rods and cones of the eyes are sensitive to changes in light intensity and wavelength.

Chemoreceptors. These respond to chemical changes associated with taste and smell and oxygen and carbon dioxide concentrations in the blood.

Anatomical Types of Receptors

For convenience the sensory endings can be classified, on a structural basis, into nonencapsulated and encapsulated receptors. Table 3-3 classifies and compares the receptor types.

NONENCAPSULATED RECEPTORS

Free Nerve Endings

Free nerve endings are widely distributed throughout the body (Fig. 3-19). They are found between the epithelial cells of the skin, the cornea, and the alimentary tract, and in connective tissues, including the dermis, fascia, ligaments, joint capsules, tendons, periosteum, perichondrium, haversian systems of bone, tympanic membrane, and dental pulp, and they are also present in muscle.

The afferent nerve fibers from the free nerve endings are either myelinated or nonmyelinated. The terminal endings are devoid of a myelin sheath and there are no Schwann cells covering their tips.

Most of these endings detect pain, while others detect crude touch, pressure, and tickle sensations, and possibly cold and heat.

Merkel's Discs

Merkel's discs are found in hairless skin, for example, the fingertips (Figs. 3-20 and 3-21)and in hair follicles. The nerve fiber passes into the epidermis and terminates as a disc-shaped expansion that is applied closely to a dark-staining epithelial cell in the deeper part of the epidermis, called the **Merkel cell**. In hairy skin, clusters of Merkel's discs, known as **tactile domes**, are found in the epidermis between the hair follicles.

Table 3–3   Classification and Comparison of Receptor Types

Type of Receptor	Location	Stimulus	Sensory Modality	Adaptability	Nerve Fibers
Nonencapsulated receptors					
Free nerve endings	Epidermis, cornea, gut, dermis, ligaments, joint capsules, bone, dental pulp, etc.	Mechanoreceptor	Pain (fast), pain (slow), touch (crude), pressure, ?heat and cold	Rapid	A delta C
Merkel's discs	Hairless skin	Mechanoreceptor	Touch	Slow	A beta
Hair follicle receptors	Hairy skin	Mechanoreceptor	Touch	Rapid	A beta
Encapsulated receptors					
Meissner's corpuscles	Dermal papillae of skin of palm and sole of foot	Mechanoreceptor	Touch	Rapid	A beta
Pacinian corpuscles	Dermis, ligaments, joint capsules, peritoneum, external genitalia, etc.	Mechanoreceptor	Vibration	Rapid	A beta
Ruffini's corpuscles	Dermis of hairy skin	Mechanoreceptor	Stretch	Slow	A beta
Neuromuscular spindles	Skeletal muscle	Mechanoreceptor	Stretch—muscle length	Fast	A alpha A beta
Neurotendinous spindles	Tendons	Mechanoreceptor	Compression—muscle tension	Fast	A alpha

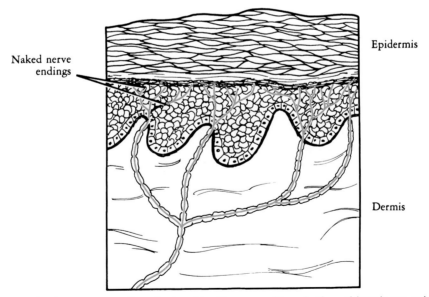

Figure 3–19   Free nerve endings in the skin. The nerve fibers in the epidermis are naked.

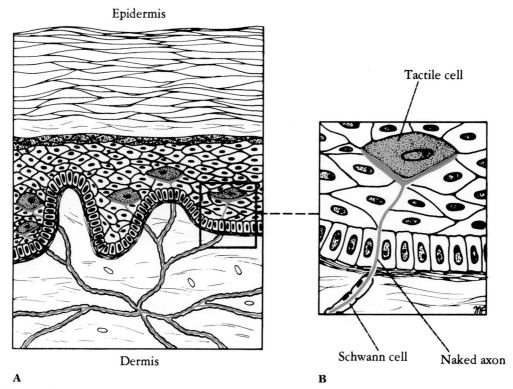

Figure 3–20 Merkel's discs in the skin. **A.** Low magnification. **B.** Merkel's disc showing the expanded ending of an axon with a stippled tactile cell.

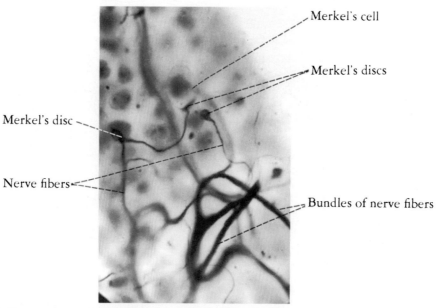

Figure 3–21 Photomicrograph of digital skin showing fine nerve terminals ending in Merkel's discs, stained by the silver method. (Courtesy Dr. N. Cauna.)

Merkel's discs are slowly adapting touch receptors that transmit information about the degree of pressure exerted on the skin, as for example, when one is holding a pen.

Hair Follicle Receptors

Nerve fibers wind around the follicle in its outer connective tissue sheath below the sebaceous gland. Some branches surround the follicle, while others run parallel to its long axis (Figs. 3-22 and 3-23). Many naked axon filaments terminate among the cells of the outer root sheath.

Bending of the hair stimulates the follicle receptor, which belongs to the rapidly adapting group of mechanoreceptors. While the hair remains bent, the receptor is silent, but when the hair is released, a further burst of nerve impulses is initiated.

ENCAPSULATED RECEPTORS

These receptors show wide variations in size and shape and the termination of the nerve is covered by a capsule.

Meissner's Corpuscles

Meissner's corpuscles are located in the dermal papillae of the skin (Figs. 3-24 and 3-25), especially that of the palm of the hand and the sole of the foot. Many also are present in the skin of the nipple and the external genitalia. Each corpuscle is ovoid in shape and consists of a stack of modified flattened Schwann cells arranged transversely across the long axis of the corpuscle. The corpuscle is enclosed by a capsule of connective tissue that is continuous with the endoneurium of the nerves that enter it. A few myelinated nerve fibers enter the deep end of the corpuscle; myelinated and unmyelinated branches decrease in size and ramify among the Schwann cells. There is a considerable reduction in the number of Meissner's corpuscles between birth and old age.

Meissner's corpuscles are very sensitive to touch and are rapidly adapting mechanoreceptors. They enable an individual to distinguish between two pointed structures when they are placed close together on the skin (two-point tactile discrimination).

Pacinian Corpuscles

Pacinian corpuscles (Figs.3-26 and 3-27) are widely distributed throughout the body and are abundant in the dermis, subcutaneous tissue, ligaments, joint capsules, pleura, peritoneum, nipples, and external genitalia. Each corpuscle is ovoid in shape, measuring about 2 mm long and about 100 to 500 μm across. It consists of a capsule and a central core containing the nerve ending. The capsule consists of numerous concentric lamellae of flattened cells. A large myelinated nerve fiber enters the corpuscle and loses its myelin sheath and then its Schwann cell covering. The naked axon, surrounded by lamellae formed of flattened cells, passes through the center of the core and terminates in an expanded end.

The pacinian corpuscle is a rapidly adapting mechanoreceptor that is particularly sensitive to vibration. It can respond to up to 600 stimuli per second.

Ruffini's Corpuscles

Ruffini's corpuscles are located in the dermis of hairy skin. Each corpuscle consists of several large unmyelinated nerve fibers ending within a bundle of collagen fibers and surrounded by a cellular capsule. These slowly adapting mechanoreceptors are stretch receptors, which respond when the skin is stretched.

Function of Cutaneous Receptors

In the past it was believed that the different histological types of receptors corresponded to specific types of sensation. It was soon pointed out that there are areas of the body that have only one or two histological types of receptors and yet they are sensitive to a variety of different stimuli. Moreover, although the body has these different receptors, all nerves only transmit nerve impulses. It is now generally agreed that the type of sensation felt is determined by the specific area of the central nervous system to which the afferent nerve fiber passes. For example, if a pain nerve fiber is stimulated by heat, cold, touch, or pressure, the individual will experience only pain.

Transduction of Sensory Stimuli Into Nerve Impulses

Transduction is the process by which one form of energy (the stimulus) is changed into another form of energy (electrochemical energy of the nerve impulse). The stimulus, when applied to the receptor, brings about a change in potential of the plasma membrane of the nerve ending. Since this process takes place in the receptor, it is referred to as the **receptor potential**. The amplitude of the receptor potential is proportional to the intensity of the stimulus. By opening more ion channels for longer time, a stronger mechanical pressure, for example, can produce a greater depolarization than does weak pressure. With chemoreceptors and photoreceptors, the receptor potential is produced by second messengers activated when the stimulus agent binds to the membrane receptors coupled to G proteins. If large enough, the receptor potential will generate an action potential that will travel along the afferent nerve fiber to the central nervous system.

Joint Receptors

Four types of sensory endings can be located in the capsule and ligaments of synovial joints. Three of these endings are encapsulated and resemble pacinian, Ruffini's, and tendon stretch receptors. They provide the central nervous system with information regarding the position and movements of the joint. A fourth type of ending is nonencapsulated and is thought to be sensitive to excessive movements and to transmit pain sensations.

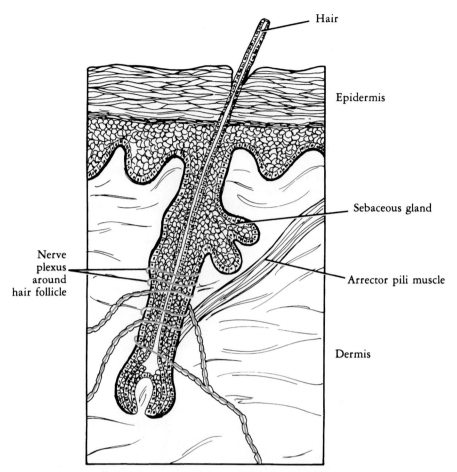

Figure 3–22   Nerve endings around a hair follicle.

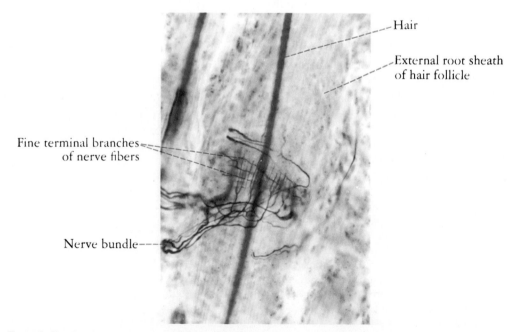

Figure 3–23   Photomicrograph of nerve endings around a hair follicle stained by the silver method. (Courtesy Dr. M. J. T. Fitzgerald.)

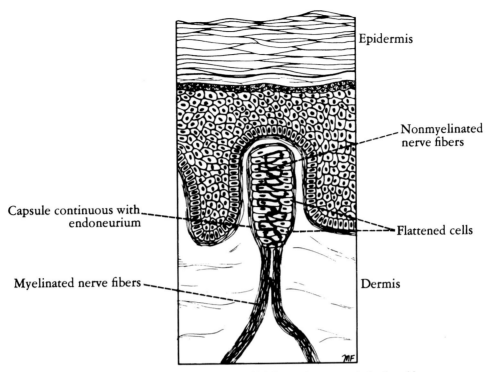

Figure 3–24   Detailed structure of Meissner's corpuscle in the skin.

Epidermis

Nonmyelinated
nerve fibers

Capsule continuous with
endoneurium

Flattened cells

Myelinated nerve fibers

Dermis

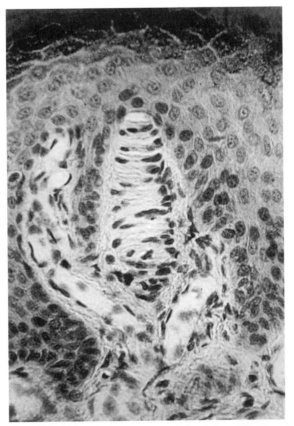

Figure 3–25   Photomicrograph of Meissner's corpuscle of the skin. (Courtesy Dr. N. Cauna.)

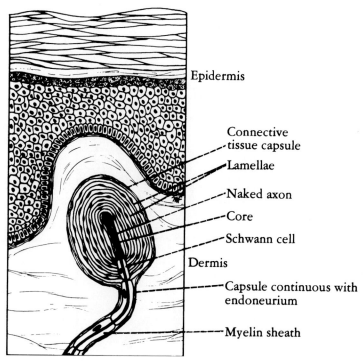

Figure 3–26 Detailed structure of a pacinian corpuscle in the skin.

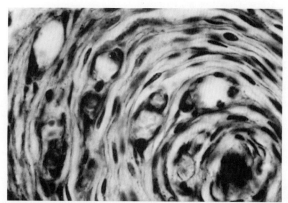

Figure 3–27 Photomicrograph of part of a pacinian corpuscle of the skin seen in transverse section, showing concentric lamellae of flattened cells. (Courtesy Dr. N. Cauna.)

Neuromuscular Spindles

Neuromuscular spindles, or muscular spindles (Figs. 3-28 and 3-29), are found in skeletal muscle and are most numerous toward the tendinous attachment of the muscle. They provide sensory information that is used by the central nervous system in the control of muscle activity. Each spindle measures about 1 to 4 mm in length and is surrounded by a fusiform capsule of connective tissue. Within the capsule are 6 to 14 slender **intrafusal muscle fibers**; the ordinary muscle fibers situated outside the spindles are referred to as **extrafusal fibers**. The intrafusal fibers of the spindles are of two types: the **nuclear bag** and **nuclear chain** fibers.

The nuclear bag fibers are recognized by the presence of numerous nuclei in the equatorial region, which consequently is expanded; also, cross-striations are absent in this region. In the nuclear chain fibers, the nuclei form a single longitudinal row or chain in the center of each fiber at the equatorial region. The nuclear bag fibers are larger in diameter than the nuclear chain fibers, and they extend beyond the capsule at each end to be attached to the endomysium of the extrafusal fibers.

There are two types of sensory innervation of muscle spindles: the annulospiral and the flower spray. The **annulospiral endings** are situated at the equator of the intrafusal fibers. As the large myelinated nerve fiber pierces the capsule, it loses its myelin sheath and the naked axon winds spirally around the nuclear bag or chain portions of the intrafusal fibers.

The **flower spray endings** are situated mainly on the nuclear chain fibers some distance away from the equatorial region. A myelinated nerve fiber slightly smaller than that for the annulospiral ending pierces the capsule and loses its myelin sheath and the naked axon branches terminally and ends as varicosities; it resembles a spray of flowers.

Stretching (elongation) of the intrafusal fibers results in stimulation of the annulospiral and flower spray endings, and nerve impulses pass to the spinal cord in the afferent neurons.

Motor innervation of the intrafusal fibers is provided by fine gamma motor fibers. The nerves terminate in small motor end-plates situated at both ends of the intrafusal fibers. Stimulation of the motor nerves causes both ends of the intrafusal fibers to contract and activate the sensory endings. The

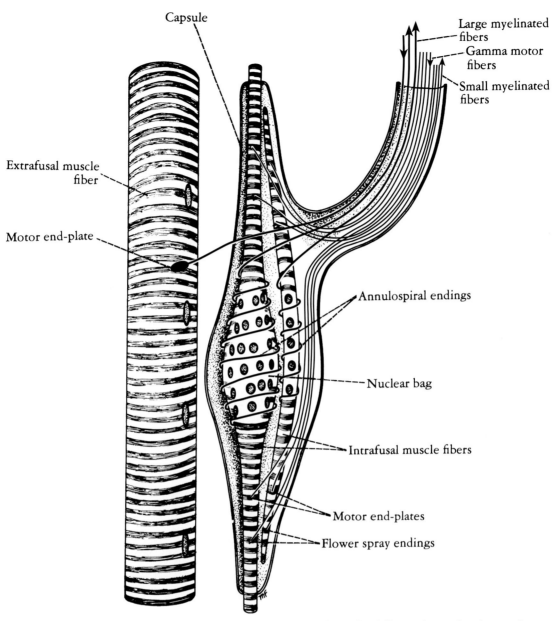

Figure 3–28 Neuromuscular spindle showing two types of intrafusal fibers: the nuclear bag and nuclear chain fibers.

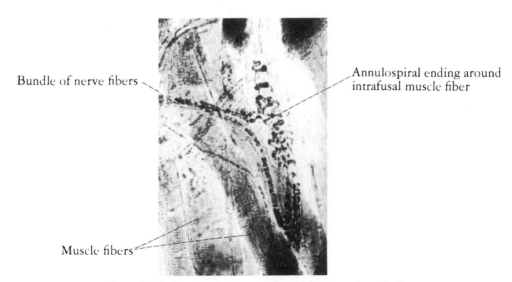

Figure 3–29 Photomicrograph of a neuromuscular spindle.

equatorial region, which is without cross-striations, is non-contractile. The extrafusal fibers of the remainder of the muscle receive their innervation in the usual way from large alpha-size axons.

Function of the Neuromuscular Spindle

Under resting conditions, the muscle spindles give rise to afferent nerve impulses all the time, and most of this information is not consciously perceived. When muscle activity occurs, either actively or passively, the intrafusal fibers are stretched and there is an increase in the rate of passage of nerve impulses to the spinal cord or brain in the afferent neurons. Similarly, if the intrafusal fibers are now relaxed due to the cessation of muscle activity, the result is a decrease in the rate of passage of nerve impulses to the spinal cord or brain. The neuromuscular spindle thus plays a very important role in keeping the central nervous system informed about muscle activity, thereby indirectly influencing the control of voluntary muscle.

STRETCH REFLEX

The neurons of the spinal cord involved in the simple stretch reflex are as follows. Stretching a muscle results in elongation of the intrafusal fibers of the muscle spindle and stimulation of the annulospiral and flower spray endings. The nerve impulses reach the spinal cord in the afferent neurons and synapse with the large alpha motor neurons situated in the anterior gray horns of the spinal cord. Nerve impulses now pass via the efferent motor nerves and stimulate the extrafusal muscle fibers and the muscle contracts.

This simple stretch reflex depends on a two-neuron arc consisting of an afferent neuron and an efferent neuron. It is interesting to note that the muscle spindle afferent impulses inhibit the alpha motor neurons supplying the antagonist muscles. This effect is called **reciprocal inhibition**.

CONTROL OF THE INTRAFUSAL FIBERS OF THE NEUROMUSCULAR SPINDLE

In the brain and spinal cord there are centers that give rise to tracts that synapse with gamma motor neurons in the spinal cord. The reticular formation, the basal ganglia, and the cerebellum are examples of such centers. It is by these means that these centers can greatly influence voluntary muscle activity. The gamma efferent motor fibers cause shortening of the intrafusal fibers, stretching the equatorial regions and stimulating the annulospiral and flower spray endings. This in turn initiates the reflex contraction of the extrafusal fibers described previously.

It is estimated that about one-third of all the motor fibers passing to a muscle are gamma efferents; the remaining two-thirds are the large alpha motor fibers. It is believed that the nuclear bag fibers are concerned with dynamic responses and are associated more with position and velocity of contraction, whereas the nuclear chain fibers are associated with slow static contractions of voluntary muscle.

Neurotendinous Spindles (Golgi Tendon Organs)

Neurotendinous spindles are present in tendons and are located near the junctions of tendons with muscles (Fig. 3-30).

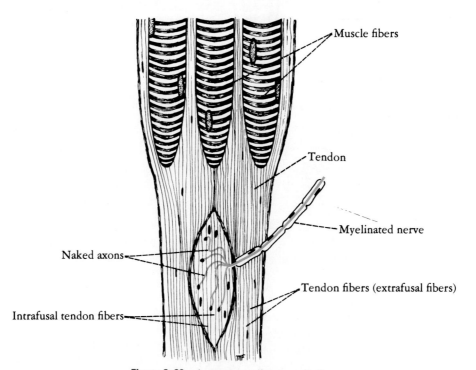

Figure 3–30 A neurotendinous spindle.

Each spindle consists of a fibrous capsule that surrounds a small bundle of loosely arranged tendon (collagen) fibers (intrafusal fibers). The tendon cells are larger and more numerous than those found elsewhere in the tendon. One or more myelinated sensory nerve fibers pierce the capsule, lose their myelin sheath, branch, and terminate in club-shaped endings.

The nerve endings are activated by being squeezed by the adjacent tendon fibers within the spindle when tension develops in the tendon. Unlike the neuromuscular spindle, which is sensitive to changes in muscle length, the neurotendinous organ detects changes in muscle tension.

FUNCTION OF THE NEUROTENDINOUS SPINDLE

Increased muscle tension stimulates the neurotendinous spindles and an increased number of nerve impulses reach the spinal cord through the afferent nerve fibers. These fibers synapse with the large alpha motor neurons situated in the anterior gray horns of the spinal cord. Unlike the muscle spindle reflex, this reflex is inhibitory and inhibits muscle contraction. In this manner the tendon reflex prevents the development of too much tension in the muscle. Although this function is probably important as a protective mechanism, its main function is to provide the central nervous system with information that can influence voluntary muscle activity.

EFFECTOR ENDINGS

Innervation of Skeletal Muscle

Skeletal muscle is innervated by one or more nerves. In the limbs and head and neck the innervation is usually single, but in the large muscles of the abdominal wall the innervation is multiple, the latter muscles having retained their embryonic segmental nerve supply.

The nerve supply and blood supply to a muscle enter it at a more or less constant position called the **neurovascular hilus.** The nerve to a muscle contains motor and sensory fibers. The motor fibers are of three types: (1) large alpha myelinated fibers, (2) small gamma myelinated fibers, and (3) fine unmyelinated C fibers. The large myelinated axons of the alpha anterior horn cells supply the extrafusal fibers that form the main mass of the muscle. The small gamma myelinated fibers supply the intrafusal fibers of the neuromuscular spindles. The fine unmyelinated fibers are postganglionic autonomic efferents that supply the smooth muscle in the walls of blood vessels.

The sensory fibers are of three main types: (1) the myelinated fibers, which originate in the annulospiral and flower spray endings of the neuromuscular spindles; (2) the myelinated fibers, which originate in the neurotendinous spindles; and (3) the myelinated and nonmyelinated fibers, which originate from a variety of sensory endings in the connective tissue of the muscle.

MOTOR UNIT

The motor unit may be defined as the single alpha motor neuron and the muscle fibers that it innervates (Fig. 3-31). The muscle fibers of a single motor unit are widely scattered throughout the muscle. Where fine, precise muscle control is required, such as in the extraocular muscles or the small muscles of the hand, the motor units possess only a few muscle fibers. However, in a large limb muscle, such as the gluteus maximus, where precise control is not necessary, a single motor nerve may innervate many hundreds of muscle fibers.

Neuromuscular Junctions In Skeletal Muscle

As each large alpha myelinated fiber enters a skeletal muscle, it branches many times. The number of branches depends on the size of the motor unit. A single branch then terminates on a muscle fiber at a site referred to as a **neuromuscular junction** or **motor end-plate** (Figs. 3-32 and 3-33). The great majority of muscle fibers are innervated by just one motor end-plate. On reaching the muscle fiber, the nerve loses its myelin sheath and breaks up into a number of fine branches. Each branch ends as a naked axon and forms the **neural element** of the motor end-plate (Fig. 3-34). The axon is expanded slightly and contains numerous mitochondria and vesicles (approximately 45 nm in diameter). At the site of the motor end-plate the surface of the muscle fiber is elevated slightly to form the **muscular element** of the plate, often referred to as the **sole plate** (Fig. 3-32). The elevation is due to the local accumulation of granular sarcoplasm beneath the sarcolemma and the presence of numerous nuclei and mitochondria.

The expanded naked axon lies in a groove on the surface of the muscle fiber. Each groove is formed by the infolding of the sarcolemma. The groove may branch many times, each branch containing a division of the axon. It is important to realize that the axons are truly naked; the Schwann cells merely serve as a cap or roof to the groove and never project into it. The floor of the groove is formed of sarcolemma, which is thrown into numerous folds, called **junctional folds;** these serve to increase the surface area of the sarcolemma that lies close to the naked axon (Fig. 3-35). The plasma membrane of the axon (the axolemma or presynaptic membrane) is separated, by a space about 30 to 50 nm wide, from the plasma membrane of the muscle fiber (the sarcolemma or postsynaptic membrane). This space constitutes the **synaptic cleft**. The synaptic cleft is filled with the basement membranes of the axon and the muscle fiber (Fig. 3-32). The motor end-plate is strengthened by the connective tissue sheath of the nerve fiber, the endoneurium, which becomes continuous with the connective tissue sheath of the muscle fiber, the endomysium.

A nerve impulse (action potential), on reaching the presynaptic membrane of the motor end-plate, causes the opening of voltage-gated Ca^{2+} channels that allow Ca^{2+} ions to enter the axon. This stimulates the fusion of some of the synaptic vesicles with the presynaptic mem-

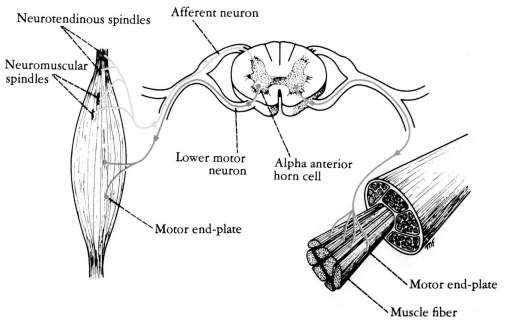

Neurotendinous spindles

Afferent neuron

Neuromuscular spindles

Lower motor neuron

Alpha anterior horn cell

Motor end-plate

Motor end-plate

Muscle fiber

Figure 3–31 Simple reflex arc consisting of an afferent neuron arising from neuromuscular spindles and neurotendinous spindles and an efferent lower motor neuron whose cell body is an alpha anterior horn cell within the spinal cord. Note that the efferent neuron terminates on muscle fibers at motor end-plates.

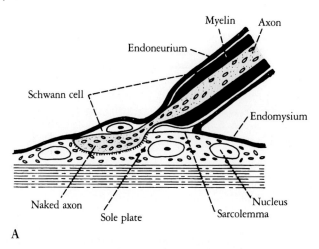

Myelin   Axon

Endoneurium

Schwann cell

Endomysium

Naked axon

Sole plate

Nucleus

Sarcolemma

A

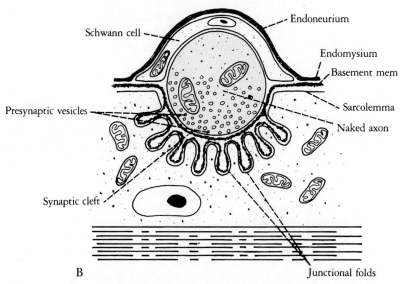

Schwann cell

Endoneurium

Endomysium

Basement mem

Presynaptic vesicles

Sarcolemma

Naked axon

Synaptic cleft

B

Junctional folds

Figure 3–32 **A.** A skeletal neuromuscular junction. **B.** Enlarged view of a muscle fiber showing the terminal naked axon lying in the surface groove of the muscle fiber.

Nerve fibers and bundles
of nerve fibers

Acetylcholinesterase
at motor end-plates

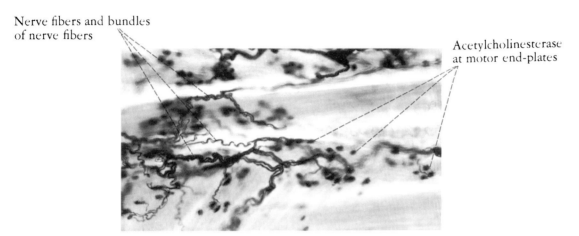

Figure 3–33   Photomicrograph showing nerve fibers terminating on skeletal muscle fibers at motor end-plates, stained histochemically for acetylcholinesterase and counterstained with silver. (Courtesy Dr. M. J. T. Fitzgerald.)

Muscle fiber

Motor end-plate

Schwann cell

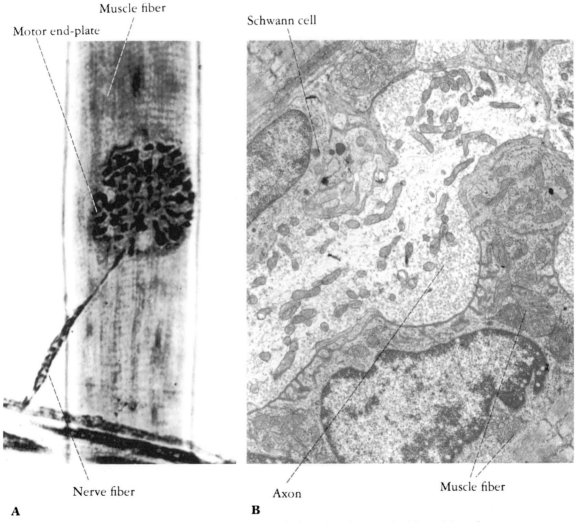

Nerve fiber

Axon

Muscle fiber

A   **B**

Figure 3–34   A. Photomicrograph of a motor end-plate showing terminal branching of a nerve fiber. **B.** Electron micrograph of a terminal axon at a motor end-plate, showing axon lying in a groove on the surface of the muscle fiber. (Courtesy Dr. J. M. Kerns.)

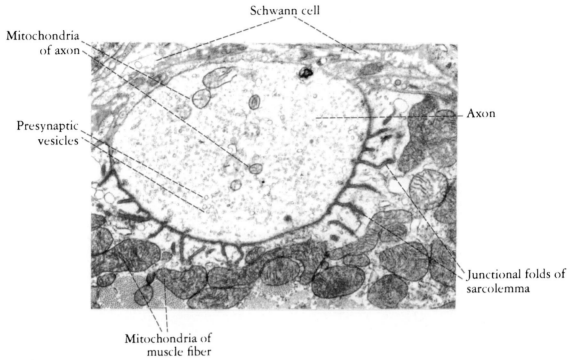

Figure 3–35 Electron micrograph of a cross section of an axon at a motor end-plate, showing the axon lying in a groove of folded sarcolemma. (Courtesy Dr. J. M. Kerns.)

brane and causes the release of acetylcholine into the synaptic cleft. The acetylcholine is thus discharged into the cleft by a process of **exocytosis** and diffuses rapidly across the cleft to reach the nicotinic type of Ach receptors on the postsynaptic membrane of the junctional folds. The postsynaptic membrane possesses large numbers of Ach-gated channels.

Once the Ach-gated channels are opened, the postsynaptic membrane becomes more permeable to Na$^+$ ions which flow into the muscle cell and a local potential called the **end-plate potential** is created. (The Ach-gated channels are also permeable to K$^+$ ions, which flow out of the cell, but to a lesser extent). If the end-plate potential is large enough, the voltage-gated channels for Na$^+$ ions are opened and an action potential will be initiated and will spread along the surface of the sarcolemma. The wave of depolarization is carried into the muscle fiber to the contractile myofibrils through the system of T tubules. This leads to the release of Ca$^+$ ions from the sarcoplasmic reticulum that in turn causes the muscle to contract.

The amount of acetylcholine released at the motor end-plate will depend on the number of nerve impulses arriving at the nerve terminal. Once the acetylcholine crosses the synaptic cleft and triggers the ionic channels on the postsynaptic membrane, it immediately undergoes hydrolysis due to the presence of the enzyme **acetylcholinesterase (AChE)** (Fig. 3-33). The enzyme is adherent to the collagen fibrils of the basement membranes in the cleft; some of the acetylcholine also diffuses away from the cleft. The acetylcholine remains for about 1 msec in contact with the postsynaptic membrane, and it is rapidly destroyed to prevent

reexcitation of the muscle fiber. After the fall in concentration of Ach in the cleft, the ionic channels close and remain closed until the arrival of more Ach.

Skeletal muscle fiber contraction is thus controlled by the frequency of the nerve impulses that arrive at the motor nerve terminal. A resting muscle fiber shows small occasional depolarizations (end-plate potentials) at the motor end-plate, which are insufficient to cause an action potential and make the fiber contract. These are believed to be due to the sporadic release of acetylcholine into the synaptic cleft from a single presynaptic vesicle.

The sequence of events that takes place at a motor end-plate upon stimulation of a motor nerve can be summarized as follows:

ACh → Nicotinic Type of ACh Receptor, Ach-gated channels opened → Na$^+$ influx → End-plate potential created.

End-plate potential (if large enough) → Na$^+$ gated channels opened → Na$^+$ influx → Action potential created.

Action potential → Increased release of Ca^{2+} → muscle fiber contraction.

Immediate hydrolysis of acetylcholine by AChE → Ach-gated channels closed → muscle fiber repolarization

If drugs having a similar chemical structure to acetylcholine were to arrive at the receptor site of a motor end-plate, they might bring about the same changes as acetylcholine and mimic its action. Two examples of such drugs are **nicotine** and **carbamylcholine**. If, on the other hand, drugs having a similar chemical structure to acetylcholine were to arrive at the receptor site of a motor end-plate and were unable to bring about the sequence of changes normally induced by acetylcholine, they would occupy the

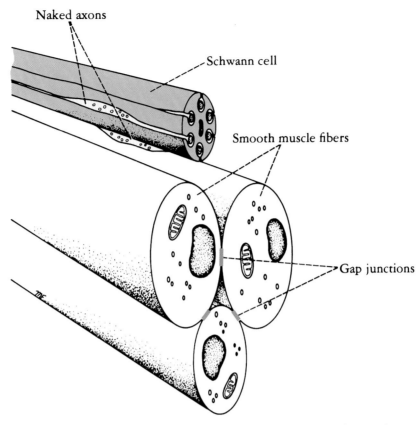

Naked axons

Schwann cell

Smooth muscle fibers

Gap junctions

Figure 3-36   Autonomic neuromuscular junction. The exposed axons are close to the smooth muscle fibers.

receptor site and block access of acetylcholine. Such drugs would be competing with acetylcholine and are called **competitive blocking agents**. An example of such a drug is ***d*-tubocurarine**, which causes skeletal muscle to relax and not contract by preventing the action of locally produced acetylcholine (see also p. 120).

Neuromuscular Junctions In Smooth Muscle

In smooth muscle, where the action is slow and widespread, such as within the wall of the intestine, the autonomic nerve fibers branch extensively, so that a single neuron exerts control over a large number of muscle fibers. In some areas, for example, the longitudinal layer of smooth muscle in the intestine, only a few muscle fibers are associated with autonomic endings, the wave of contraction passing from one muscle cell to another by means of gap junctions (Fig. 3-36).

In smooth muscle, in which the action is fast and precision is required, such as in the iris, the branching of the nerve fibers is less extensive, so that a single neuron exerts control over only a few muscle fibers.

The autonomic nerve fibers, which are postganglionic, are nonmyelinated and terminate as a series of varicosed branches. An interval of 10 to 100 nm may exist between the axon and the muscle fiber. At the site where transmission is to occur, the Schwann cell is retracted so that the axon lies within a shallow groove on its surface (Fig. 3-36). Part of the axon thus is naked, permitting free diffusion of the transmitter substance from the axon to the muscle cell (Fig. 3-36). Here the axoplasm contains numerous vesicles similar to those seen at the motor end-plate of skeletal muscle.

Smooth muscle is innervated by sympathetic and parasympathetic parts of the autonomic system. Those nerves that are cholinergic liberate acetylcholine at their endings by a process of exocytosis, the acetylcholine being present in the vesicles at the nerve ending. Those nerves that are noradrenergic liberate **norepinephrine** at their endings by a process of exocytosis, the norepinephrine being present in dark-cored vesicles at the nerve endings. Both the acetylcholine and norepinephrine bring about depolarization of the muscle fibers innervated, which thereupon contract. The fate of these neurotransmitter substances differs. The acetylcholine is hydrolyzed in the presence of acetylcholinesterase in the synaptic cleft of the muscle fiber and the norepinephrine is taken up by the nerve endings. It is important to note that in some areas of the body (e.g., bronchial muscle) the norepinephrine liberated from postganglionic sympathetic fibers causes smooth muscle to relax and not contract.

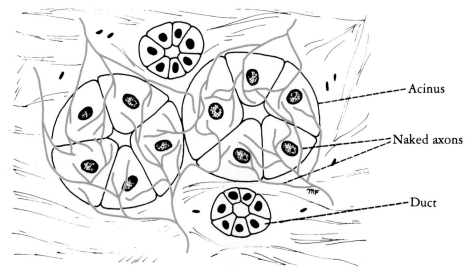

Figure 3–37   Nerve fibers ending around glandular acini.

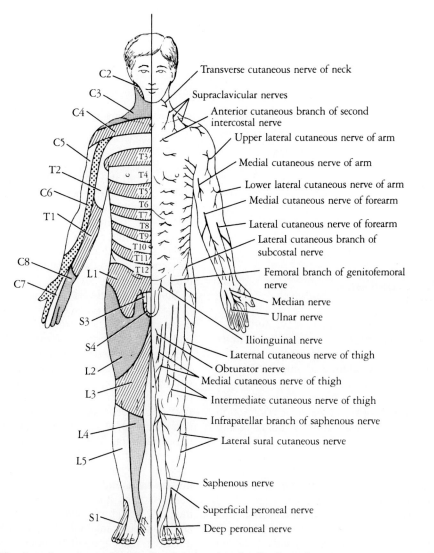

Figure 3–38   Anterior aspect of the body, showing the distribution of cutaneous nerves on the left side and dermatomes on the right side.

Neuromuscular Junctions In Cardiac Muscle

Nonmyelinated postganglionic autonomic nerves extend into the connective tissue between the muscle fibers and terminate in close proximity to the individual cardiac muscle fibers. At the site where transmission takes place, the axon becomes naked because of the retraction of the Schwann cell. This permits free diffusion of the neurotransmitter substance from the axon to the muscle fiber. Because of the presence of intermittent desmosomes and gap junctions between abutting muscle fibers, excitation and contraction of one muscle fiber rapidly spreads from fiber to fiber.

Nerve Endings on Secretory Cells of Glands

Nonmyelinated postganglionic autonomic nerves extend into the connective tissue of glands and branch close to the secretory cells (Fig. 3-37). In many glands the nerve fibers have been found to innervate only the blood vessels.

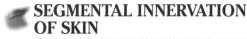

SEGMENTAL INNERVATION OF SKIN

The area of skin supplied by a single spinal nerve, and, therefore, a single segment of the spinal cord, is called a **dermatome**. On the trunk the dermatomes extend round the body from the posterior to the anterior median plane. Adjacent dermatomes overlap considerably, so that to produce a region of complete anesthesia at least three contiguous spinal nerves have to be sectioned. It should be noted that the area of tactile loss is always greater than the area of loss of painful and thermal sensations. The reason for this difference is that the degree of overlap of fibers carrying pain and thermal sensations is much more extensive than the overlap of fibers carrying tactile sensations. Dermatomal charts for the anterior and posterior surfaces of the body are shown in Figures 3-38 and 3-39.

In the limbs the arrangement of the dermatomes is more complicated, and the reason for this is the embryological rotation of the limbs as they grow out from the trunk. (For details, see Figs. 3-38 and 3-39).

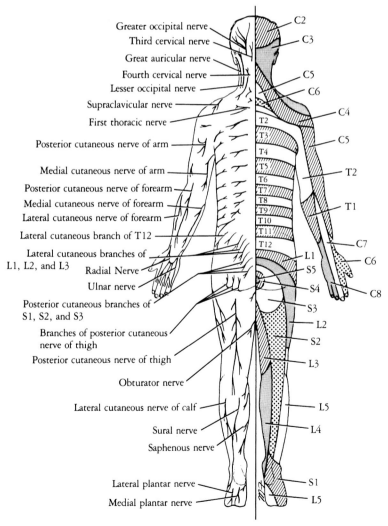

Figure 3–39 Posterior aspect of the body, showing the distribution of cutaneous nerves on the left side and dermatomes on the right side.

In the face, the divisions of the trigeminal nerve supply a precise area of skin and there is little or no overlap to the cutaneous area of another division.

SEGMENTAL INNERVATION OF MUSCLES

Skeletal muscle also receives a segmental innervation. Most of these muscles are innervated by more than one spinal nerve and, therefore, by the same number of segments of the spinal cord. Thus, to paralyze a muscle completely it would be necessary to section several spinal nerves or destroy several segments of the spinal cord.

To learn the segmental innervation of all the muscles of the body is an impossible task. Nevertheless, the segmental innervation of the following muscles should be known, because it is possible to test them by eliciting simple muscle reflexes in the patient (Fig. 3-40):

Biceps brachii tendon reflex C5-6 (flexion of the elbow joint by tapping the biceps tendon).

Triceps tendon reflex C6-7, and **8** (extension of the elbow joint by tapping the triceps tendon).

Brachioradialis tendon reflex C5-6, and 7 (supination of the radioulnar joints by tapping the insertion of the brachioradialis tendon).

Abdominal superficial reflexes (contraction of underlying abdominal muscles by stroking the skin). Upper abdominal skin T6-7; middle abdominal skin T8-9; lower abdominal skin T10-12.

Patellar tendon reflex (knee jerk) L2, 3, and **4** (extension of knee joint on tapping the patellar tendon).

Achilles tendon reflex (ankle jerk) S1 and 2 (plantar flexion of ankle joint on tapping the Achilles tendon—tendo calcaneus).

MUSCLE TONE AND MUSCLE ACTION

A **motor unit** consists of a motor neuron in the anterior gray column (horn) of the spinal cord and all the muscle fibers it supplies (Fig. 3-41). In a large buttock muscle, such as the gluteus maximus, where fine control is unnecessary, a given motor neuron may supply as many as 200 muscle fibers. In contrast, in the small muscles of the hand or the extrinsic muscles of the eyeball, where fine control is required, one nerve fiber supplies only a few muscle fibers.

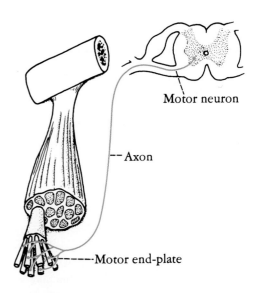

Bundle of muscle fibers

Figure 3–41   Components of a motor unit.

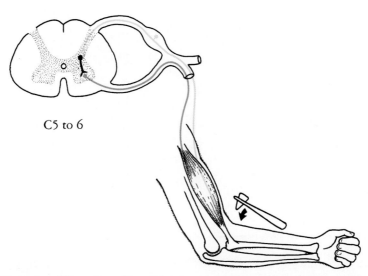

Figure 3–40   Biceps brachii tendon reflex. Note that the reflex arc passes through the fifth and sixth cervical segments of the spinal cord. This is usually monosynaptic, the internuncial neuron (black) being absent.

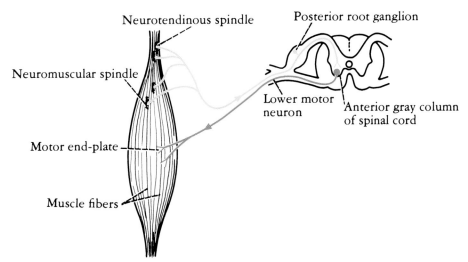

Figure 3–42 Simple reflex arc consisting of an afferent neuron arising from neuromuscular spindles and neurotendinous spindles, and an efferent neuron whose cell body lies in the anterior gray column (horn) of the spinal cord. Note that for simplicity the afferent fibers from the neurotendinous spindle and the neuromuscular spindle are shown as one pathway; in fact, the neurotendinous receptor is inhibitory and reduces tone whereas the neuromuscular spindle is excitatory and increases tone.

Every skeletal muscle, while resting, is in a partial state of contraction. This condition is referred to as **muscle tone**. Since there is no intermediate stage, muscle fibers are either fully contracted or relaxed; it follows that a few muscle fibers within a muscle are fully contracted all the time. To bring about this state, and to avoid fatigue, different groups of motor units, and thus different groups of muscle fibers, are brought into action at different times. This is accomplished by the asynchronous discharge of nervous impulses in the motor neurons in the anterior gray horn of the spinal cord.

Basically, muscle tone is dependent on the integrity of a simple monosynaptic reflex arc composed of two neurons in the nervous system (Fig. 3-42). The lengthening and shortening in a muscle are detected by sensitive sensory endings called **muscle spindles** (see p. 96) and the tension is detected by **tendon spindles** (see p. 98). The nervous impulses travel in the large afferent fibers to the spinal cord. There, they synapse with the motor neurons situated in the anterior gray column, which, in turn, send impulses down their axons to the muscle fibers (see Fig. 3-42). The muscle spindles themselves are innervated by small gamma efferent fibers that regulate the response of the muscle spindles, acting synergically with external stretch. In this manner, muscle tone is maintained reflexly and adjusted to the needs of posture and movement.

Should the afferent or efferent pathways of the reflex arc be cut, the muscle would lose its tone immediately and become flaccid. A flaccid muscle, on palpation, feels like a mass of dough and has completely lost its resilience. It quickly atrophies and becomes reduced in volume. It is important to realize that the degree of activity of the motor anterior column cells, and therefore the degree of muscle tone, depends on the summation of the nerve impulses received by these cells from other neurons of the nervous system.

Muscle movement is accomplished by bringing into action increasing numbers of motor units and, at the same time, reducing the activity of the motor units of muscles that will oppose or antagonize the movement. When the maximum effort is required, all the motor units of a muscle are thrown into action.

SUMMATION OF MOTOR UNITS

When a muscle begins to contract, the smaller motor units are stimulated first. The reason for this is that the smaller motor units are innervated by smaller neurons in the spinal cord and brainstem and they have a lower threshold of excitability. As the contraction increases, progressively larger motor units are brought into action. This phenomenon causes a gradual increase in muscle strength as the muscle contracts.

MUSCLE FATIGUE

The progressive loss of strength of a muscle with prolonged strong contraction is due to the reduction in the amounts of adenosine triphosphate (ATP) within the muscle fibers. Nerve impulses continue to arrive at the neuromuscular junction and normal depolarization of the plasma membrane of the muscle fiber occurs.

POSTURE

Posture may be defined as the position adopted by the individual within his or her environment. In the standing position the line of gravity passes through the odontoid process of the axis, behind the centers of the hip joints, and in front

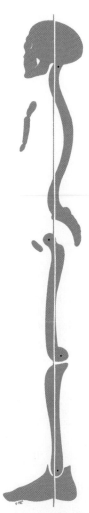

Figure 3–43 Lateral view of the skeleton, showing the line of gravity. Since the greater part of body weight lies anterior to the vertebral column, the deep muscles of the back are important in maintaining normal postural curves of the vertebral column in the standing position.

of the knee and ankle joints (Fig. 3-43). In order to stabilize the body and prevent it from collapsing, it is not surprising to find that in humans the antigravity muscles are well developed and exhibit the greatest degree of tone. One can therefore say that posture depends on the degree and distribution of muscle tone, which in turn depends on the normal integrity of simple reflex arcs centered in the spinal cord.

An individual may assume a particular posture (sitting or standing) over long periods of time with little evidence of fatigue. The reason for this is that muscle tone is maintained through different groups of muscle fibers contracting in relays, only a small number of muscle fibers within a muscle being in a state of contraction at any one time. The active muscle fiber groups are scattered throughout the muscle.

In order to maintain posture, the simple muscle reflex, upon which muscle tone is dependent, must receive ade-

quate nervous input from higher levels of the nervous system (Fig. 3-44). For example, impulses arising from the labyrinths and neck muscles, information arising from the cerebellum, midbrain, and cerebral centers, general information arising from other muscle groups, joints, and even skin receptors will result in nervous impulses impinging on the large anterior gray column cells (i.e., the final common pathway) controlling the muscle fibers.

When an individual assumes a given posture, the tone of the muscles controlling that posture is constantly undergoing fine adjustments so that the posture is maintained. Normal posture thus depends not only on the integrity of the reflex arc but also on the summation of the nervous impulses received by the motor anterior gray column cells from other neurons of the nervous system (Fig. 3-45). The detail of the different nervous pathways involved in bringing the information to the anterior gray column cells is dealt within Chapter 4.

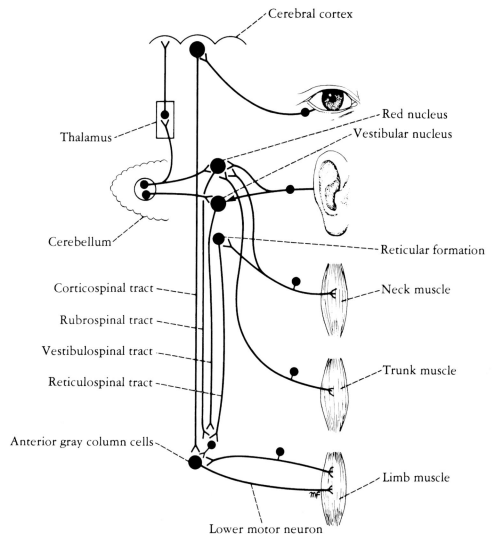

Figure 3–44 Nervous input from higher levels of the central nervous system, which can influence the activity of the anterior gray column (horn) cells of the spinal cord.

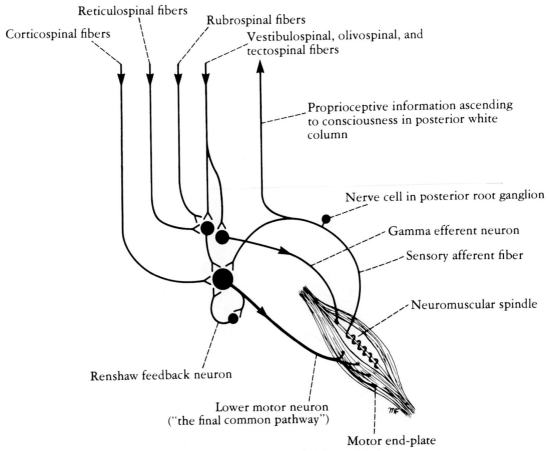

Figure 3–45 Normal postural tone of skeletal muscle is dependent not only on the integrity of the reflex arc, but also on the summation of the nervous impulses received by the motor anterior gray column (horn) cells from other neurons of the nervous system.

CLINICAL NOTES

RESPONSE OF NEURONS TO INJURY

The survival of the cytoplasm of a neuron depends on its being connected, however indirectly, with the nucleus. The nucleus plays a key role in the synthesis of proteins, which pass into the cell processes and replace proteins that have been metabolized by cell activity. Thus, the cytoplasm of axons and dendrites will undergo degeneration quickly if these processes are separated from the nerve cell body.

Injury of the Nerve Cell Body

Severe damage of the nerve cell body due to trauma, interference with the blood supply, or disease may result in degeneration of the entire neuron, including its dendrites and synaptic endings. In the brain and spinal cord, the neuronal debris and the fragments of myelin (if the processes are myelinated) are engulfed and phagocytosed by the microglial cells. Later, the neighboring astrocytes proliferate and replace the neuron with scar tissue.

In the peripheral nervous system, the tissue macrophages remove the debris and the local fibroblasts replace the neuron with scar tissue.

Injury of the Nerve Cell Process

If the axon of the nerve cell is divided, degenerative changes will take place in (1) the distal segment that is separated from the cell body, (2) a portion of the axon proximal to the injury, and (3) possibly the cell body from which the axon arises.

CHANGES IN THE DISTAL SEGMENT OF THE AXON
The changes spread distally from the site of the lesion (Fig. 3-46) and include its terminations; the process is referred to as **wallerian degeneration**. In the peripheral nervous system, on the first day the axon becomes swollen and irregular, and by the third or fourth day the axon is broken into fragments (Fig. 3-46) and the debris

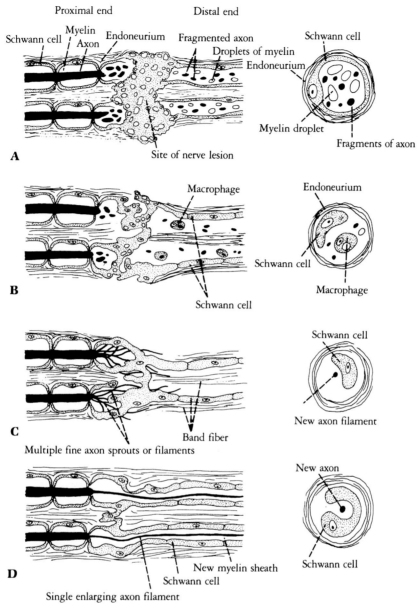

Proximal end   Distal end

Figure 3–46 **A, B, C,** and **D.** Degeneration and regeneration in a divided nerve.

is digested by the surrounding Schwann cells and tissue macrophages. The entire axon is destroyed within a week.

Meanwhile, the myelin sheath slowly breaks down and lipid droplets appear within the Schwann cell cytoplasm (Fig. 3-46). Later, the droplets are extruded from the Schwann cell and subsequently are phagocytosed by tissue macrophages. The Schwann cells now begin to proliferate rapidly and become arranged in parallel cords within the persistent basement membrane. The endoneurial sheath and the contained cords of Schwann cells are sometimes referred to as a **band fiber**. If regeneration does not occur, the axon and the Schwann cells are replaced by fibrous tissue produced by local fibroblasts.

In the central nervous system, degeneration of the axons and the myelin sheaths follows a similar course, and the debris is removed by the phagocytic activity of the microglial cells. Little is known about the role of oligodendrocytes in this process. The astrocytes now proliferate and replace the axons.

CHANGES IN THE PROXIMAL SEGMENT OF THE AXON

The changes in the proximal segment of the axon are similar to those that take place in the distal segment (Fig. 3-46) but extend only proximally above the lesion as far as the first node of Ranvier. The proliferating cords of Schwann cells in the peripheral nerves bulge from the cut surfaces of the endoneurial tubes.

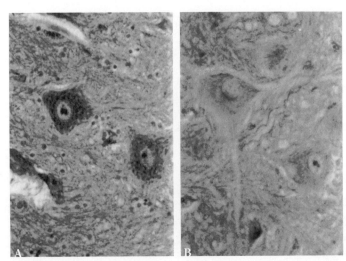

Figure 3–47 Photomicrographs of motor neurons of the anterior gray column of the spinal cord. **A.** Nissl substance in normal neurons. **B.** Following section of anterior roots of spinal nerve, showing chromatolysis.

CHANGES IN THE NERVE CELL BODY FROM WHICH THE AXON ARISES

The changes that occur in the cell body following injury to its axon are referred to as **retrograde degeneration**; the changes that take place in the proximal segment of the axon commonly are included under this heading. The possible reason for these changes is that section of the axon cuts off the cell body from its supply of trophic factors derived from the target organs at the distal end of the axon.

The most characteristic change occurs in the cell body within the first 2 days following injury and reaches its maximum within 2 weeks. The Nissl material becomes fine, granular (Figs. 3-47 and 3-48), and dispersed throughout the cytoplasm, a process known as **chromatolysis.** Chromatolysis begins near the axon hillock and spreads to all parts of the cell body. In addition, the nucleus moves from its central location toward the periphery of the cell and the cell body swells and becomes rounded (Fig. 3-48). The degree of chromatolysis and the degree of swelling of the cell are greatest when the injury to the axon is close to the cell body. In some neurons, very severe damage to the axon close to the cell body may lead to death of the neuron. On the other hand, damage to the most distal process may lead to little or no detectable change in the cell body. The dispersal of the Nissl material, that is, the cytoplasmic RNA, and the swelling of the cell are caused by cellular edema. The apparent loss of staining affinity of the Nissl material is due to the wide dispersal of the cytoplasmic RNA. The movement of the nucleus away from the center of the cell may be due to the cellular edema.

Synaptic terminals are seen to withdraw from the surface of the injured nerve cell body and its dendrites and are replaced by Schwann cells in the peripheral nervous system and microglial cells or astrocytes in the central nervous system. This process is called **synaptic stripping.** The possible causes of synaptic stripping are (1) Loss of plasma membrane adhesiveness following injury, (2) The supporting cells are stimulated by chemicals released from the injured neuron. If the injury is sufficiently great the cells of the immune system, namely, monocytes and macrophages, may migrate into the area.

RECOVERY OF NEURONS FOLLOWING INJURY

In contrast to the rapid onset of retrograde degeneration, the recovery of the nerve cell body and regeneration of its processes may take several months.

Recovery of the Nerve Cell Body

The nucleolus moves to the periphery of the nucleus and polysome clusters reappear in the cytoplasm. This indicates that RNA and protein synthesis is being accelerated in preparation for the reformation of the axon. Thus, there is a reconstitution of the original Nissl structure, a decrease in the swelling of the cell body, and a return of the nucleus to its characteristic central position (Fig. 3-48).

Regeneration of Axons in Peripheral Nerves

Regrowth of the axons (motor, sensory, and autonomic) is possible in peripheral nerves and appears to depend on the presence of endoneurial tubes and the special qualities possessed by Schwann cells. Sprouts from the axons grow from the proximal stump and into the distal stump toward the nerve's end organs. The following mechanisms are thought to be involved: (1) The axons are attracted by chemotropic factors secreted by the Schwann cells in the distal stump, (2) Growth stimulating factors exist within the distal stump, and (3) Inhibitory factors are present in the perineurium to inhibit the axons from leaving the nerve.

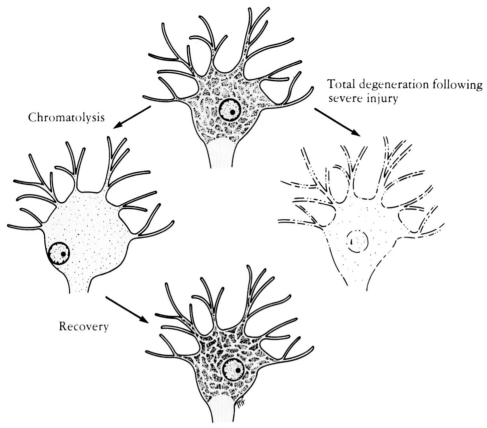

Chromatolysis

Total degeneration following
severe injury

Recovery

Figure 3–48 The changes that may take place in a nerve cell body following division of one of its processes.

The satisfactory regeneration of axons and the return of normal function depend on the following factors:

1. In crush nerve injuries, where the axon is divided or its blood supply has been interfered with but the endoneurial sheaths remain intact, the regenerative process may be very satisfactory.
2. In nerves that have been completely severed there is much less chance of recovery, because the regenerating fibers from the proximal stump may be directed to an incorrect destination in the distal stump, that is, cutaneous fibers entering incorrect nerve endings or motor nerves supplying incorrect muscles.
3. If the distance between the proximal and distal stumps of the completely severed nerve is greater than a few millimeters, or the gap becomes filled with proliferating fibrous tissue or is simply filled by adjacent muscles that bulge into the gap, then the chances of recovery are very poor. The outgrowing axonal sprouts escape into the surrounding connective tissue and form a tangled mass or **neuroma**. In these cases, early close surgical approximation of the severed ends, if possible, greatly facilitates the chances of recovery.
4. When mixed nerves (those containing sensory, motor, and autonomic fibers) are completely severed, the chances of a good recovery are very much less than when the nerve is purely sensory or purely motor. The reason for this is that the regenerating fibers from the proximal stump may be guided to an incorrect destination in the distal stump; for example, cutaneous fibers may enter motor endoneurial tubes and vice versa.
5. Inadequate physiotherapy to the paralyzed muscles will result in their degenerating before the regenerating motor axons have reached them.
6. The presence of infection at the site of the wound will seriously interfere with the process of regeneration.

If one assumes that the proximal and distal stumps of the severed nerve are in close apposition, the following regenerative processes take place (Fig. 3-46). The Schwann cells, having undergone mitotic division, now fill the space within the basal lamina of the endoneurial tubes of the proximal stump as far proximally as the next node of Ranvier, and in the distal stump as far distally as the end-organs. Where a small gap exists between the proximal and distal stumps, the multiplying Schwann cells form a number of cords to bridge the gap.

Each proximal axon end now gives rise to multiple fine sprouts or filaments with bulbous tips. These filaments, as they grow, advance along the clefts between the Schwann cells and thus cross the interval between the proximal and distal nerve stumps. Many such filaments now enter the prox-

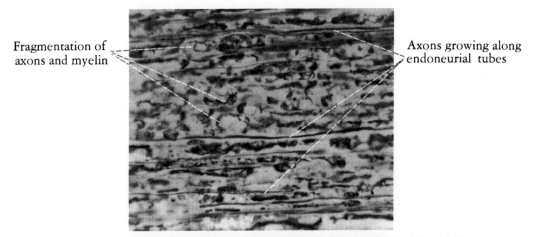

Fragmentation of axons and myelin

Axons growing along endoneurial tubes

Figure 3–49 Photomicrograph of a longitudinal section of the distal stump of the sciatic nerve, showing evidence of degeneration and axon regeneration following injury. (Courtesy Dr. M. J. T. Fitzgerald.)

imal end of each endoneurial tube and grow distally in contact with the Schwann cells (Fig. 3-49). It is clear that the filaments from many different axons may enter a single endoneurial tube. However, only one filament persists, the remainder degenerating, and that one filament grows distally to reinnervate a motor or sensory end-organ. While crossing the gap between the severed nerve ends, many filaments fail to enter an endoneurial tube and grow out into the surrounding connective tissue. It is interesting to note that the formation of multiple sprouts or filaments from a single proximal axon greatly increases the chances that a neuron will become connected to a sensory or motor ending. It is not known why one filament within a single endoneurial tube should be selected to persist while the remainder degenerate.

Once the axon has reached the end-organ, the adjacent Schwann cells start to lay down a myelin sheath. This process begins at the site of the original lesion and extends in a distal direction. By this means, the nodes of Ranvier and the Schmidt-Lanterman incisures are formed.

Many months may elapse before the axon reaches its appropriate end-organ, depending on the site of the nerve injury. The rate of growth has been estimated to be of the order of 2 to 4 mm per day. If, however, one takes into consideration the almost certain delay incurred by the axons as they cross the site of the injury, an overall regeneration rate of 1.5 mm per day is a useful figure to remember for clinical use. Even if all the difficulties outlined above are overcome and a given neuron reaches the original end-organ, the enlarging axonal filament within the endoneurial tube reaches only about 80 percent of its original diameter. For this reason the conduction velocity will not be as great as that of the original axon. Moreover, a given motor axon tends to innervate more muscle fibers than formerly, so that the control of muscle is less precise.

Regeneration of Axons in the Central Nervous System

In the central nervous system there is an attempt at regeneration of the axons, as evidenced by sprouting of the axons, but the process ceases after about 2 weeks. Long distance regeneration is rare and the injured axons make few new synapses. There is no evidence that restoration of function takes place. The regeneration process is aborted by the absence of endoneurial tubes (which are necessary to guide the regenerating axons), the failure of oligodendrocytes to serve in the same manner as Schwann cells, and the laying down of scar tissue by the active astrocytes. It has also been suggested that there is an absence of nerve growth factors in the central nervous system or that the neuroglial cells may produce nerve growth-inhibiting factors.

Research has shown that the Schwann cell basal laminae contain laminin and cell adhesion molecules of the immunoglobulin family, both of which stimulate axon growth. The central nervous system contains only low concentrations of these molecules. In the embryo when axon growth actively takes place in both the central and peripheral nervous systems, growth promoting factors are present in both systems. Later in development, these factors disappear in the central nervous system. Myelin in the central nervous system inhibits axonal growth and it is interesting to note that myelination in the central nervous system occurs late in the development process when growth of the main nervous pathways is complete.

Central axons may not be as good at regeneration as peripheral axons. In tissue culture, peripheral axons are more successful at growth than central axons. Moreover, central axon ability to grow decreases with age.

NEUROBIOLOGICAL RESEARCH INTO CENTRAL NERVOUS SYSTEM REGENERATION

Because traumatic injury to the central nervous system produces such devastating disabilities that are largely irreversible, neurobiologists are now enthusiastically pressing forward with research in this area. It is no longer doubted that differences exist between the environment in the central and peripheral systems. Moreover, the ability of central axons in lower vertebrates, such as frogs, to regenerate provides an enormous stimulus for future work.

Research has taken the following directions:

(1) Molecules present in the peripheral nervous system, such as laminins and neurotropins, have been introduced into the central nervous system at the site of injury to promote axon growth.
(2) Schwann cells have been grafted into the central nervous system and it has been found that central axons will grow into the graft.
(3) Attempts have been made to reduce the inhibitory factors present in the central nervous system. Infusion of antibodies at the site of injury has been carried out with some success.
(4) The introduction of anti-inflammatory agents to suppress the neuroglial and monocyte response has been used with success. **Methylprednisolone** is now commonly used as soon as possible after the incident in all patients with spinal cord injuries.

Although a vast amount of research still needs to be done, a combination of treatments may provide the return of some function to these patients with central nervous system injuries.

TRANSNEURONAL DEGENERATION

The responses of a single neuron to injury were considered in the previous section. In the central nervous system, if one group of neurons is injured, then a second group farther along the pathway, serving the same function, may also show degenerative changes. This phenomenon is referred to as **anterograde transneuronal degeneration**. For example, if the axons of the ganglion cells of the retina are severed, not only do the distal ends of the axons that go to the lateral geniculate bodies undergo degeneration, but also the neurons in the lateral geniculate bodies with which these axons form synapses undergo degeneration. In fact, a further set of neurons may be involved in the degenerative process in the visual cortex.

In situations in the central nervous system in which multiple neurons synapse with a single distal neuron, injury to one of the proximal neurons is not followed by degeneration of the distal neuron.

Experimentation on animals with artificial lesions of the central nervous system has shown that **retrograde transneuronal degeneration** may occur in certain situations.

NEURONAL DEGENERATION ASSOCIATED WITH SENESCENCE

Many neurons degenerate and disappear during fetal development. This process is believed to be due to their failure to establish adequate functional connections. During postnatal life further gradual neuronal degeneration continues to occur. It has been estimated that in old age an individual may have lost up to 20 percent of the original number of neurons. This may account to some extent for the loss of efficiency of the nervous system that is associated with senescence.

ATROPHY OF VOLUNTARY MUSCLE AND OTHER END-ORGANS FOLLOWING PERIPHERAL NERVE DEGENERATION

Voluntary muscle undergoes degenerative changes following motor nerve section. First, there is an altered response to acetylcholine, followed by gradual wasting of the sarcoplasm, and finally loss of the fibrils and striations. Eventually the muscle completely atrophies and is replaced by fibrous tissue. Reinnervation of the muscle halts its degeneration, and if the muscle atrophy is not too advanced, normal structure and function return.

Furthermore, if the motor nerve that supplies fast white voluntary muscle fibers is exchanged for a motor nerve that supplies slow red voluntary muscle fibers, the muscle fibers change their structural and functional properties to comply with the new type of innervation. This experimental result strongly suggests that not only are voluntary muscle cells dependent on the presence of intact motor nerves, but also the nerve has some trophic influence on the muscle and even determines the type of muscle that it innervates.

Another end-organ, the taste bud, also depends on the integrity of the sensory nerve. If the nerve is sectioned, the taste bud quickly atrophies. Once the sensory nerve regenerates into the mucous membrane, new taste buds develop.

TRAUMATIC LESIONS OF PERIPHERAL NERVES

Seddon (1944) described three clinical types of nerve injury:

- **Neuropraxia** is the term applied to a transient block. The paralysis is incomplete, recovery is rapid and complete, and there is no microscopic evidence of nerve degeneration. Pressure is the most common cause. It is essentially a temporary interference in function.
- **Axonotmesis** is the term applied to a nerve lesion in which the axons are damaged but the surrounding connective tissue sheaths remain more or less intact. Wallerian degeneration occurs peripherally. Functional recovery is more rapid and more complete than after complete section of the nerve trunk. The explanation of the more rapid and more complete recovery is that the nerve fibers, although severely damaged, for the most part retain their normal anatomical relationships to one another, owing to the preservation of the connective tissue sheaths. Crush injuries, traction, and compression are the most common causes.
- **Neurotmesis** is the term applied to complete section of the nerve trunk.

Symptoms and Signs of Neurotmesis

MOTOR CHANGES
The muscles innervated show flaccid paralysis and rapidly waste. The reflexes in which the muscles participate are lost. The paralyzed muscle ceases to respond to faradic stimulation after 4 to 7 days. After 10 days the muscle responds only sluggishly to galvanic stimulation and the strength of the current must be greater than that required for a normal innervated muscle. This altered response of muscle to electrical stimulation is known as **the reaction of degeneration.**

SENSORY CHANGES

There is a total loss of cutaneous sensibility over the area exclusively supplied by the nerve. This area is surrounded by a zone of partial sensory loss where adjacent sensory nerves overlap. The skin area in which the sensation of light touch is lost is much greater than the area lost to pinprick.

VASOMOTOR, SUDOMOTOR, AND TROPHIC CHANGES

Section of a peripheral nerve results in the interruption of postganglionic sympathetic fibers traveling in the nerve. As a result of the loss of vascular control, the skin area at first becomes red and hot. Later, the affected area becomes blue and colder than normal, especially in cold weather. Because of the loss of sudomotor control, the sweat glands cease to produce sweat and the skin becomes dry and scaly. Nail growth becomes retarded as the direct result of poor peripheral circulation. If a large area of the body is denervated, as, for example, in cases in which the sciatic nerve is sectioned, the bones undergo decalcification as a result of disuse and loss of circulatory control.

Symptoms and Signs of Recovery Following Neurotmesis

Assuming that the divided peripheral nerve has been carefully sutured together, a physician must be aware of the symptoms and signs of recovery and their sequence.

MOTOR RECOVERY

Regenerating motor axons grow at an average rate of about 1.5 mm per day. The proximal muscles will recover first and the distal muscles later. The muscles may respond to faradic stimulation before voluntary control returns.

SENSORY RECOVERY

Sensory recovery occurs before there is a return of voluntary movement. The part of the nerve distal to the section becomes very sensitive to mechanical stimulation once the regenerating sensory axons have entered the distal segment. Simple tapping of the distal nerve trunk gives rise to a tingling sensation in the area of cutaneous distribution of the nerve. This sign is referred to as **Tinel's sign**. Recovery of deep cutaneous sensibility, that is, pain caused by deep pressure, is the first sign of recovery. This is followed by the return of poorly localized, superficial cutaneous pain. Vasomotor control also returns at about this time. Later, the sensations of heat and cold are recovered. Light touch and tactile discrimination are the last sensations to return, many months later, and they are often incomplete.

Specific Spinal Nerve Injuries

While a detailed description of the neurological deficits following the many spinal nerve injuries seen in clinical practice is beyond the scope of this book, it seems appropriate to include a table that summarizes the important features found in cervical and lumbosacral root syndromes (Table 3-4). Tables that summarize the branches of the brachial (Table 3-5) and lumbar and sacral (Table 3-6) plexuses and their distribution are also included. These tables can assist the reader in determining the specific nerve lesion associated with a particular motor or sensory deficit in the upper or lower limbs.

Cranial nerve injuries are considered in Chapter 11.

Table 3–4   Important Features Found in Cervical and Lumbosacral Root Syndromes

Root Injury	Dermatome Pain	Muscles Supplied	Movement Weakness	Reflex Involved
C5	Lateral side of upper part of arm	Deltoid and biceps brachii	Shoulder abduction, elbow flexion	Biceps
C6	Lateral side of forearm	Extensor carpi radialis longus and brevis	Wrist extensors	Brachioradialis
C7	Middle finger	Triceps and flexor carpi radialis	Extension of elbow and flexion of wrist	Triceps
C8	Medial side of forearm	Flexor digitorum superficialis and profundus	Finger flexion	None
L1	Groin	Iliopsoas	Hip flexion	Cremaster
L2	Anterior part of thigh	Iliopsoas, sartorius, hip adductors	Hip flexion, hip adduction	Cremaster
L3	Medial side of knee	Iliopsoas, sartorius, quadriceps, hip adductors	Hip flexion, knee extension, hip adduction	Patellar
L4	Medial side of calf	Tibialis anterior, quadriceps	Foot inversion, knee extension	Patellar
L5	Lateral side of lower leg and dorsum of foot	Extensor hallucis longus, extensor digitorum longus	Toe extension, ankle dorsiflexion	None
S1	Lateral edge of foot	Gastrocnemius, soleus	Ankle plantar flexion	Ankle jerk
S2	Posterior part of thigh	Flexor digitorum longus, flexor hallucis longus	Ankle plantar flexion, toe flexion	None

Table 3–5   Branches of the Brachial Plexus and Their Distribution

Branches	Distribution
Roots	
Dorsal scapular nerve (C5)	Rhomboid minor, rhomboid major, levator scapulae muscles
Long thoracic nerve (C5, C6, C7)	Serratus anterior muscle
Upper trunk	
Suprascapular nerve (C5, C6)	Supraspinatus and infraspinatus muscles
Nerve to subclavius (C5, C6)	Subclavius
Lateral cord	
Lateral pectoral nerve (C5, C6, C7)	Pectoralis major muscle
Musculocutaneous nerve (C5, C6, C7)	Coracobranchialis, biceps brachii, brachialis muscles; supplies skin along lateral border of forearm when it becomes the lateral cutaneous nerve of forearm
Lateral root of median nerve (C[5], C6, C7)	See Medial root of median nerve
Posterior cord	
Upper subscapular nerve (C5, C6)	Subscapularis muscle
Thoracodorsal nerve (C6, C7, C8)	Latissimus dorsi muscle
Lower subscapular nerve (C5, C6)	Subscapularis and teres major muscles
Axillary nerve (C5, C6)	Deltoid and teres minor muscles; upper lateral cutaneous nerve of arm supplies skin over lower half of deltoid muscle
Radial nerve (C5, C6, C7, C8, T1)	Triceps, anconeus, part of brachialis, brachioradialis, extensor carpi radialis longus; via deep radial nerve branch supplies extensor muscles of forearm: supinator, extensor carpi radialis brevis, extensor carpi ulnaris, extensor digitorum, extensor digiti minimi, extensor indicis, abductor pollicis longus, extensor pollicis longus, extensor pollicis brevis; skin, lower lateral cutaneous nerve of arm, posterior cutaneous nerve of arm, and posterior cutaneous nerve of forearm; skin on lateral side of dorsum of hand and dorsal surface of lateral $3\frac{1}{2}$ fingers; articular branches to elbow, wrist, and hand
Medial cord	
Medial pectoral nerve (C8, T1)	Pectoralis major and minor muscles
Medial cutaneous nerve of arm joined by intercostal brachial nerve from second intercostal nerve (C8, T1, T2)	Skin of medial side of arm
Medial cutaneous nerve of forearm (C8, T1)	Skin of medial side of forearm
Ulnar nerve (C8, T1)	Flexor carpi ulnaris and medial half of flexor digitorum profundus, flexor digiti minimi, opponens digiti minimi, abductor digiti minimi, adductor pollicis, third and fourth lumbricals, interossei, palmaris brevis, skin of medial half of dorsum of hand and palm, skin of palmar and dorsal surfaces of medial $1\frac{1}{2}$ fingers
Medial root of median nerve (with lateral root) forms median nerve (C5, C6, C7, C8, T1)	Pronator teres, flexor carpi radialis, palmaris longus, flexor digitorum superficialis, abductor pollicis brevis, flexor policis brevis, opponens pollicis, first two lumbricals (by way of anterior interosseous branch), flexor pollicis longus, flexor digitorum profundus (lateral half), pronator quadratus; palmar cutaneous branch to lateral half of palm and digital branches to palmar surface of lateral $3\frac{1}{2}$ fingers; articular branches to elbow, wrist, and carpal joints

Table 3–6 Branches of the Lumbar and Sacral Plexuses and Their Distribution

Branches	Distribution
Femoral nerve (L2, L3, L4)	Iliacus, pectineus, sartorius, quadriceps femoris muscles; skin, medial cutaneous and intermediate cutaneous nerves of thigh, saphenous nerve to medial side of leg, medial side of foot as far as ball of big toe; articular branches to hip and knee joints
Obturator nerve (L2, L3, L4)	Pectineus, adductor longus, adductor brevis, adductor magnus (adductor portion), gracilis muscles; skin, medial side of thigh; articular branches to hip and knee joints
Sciatic nerve (L4, L5, S1, S2, S3)	
Common peroneal nerve	Biceps femoris muscle (short head); skin, lateral cutaneous nerve of calf, sural communicating branch to lateral side of leg, lateral side of foot, and little toe
Superficial peroneal nerve	Peroneus longus and brevis muscles; skin, lower leg, and dorsum of foot
Deep peroneal nerve	Tibialis anterior, extensor hallucis longus, extensor digitorum longus, peroneus tertius, extensor digitorum brevis muscles; skin, cleft between first second toes; articular branches to tibiofibular, ankle, and foot joints
Tibial nerve	Semitendinosus, biceps femoris (long head), semimembranosus, adductor magnus (hamstring part), gastrocnemius, soleus, plantaris, popliteus, tibialis posterior, flexor digitorum longus, flexor hallucis longus muscles; skin, medial side of ankle; articular branches to hip, knee, and ankle joints
Medial plantar nerve	Abductor hallucis, flexor digitorum brevis, flexor hallucis brevis, first lumbrical muscles; skin, medial side of sole of foot; articular branches to foot joints
Lateral plantar nerve	Flexor accessorius, abductor digiti minimi, flexor digiti minimi brevis, second, third, and fourth lumbricals, adductor hallucis, all interossei muscles; skin of lateral side of sole of foot

SOME BASIC CLINICAL PRINCIPLES UNDERLYING PERIPHERAL NERVE INJURIES

In open, dirty wounds, where there is a high risk of infection, the sectioned nerve should be ignored and the wound infection should be treated. Later, when the wound has healed satisfactorily, the nerve should be explored and the cut ends of the nerve sutured together.

For a patient with a healed wound and no evidence of nerve recovery, the treatment should be conservative. Sufficient time should be allowed to elapse to enable the regenerating nerve fibers to reach the proximal muscles. If recovery fails to occur, the nerve should be explored surgically.

In those cases in which connective tissue, bone fragments, or muscles come to lie between the cut ends of a severed nerve, the nerve should be explored and, if possible, the cut ends of the nerve should be brought together and sutured.

The nutrition of the paralyzed muscles must be maintained with adequate physiotherapy. Warm baths, massage, and warm clothing help to maintain adequate circulation.

The paralyzed muscles must not be allowed to be stretched by antagonist muscles or by gravity. Moreover, excessive shortening of the paralyzed muscles leads to contracture of these muscles.

Mobility must be preserved by daily passive movements of all joints in the affected area. Failure to do this results in the formation of adhesions and consequent limitation of movement.

Once voluntary movement returns in the most proximal muscles, the physiotherapist can assist the patient in performing active exercises. This not only aids in the return of a normal circulation to the affected part but also helps the patient to learn once again the complicated muscular performance of skilled movements.

NERVE TRANSPLANTATION

Nerve grafts have been used with some success to restore muscle tone in facial nerve palsy. In mixed nerve injuries nerve grafts have succeeded only in restoring some sensory function and slight muscle activity. The presence of two suture lines and the increased possibility of mixing the nerve fibers is probably the reason for the lack of success with nerve grafts. In most nerve injuries, even when the gap between the proximal and distal ends is as great as 10 cm, it is usually possible to mobilize the nerve or alter its position in relation to joints so that the proximal and distal ends may be brought together without undue tension; the ends are then sutured together.

TUMORS OF PERIPHERAL NERVES

A peripheral nerve consists essentially of nerve fibers (axons), each of which is associated with Schwann cells; the fibers are either myelinated or nonmyelinated. The nerve fibers are arranged in parallel bundles and are surrounded by connective tissue sheaths.

A **benign fibroma** or a **malignant sarcoma** may arise in the connective tissue of the nerve and does not differ from similar tumors elsewhere. **Neurilemmomas** are believed to arise from Schwann cells. They arise from any nerve trunk, cranial or spinal, and in any part of its course. Primary tumors of the axons are very rare.

BLOOD VESSELS, LYMPHATICS, AND ENDONEURIAL SPACES WITHIN PERIPHERAL NERVES

Peripheral nerves receive branches from arteries in the regions through which they pass. The anastomotic network that exists within a nerve is considerable and local ischemia does not occur should a single artery be obstructed.

A plexus of lymph vessels lies within the epineurial connective tissues and this drains to regional lymph nodes.

As the result of experiments in which dyes have been injected into peripheral nerves, spaces have been demonstrated between individual nerve fibers. There seems to be little doubt that these endoneurial spaces provide a potential route for the ascent of **tetanus toxin** to the spinal cord.

ACTION OF LOCAL ANESTHETICS ON NERVE CONDUCTION

Local anesthetics are drugs that block nerve conduction when applied locally to a nerve fiber in suitable concentrations. Their site of action is the axolemma and they interfere with the transient increase in permeability of the axolemma to Na^+, K^+, and other ions. The sensitivity of nerve fibers to local anesthetics is related to the size of the nerve fibers (see Table 3-2). Small nerve fibers are more susceptible than are large fibers; small fibers are also slower to recover.

Cocaine has been used clinically to block nerve conduction. Unfortunately, it is a strong stimulant of the cerebral cortex and readily causes addiction. **Procaine** is a synthetic compound that is widely used as a local anesthetic agent.

APPARENT RECOVERY OF FUNCTION OF THE CENTRAL NERVOUS SYSTEM FOLLOWING INJURY

Axon regeneration in the brain and spinal cord is minimal following a lesion, and yet considerable functional recovery often occurs. Several explanations exist and more than one mechanism may be involved.

1. The function of nerve fibers may be interfered with as the result of compression by edema fluid. Once the edema subsides, a substantial recovery may take place.
2. The damaged nerve fiber proximal to the lesion may form new synapses with neighboring normal neurons.
3. Following a lesion of an afferent neuron, an increased number of receptor sites may develop on a postsynaptic membrane. This may result in the second neuron responding to neurotransmitter substances from neighboring neurons.
4. Nonfunctioning neurons may take over the function of damaged neurons.
5. It is possible with intensive physiotherapy for patients to be trained to use other muscles to compensate for the loss of paralyzed muscles.

HERPES ZOSTER

Herpes zoster or shingles is a relatively common condition caused by the reactivation of the latent varicella-zoster virus in a patient who has previously had chickenpox. The infection is found in the first sensory neuron in a cranial or spinal nerve. The lesion is seen as an inflammation and degeneration of the sensory neuron with the formation of vesicles with inflammation of the skin. The first symptom is pain in the distribution of the sensory neuron followed in a few days by a skin eruption. The condition occurs most frequently in patients over the age of 50.

POLYNEUROPATHY

Polyneuropathy is an impairment of function of many peripheral nerves simultaneously. There are many causes, including infection (endotoxin of diphtheria, Guillain-Barré syndrome [see Clinical Example at beginning of chapter]), metabolic disorders (vitamin B_1 and B_{12} deficiency, poisoning by heavy metals, drugs), and endocrine disorders (diabetes). Axon degeneration and/or segmental demyelination may take place and the neuron cell body may be involved. In mild cases the condition is reversible, but in severe cases it may be permanent. Both sensory and motor symptoms and signs may be evident.

Receptors

Sensory endings are found throughout the body in both somatic and visceral areas. It is fortunate that they are so widely distributed, because they enable the human subject to react to changes in the external and internal environment.

A physician, to make a diagnosis or study the effect of treatment on a disease process, relies almost entirely on the patient's ability to describe changes in subjective sensations, or to respond to specific stimuli during a physical examination. Such descriptions as "knifelike pain," "dull aching pain," "colicky pain," "pins and needles," and "cannot feel anything, doctor," are very familiar to the practicing physician. Each main type of sensation that can be experienced, such as pain, temperature, and touch and pressure, is called a **modality** of sensation. The type of modality felt by a patient from a particular part of the body is determined by the specific area of the central nervous system to which the afferent nerve fiber passes. However, it is clinically useful to remember that axons that carry specific modalities are associated with one or more anatomically distinct receptors.

Receptor	Associated Function
Free nerve endings	Pain, touch, pressure, tickle Sensations,? cold and heat
Merkel's discs	Touch and pressure
Hair follicle receptor	Touch
Meissner's corpuscles	Touch (two-point tactile discrimination)
Pacinian corpuscles	Pressure and vibration
Ruffini's corpuscles	Stretch
Neuromuscular spindles	Elongation of muscle (stretch)
Neurotendinous spindles	Tension

Sensory Receptors And Age

With life expectancy increasing, many patients now reach the age when sensory receptor degeneration can cause disequilibrium. This critical age varies in different individuals, but once it starts, there is a progressive deterioration in the sensory systems, involving not only visual and auditory systems but also proprioception and the ability to integrate the afferent information entering the central nervous system.

EXAMINATION OF INDIVIDUAL SENSORY MODALITIES

An accurate physical examination may enable the neurologist to make a precise diagnosis. He or she may be able to determine whether a particular sensation can or cannot be appreciated, or whether it is less than normal. The physician will be able to determine the precise area over the surface of the body where impairment of sensation is found. The following sensations are usually tested:

1. **Light touch**. This is tested by gently touching the skin with a wisp of cotton; the patient has the eyes closed and responds "yes" whenever he or she feels the stimulus. It is important to realize that different areas of the skin normally exhibit different thresholds for touch. The back and buttocks are less sensitive than the face or fingertips. On hairy surfaces, the slightest movement of a hair usually can be felt.
2. **Localization of touch**. After the patient has detected the light touch with the eyes closed, he or she is asked to place a finger on the exact site touched. Failure to accomplish this may be due to damage to the cerebral cortex.
3. **Two-point tactile discrimination**. Two blunt points are applied to the skin surface while the patient's eyes are closed. Gradually the points are brought closer together until the patient is unable to distinguish two definite points. A normal person is able to distinguish two separate points on the tip of the index finger when they are separated by a distance greater than about 3 mm. On the back, however, they have to be separated by as much as 3 to 4 cm.
4. **Pain**. The skin may be touched with the sharp end of a pin. First the pain threshold is established, and the areas of diminished or lost pain sensation are mapped out. It is advisable to apply the stimulus in an irregular manner, first using the sharp end of the pin, and then the dull head, the patient responding "sharp" or "dull." In certain diseases, such as tabes dorsalis or polyneuropathy (polyneuritis), there is a delay of up to 3 seconds before the patient recognizes the sharp pain.
5. **Pressure pain**. This poorly localized pain is perceived by deep pressure on a muscle or by squeezing a tendon.
6. **Temperature testing**. Test tubes filled with hot or cold water may be used. When they are applied to the skin, the patient responds with either "warm" or "cold." First the temperature threshold is established and then the areas of diminished or lost temperature sensation are mapped out.
7. **Vibration.** When the handle of a vibrating tuning fork is applied to the skin over bone (e.g., the medial malleolus of the tibia or the olecranon process of the ulna), a tingling sensation is felt. This is due to the stimulation of superficial and deep pressure receptors. The patient is asked to respond when he or she first feels the vibration and when he or she no longer can detect the vibration. The perception of vibration in the legs is usually diminished after the age of 60.
8. **Appreciation of form (stereognosis).** With the patient's eyes closed, the examiner places common objects such as coins or keys in the patient's hands. The patient normally should be able to identify objects by moving them around in the hand and feeling them with the fingers.
9. **Passive movements of joints**. This test may be carried out on the fingers or toes. With the patient completely relaxed and in the supine position with eyes closed, the digit is flexed or extended irregularly. After each movement, the patient is asked, "Is the digit 'up' or 'down'?" A normal individual not only can determine that passive movement is taking place but also is aware of the direction of the movement.
10. **Postural sensibility**. This is the ability to describe the position of a limb when it is placed in that position while the patient's eyes are closed. Another way to perform the test is to ask the patient, with his or her eyes closed, to place the limb on the opposite side in the same position as the other limb. The application and interpretation of the results of these tests will be understood more fully when the afferent or sensory pathways have been discussed (see p. 145).

PHANTOM LIMB

Wherever a particular sensory pathway is stimulated along its course from the receptor to the sensory cortex of the brain, the sensation experienced by the individual is referred to the site of the receptor. For example, if the pain fibers from the receptors in the little finger are stimulated in the ulnar nerve at the elbow, the individual will experience pain in the little finger and not at the elbow.

Following the amputation of a limb, the patient may experience severe pain in the absent limb due to pressure on the nerve fibers at the end of the stump. This phenomenon is referred to clinically as **phantom limb**.

ACTION OF DRUGS AND OTHER AGENTS ON SKELETAL NEUROMUSCULAR JUNCTIONS

Table 3-7 gives some examples of drugs and diseases affecting the motor end-plates in skeletal muscle.

Neuromuscular Blocking Agents

d-**Tubocurarine** produces flaccid paralysis of skeletal muscle, first affecting the extrinsic muscles of the eyes and then those of the face, the extremities, and finally the diaphragm. **Dimethyltubocurarine**, **gallamine**, and **benzoquinonium** have similar effects.

These drugs combine with the receptor sites at the postsynaptic membrane normally used by acetylcholine, and thus block the neurotransmitter action of acetylcholine. They are therefore referred to as competitive blocking agents, since they are competing for the same receptor site

Table 3–7 Drugs and Diseases Affecting the Motor End-Plates in Skeletal Muscle

Drug or Disease	Increasing ACh Release	Decreasing ACh Release	Acting on ACh Receptors		AChE Inhibition
			Depolarizing Blockade	ACh Receptor Blockade	
Drug					
4-Aminopyridines	Yes				
Guanidine hydrochloride	Yes				
Succinylcholine			Yes		
d-Tubocurarine,				Yes	
dimethyltubocurarine,				Yes	
gallamine,				Yes	
benzoquinonium				Yes	
Physostigmine,					Yes
neostigmine					Yes
Disease					
Botulinum toxin		Yes			
Myasthenia gravis			Destruction of receptors		

ACh = acetylcholine; AChE = acetylcholinesterase.

as does acetylcholine. As these drugs are slowly metabolized, the paralysis passes off.

Decamethonium and **succinylcholine** also paralyze skeletal muscle, but their action differs from that of competitive blocking agents because they produce their effect by causing depolarization of the motor end-plate. Acting like acetylcholine, they produce depolarization of the postsynaptic membrane and the muscle contracts once. This is followed by a flaccid paralysis and a blockage of neuromuscular activity. Although the blocking action endures for some time, the drugs are metabolized and the paralysis passes off. The actual paralysis is produced by the continued depolarization of the postsynaptic membrane. It must be remembered that continuous depolarization does not produce continuous skeletal muscle contraction. Repolarization has to take place before further depolarization can occur.

Neuromuscular blocking agents are commonly used with general anesthetics to produce the desired degree of muscle relaxation without using larger doses of general anesthetics. Because the respiratory muscles are paralyzed, facilities for artificial respiration are essential.

Anticholinesterases

Physostigmine and **neostigmine** have the capacity to combine with acetylcholinesterase and prevent the esterase from inactivating acetylcholine. In addition, neostigmine has a direct stimulating action on skeletal muscle. The actions of both drugs are reversible and they have been used with success in the treatment of myasthenia gravis.

Bacterial Toxins

Clostridium botulinum, the causative organism in certain cases of food poisoning, produces a toxin that inhibits the release of acetylcholine at the neuromuscular junction. Death results from paralysis of the respiratory muscles. The

course of the disease can be improved by the administration of calcium gluconate or guanidine which promote the release of Ach from the nerve terminals.

MOTOR NERVE AND SKELETAL MUSCLE

Not only does the motor nerve control the activity of the muscle it supplies, but its integrity is essential for the muscle's normal maintenance. Following section of a motor nerve, the muscle fibers rapidly atrophy and are replaced by connective tissue. The total bulk of the muscle may be reduced by three-fourths in as little as 3 months. This degree of atrophy does not occur if the muscle simply is immobilized; that is, it is not just disuse atrophy. It is apparent that the maintenance of normal muscle is dependent on the continued reception of acetylcholine at the postsynaptic membrane at the neuromuscular junction.

DENERVATION SUPERSENSITIVITY OF SKELETAL MUSCLE

After approximately 2 weeks of denervation, skeletal muscle fibers respond to externally applied acetylcholine at sites other than the neuromuscular junctions. This supersensitivity could be explained on the basis that many new acetylcholine receptors have developed along the length of the muscle fibers following denervation.

MYASTHENIA GRAVIS

Myasthenia gravis is a disease characterized by drooping of the upper eyelids (ptosis), double vision (diplopia), difficulty in swallowing (dysphagia), difficulty in talking (dysarthria), and general muscle weakness and fatigue. Initially, the disease most commonly involves the muscles of the eye and the pharynx and the symptoms can be relieved with rest. In the progressive form of the disease, the weakness becomes steadily worse and ultimately death occurs.

The condition is an autoimmune disorder in which antibodies are produced against the nicotinic acetylcholine receptors on the postsynaptic membrane. The antibodies interfere with the synaptic transmission by reducing the number of receptors or by blocking the interaction of Ach with its receptors. The size of the junctional folds is also reduced and the width of the synaptic cleft is increased. Together these changes result in a reduced amplitude in end-plate potentials. The condition can be temporarily relieved by anticholinesterase drugs such as **neostigmine**, which potentiates the action of acetylcholine.

A rare congenital form of myasthenia gravis may exist from birth and in this form there is no abnormal antibody present. The causes of the congenital disease include a deficiency of acetylcholinesterase at the motor end plates, impaired release of Ach, impaired capacity of the receptors to interact with Ach, or a reduced number of Ach receptors.

HYPOKALEMIC PERIODIC PARALYSIS AND HYPERKALEMIC PARALYSIS

These are diseases due to decreased or increased blood potassium levels. It is known that the ability of acetylcholine to initiate electrical changes in the postsynaptic membrane of the neuromuscular junction can be greatly influenced by the level of blood potassium, and it is this blood change that is responsible for the paralysis in these patients.

ACTION OF DRUGS ON NEUROMUSCULAR JUNCTIONS IN SMOOTH MUSCLE, CARDIAC MUSCLE, AND NERVE ENDINGS ON SECRETORY CELLS

It has been stated that, in normal body physiology, acetylcholine released from postganglionic parasympathetic fibers can bring about depolarization and resulting contraction of smooth muscle fibers. Acetylcholine, however, is a useless drug to be administered by the physician, because it is rapidly destroyed by the **cholinesterases**, and because its actions are so widespread it cannot be used selectively. By slightly changing the structure, as in the case of **methacholine chloride** or **carbachol**, the drugs are less susceptible to destruction by the cholinesterases but still possess the ability to react with the receptors.

Atropine and **scopolamine** are drugs that compete with acetylcholine for the same receptors. These drugs are competitive antagonists of acetylcholine at receptor sites of smooth muscle, cardiac muscle, and various secretory cells.

Norepinephrine is released from postganglionic sympathetic fibers and can bring about depolarization of smooth muscle in the walls of arteries, for example, resulting in their contraction. At other sites, such as the bronchi, it causes smooth muscle relaxation. Sympathetic receptors have been classified as alpha and beta. The functions associated with alpha receptors are vasoconstriction, mydriasis (dilation of pupil), and relaxation of the smooth muscle of the intestine. Beta receptors are associated with vasodilatation, cardioacceleration, bronchial relaxation, and intestinal relaxation.

Phenoxybenzamine has been found to block alpha receptors while **propranolol** blocks beta receptors. The structure of these receptors is not known.

ABNORMALITIES IN SENSORY PERCEPTION

Abnormalities in sensory perception should be looked for on the face, trunk, and limbs. Areas of diminished pain sensation (**hypalgesia**) or touch sensation (**hypesthesia**) or heightened sensation (**hyperesthesia**) should be identified. Abnormal sensations (**paresthesia)**, such as pins and needles, may be experienced by a patient who has a lesion located anywhere along the sensory pathway from the peripheral nerve to the cerebral cortex. The areas of sensory abnormality should be precisely defined and recorded, each modality being recorded separately.

Testing sensory function requires practice and experience. Many patients have difficulty in responding to a physician's examination of the sensory system. Some individuals try to assist the examiner by wrongly anticipating the correct response. This problem can largely be overcome by testing for cutaneous sensibility with the patient's eyes closed. In this way the patient cannot see which areas of skin are being tested. Other patients find it difficult to understand exactly what information is required of them. Some intelligent patients respond more to differences in intensity of stimulation rather than giving a simple "yes" or "no" answer to the question "Can you feel anything?" The physician must always be aware of the possibility of hysteria, which is when a patient complains of sensory loss that has no neuroanatomical explanation. For example, a total loss of skin sensation on one side of the face, including the angle of the jaw, would infer that the patient has a lesion involving the fifth cranial nerve in the pons and the greater auricular nerve (C2 and 3), which is anatomically very unlikely. Patience and objectivity are required and if doubt exists as to the accuracy of the assessment, the patient should be reexamined on another occasion.

SEGMENTAL INNERVATION OF THE SKIN

Because large nerve plexuses are present at the roots of the upper and lower limbs, it follows that a single spinal nerve may send both motor and sensory fibers to several peripheral nerves, and, conversely, a single peripheral nerve may receive nerve fibers from many spinal nerves. Moreover, it follows that a lesion of a segment of the spinal cord, or posterior root, or spinal nerve will result in a sensory loss that is different from that occurring after a lesion of a peripheral nerve.

The area of skin supplied by a single spinal nerve, and, therefore, a single segment of the spinal cord, is called a **dermatome**. A physician should remember that dermatomes overlap and that in the trunk at least three contiguous spinal nerves have to be sectioned to produce a region of complete anesthesia. A physician should remember also that the degree of overlap for painful and thermal sensations is much greater than that for tactile sensation. A physician should have a working knowledge of the segmental (dermatomal) innervation of skin, since with the help of a pin or a piece of cotton he or she can determine whether or not the sensory function of a particular spinal nerve or segment of the spinal cord is normal. When examining the dermatomal charts, one should note that because of the development of the upper limbs the anterior rami of the lower cervical and first thoracic spinal nerves have lost their cutaneous innervation of the trunk anteriorly, and at the level of the second costal cartilage the fourth cervical dermatome is contiguous with the second thoracic dermatome. In the sensory innervation of the head, the trigeminal (fifth cranial) nerve supplies a large area of the face and scalp, and its cutaneous area is contiguous with that of the second cervical segment.

Since the dermatomes run longitudinally along the long axis of the upper limbs, sensation should be tested by dragging a wisp of cotton or a pin along the long axis of the medial and lateral borders of the limbs. On the trunk the dermatomes run almost horizontally, so the stimulus should be applied by moving in a vertical direction.

SEGMENTAL INNERVATION OF THE MUSCLES

It is important to remember that most skeletal muscles are innervated by more than one spinal nerve and, therefore, by the same number of segments of the spinal cord. Complete destruction of one segment of the spinal cord as the result of trauma or pressure from a tumor will cause weakness of all the muscles that are innervated from that segment. To paralyze a muscle completely, several adjacent segments of the spinal cord have to be destroyed.

Because of the presence of the cervical, brachial, and lumbosacral plexuses the axons of motor anterior gray column cells are redistributed into a number of peripheral nerves. A physician, knowing this, is able to distinguish between a lesion of a segment of the spinal cord, an anterior root, or a spinal nerve, on the one hand, and a lesion of a peripheral nerve on the other. For example, the musculocutaneous nerve of the arm, which receives nerve fibers from the fifth, sixth, and seventh cervical segments of the spinal cord, supplies a finite number of muscles, namely, the biceps brachii, the brachialis, and the coracobrachialis muscles, and section of that nerve would result in total paralysis of these muscles; a lesion of the fifth, sixth, and seventh cervical spinal segments, or their anterior roots, or their spinal nerves, would result in paralysis of these muscles; a lesion of the fifth, sixth, and seventh cervical spinal segments, or their anterior roots, or their spinal nerves, would result in paralysis of these muscles and also partial paralysis of many other muscles, including the deltoid, supraspinatus, teres minor, and infraspinatus.

The segmental innervation of the biceps brachii, triceps, brachioradialis, muscles of the anterior abdominal wall, quadriceps femoris, gastrocnemius, and soleus should be memorized, because it is possible to test them easily by eliciting their reflex contraction (for details, see p. 106).

MUSCLE TONE

Skeletal muscle tone is due to the presence of a few muscle fibers within a muscle being in a state of full contraction all the time. Muscle tone is controlled reflexly from afferent nerve endings situated in the muscle itself. It follows, therefore, that any disease process that interferes with any part of the reflex arc will abolish the muscle tone. Some examples are syphilitic infection of the posterior root (tabes dorsalis); destruction of the motor anterior gray column cells, as in poliomyelitis or syringomyelia; destruction of a segment of the spinal cord by trauma or pressure from a tumor; section of an anterior root; pressure on a spinal nerve by a prolapsed intervertebral disc; and section of a peripheral nerve, as in a stab wound. All these clinical conditions will result in loss of muscle tone.

Although it has been emphasized that the basic mechanism underlying muscle tone is the integrity of the spinal segmental reflex, it must not be forgotten that this reflex activity is influenced by nervous impulses received by the anterior horn cells from all levels of the brain and spinal cord. Spinal shock, which follows injury to the spinal cord and is caused by loss of functional activity of neurons, will result in diminished muscle tone. Cerebellar disease also results in diminished muscle tone, because the cerebellum facilitates the stretch reflex. The reticular formation normally tends to increase muscle tone, but its activity is inhibited by higher cerebral centers. Therefore, it follows that if the higher cerebral control is interfered with by trauma or disease, the inhibition is lost and the muscle tone is exaggerated (decerebrate rigidity). It must not be forgotten that primary degeneration of the muscles themselves (myopathies) can cause loss of muscle tone.

POSTURE

The posture of an individual depends on the degree and distribution of muscle tone and, therefore, on the activity of the motor neurons that supply the muscles. The motor neurons in the anterior gray columns of the spinal cord are the points upon which converge the nervous impulses from many posterior nerve roots, and the descending fibers from many different levels of the brain and spinal cord. The successful coordination of all these nervous influences results in a normal posture.

When one is in the standing posture, there is remarkably little muscular activity taking place in the muscles of the limbs and trunk. The reason for this is that the center of gravity of any part of the body is mainly above the joints upon which its weight is directed. Moreover, in many joints, for example, the hip and the knee, the ligaments are very strong and support the body in the erect posture. However, it must be stressed that a person cannot remain standing if all muscles are paralyzed. Once a person starts to fall, either forward, backward, or laterally, the muscle spindles and other stretch receptors immediately increase their activity and the reflex arcs come into play, so that reflex compensatory muscle contractions take place to restore the state of balance. The eyes and the receptors in the membranous labyrinth also play a vital part in the maintenance of balance. The importance of the eyes in maintaining the erect position can easily be tested in a normal person. Once the eyes are closed, the person shows a tendency to sway slightly, because he or she now must rely exclusively on muscle and labyrinthine receptors to preserve his or her balance.

It follows that a pathological alteration in muscle tone will affect posture. For example, in hemiplegia or in Parkinson's disease, in which there is hypertonicity, posture will be changed. As with cerebellar disease, hypotonicity will cause drooping of the shoulder on the affected side. Lesions involving peripheral nerves that innervate antigravity muscles will produce wristdrop (radial nerve) and footdrop (common peroneal nerve).

CLINICAL OBSERVATION OF MUSCULAR ACTIVITY

Muscular Power

Ask the patient to perform movements for which the muscle under examination is primarily responsible. Next, ask the patient to perform each movement against resistance and compare the strengths of the muscles on the two sides of the body. Section of the peripheral nerve that supplies the muscle or disease affecting the anterior gray column cells (e.g., poliomyelitis) will clearly reduce the power of or paralyze the muscles involved.

Muscle Wasting

This occurs within 2 to 3 weeks after section of the motor nerve. In the limbs it is easily tested by measuring the diameter of the limbs at a given point over the involved muscle and comparing the measurement obtained with that at the same site on the opposite limb.

Muscular Fasciculation

Twitching of groups of muscle fibers is seen most often in patients with chronic disease that affects the anterior horn cells—for example, progressive muscular atrophy.

Muscular Contracture

Muscular contracture occurs most commonly in the muscles that normally oppose paralyzed muscles. The muscles contract and undergo permanent shortening.

Muscle Tone

A muscle without tone, that is, one in which the simple spinal reflex arcs are not functioning, is noncontractile and is doughlike on palpation. Degrees of loss of tone may be tested by passively moving the joints and comparing the resistance to the movements by the muscles on the two sides of the body. Increase in muscle tone can occur following the removal of the cerebral inhibition on the reticular formation (see p. 170).

Muscular Coordination

Ask the patient to touch, with the eyes open, the tip of the nose with the tip of the forefinger, and then ask him or her to repeat the process with the eyes closed. A similar test of the lower limbs may be carried out with the patient lying down. Ask the patient to place one heel on the opposite knee, with the eyes open, and then ask him or her to repeat the process with the eyes closed.

Another test is to ask the patient to quickly supinate and pronate both forearms simultaneously. Disease of the cerebellum, for example, which coordinates muscular activity, would result in impaired ability to perform these rapid repetitive movements.

INVOLUNTARY MOVEMENT OF MUSCLES

Tic. This is a coordinated, repetitive movement involving one or more muscles.

Choreiform movements. These are quick, jerky, irregular movements that are nonrepetitive. Swift grimaces and sudden movements of the head or limbs are examples of this condition.

Athetosis. This consists of slow, sinuous, writhing movements that most commonly involve the distal segments of the limbs.

Tremor. This is the alternating contraction of the agonists and antagonists of a joint.

Myoclonus. This consists of shocklike muscular contractions of a portion of a muscle, or an entire muscle, or a group of muscles.

Tonic spasm. This term refers to a sustained contraction of a muscle or group of muscles, as in the tonic phase of an epileptic seizure.

NEUROLOGICAL SENSORY AND MOTOR SYMPTOMS—ARE THEY ALWAYS OF PRIMARY NEUROLOGICAL ORIGIN?

A neurological diagnosis depends on determining the site of the lesion and the nature of the pathology causing the disease. The physician cannot consider the nervous system in isolation, for the neurological symptoms and signs may depend on disorders mainly involving another system. For example, a cerebral embolism may follow the formation of a blood clot on the ventricular wall of a patient with coronary thrombosis. A cerebral abscess may follow the formation of a lung abscess. It follows that a neurological examination in many patients should be accompanied by a more general physical examination involving other systems.

Clinical Problem Solving

1. A 20-year-old man was seen in the emergency department following an automobile accident. A diagnosis of fracture dislocation of the fourth thoracic vertebra was made, with injury to the spinal cord as a complication. A laminectomy was performed to decompress the spinal cord in order to avoid permanent injury to the tracts of the cord. What is a nerve tract in the spinal cord? How does this differ in structure from a peripheral nerve?

2. Multiple sclerosis is an example of a demyelinating disease of the nervous system. Many other diseases of the nervous system also have the common pathological feature of destruction of the myelin sheaths of nerve fibers. How does myelination normally take place in (a) peripheral nerves and (b) central nervous system tracts? When does myelination of nerves normally take place?

3. The myelin sheath is said to be formed in the peripheral nervous system by the rotation of Schwann cells on the axon so that the plasma membrane becomes wrapped around and around the axon in a spiral. In the central nervous system, do the oligodendrocytes rotate on the axons in a similar manner to form myelin?

4. A 26-year-old man was involved in a street brawl and received a knife wound of the right arm at about the midhumeral level. Physical examination revealed that the median nerve had been sectioned. Motor loss consisted of paralysis of the pronator muscles of the forearm and the long flexor muscles of the wrist and fingers, with the exception of the flexor carpi ulnaris and the medial half of the flexor digitorum profundus. As a result of this, the right forearm was kept in the supine position; wrist flexion was weak and was accompanied by adduction. The latter deviation was due to the paralysis of the flexor carpi radialis and the strength of both the flexor carpi ulnaris and the medial half of the flexor digitorum profundus. No flexion was possible at the interphalangeal joints of the index and middle fingers, although weak flexion of the metacarpophalangeal joints of these fingers was attempted by the interossei. When the patient was asked to make a fist of his right hand, the index and, to a lesser extent, the middle fingers tended to remain straight, while the ring and little fingers flexed. The latter two fingers were weakened by the loss of the flexor digitorum superficialis. Flexion of the terminal phalanx of the thumb was lost due to paralysis of the flexor pollicis longus. The muscles of the thenar eminence were paralyzed and the right thumb was laterally rotated and adducted.

   Sensory loss of the skin of the right hand involved the lateral half of the palm and the palmar aspect of the lateral three and one-half fingers. There was also sensory loss of the skin of the distal parts of the dorsal surfaces of the lateral three and one-half fingers.

   The skin areas involved in sensory loss became warmer and drier than normal, evidencing vasomotor changes. This was due to arteriolar dilatation and absence of sweating resulting from loss of sympathetic nervous control.

   (a) Describe the changes that would take place in the median nerve proximal and distal to the site of section. (b) How would you treat this case? (c) What will be the first signs and symptoms to indicate that the nerve is regenerating adequately? (d) Which function will return first, sensory or muscular? (e) About how long will it take for the nerve to regenerate and reach its end-organs?

5. A 45-year-old woman with a right-sided facial palsy was examined. When questioned, she said that 3 years previously she had experienced a weakness of the right side of the face and some degree of loss of taste sensation following a ride in an open car on a cold day. A diagnosis of Bell's palsy was made. What is Bell's palsy? How would you treat this patient?

6. A family with five small children moved into an old house. Six months later the mother noticed that her 1-year-old son was becoming somnolent and quiet. Whereas previously he was very active and crawled around the house, he now tended to lie about the floor, uninterested in his toys. He had also stopped eating well and was very constipated. The mother decided to take him to a pediatrician when, as she put it, the child suddenly "threw a fit." On examination, there was an absence of positive physical signs except for a dark line between the gums and teeth. When questioned further, the mother admitted that the child liked sucking the peeling paint on the railings outside the house. A diagnosis of chronic lead poisoning was made. This was confirmed by finding that the blood lead level was in excess of 50 µg per 100 ml. What effect does lead have on the nervous system?

7. A 54-year-old man suddenly developed severe pain down both legs in the distribution of the sciatic nerve. He also noticed numbness in the buttocks and perineum and recently noted that he could not feel the passage of urine or feces. A diagnosis was made of central protrusion posteriorly of the intervertebral disc between the third and fourth lumbar vertebrae. From the symptoms it was clear that the cauda equina was being pressed upon. Can regeneration occur in the cauda equina?

8. By what anatomical route is tetanus toxin believed to pass from a wound to the central nervous system?

9. Following an automobile accident, a 35-year-old man was seen in the emergency department with fractures of the fifth and sixth ribs on the right side. In order to relieve the pain and discomfort experienced by the patient when breathing, the physician decided to block

the right fifth and sixth intercostal nerves by injecting a local anesthetic, lidocaine (Xylocaine), around the nerve trunks. What is the effect of the local anesthetic agent on the nerve fibers? Are the large-diameter or the small-diameter nerve fibers more susceptible to the action of the drug?

10. A 65-year-old man, on returning home from a party, found that he could not climb the stairs. He had consumed a large amount of whiskey and seemed to have lost control of his legs. He sat down on a chair in the hallway and was soon in a deep, stuporous sleep, with his right arm suspended over the back of the chair. Next morning he awoke with a severe headache and loss of the use of his right arm and hand. During examination in the emergency department, it was found that the patient had severe paralysis involving branches of the medial cord of the brachial plexus and the radial nerve. The diagnosis was neuropraxia, which occurred as the result of the pressure of the back of the chair on the involved nerves. What is neuropraxia? How does this differ from axonotmesis and neurotmesis? What is the prognosis in this patient? How would you treat this case?

11. A well-known politician was attending a rally when a youth suddenly stepped forward and shot him in the back. During examination in the emergency department, it was found that the bullet had entered the back obliquely and was lodged in the vertebral canal at the level of the eighth thoracic vertebra. The patient could not feel anything below this level and was paralyzed from the waist downward. At the operation a laminectomy was performed and the bullet was removed. Considerable damage to the spinal cord was noted. What changes take place in the spinal cord when the nerve fibers are damaged? Does regeneration take place in the central nervous system?

12. An 18-year-old woman visited her physician because she had burns, which she had not felt, on the tips of the fingers of the right hand. She also mentioned that she had weakness of her right hand. On physical examination severe scarring of the fingers of the right hand was noted. Obvious atrophy of the small muscles of the right hand was also found. Testing the sensory modalities of the skin of the entire patient showed total loss of pain and temperature sensation of the distal part of the right upper limb. There was diminished sensibility to pain and temperature of the left hand. Definite muscular weakness was demonstrated in the small muscles of the right hand and a small amount of weakness also was found in the muscles of the left hand. A diagnosis of syringomyelia was made. (a) Using your neuroanatomical knowledge, describe the type of sensory nerve endings that are sensitive to pain and temperature. (b) How would you examine a patient to determine if there is cutaneous pain and temperature sensory loss?

13. A 35-year-old man, while walking past some workmen who were digging a hole in the road, suddenly became aware of a foreign body in his left eye. Since the cornea is extremely sensitive, he suffered considerable discom-

fort. What sensory endings are present in the cornea? Is the cornea sensitive to stimuli other than pain?

14. A 60-year-old man visited his physician because for the past 3 months he had been experiencing an agonizing stabbing pain over the middle part of the right side of his face. The stabs would last a few seconds but might be repeated several times. "The pain is the worst I have ever experienced," he told his physician. He had noticed particularly that a draft of cold air on his face or the touching of a few scalp hairs in the temporal region could trigger the pain. Physical examination revealed no sensory or motor loss of the trigeminal nerve. A diagnosis of trigeminal neuralgia was made. Using your knowledge of neuroanatomy, explain why hairs are so sensitive to touch.

15. A 50-year-old man was diagnosed as suffering from tabes dorsalis. On physical examination, many signs of the syphilitic disease were present, including a total lack of deep sensation to pain. Intense squeezing of the tendo calcaneus or the testicles produced no response. Using your knowledge of neuroanatomy, explain how deep pain sensation is normally experienced.

16. While carrying out a physical examination of a patient, the physician asked the patient to cross his knees and relax his leg muscles. The left ligamentum patellae was then struck smartly with a reflex hammer, and this immediately produced an involuntary partial extension of the left knee joint (the knee-jerk test was positive). How does the central nervous system receive nervous information from the quadriceps femoris muscle in order that it may respond reflexly by extending the knee?

17. A 55-year-old man suffering from syphilis of the spinal cord presented characteristic symptoms and signs of tabes dorsalis. He had experienced severe stabbing pains in the abdomen and legs for the last 6 months. When asked to walk, the patient was seen to do so with a broad base, slapping the feet on the ground. How would you test the patient's ability to perceive the position of his lower extremities and his vibratory sense? Using your knowledge of neuroanatomy, explain how a normal individual is able to perceive the position of the extremities and detect vibrations.

18. Using your knowledge of pharmacology, name two drugs that act as competitive blocking agents on skeletal neuromuscular junctions. Name the chemical substance against which these agents are competing. Name the sites at which the blocking agents are believed to act.

19. Name a drug that will bring about flaccid paralysis of skeletal muscle by causing depolarization of the postsynaptic membrane.

20. In cases of severe food poisoning the organism *Clostridium botulinum* may be found to be responsible. How does this organism cause paralysis of the respiratory muscles?

21. An orthopedic surgeon stated, during a ward round, that the degree of muscular atrophy that occurs in a limb immobilized in a cast is totally different from the

degree of muscular atrophy that follows section of the motor nerve supply to muscles. The surgeon asked a medical student to explain this difference. How would you account for this difference in the degree of muscular atrophy?

22. A 57-year-old man visited his physician because of pain in the right buttock that extended down the right leg, the back of the thigh, the outer side and back of the calf, and the outer border of the foot. The patient gave no history of previous injury, but stated that the pain started about 3 months ago as a dull, low backache. Since that time the pain has increased in intensity and has spread down the right leg. When asked if the pain had ever disappeared, he replied that on two separate occasions the pain had diminished in intensity, but his back remained "stiff" all the time. He said the pain was aggravated by stooping or by coughing and sneezing. Sometimes he experienced pins and needles along the outer border of his right foot. After a complete physical examination, a diagnosis was made of herniation of a lumbar intervertebral disc. Using your knowledge of anatomy, state which intervertebral disc is most likely to have been herniated.

23. A 61-year-old woman was seen by her physician because she was experiencing a shooting, burning pain in the left side of her chest. Three days later a group of localized papules appeared on the skin covering the left fifth intercostal space. One day later the papules became vesicular; a few days later the vesicles dried up into crusts, and these later separated, leaving small permanent scars. The patient also noticed that there was some loss of sensibility over the left side of the chest. A diagnosis of herpes zoster was made. Using your knowledge of anatomy, state the segment of the spinal cord involved with the disease.

24. While examining the sensory innervation of the skin of the head and neck in a patient, a medical student had difficulty remembering the dermatomal pattern at the junction of the head with the neck and at the junction of the neck with the thorax. Are the dermatomes arranged in a special manner in these areas? If so, what is the underlying reason for this?

25. A 30-year-old man was found, on physical examination, to have weakness and diminished tone of the rhomboid muscles, deltoids, and biceps brachii on both sides of the body. The degree of weakness was greater on the right side. The biceps tendon jerk was absent on the right side and diminished on the left side. The triceps jerks were normal on both sides of the body. The muscles of the trunk and lower limb showed increased tone and exhibited spastic paralysis. Radiology of the vertebral column revealed the presence of vertebral destruction due to a tumor arising within the vertebral canal. Using your knowledge of anatomy, answer the following questions: (a) Which vertebra is likely to have the tumor within the vertebral canal? (b) Name the segments of the spinal cord that are being pressed upon by the tumor. (c) Which segments of the spinal cord participate in the reflex arcs responsible for the biceps brachii

tendon jerk? (d) Why do the rhomboid and deltoid muscles exhibit diminished muscle tone, whereas the muscles of the lower limb exhibit increased tone?

26. Name three clinical conditions that could result in a loss of tone of skeletal muscle.

27. A 69-year-old man with advanced tabes dorsalis was asked to stand with his toes and heels together and his eyes closed. He immediately started to sway violently and if the nurse had not held on to his arm he would have fallen to the ground (positive Romberg test). Why was it vital for this patient to keep his eyes open in order to remain upright?

28. A 63-year-old man with moderately advanced Parkinson's disease was disrobed and asked to walk in a straight line in the examining room. The physician observed that the patient had his head and shoulders stooped forward, the arms slightly abducted, the elbow joints partly flexed, and the wrists slightly extended with the fingers flexed at the metacarpophalangeal joints and extended at the interphalangeal joints. It was noted that on starting to walk, the patient leaned forward and slowly shuffled his feet. The farther he leaned forward the more quickly he moved his legs, so that by the time he had crossed the room he was almost running. The patient's face was masklike and exhibited few emotional movements. The hands showed a coarse tremor and the muscles of the upper and lower limbs showed increased tone in the opposing muscle groups when the joints were passively moved. Parkinson's disease, or the parkinsonian syndrome, can be caused by a number of pathological conditions but they usually interfere in the normal function of the corpus striatum or the substantia nigra or both. Using your knowledge of the anatomy and physiology of muscle action, explain the different signs seen in this important syndrome.

29. A 10-year-old girl was taken to a neurologist because of a 6-month history of epileptic attacks. The parents described the attacks as starting with sudden involuntary movements of the trunk, arms, or legs. Sometimes the muscle movements were slight, but at other times they were so violent that she had been known to throw an object in her hand across the room. At other times the patient just fell to the ground, as the result of a sudden loss of muscle tone. Having hit the ground, the patient would immediately rise to her feet. On one occasion she severely bruised her head and shoulder by striking a chair and a table. One month ago the parents noticed that their daughter appeared to lose consciousness briefly. At the time, she was carrying on a normal conversation, when she suddenly stopped and her gaze became fixed. After a few seconds she became alert and continued her conversation. This patient is suffering from a form of epilepsy known as petit mal. What is the correct term for the sudden involuntary contraction of the muscles of the trunk or extremities? Name the condition of a patient who suddenly loses all muscle tone and falls to the ground?

30. A 45-year-old man suffering from amyotrophic lateral sclerosis was examined by a third-year medical student.

The student found that the flexor and extensor muscles of the knee and ankle joints of the right leg were weaker than those of the left leg. However, she was of the opinion that the muscles of the left leg also were somewhat weaker than normal. On palpation of the extensor muscles of the right thigh it was possible to detect a twitching of the muscle fibers in the quadriceps muscle. Marked atrophy of the muscles of both legs also was noted. There was no evidence of cutaneous sensory loss in either limb. Amyotrophic lateral sclerosis is a condition in which there is degeneration of the motor anterior horn cells of the spinal cord and brainstem with secondary degeneration of the nervous tracts in the lateral and anterior portions of the spinal cord. Why do you think this patient had weakness and atrophy of the muscles of the lower limbs? What is the correct clinical term for the twitching of the muscle fibers in the extensor muscles of the right knee?

31. A 12-year-old girl was diagnosed as suffering from a medulloblastoma of the cerebellum. Clinical and radiological examinations revealed that the tumor was predominantly invading the right cerebellar hemisphere. Knowing that the cerebellum is concerned with the coordination of motor activity so that complex voluntary movements involving antagonistic muscle groups can take place in a precise manner, what should you test for to demonstrate loss of cerebellar function? Describe the test for each parameter.

Answers to Clinical Problem Solving

1. Nervous tracts are bundles of nerve fibers found in the brain and spinal cord, most of which are myelinated. Some of the main structural differences between a myelinated nerve tract and a myelinated peripheral nerve fiber are as follows:

Nerve Tract
      Oligodendrocyte
      Mesaxon absent
      Schmidt-Lanterman incisures present
      Nerve fibers supported by neuroglia

Peripheral Nerve Fiber
      Schwann cell
      Mesaxon present
      Schmidt-Lanterman incisures present
      Nerve fibers supported by connective tissue sheaths, endoneurium, perineurium, and epineurium

2. Myelination is fully described on page 75. Myelin sheaths begin to be formed during fetal development and during the first year postnatally.

3. No. In the central nervous system a single oligodendrocyte may be responsible for the formation of myelin for as many as 60 nerve fibers. Clearly, it would not be possible for an oligodendrocyte to rotate on each axon as does the Schwann cell in the peripheral nervous system. It is believed that in the central nervous system the process of the oligodendrocyte grows in length and wraps itself around the axon.

4. (a) The microscopic changes that occur in the proximal and distal segments of a divided peripheral nerve are fully described on page 110. Remember that in the proximal segment the changes occur only as far proximally as the next node of Ranvier, whereas the changes spread distally from the site of the lesion and include its terminations. (b) If one bears in mind the considerations outlined on pages 112 to 114 and that the surgeon has the experience to perform nerve suture, the following treatment should be instituted. If the knife was clean, the nerve should be immediately sutured and any arterial damage repaired. On the other hand, if the knife was contaminated or the wound was more than 6 hours old, the wound should be treated and the nerve ignored. In the latter case, when the wound has healed and there is no sign of residual infection, the nerve ends should be explored and sutured together without tension. In either case, the paralyzed muscles are protected with a suitable splint and the joints are gently exercised daily. (c) Once the regenerating axons have entered the distal segment, the nerve distal to the section becomes very sensitive to mechanical stimulation (Tinel's sign). (d) Sensory recovery occurs first. Deep pressure sensation is the first sign of recovery. This is followed by the return of superficial cutaneous pain and vasomotor control of blood vessels, later the sensations of heat and cold return, and later still light touch and tactile discrimination reappear. Sensory recovery occurs before there is return of voluntary movement. (e) For clinical purposes a figure of 1.5 mm per day is the average rate of regeneration. It is possible, using this figure, to determine approximately how long it will take for a regenerating nerve to reach its end-organs.

5. Bell's palsy is produced by swelling of the seventh cranial nerve (facial nerve) in the facial nerve canal of the skull. Its cause is unknown, although it often follows exposure to cold. Since the facial canal is bony, the nerve cannot expand and consequently becomes compressed and ischemic. In severe cases the muscles of facial expression are paralyzed on one side of the face and there is loss of taste sensation in the anterior part of the tongue on the same side. Massage of the paralyzed muscles should be undertaken to preserve their integrity until nerve function returns. The majority of patients recover completely. There existed in this patient a serious residual palsy after 3 years. A treatment that has been successful in many cases is to section the hypoglossal nerve below and behind the angle of the mandible and to anastomose its proximal end to the

distal end of the facial nerve. Although the right half of the tongue would be paralyzed, this causes little disability. A reasonable return of facial movement can be expected. The patient learns to move the face instead of the tongue by practicing in front of a mirror. Note that both the hypoglossal and facial nerves are peripheral nerves and therefore regeneration is possible. The prognosis is especially good since the hypoglossal nerve is purely a motor nerve.

6. Lead causes neuronal degeneration in the central nervous system and demyelination in the tracts of the spinal cord and peripheral nerves. The treatment is to remove the child from the source of the lead and to aid rapid excretion by administering a chelating agent, calcium disodium versenate. Nontoxic lead versenate is excreted in the urine.

7. Yes. The cauda equina consists of the anterior and posterior roots of the spinal nerves below the level of the first lumbar segment of the spinal cord. These are peripheral nerves with endoneurial sheaths and Schwann cells and therefore regeneration will take place if adequate treatment is promptly instituted.

8. As the result of experiments in which dyes have been injected into peripheral nerves, spaces have been demonstrated between individual nerve fibers in the endoneurium. These spaces are believed to provide the route for the ascent of the tetanus toxin to the spinal cord.

9. Lidocaine is a local anesthetic that, when applied to a nerve fiber, blocks nerve conduction. The anesthetic acts on the axolemma and interferes with the transient increase in permeability of the axolemma to Na^+ ions and in the resting axon reduces the permeability of the axolemma to Na^+, K^+, and other ions. The small-diameter pain fibers are more susceptible to the action of this drug.

10. *Neuropraxia* is the term applied to a transient nerve block. Pressure is the most common cause and this case was due to the pressure of the upper edge of the chair back on the brachial plexus in the axilla. The loss of function is probably caused by ischemia of the nerve fibers. There is no microscopic evidence of degeneration. Axonotmesis is the term applied to a nerve lesion where the axons are damaged but the surrounding connective tissue sheaths remain intact. Neurotmesis is the term applied to complete section of the nerve trunk.

The prognosis in this patient is excellent for rapid, complete recovery. It is important that the paralyzed muscles not be stretched by antagonist muscles or by gravity. Therefore, suitable splints should be applied and gentle passive movement of the joints should be performed once daily.

11. Degeneration in the central nervous system occurs in a manner similar to that found in the peripheral nervous system. The axon breaks up into small fragments and the debris is digested by the neighboring microglial cells. The myelin sheath is broken down into lipid droplets, which are also phagocytosed by the microglial cells.

There is an attempt at regeneration of the axons as evidenced by sprouting of the axons, but there is no evidence that restoration of function ever occurs. The reasons for the failure of regeneration are fully described on page 114.

12. Syringomyelia is a chronic disease of the spinal cord and is due to a developmental abnormality in the formation of the central canal. It is characterized by the appearance of a fluid-filled cavity within the spinal cord that gradually enlarges, causing destruction of surrounding nervous tissue. In this patient, the cavity or syrinx was located in the lower cervical and upper thoracic segments of the cord, causing destruction of the ascending tracts that serve pain and temperature from the upper limbs. The cavity was encroaching on the motor anterior horn cells of both sides also, causing weakness of the small muscles of the hands.

(a) It is now generally accepted that the type of sensation felt is determined not by a specific receptor but by the specific area of the central nervous system to which the afferent nerve fiber passes. Free nerve endings are commonly associated with axons serving pain and temperature. (b) The examination of a patient to test different sensory modalities is discussed on page 119.

13. The only sensory receptors present in the cornea are free nerve endings. The cornea is sensitive to touch and temperature changes in addition to pain.

14. All hair follicles possess a rich innervation. Free nerve endings are found as a branching network that winds around the follicle below the entrance of the sebaceous duct. Merkel's discs also are found in the epidermis of the follicle. The hair shaft acts as a lever, so that the slightest movement of the hair readily stimulates the nerve endings in the hair follicle. In this patient suffering from trigeminal neuralgia, the temporal region of the scalp was the trigger area, which on stimulation initiated the intense stabs of pain in the distribution of the maxillary division of the trigeminal nerve.

15. Numerous free nerve endings are found in the connective tissue of tendons and the testes. Normally, squeezing of these structures elicits an aching type of pain. In tabes dorsalis the disease process affects the sensory neurons in the posterior roots of the spinal nerves.

16. Striking the ligamentum patellae with a reflex hammer causes elongation of the intrafusal fibers of the muscle spindles of the quadriceps muscle and stimulation of the annulospiral and flower spray endings. The nerve impulses reach the spinal cord in the afferent neurons within the femoral nerve and enter the cord at the level of L2, 3, and 4. The afferent neurons synapse with the large alpha motor neurons in the anterior gray horns of the spinal cord. Nerve impulses now pass via the efferent motor neurons in the femoral nerve and stimulate the extrafusal muscle fibers of the quadriceps muscle, which then contracts. The muscle spindle afferent impulses inhibit the motor neurons of the antagonist muscles (see reciprocal inhibition, p. 98).

17. To test position sense, the patient is placed in the supine position and asked to close the eyes. The big toe is grasped at the sides between the thumb and index finger and extended and flexed. The patient is asked, on completion of each movement, "Is the toe pointing up or down?" Another simple test is to ask the patient, again with the eyes closed, to place the right heel on the left shin and run it down the shin to the dorsum of the left foot. The patient is then asked to repeat the performance with the left heel on the right shin.

Vibratory sense can be tested by placing the handle of a vibrating tuning fork on the tibial tuberosity, the anterior border of the tibia, and the medial or lateral malleoli. The patient is asked to indicate when he or she first feels the vibration and when it ceases. Symmetrical points on the two limbs may be compared and the physician can use his or her own limbs as a control. In the normal individual, the sense of position depends on the central nervous system's receiving adequate information from the pressure receptors (pacinian corpuscles) in the joint capsules and ligaments, touch receptors (free nerve endings) in the tissues in and around joints, and the stretch receptors in the muscles and tendons (especially the neurotendinous spindles).

Vibration sense is normally believed to be due to the stimulation of superficial and deep pressure receptors (pacinian corpuscles).

The appreciation of the passive movements of joints, postural sensibility, and vibration sense are often lost in tabes dorsalis due to syphilitic destruction of the posterior columns of the spinal cord and degeneration of the posterior roots.

18. *d*-Tubocurarine, dimethyltubocurarine, gallamine, and benzoquinonium are examples of competitive blocking agents. These drugs compete with the neurotransmitter acetylcholine. The competitive blocking agents are believed to combine with the same sites at the postsynaptic membrane (sarcolemma) of the motor end-plate normally used by acetylcholine.

19. Decamethonium and succinylcholine paralyze skeletal muscle by causing depolarization of the motor end-plate.

20. *C. botulinum* produces a toxin that inhibits the release of acetylcholine at the motor end-plate. Death results from paralysis of the respiratory muscles.

21. Skeletal muscles that are not used, for example in a limb fitted with a splint immobilizing a fracture, undergo disuse atrophy. The longer the muscles are not used, the greater the degree of atrophy, and in severe cases, it may amount to as much as one-fourth of the muscle mass. The muscle fibers rapidly atrophy following section of a motor nerve, so that the total mass of the muscle may be reduced by as much as three-fourths in as little as 3 months. The precise reason for this severe atrophy is not understood. Apparently the maintenance of normal muscle depends on the continued reception of acetylcholine and trophic substances from the nerve terminals at the postsynaptic membrane at the neuromuscular junction. The latter mechanism

would be impossible if the motor nerve were sectioned and the distal end had degenerated.

22. Your knowledge of the dermatomes of the lower limb will enable you to ascertain that the patient's pain was felt in the area of distribution of the fifth lumbar and first sacral nerve roots. The involvement of these roots is usually due to herniation of the fourth or fifth lumbar intervertebral disc.

23. Herpes zoster is a viral infection of the posterior root ganglia (or sensory ganglia of the cranial nerves), the posterior root, or the posterior gray horn of the spinal cord. This patient experienced pain and had a skin eruption in the area of distribution of the fifth left intercostal nerve. The virus was producing an acute inflammation at some point along the course of the sensory neurons of the fifth segment of the spinal cord on the left side.

24. The trigeminal (fifth cranial) nerve innervates the skin of the greater part of the face. The next dermatome that occurs inferior to this is that of the second cervical nerve. The sixth to the twelfth cranial nerves do not innervate the skin of the face. At the junction of the neck with the thorax, the fourth cervical dermatome is contiguous with the second thoracic dermatome; the anterior rami of the lower cervical and first thoracic spinal nerves lose their cutaneous distribution on the neck and trunk during the development of the upper limb.

25. (a) The physical examination revealed weakness of the rhomboid, deltoid, and biceps brachii muscles, which are innervated by the fifth and sixth cervical segments of the spinal cord. These spinal cord segments lie within the vertebral foramina of the sixth and seventh cervical vertebrae, respectively. (b) The fifth and sixth cervical segments of the spinal cord are being pressed upon. (c) The biceps brachii reflex arc involves the fifth and sixth segments of the spinal cord. (d) The rhomboid and deltoid muscles show diminished muscle tone because the reflex arcs upon which their tone depends travel through the compressed segments of the spinal cord; that is, the reflex arcs were no longer functioning normally. Because of the pressure of the tumor on the cervical region of the spinal cord, the nervous pathways passing down to lower segments of the spinal cord were interrupted. This resulted in the motor anterior gray column cells of the segments of the cord below the level of compression receiving diminished information from the higher centers, with a consequent increase in muscle tone.

26. Any disease process that can interrupt the normal functioning of the basic spinal reflex arc upon which skeletal muscle tone is dependent will cause loss of muscle tone. Some examples are spinal shock following trauma to the spinal cord; section of or pressure upon a spinal nerve, a posterior root, or an anterior root; syringomyelia; and poliomyelitis.

27. Tabes dorsalis, which is a syphilitic infection of the brain and spinal cord, produces degeneration of the central processes of the posterior root ganglion cells and also,

usually, the ganglion cells themselves. The lower thoracic and lumbar sacral segments of the cord are involved first, and the interruption of the proprioceptive fibers results in impairment of appreciation of posture, and the tendency to fall down if one closes the eyes while standing. Eyesight in this patient compensated for lack of proprioception.

28. In a normal individual, standing and walking are largely automatic but, as you have read in this chapter, these activities are highly complex and require the proper integration of neural mechanisms at all levels of the spinal cord and brain. The basic mechanism underlying muscle tone is the spinal segmental reflex. In order to maintain normal posture, these reflex arcs must receive adequate nervous input from higher levels of the nervous system. Diseases involving the corpus striatum (caudate and lentiform nuclei) or the substantia nigra result in an alteration in the pattern of nervous impulses impinging on the anterior horn cells of the spinal cord, hence the abnormal muscle tone. The increased tone is equal in extent in opposing muscle groups. The tremor of the parkinsonian syndrome is produced by the alternating movements of the agonist and antagonist muscles of a joint. The tremor is most prominent when the limb is at rest, ceases temporarily when voluntary movement is performed, and then starts again when the movement is completed. The tremor ceases when the patient is asleep. In Parkinson's disease there is a neuronal degeneration in the substantia nigra, resulting in the loss of inhibitory control of the substantia nigra over the lentiform nucleus, putamen, and caudate nucleus.

29. The syndrome of petit mal commonly has three sets of symptoms: (a) myoclonic jerks, in which the patient experiences sudden involuntary contraction of the muscles of the trunk and extremities; (b) akinetic seizures, in which there is a sudden loss of tone in all muscles of the body; and (c) brief losses of consciousness, in which the patient loses contact with the environment for a few seconds.

30. Destruction of the anterior gray column cells in the lumbar and sacral regions of the spinal cord resulted in paralysis and atrophy of the muscles of both legs. The twitching of groups of muscle fibers is referred to as muscular fasciculation and is commonly seen in patients with chronic disease affecting the anterior horn cells.

31. (a) Muscular hypotonia, which is present on the same side of the body as the lesion. Passively move the joints on the right side of the body and then on the left side and compare the resistance to these movements by the muscles on the two sides of the body. (b) Posture. The shoulder girdle on the affected side drops, because of loss of muscle tone. With the patient disrobed ask her to stand up straight with her back toward you. With a unilateral cerebellar lesion the shoulder on the affected side may be lower than that on the opposite, normal side. (c) Disorders of voluntary movement (ataxia) due to loss of muscle coordination. The finger-nose test and the heel-knee test are described on page 124. These tests will reveal ataxia on the side of the body in which the lesion is situated. (d) Nystagmus. This may be defined as an involuntary to-and-fro movement of the eyes. It is commonly demonstrated in cerebellar disease and is due to lack of muscle coordination. When the eyes are turned horizontally laterally there are quick, rhythmic jerks in the direction of gaze. In unilateral cerebellar lesions, the amplitude of nystagmus is greater and its rate slower when the eyes are rotated toward the side of the lesion than when they are displaced to the opposite side.

Review Questions

Directions: Each of the numbered items in this section is followed by answers that are positively phrased. Select the ONE lettered answer that is an EXCEPTION.

1. The following statements concerning nerves are correct **except:**
   (a) A nerve tract is the name given to a nerve fiber in the central nervous system.
   (b) The supporting cell of a myelinated nerve fiber in the central nervous system is called an oligodendrocyte.
   (c) A node of Ranvier in peripheral nerves is where two Schwann cells terminate and the plasma membrane of the axon is exposed.
   (d) Nodes of Ranvier are absent from myelinated nerve fibers in the central nervous system.
   (e) The major dense line of myelin consists of two inner protein layers of the plasma membrane that are fused together.

2. The following statements concerning nerves are correct **except:**
   (a) The minor dense line of myelin is made up of lipid.
   (b) The incisures of Schmidt-Lanterman are caused by the mesaxons of the Schwann cells.
   (c) As many as 15 or more unmyelinated axons may share a single Schwann cell in the peripheral nervous system.

(d) The node of Ranvier is the site of nerve activity.

(e) Chromatolysis is the term used to describe the changes in the arrangement of Nissl material within the neuronal cytoplasm following injury.

3. The following statements concerning an oligodendrocyte are true **except:**

(a) A single oligodendrocyte may be associated with several segments of myelin on a single axon.

(b) A single oligodendrocyte may be associated with the myelin sheaths of as many as 60 axons.

(c) Myelination in the central nervous system occurs by the growth in length of the oligodendrocytic process and the wrapping of it around the axon.

(d) A nonmyelinated axon in the central nervous system has a special relationship with the oligodendrocyte.

(e) The incisures of Schmidt-Lanterman are present in the myelinated fibers of the central nervous system.

4. The following statements concerning spinal nerves are true **except:**

(a) There are 31 pairs.

(b) They are formed by the union of anterior and posterior nerve roots.

(c) The posterior ramus contains only sensory axons.

(d) The anterior root contains only motor axons.

(e) The posterior root ganglion contains unipolar neurons enveloped in capsular cells.

5. The following statements concerning peripheral nerve plexuses are true **except:**

(a) They are formed by a network of nerve fibers.

(b) Bundles of nerve fibers branch, but in most instances the individual nerve fibers do not branch.

(c) The plexuses at the roots of the limbs are formed from posterior rami of spinal nerves.

(d) The plexuses of the autonomic nervous system possess a network of nerve fibers and nerve cells.

(e) A plexus situated at the root of a limb permits nerve fibers from different segments of the spinal cord to become rearranged so that they more easily travel to different parts of the limb.

6. The following statements concerning nerve conduction are correct **except:**

(a) An adequate stimulus alters the permeability of the axolemma to Na^+ ions at the point of stimulation.

(b) A typical action potential is about +40 mV.

(c) As the action potential moves along the axon, the entry of Na^+ ions into the axon increases and the permeability to K^+ ions decreases.

(d) During the refractory period, no stimulus, no matter how strong, will excite the nerve fiber.

(e) In the resting unstimulated nerve fiber the interior of the axolemma is negative to the exterior.

7. The following statements concerning the propagation of a nerve impulse are correct **except:**

(a) The conduction velocity is greatest in nerve fibers having a large cross-sectional diameter.

(b) In nonmyelinated nerve fibers the action potential occurs along the length of the fiber.

(c) A myelinated nerve fiber can be stimulated only at the nodes of Ranvier, where the axon is naked.

(d) Saltatory conduction occurs only in the central nervous system.

(e) The action potential at a node of Ranvier sets up a current in the surrounding tissue fluid.

8. The following statements concerning wallerian degeneration are correct **except:**

(a) The myelin breaks down into droplets that are phagocytosed by the Schwann cells.

(b) The axon is broken down into fragments.

(c) The Schwann cells multiply.

(d) In the central nervous system the debris is removed by the microglial cells.

(e) In the peripheral nervous system the tissue macrophages play no part in the digestion of the nerve fragments.

9. The following statements concerning the failure of regeneration of nerve fibers in the central nervous system are correct **except:**

(a) Endoneurial tubes are absent.

(b) Oligodendrocytes have a basement membrane.

(c) Oligodendrocytes fail to multiply and form a band fiber as do Schwann cells in the peripheral nervous system.

(d) The blood supply is usually adequate.

(e) There are no nerve growth factors.

10. The following factors may explain the partial return of function following injury to the spinal cord **except:**

(a) The edema subsides at the site of injury.

(b) Nonfunctional neurons take over the function of damaged neurons.

(c) An increased number of receptor sites may develop on postsynaptic membranes.

(d) Some of the axons completely regenerate.

(e) With training the patient may use other muscles to compensate for the loss of paralyzed muscles.

11. The following statements concerning receptor endings are correct **except:**

(a) The rods and cones of the eyes are examples of electromagnetic receptors.

(b) The taste and smell endings are chemoreceptors.

(c) Free nerve endings have no Schwann cells covering their tips.

(d) Merkel's discs are slow-adapting touch receptors.

(e) Meissner's corpuscles are absent from the skin of the palm of the hand and the sole of the foot.

12. The following statements concerning receptor endings are correct **except:**

(a) The pacinian corpuscle is a slowly adapting mechanoreceptor.

(b) There is a considerable reduction in the number of Meissner's corpuscles between birth and old age.

(c) Each pacinian corpuscle has a lamellated capsule and a central core containing the nerve ending.

(d) The annulospiral endings in skeletal muscle possess intrafusal muscle fibers.

(e) Ruffini's corpuscles are slowly adapting stretch receptors found in the dermis of hairy skin.

13. The following statements concerning cutaneous receptors are true **except:**
    (a) Although there are a variety of histological types of receptors, nerves only transmit nerve impulses.
    (b) The type of sensation felt is determined by the specific area of the central nervous system to which the sensory nerve fiber passes.
    (c) Transduction at the receptor is the process by which the energy of the stimulus is changed into electrochemical energy of the nerve impulse.
    (d) When applied to the receptor, the stimulus brings about a change in the potential of the plasma membranes of the capsule cells and not the nerve ending.
    (e) If large enough, the receptor potential will generate an action potential in the afferent sensory nerve fiber.

14. The following statements concerning the function of a neuromuscular spindle are true **except:**
    (a) It gives rise to afferent nerve impulses all the time.
    (b) When active or passive muscle movement occurs, there is an increase in the rate of passage of nerve impulses in the afferent nerve fiber.
    (c) The neuromuscular spindle keeps the central nervous system informed about muscle activity.
    (d) The neuromuscular spindle indirectly influences the control of voluntary movement.
    (e) The flower spray endings are situated mainly on the nuclear bag fibers close to the equatorial region.

15. The following statements concerning the neurotendinous spindles are correct **except:**
    (a) They are situated in tendons close to the musculotendinous junction.
    (b) Each has a fibrous capsule, loosely arranged collagen fibers, and tendon cells.
    (c) The nerve ends by branching and terminating in club-shaped endings.
    (d) Neurotendinous spindles are found only in slow-acting muscles.
    (e) The neurotendinous spindle is activated by changes in muscle tension and inhibits muscle contraction.

16. The following statements concerning the neuromuscular junctions in skeletal muscle are correct **except:**
    (a) Each terminal branch of the motor nerve ends as a naked axon.
    (b) Each axon lies in a groove on the surface of the muscle fiber formed by the infolding of the sarcolemma.
    (c) Having caused depolarization of the postsynaptic membrane, acetylcholine is reabsorbed into the axon terminal.

(d) Acetylcholine is released from the axon terminal when the nerve impulse reaches the neuromuscular junction.

(e) The Schwann cell forms a cap or roof for the groove on the surface of the muscle fiber.

17. The following statements concerning the neuromuscular junctions on smooth and cardiac muscle are correct **except:**
    (a) In smooth muscle the autonomic nerve fiber exerts control over several muscle fibers.
    (b) The autonomic nerve fibers terminate on smooth muscle as unmyelinated fibers.
    (c) In cardiac muscle the wave of contraction spreads rapidly from one muscle fiber to another by way of desmosomes and gap junctions.
    (d) In smooth muscle the wave of contraction passes from one muscle fiber to another by means of gap junctions.
    (e) At the site of the neuromuscular junction, the axon is completely surrounded by Schwann cells.

18. The following statements concerning skin sensations and dermatomes is correct **except:**
    (a) To produce on the trunk a region of complete anesthesia, at least three segments of the spinal cord have to be damaged.
    (b) When contiguous spinal nerves are sectioned, it is noted that the area of tactile loss is always greater than the area of loss of painful and thermal sensations.
    (c) The dermatome present on the medial side of the wrist is C8.
    (d) The dermatomes present on the point of the shoulder are C3 and C4.
    (e) The dermatomes for the limbs run almost horizontally.

19. The following statements concerning muscle reflexes are correct **except:**
    (a) The biceps brachii tendon reflex involves C5 and C6 segments of the spinal cord.
    (b) The triceps tendon reflex involves the T1 segment of the spinal cord.
    (c) The patellar tendon reflex (knee jerk) involves L2,3,and 4 segments of the spinal cord.
    (d) A tumor pressing on the first and second sacral segments of the spinal cord is likely to interfere with the ankle jerk.
    (e) The abdominal superficial reflexes involve T6-12 segments of the spinal cord.

20. The following statements concerning the dermatomes of the trunk and lower limbs are true **except:**
    (a) The T10 dermatome includes the skin of the umbilicus.
    (b) The L1 dermatome lies over the inguinal ligament.
    (c) The L2 dermatome lies over the medial side of the knee joint.
    (d) The S1 dermatome runs along the lateral side of the foot.

(e) The L3 and 5 dermatomes lie over the lateral side of the knee joint.

21. The following statements concerning muscle innervation are correct **except:**
    (a) A motor unit consists of the posterior root ganglion and all the neuromuscular spindles it is connected to.
    (b) In the small muscles of the hand one nerve fiber supplies only a few muscle fibers.
    (c) Neurotendinous spindles are innervated by myelinated nerve fibers.
    (d) Muscle tone is dependent on the integrity of a simple monosynaptic reflex arc.
    (e) The gamma motor efferent fibers innervate the intrafusal fibers of a muscle spindle.

22. The following statements concerning skeletal muscle action are correct **except:**
    (a) When a muscle begins to contract, the smaller motor units are stimulated first.
    (b) Muscle fatigue is caused by an exhaustion of the presynaptic vesicles at the neuromuscular junction.
    (c) When a prime mover contracts, the antagonistic muscles are inhibited.
    (d) When a muscle is paralyzed, it immediately loses its normal tone.
    (e) To paralyze a muscle completely, it is usually necessary to destroy several adjacent segments of the spinal cord or their nerve roots.

23. The following statements concerning posture are correct **except:**
    (a) In the standing position, the line of gravity passes through the odontoid process of the axis, behind the centers of the hip joints, and in front of the knee and ankle joints.
    (b) Posture depends on the degree and distribution of muscle tone.
    (c) A particular posture can often be maintained for long periods by different groups of muscle fibers in a muscle contracting in relays.
    (d) The cerebral cortex makes an important contribution to the maintenance of normal posture.
    (e) Nerve impulses arising in the eyes and ears cannot influence posture.

24. The following clinical observations on muscle activity can be made **except:**
    (a) Muscle contracture is a condition in which the muscle contracts for a long period of time.
    (b) Muscle fasciculation is seen with chronic disease that affects anterior horn cells or the motor nuclei of cranial nerves.
    (c) Muscle atrophy takes place when a limb is immobilized in a splint.
    (d) Muscle wasting can occur if only the efferent motor nerve fibers to a muscle are sectioned.
    (e) Wasting occurs in the muscles acting on the shoulder joint in patients with painful pericapsulitis involving that joint.

Directions: Read the case histories then answer the questions. You will be required to select ONE BEST lettered answer.

A 35-year-old woman caught her hand in a machine at work and suffered multiple skin lacerations on the hand. It was decided to suture the lacerations after performing a complete block of all the nerves supplying the hand above the wrist.

25. Which of the following nerves does **not** supply the skin of the hand?
    (a) Musculocutaneous nerve
    (b) Median nerve
    (c) Radial nerve
    (d) Ulnar nerve
    (e) Posterior cutaneous branch of the ulnar nerve

26. Which of the following nerve fibers is **first** blocked by the local anesthetic?
    (a) Motor fibers
    (b) Large pain sensory fibers
    (c) Sensory touch fibers
    (d) Small deep pain sensory fibers
    (e) Vibration sensory fibers

27. Which of the following nerve fibers recovers **first** as the effect of the anesthetic wears off?
    (a) C fibers
    (b) A alpha fibers
    (c) B fibers
    (d) A beta fibers
    (e) A delta fibers

A 26-year-old woman attended a neighborhood party celebrating the safe return of her husband from Bosnia. Forty-eight hours later she awoke in the middle of the night with severe nausea, which was quickly followed by vomiting and diarrhea. By morning she noticed that she had sagging of her upper eyelids (ptosis) and difficulty in moving her eyes. Later, during the day she experienced weakness of the jaw muscles and had difficulty in swallowing (dysphagia). Two friends who had also attended the party telephoned her and said that they were experiencing similar symptoms.

After a thorough examination in the emergency department, the diagnosis of acute botulism was made.

28. The following statements concerning the botulinum toxin are correct **except:**
    (a) The toxin causes weakness in both striated and smooth muscle.
    (b) The toxin impairs the release of acetylcholine at all peripheral nerve synapses.
    (c) The toxin acts at the motor end-plates of skeletal muscle by inhibiting the release of acetylcholine.
    (d) The toxin acts at the motor end-plates of skeletal muscle by stimulating cholinesterase activity.
    (e) The toxin does not act at the motor end-plates of skeletal muscle by causing an acetylcholine blockade.

Answers to Review Questions

1. D	19. B
2. B	20. C
3. D	21. A
4. C	22. B
5. C	23. E
6. C	24. A
7. D	25. A. The musculocutaneous nerve becomes the lateral cutaneous nerve of the forearm, which supplies the skin on the anterior and posterior surfaces of the forearm down as far as the wrist.
8. E	
9. B	
10. D	26. D. In a mixed peripheral nerve, the smallest-diameter nerve fibers are blocked first by the local anesthetic and the largest-diameter fibers are blocked last.
11. E	
12. A	
13. D	27. B. In a mixed peripheral nerve, the largest-diameter nerve fibers are the first to recover from a local anesthetic and the smallest fibers are the last to recover.
14. E	
15. D	
16. C	28. D
17. E	
18. E	

ADDITIONAL READING

Aguayo, A. J., Benfey, M., and David, S. A potential for axonal regeneration in neurons of the adult mammalian nervous system. *Birth Defects* 19(4):327, 1983.

Andersen, O.S., Koeppe, R.E. II. Molecular determinants of channel function. *Physiol. Rev.* 72: S89-S158,1992.

Angle, C. R. Childhood lead poisoning and its treatment. *Ann. Rev. Pharmacol. Toxicol.* 32:409, 1993.

Armstrong, C.M. Voltage-dependent ion channels and their gating. *Physiol. Rev.* 72:S5-13,1992.

Armstrong, C.M.,Hille, B. Voltage-gated ion channels and electrical excitability. *Neuron* 20:371-380,1998.

Asbury, A. K., McKhann, G. M., and McDonald, W. I. (eds.), *Diseases of the Nervous System: Clinical Neurobiology.* Vol. 1. Philadelphia: Saunders, 1992. pp. 123-353.

Bannister, L. H. Sensory Terminals of Peripheral Nerves. In D. N. Landon (ed.), *The Peripheral Nerve.* London: Chapman and Hall, 1976. P. 396.

Boyd,I.A.,Smith,R.S. The muscle spindle. In: P.J Dyck,P.K. Thomas, E.H. Lambert, R. Bunge (eds). *Peripheral Neuropathy, 2nd ed.,1:171-202 Philadelphia:Saunders,1984.*

Brazis, P. W., Masdeu, J. C., and Biller, J. *Localization in Clinical Neurology* (2nd ed.). Boston: Little, Brown, 1990.

Catterall, W.A. Structure and function of voltage-gated ion channels. *Trends Neurosci.* 16:500-506,1993.

Cauna, N. The free penicillate nerve endings of the human hairy skin. *J. Anat.* 115:277, 1973.

Cauna, N., and Mannan, G. The structure of human digital pacinian corpuscles (corpusculae lamellosae) and its functional significance. *J. Anat.* 92:1, 1958.

Cauna, N., and Ross, L. L. The fine structure of Meissner's touch corpuscle of human fingers. *J. Biophys. Biochem. Cytol.* 8:467, 1960.

Cherington, M. Clinical spectrum of botulism. *Muscle Nerve* 21:701-710, 1998.

Craig, C. R., and Stitzel, R. E. *Modern Pharmacology* (4th ed.), Boston: Little, Brown, 1994.

Couteaux, R. Localization of cholinesterase at neuromuscular junctions. *Int. Rev. Cytol.* 4:335, 1955.

Cunningham, F. O., and Fitzgerald, M. J. T. Encapsulated nerve endings in hairy skin. *J. Anat.* 112:93, 1972.

Dawson, D. M., Hallett, M., and Millender, L. H. *Entrapment Neuropathies* (2nd ed.). Boston: Little, Brown, 1990.

Doyle, D.A., Cabral, J.M., Pfuetzner,R.A., Kuo, A, Gulbis, J.M., Cohen, S.L., Chait, B.T., Mackinnon, R. The structure of the potassium channel: molecular basis of K + conduction and selectivity. *Science* 280:69-77,1998.

Drachman, D.B. Myasthenia gravis: biology and treatment. *Ann. N.Y. Acad. Sci.* 505:1-914,1987.

Drachman, D.B. Myasthenia gravis. *N. Engl. J. Med.* 330:1797-1810,1994.

Engel, A.G.,(ed). *Myasthenia gravis and Myasthenic syndromes.* New York: Oxford Univ. Press,1999.

Grafstein, B. Axonal transport:function and mechanisms. In: S.G.Waxman, J.D.Kocsis, P.K. Stys (eds). *The Axon:Structure, Function and Pathophysiology,* pp. 185-199. New York:Oxford Univ. Press,1995.

Halata, Z., and Munger, B. L. Identification of the Ruffini corpuscle in human hairy skin. *Cell Tissue Res.* 219:437, 1981.

Hille, B. *Ionic Channels of Excitable Membranes,* 2nd ed. Sunderland, M.A.: Sinauer,1992.

Hodgkin, A. L., and Huxley, A. F. Movement of sodium and potassium ions during nervous activity. *Cold Spring Harbor Symp. Quant. Biol.* 17:43, 1952.

Kelly, R.B. Storage and release of neurotransmitters. *Cell/Neuron* 72/10:43-53,1993.

Kukuljan, M., Labarca, P., Latorre, R. Molecular determinants of ion conduction and inactivation in K+ channels. *Am. J. Physiol.* 268:C535-C556, 1995.

Lemke, G. Myelin and myelination. In: Z.Hall(ed). *An Introduction to Molecular Neurobiology,* pp. 281-312. Sunderland,M.A.: Sinauer,1992.

Lewis, R.A., Selwa, J.F., Lisak, R.P. Myasthenia gravis:immunological mechanisms and immunotherapy. *Ann. Neurol.* 37:(Suppl 1):S51-S62,1995.

Numa, S. Molecular structure and function of acetylcholine receptors and sodium channels. In:S Chien (ed). *Molecular Biology in Physiology,* pp. 93-118. New York: Raven,1989.

Peters, A., Palay, S. L., and Webster, H. *The Fine Structure of the Nervous System:The Neurons and Supporting Cells, 3rd* ed. New York:Oxford Univ. Press,1991.

Rhoades, R. A., and Tanner, G. A. (eds.). *Medical Physiology.* Boston: Little, Brown, 1995.

Risling, M., Dalsgaard, C. J., Cukierman, A., and Cuello, A. C. Electron microscopic and immunohistochemical evidence that unmyelinated ventral root axons make U-turns or enter the spinal pia mater. *J. Comp. Neurol.* 225:53, 1984.

Rothwell, J., *Control of Human Voluntary Movement,* 2nd ed. London: Chapman & Hall,1994.

Seddon, H. J. Three types of nerve injury. *Brain* 66:237, 1944.

Seddon, H. J. *Surgical Disorders of Peripheral Nerves.* Edinburgh and London: Longman, 1972.

Seybold, M.E. Myasthenia gravis: diagnosis and therapeutic perspectives in the 1990s. *Neurologist* 1:345-360,1995.

Siegel, G.J., Agranoff, B.W., Albers, R.W.(eds). *Basic Neurochemistry: Molecular, Cellular, and Medical Aspects,* 6th ed. Philadelphia: Lippincott-Raven,1999.

Snell, R. S., and McIntyre, N. Changes in the histochemical appearances of cholinesterase at the motor end-plate following denervation. *Br. J. Exp. Pathol.* 37:44, 1956.

Snell, R. S. Changes in the histochemical appearances of cholinesterase in a mixed peripheral nerve following nerve section and compression injury. *Br. J. Exp. Pathol.* 38:34, 1957.

Snell, R. S., and Smith, M. S. *Clinical Anatomy for Emergency Medicine.* St. Louis: Mosby, 1993.

Sunderland, S. *Nerves and Nerve Injuries* (2nd ed.). Edinburgh: Churchill Livingstone, 1979.

Swash, M., and Fox, K. P. Muscle spindle innervation in man. *J. Anat.* 112:61, 1972.

Thomas, P. K., and King, R. H. M. The degeneration of unmyelinated axons following nerve section: An ultrastructural study. *J. Neurocytol.* 3:497, 1974.

Tracey, D. J. Joint receptors and the control of movement. *Trends Neurosci.* 2:253, 1980.

Trojaborg, W. Rate of recovery in motor and sensory fibers of the radial nerve: Clinical and electrophysiological aspects. *J. Neurol. Neurosurg. Psychiatry* 33:625, 1970.

Unwin, N. Neurotransmitter action: opening of ligand-gated ion channels. *Cell* 72(Supp.l):31-41,1993.

Veraa, R. P., and Grafstein, B. Cellular mechanisms for recovery from nervous system injury. *Exp. Neurol.* 71:6, 1981.

Westmoreland, B. F., Benarroch, E. E., Daube, J. R., Reagan, T. J., and Sandok, B. A. *Medical Neurosciences* (3rd ed.). Boston: Little, Brown, 1994.

Williams, P. L., et al. *Gray's Anatomy* (38th ed.). Philadelphia: Churchill Livingstone, 1995.

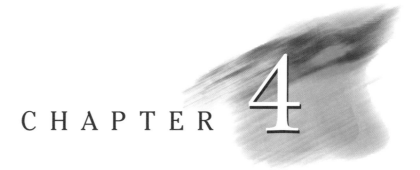

CHAPTER 4

The Spinal Cord and the Ascending and Descending Tracts

A 35-year-old man was galloping his horse when he attempted to jump over a farm gate. His horse refused to jump and he was thrown to the ground. His head struck a log and his head and neck were excessively flexed. On initial evaluation in the emergency department after he had regained consciousness, he was found to have signs and symptoms of severe neurological deficits in the upper and lower extremities. A lateral radiograph of the cervical region of the spine showed fragmentation of the body of the fourth cervical vertebra with backward displacement of a large bony fragment on the left side.

After stabilization of the vertebral column by using skeletal traction to prevent further neurological damage, a complete examination revealed that the patient had signs and symptoms indicating incomplete hemisection of the spinal cord on the left side.

Any medical personnel involved in the evaluation and treatment of a patient with spinal cord injuries must know the structure of the spinal cord and the arrangement and functions of the various nerve tracts passing up and down this vital conduit in the central nervous system. Because of the devastating nature of spinal cord injuries and the prolonged disability that results, it is vital that all concerned with the care of such patients are trained to prevent any additional cord injury and provide the best chance for recovery. All medical personnel must have a clear picture of the extent of the cord lesion and the possible expectations for the return of function.

GROSS APPEARANCE OF THE SPINAL CORD

The spinal cord is roughly cylindrical in shape. It begins superiorly at the foramen magnum in the skull, where it is continuous with the **medulla oblongata** of the brain, and it terminates inferiorly in the adult at the level of the **lower border of the first lumbar vertebra**. In the young child, it is relatively longer and usually ends at the upper border of the third lumbar vertebra. Thus it occupies the upper two-thirds of the **vertebral canal** of the vertebral column and is surrounded by the three meninges, the **dura mater**, the arachnoid mater, and the **pia mater**. Further protection is provided by the **cerebrospinal fluid**, which surrounds the spinal cord in the **subarachnoid space**.

In the cervical region, where it gives origin to the brachial plexus, and in the lower thoracic and lumbar regions, where it gives origin to the lumbosacral plexus, the spinal cord is fusiformly enlarged; the enlargements are referred to as the **cervical and lumbar enlargements** (Fig. 4-1). Inferiorly, the spinal cord tapers off into the **conus medullaris**, from the apex of which a prolongation of the pia mater, the **filum terminale,** descends to be attached to the posterior surface of the coccyx. The cord possesses, in the midline anteriorly, a deep longitudinal fissure, the **anterior median fissure**, and on the posterior surface, a shallow furrow, the **posterior median sulcus** (Fig. 4-1).

Along the entire length of the spinal cord are attached 31 pairs of spinal nerves by the **anterior or motor roots** and the **posterior or sensory roots** (Fig. 4-1). Each root is attached to the cord by a series of rootlets, which extend the whole length of the corresponding segment of the cord.

Each posterior nerve root possesses a **posterior root ganglion**, the cells of which give rise to peripheral and central nerve fibers.

STRUCTURE OF THE SPINAL CORD

The spinal cord is composed of an inner core of gray matter, which is surrounded by an outer covering of white matter (Figs. 4-2 through 4-6); there is no indication that the cord is segmented.

For a comparison of the structural details in different regions of the spinal cord, see Table 4-1.

Gray Matter

On cross section, the gray matter is seen as an H-shaped pillar with **anterior** and **posterior gray columns**, or **horns,** united by a thin **gray commissure** containing the small **central canal** (Fig. 4-2). A small **lateral gray column** or **horn** is present in the thoracic and upper lumbar segments of the cord. The amount of gray matter present at any given level of the spinal cord is related to the amount of muscle innervated at that level. Thus, its size is greatest within the cervical and lumbosacral enlargements of the cord, which innervate the muscles of the upper and lower limbs, respectively (Figs. 4-2 through 4-6).

STRUCTURE

As in other regions of the central nervous system, the gray matter of the spinal cord consists of a mixture of nerve cells and their processes, neuroglia, and blood vessels. The nerve cells are multipolar and the neuroglia forms an intricate network around the nerve cell bodies and their neurites.

Nerve Cell Groups in the Anterior Gray Columns

Most nerve cells are large and multipolar, and their axons pass out in the anterior roots of the spinal nerves as **alpha**

Since much of the early neurobiological research was performed on animals, many investigators refer to the posterior roots and anterior roots as dorsal roots and ventral roots, respectively. This designation results in confusion, especially because, regarding the gray and white matter of the spinal cord in humans, reference is generally made to anterior gray columns, posterior white columns, and so on. For this reason the terminology used for spinal nerve roots in this section will be followed throughout this text.

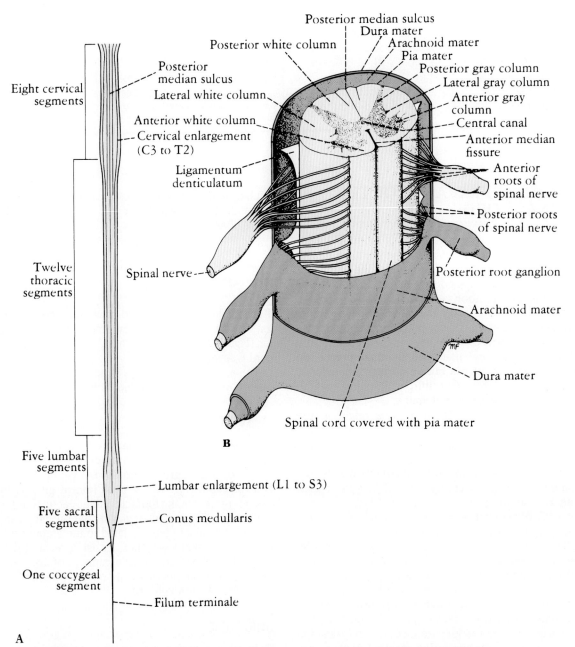

Figure 4–1   Spinal cord. **A.** Posterior view, showing cervical and lumbar enlargements. **B.** Three segments of the spinal cord, showing the coverings of dura mater, arachnoid mater, and pia mater.

			Gray Matter		
Region	Shape	White Matter	Anterior Gray Column	Posterior Gray Column	Lateral Gray Column
Cervical	Oval	Fasciculus cuneatus and fasciculus gracilis present	Medial group of cells for neck muscles; central group of cells for accessory nucleus (C1–5) and phrenic nucleus (C3, 4, and 5); lateral group of cells for upper limb muscles	Substantia gelatinosa present, continuous with Sp.N. of cranial nerve V at level C2; nucleus proprius present; nucleus dorsalis (Clark's column) absent	Absent
Thoracic	Round	Fasciculus cuneatus (T1–6) and fasciculus gracilis present	Medial group of cells for trunk muscles	Substantia gelatinosa, nucleus proprius, nucleus dorsalis (Clark's column), and visceral afferent nucleus present	Present; gives rise to preganglionic sympathetic fibers
Lumbar	Round to oval	Fasciculus cuneatus absent; fasciculus gracicilis present	Medial group of cells for lower limb muscles; central group of cells for lumbosacral nerve	Substantia gelatinosa, nucleus proprius, nucleus dorsalis (Clark's column) at L1–4, and visceral afferent nucleus present	Present (L1–2 [3]); gives rise to preganglionic sympathetic fibers
Sacral	Round	Small amount; fasciculus cuneatus absent; fasciculus gracilis present	Medial group of cells for lower limb and perineal muscles	Substantia gelatinosa and nucleus proprius present	Absent; group of cells present at S2–4, for parasympathetic outflow

Table 4–1 Comparison of Structural Details in Different Regions of the Spinal Cord*

*The information in this table is useful for identifying the specific level of the spinal cord from which a section has been taken.

efferents, which innervate skeletal muscles. The smaller nerve cells are also multipolar and the axons of many of these pass out in the anterior roots of the spinal nerves as **gamma efferents**, which innervate the intrafusal muscle fibers of neuromuscular spindles.

For practical purposes, the nerve cells of the anterior gray column may be divided into three basic groups or columns—medial, central, and lateral (see Fig. 4-2).

The medial group is present in most segments of the spinal cord and is responsible for innervating the skeletal muscles of the neck and trunk, including the intercostal and abdominal musculature.

The central group is the smallest and is present in some cervical and lumbosacral segments (Figs. 4-2 and 4-3). In the cervical part of the cord some of these nerve cells (segments C3, 4, and 5) specifically innervate the diaphragm and are collectively referred to as the phrenic nucleus (Fig. 4-2). In the upper five or six cervical segments, some of the nerve cells innervate the sternocleidomastoid and trapezius

muscles and are referred to as the **accessory nucleus** (Figs. 4-2 and 4-3). The axons of these cells form the spinal part of the accessory nerve. The **lumbosacral nucleus** present in the second lumbar down to the first sacral segment of the cord is made up of nerve cells whose axons have an unknown distribution.

The lateral group is present in the cervical and lumbosacral segments of the cord and is responsible for innervating the skeletal muscles of the limbs (Figs. 4-2, 4-3, 4-5, and 4-6).

Nerve Cell Groups in the Posterior Gray Columns

There are four nerve cell groups of the posterior gray column, two that extend throughout the length of the cord and two that are restricted to the thoracic and lumbar segments.

The **substantia gelatinosa group** is situated at the apex of the posterior gray column throughout the length of the spinal cord (Figs. 4-2 through 4-6). It is largely composed of Golgi type II neurons and receives afferent fibers concerned with pain, temperature, and touch from the posterior root. Furthermore, it receives input from descending fibers from supraspinal levels. It is believed that the inputs of the sensations of pain and temperature are modified by excitatory or inhibitory information from other sensory inputs and by information from the cerebral cortex.

In thick sections of the spinal cord, the gray matter appears to have a laminar (layered) appearance. Rexed (1954) described 10 layers of neurons in the cat spinal cord. This detailed cytoarchitectural lamination is useful for researchers but of little value to the practicing neurologist.

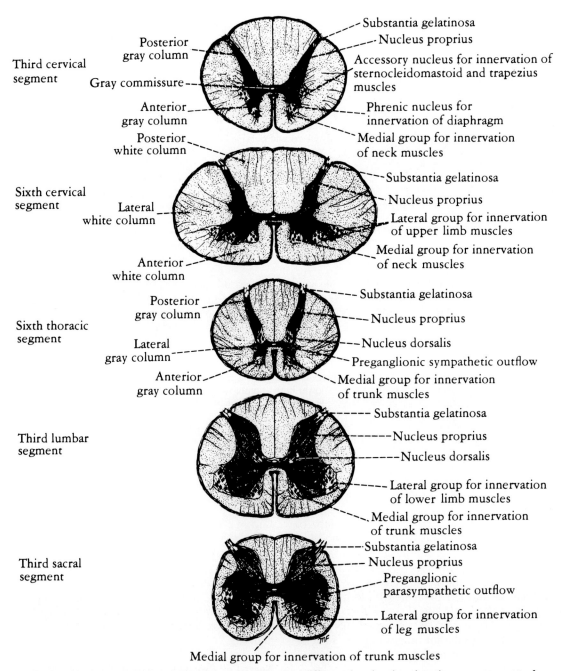

Figure 4–2 Transverse sections of the spinal cord at different levels, showing the arrangement of the gray matter and white matter.

The **nucleus proprius** is a group of large nerve cells situated anterior to the substantia gelatinosa throughout the spinal cord (Figs. 4-2 through 4-6). This nucleus constitutes the main bulk of cells present in the posterior gray column and receives fibers from the posterior white column that are associated with the senses of position and movement (proprioception), two-point discrimination, and vibration.

The **nucleus dorsalis (Clark's column)** is a group of nerve cells situated at the base of the posterior gray column and extending from the eighth cervical segment caudally to the third or fourth lumbar segment (Figs. 4-2, 4-4, and 4-5). Most of the cells are comparatively large and are associated with proprioceptive endings (neuromuscular spindles and tendon spindles).

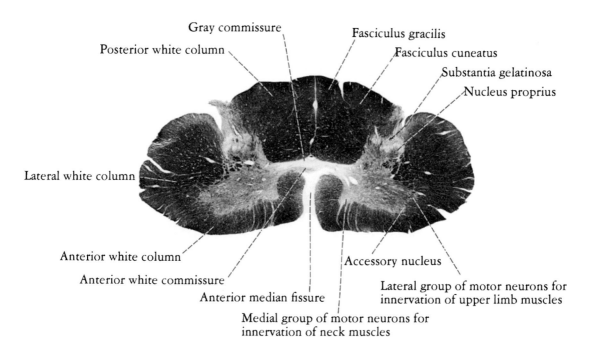

Gray commissure

Posterior white column

Fasciculus gracilis

Fasciculus cuneatus

Substantia gelatinosa

Nucleus proprius

Lateral white column

Anterior white column

Anterior white commissure

Anterior median fissure

Accessory nucleus

Lateral group of motor neurons for
innervation of upper limb muscles

Medial group of motor neurons for
innervation of neck muscles

Figure 4–3   Transverse section of the spinal cord at the level of the fifth cervical segment. (Weigert stain.)

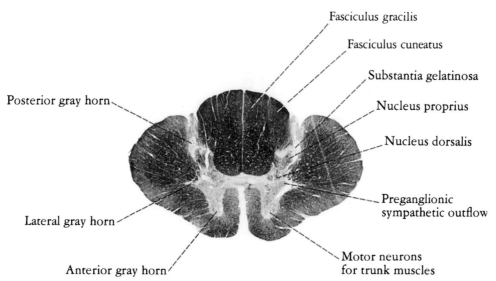

Fasciculus gracilis

Fasciculus cuneatus

Substantia gelatinosa

Nucleus proprius

Nucleus dorsalis

Posterior gray horn

Preganglionic
sympathetic outflow

Lateral gray horn

Motor neurons
for trunk muscles

Anterior gray horn

Figure 4–4   Transverse section of the spinal cord at the level of the second thoracic segment. (Weigert stain.)

The **visceral afferent nucleus** is a group of nerve cells of medium size situated lateral to the nucleus dorsalis; it extends from the first thoracic to the third lumbar segment of the spinal cord. It is believed to be associated with receiving visceral afferent information.

Nerve Cell Groups in the Lateral Gray Columns

The intermediolateral group of cells form the small lateral gray column, which extends from the first thoracic to the second or third lumbar segment of the spinal cord (Figs. 4-2 and 4-4). The cells are relatively small and give rise to preganglionic sympathetic fibers.

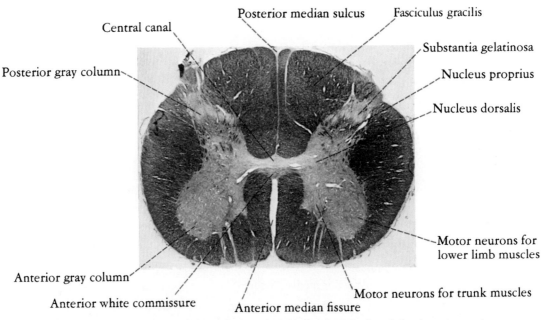

Figure 4–5 Transverse section of the spinal cord at the level of the fourth lumbar segment. (Weigert stain.)

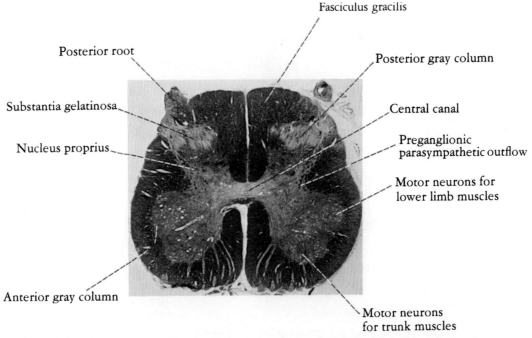

Figure 4–6 Transverse section of the spinal cord at the level of the second sacral segment. (Weigert stain.)

A similar group of cells found in the second, third, and fourth sacral segments of the spinal cord give rise to preganglionic parasympathetic fibers (Figs. 4-2 and 4-6).

The Gray Commissure and Central Canal

In transverse sections of the spinal cord, the anterior and posterior gray columns on each side are connected by a transverse **gray commissure**, so that the gray matter resembles the letter H (Figs. 4-2 through 4-6). In the center of the gray commissure is situated the **central canal**. The part of the gray commissure that is situated posterior to the central canal is often referred to as the **posterior gray commissure**; similarly, the part that lies anterior to the canal is called the **anterior gray commissure**.

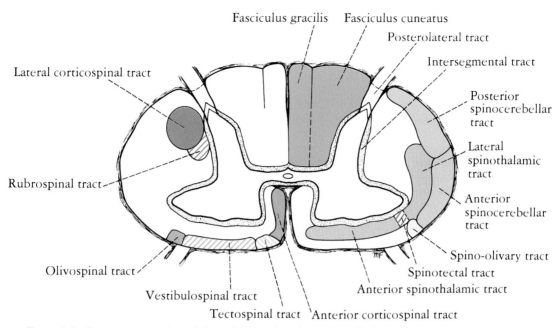

Figure 4–7   Transverse section of the spinal cord at the midcervical level, showing the general arrangement of the ascending tracts on the right and the descending tracts on the left.

The central canal is present throughout the spinal cord (Figs. 4-2 through 4-6). Superiorly, it is continuous with the central canal of the caudal half of the medulla oblongata and above this it opens into the cavity of the fourth ventricle. Inferiorly in the conus medullaris, it expands into the fusiform **terminal ventricle** and terminates below within the root of the filum terminale. It is filled with cerebrospinal fluid and is lined with ciliated columnar epithelium, the **ependyma**. Thus the central canal is closed inferiorly and opens superiorly into the fourth ventricle.

White Matter

The white matter, for purposes of description, may be divided into **anterior**, **lateral**, and **posterior white columns** or **funiculi** (Figs. 4-1 through 4-6). The anterior column on each side lies between the midline and the point of emergence of the anterior nerve roots; the lateral column lies between the emergence of the anterior nerve roots and the entry of the posterior nerve roots; the posterior column lies between the entry of the posterior nerve roots and the midline.

STRUCTURE

As in other regions of the central nervous system, the white matter of the spinal cord consists of a mixture of nerve fibers, neuroglia, and blood vessels. It surrounds the gray matter and its white color is due to the high proportion of myelinated nerve fibers.

Arrangement of Nerve Fiber Tracts

The arrangement of the nerve fiber tracts within the spinal cord has been deduced as the result of animal experimentation and study of the human spinal cord for degenerative nerve fibers resulting from injury or disease. Although some nerve tracts are concentrated in certain areas of the white matter, it is now generally accepted that considerable overlap is present. For purposes of description, the spinal tracts are divided into ascending, descending, and intersegmental tracts and their relative positions in the white matter are described below. A simplified diagram, showing the general arrangement of the major tracts, is shown in Figure 4-7.

THE ASCENDING TRACTS OF THE SPINAL CORD

On entering the spinal cord, the sensory nerve fibers of different sizes and functions are sorted out and segregated into nerve bundles or **tracts** in the white matter(Figs. 4-7 and 4-8). Some of the nerve fibers serve to link different segments of the spinal cord, while others ascend from the spinal cord to higher centers and, thus, connect the spinal cord with the brain. It is the bundles of the ascending fibers that are referred to as the **ascending tracts**.

The ascending tracts conduct afferent information, which may or may not reach consciousness. The information may be divided into two main groups: (1) **exteroceptive** information, which originates from outside the body, such as pain, temperature, and touch, and (2) **propriocep-**

tive information, which originates from inside the body, for example, from muscles and joints.

ANATOMICAL ORGANIZATION

General information from the peripheral sensory endings is conducted through the nervous system by a series of neurons. In its simplest form, the ascending pathway to consciousness consists of three neurons (Fig. 4-8). The first neuron, the **first-order neuron**, has its cell body in the **posterior root ganglion** of the spinal nerve. A peripheral process connects with a sensory receptor ending, whereas

a central process enters the spinal cord through the posterior root to synapse on the second-order neuron. The **second-order neuron** gives rise to an axon that decussates (crosses to the opposite side) and ascends to a higher level of the central nervous system, where it synapses with the **third-order neuron** (Fig. 4-8). The third-order neuron is usually in the thalamus and gives rise to a projection fiber that passes to a sensory region of the cerebral cortex (Fig. 4-8). The three-neuron chain described is the most common arrangement, but some afferent pathways use more or fewer neurons. Many of the neurons in the ascending pathways branch and give a major input into the reticular formation, which in turn activates the cerebral cortex, maintaining wakefulness. Other branches pass to motor neurons and participate in reflex muscular activity.

FUNCTIONS OF THE ASCENDING TRACTS

Painful and thermal sensations ascend in the lateral spinothalamic tract; light (crude) touch and pressure ascend in the anterior spinothalamic tract (Fig. 4-9). Discriminative touch, that is, the ability to localize accurately the area of the body touched and also to be aware that two points are touched simultaneously, even though they are close together (two-point discrimination), ascends in the posterior white columns (Fig. 4-9). Also ascending in the posterior white columns is information from muscles and joints pertaining to movement and position of different parts of the body. In addition, vibratory sensations ascend in the posterior white column. Unconscious information from muscles, joints, the skin, and subcutaneous tissue reaches the cerebellum by way of the anterior and posterior spinocerebellar tracts and by the cuneocerebellar tract (Fig. 4-9). Pain, thermal, and tactile information is passed to the superior colliculus of the midbrain through the spinotectal tract for the purpose of spinovisual reflexes (Fig. 4-9). The spinoreticular tract provides a pathway from the muscles, joints, and skin to the reticular formation, while the spinoolivary tract provides an indirect pathway for further afferent information to reach the cerebellum (Fig. 4-9).

Pain And Temperature Pathways
LATERAL SPINOTHALAMIC TRACT

The pain and thermal receptors in the skin and other tissues are free nerve endings. The pain impulses are transmitted to the spinal cord in fast-conducting delta A-type fibers and slow-conducting C-type fibers. The fast-conducting fibers alert the individual to initial sharp pain, and the slow-conducting fibers are responsible for prolonged burning,

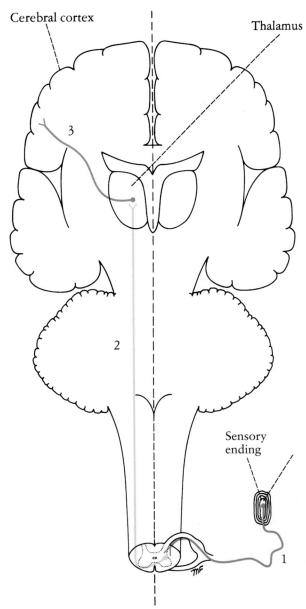

Figure 4–8   Simplest form of the ascending sensory pathway from the sensory nerve ending to the cerebral cortex. Note the three neurons involved.

Many accounts of the ascending tracts now combine the lateral and anterior spinothalamic tracts as one tract since they lie alongside one another; the combined pathway is known as the anterolateral system. The ascending tracts in the posterior white column have also been called the lemniscal system.

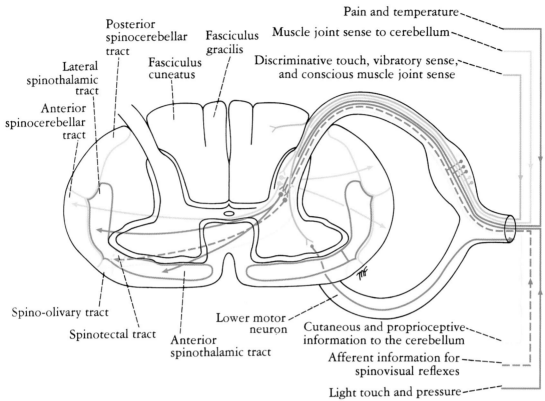

Figure 4–9 Transverse section of the spinal cord, showing the origin of the main ascending sensory tracts. Note that the sensations of pain and temperature ascend in the lateral spinothalamic tract, and light touch and pressure ascend in the anterior spinothalamic tract.

aching pain. The sensations of heat and cold also travel by delta A and C fibers.

The axons entering the spinal cord from the posterior root ganglion proceed to the tip of the posterior gray column and divide into ascending and descending branches (Fig. 4-10). These branches travel for a distance of one or two segments of the spinal cord and form the **posterolateral tract of Lissauer** (Fig. 4-10). These fibers of the first-order neuron terminate by synapsing with cells in the posterior gray column, including cells in the substantia gelatinosa. Substance P, a peptide, is thought to be the neurotransmitter at these synapses.

The axons of the second-order neurons now **cross obliquely to the opposite side in the anterior gray and white commissures within one spinal segment of the cord**, ascending in the contralateral white column as the lateral spinothalamic tract (Fig. 4-10). The lateral spinothalamic tract lies medial to the anterior spinocerebellar tract. As the lateral spinothalamic tract ascends through the spinal cord, new fibers are added to the anteromedial aspect of the tract, so that in the upper cervical segments of the cord the sacral fibers are lateral and the cervical segments are medial. The fibers carrying pain are situated slightly anterior to those conducting temperature.

As the lateral spinothalamic tract ascends through the medulla oblongata, it lies near the lateral surface and between

the inferior olivary nucleus and the nucleus of the spinal tract of the trigeminal nerve. It is now accompanied by the anterior spinothalamic tract and the spinotectal tract; together they form the **spinal lemniscus** (Fig. 4-10).

The spinal lemniscus continues to ascend through the posterior part of the pons (Fig. 4-10). In the midbrain it lies in the tegmentum lateral to the medial lemniscus. Many of the fibers of the lateral spinothalamic tract end by synapsing with the third-order neuron in the ventral posterolateral nucleus of the thalamus (Fig. 4-10). It is believed that here crude pain and temperature sensations are appreciated and emotional reactions are initiated.

The axons of the third-order neurons in the ventral posterolateral nucleus of the thalamus now pass through the posterior limb of the internal capsule and the corona radiata to reach the somesthetic area in the postcentral gyrus of the cerebral cortex (Fig. 4-10). The contralateral half of the body is represented as inverted, with the hand and mouth situated inferiorly and the leg situated superiorly, and with the foot and anogenital region on the medial surface of the hemisphere. (For details, see p. 288 and 289.) From here, the information is transmitted to other regions of the cerebral cortex to be used by motor areas and the parietal association area. The role of the cerebral cortex is interpreting the quality of the sensory information at the level of consciousness.

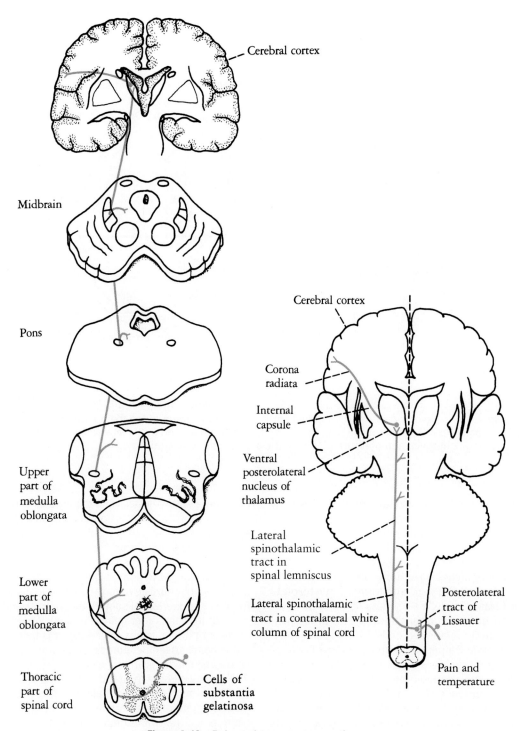

Figure 4–10 Pain and temperature pathways.

Pain Reception

The perception of pain is a complex phenomenon that is influenced by the emotional state and past experiences of the individual. Pain is a sensation that warns of potential injury and alerts the person to avoid or treat it.

Pain can be divided into two main types **fast pain** and **slow pain**. Fast pain is experienced within about 0.1 second after the pain stimulus is applied; slow pain is felt 1 second or later after the stimulation. Fast pain is described by the patient as sharp pain, acute pain, or pricking pain and is the type of pain felt after pricking the finger with a needle. Fast pain is almost confined to the skin.

Slow pain is described as burning pain, aching pain, throbbing pain and is produced when there is tissue destruction, as for example, in the development of an abscess or in severe arthritis. Slow pain can occur in any tissue of the body.

All types of pain reception takes place in free nerve endings. Fast pain is experienced by mechanical or thermal types of stimuli and slow pain may be elicited by mechanical, thermal and chemical stimuli.

Many chemical substances have been found in extracts from damaged tissue that will excite free nerve endings. These include **serotonin, histamine, bradykinin, acids, such as lactic acid, and K ions**. The threshold for pain endings can be lowered by prostaglandins and substance P but they cannot directly by themselves stimulate the endings.

The individual should be aware of the existence of stimuli , that if allowed to persist ,will bring about tissue destruction; pain receptors have little or no adaptation.

CONDUCTION OF PAIN TO THE CENTRAL NERVOUS SYSTEM

Fast pain travels in peripheral nerves in large diameter A delta axons at velocities of between 6 and 30 M/sec. Slow pain travels in the small diameter C fibers at velocities between O.5 and 2 M /sec. The fast pain impulses reach consciousness first to alert the individual to danger so that a suitable protective response may take place. Slow pain is appreciated later and lasts much longer.

CONDUCTION OF PAIN IN THE CENTRAL NERVOUS SYSTEM

The afferent pain fibers enter the spinal cord, for example, in the posterior roots of a spinal nerve and terminate predominantly in the superficial layers of the posterior gray horn. The main excitatory neurotransmitter released by the A delta fibers and the C fibers is the amino acid **glutamate**. Substance P, a neuropeptide, is also released from the C fibers. Whereas, glutamide is a fast acting localized neurotransmitter, substance P has a slow release and diffuses widely in the posterior horn and can influence many neurons.

The initial sharp, pricking, fast acting pain fibers stimulate the second order neurons of the lateral spinothalamic tract. The axons immediately cross to the opposite side of the spinal cord and ascend to the thalamus where they are relayed to the sensory post central gyrus.

The burning, aching, slow acting pain fibers also stimulate the second order neurons of the lateral spinal thalamic tract in the posterior gray horn and ascend with the axons of the fast acting pain fibers. It now believed, however, that most of the incoming slow fibers to the spinal cord take part in additional relays involving several neurons in the posterior horn before ascending in the spinal cord. The repeated

arrival of noxious stimuli through the C fibers in the posterior gray horn during severe injury results in an increased response of the second order neurons. This **winding up** phenomenon is attributed to the release of the neurotransmitter glutamate from the C fibers.

The fast type of pain is precisely localized. For example, if one hits the thumb with a hammer there is no doubt where the injury has occurred. Slow type of pain is only poorly localized. For example, in a patient with osteoarthritis of the hip joint the individual can only vaguely localize the pain to the hip area and not to the specific site of the disease. This may explained by the fact that fast pain fibers directly ascend the spinal cord in the lateral spinothalamic tract whereas the slow pain fibers take part in multiple relays in the posterior gray horn before ascending to higher centers.

OTHER TERMINATIONS OF THE LATERAL SPINOTHALAMIC TRACT

It is now generally agreed that the fast pain impulses travel directly up to the ventral posterolateral nucleus of the thalamus and are then relayed to the cerebral cortex.

The majority of the slow pain fibers in the lateral spinothalamic tract terminate in the reticular formation which then activates the entire nervous system. It is in the lower areas of the brain that the individual becomes aware of the chronic, nauseas, suffering type of pain.

As the result of research using the PET scan, the postcentral gyrus, the cingulate gyrus of the limbic system, and the insular gyrus are sites concerned with the reception and interpretation of the nociceptor information. The postcentral gyrus is responsible for the interpretation of pain in relation to past experiences. The cingulate gyrus is involved with the interpretation of the emotional aspect of pain. Whereas the insular gyrus is concerned with the interpretation of pain stimuli from the internal organs of the body and brings about an autonomic response.

The reception of pain information by the central nervous system can be modulated firstly in the posterior gray horns of the spinal cord and at other sites at higher levels.

Pain Control in the Central Nervous System
THE GATING THEORY

Massage and the application of liniments to painful areas in the body can relieve pain. The technique of acupuncture, which was discovered several thousand years ago in China, is also beneficial in relieving pain. Low-frequency electrical stimulation of the skin also relieves pain in certain cases. Although the precise mechanism for these phenomena is not understood, the gating theory was proposed some years ago. It was suggested that at the site where the pain fiber enters the central nervous system, inhibition could occur by means of connector neurons excited by large, myelinated afferent fibers carrying information of nonpainful touch and pressure. The excess tactile stimulation, produced by massage, for example, "closed the gate" for pain. Once the nonpainful tactile stimulation ceased, however, "the gate was opened" and information on the painful stimuli ascended the lateral spinothalamic tract. Although the gate theory may partially explain the phenomena, the analgesia system is probably involved with the liberation of enkephalins and endorphins in the posterior gray columns.

THE ANALGESIA SYSTEM

Stimulation of certain areas of the brainstem can reduce or block sensations of pain. These areas include the periventricular area of the diencephalon, the periaqueductal gray matter of the midbrain, and midline nuclei of the brainstem. It is believed that fibers of the reticulospinal tract pass down to the spinal cord and synapse on cells concerned with pain sensation in the posterior gray column. The analgesic system can suppress both sharp pricking pain and burning pain sensations.

Recently two compounds with morphine-like actions, called the **enkephalins** and the **endorphins**, have been isolated in the central nervous system. These compounds and serotonin serve as neurotransmitter substances in the analgesic system of the brain and that they may inhibit the release of substance P in the posterior gray column.

Light (Crude) Touch And Pressure Pathways

ANTERIOR SPINOTHALAMIC TRACT

The axons enter the spinal cord from the posterior root ganglion and proceed to the tip of the posterior gray column, where they divide into ascending and descending branches (Fig. 4-11). These branches travel for a distance of one or two segments of the spinal cord, contributing to the posterolateral tract of Lissauer. It is believed that these fibers of the first-order neuron terminate by synapsing with cells in the substantia gelatinosa group in the posterior gray column (Fig. 4-11).

The axons of the second-order neuron now **cross very obliquely to the opposite side in the anterior gray and white commissures within several spinal segments**, and ascend in the opposite anterolateral white column as the anterior spinothalamic tract (Fig. 4-11). As the anterior spinothalamic tract ascends through the spinal cord, new fibers are added to the medial aspect of the tract, so that in the upper cervical segments of the cord the sacral fibers are mostly lateral and the cervical segments are mostly medial.

As the anterior spinothalamic tract ascends through the medulla oblongata, it accompanies the lateral spinothalamic tract and the spinotectal tract, all of which form the **spinal lemniscus** (Fig. 4-11).

The spinal lemniscus continues to ascend through the posterior part of the pons, and the tegmentum of the midbrain and the fibers of the anterior spinothalamic tract terminate by synapsing with the third-order neuron in the ventral posterolateral nucleus of the thalamus (Fig. 4-11). Crude awareness of touch and pressure is believed to be appreciated here.

The axons of the third-order neurons in the ventral posterolateral nucleus of the thalamus pass through the posterior limb of the **internal capsule** (Fig. 4-11) and the **corona radiata** to reach the somesthetic area in the postcentral gyrus of the cerebral cortex. The contralateral half of the body is represented inverted, with the hand and mouth situated inferiorly, as described previously. (For details, see p. 288 and 289.) The conscious appreciation of touch and pressure depends on the activity of the cerebral cortex. The sensations can be only crudely localized, and very little discrimination of intensity is possible.

Discriminative Touch, Vibratory Sense, And Conscious Muscle Joint Sense

POSTERIOR WHITE COLUMN: FASCICULUS GRACILIS AND FASCICULUS CUNEATUS

The axons enter the spinal cord from the posterior root ganglion and pass directly to the posterior white column of the same side (Fig. 4-12). Here the fibers divide into long ascending and short descending branches. The descending branches pass down a variable number of segments, giving off collateral branches that synapse with cells in the posterior gray horn, with internuncial neurons, and with anterior horn cells (Fig. 4-12). It is clear that these short descending fibers are involved with intersegmental reflexes.

The long ascending fibers may also end by synapsing with cells in the posterior gray horn, with internuncial neurons, and with anterior horn cells. This distribution may extend over numerous segments of the spinal cord (Fig. 4-12). As in the case of the short descending fibers, they are involved with intersegmental reflexes.

Many of the long ascending fibers travel upward in the posterior white column as the **fasciculus gracilis** and **fasciculus cuneatus** (Fig. 4-12). The fasciculus gracilis is present throughout the length of the spinal cord and contains the long ascending fibers from the sacral, lumbar, and lower six thoracic spinal nerves. The fasciculus cuneatus is situated laterally in the upper thoracic and cervical segments of the spinal cord and is separated from the fasciculus gracilis by a septum. The fasciculus cuneatus contains the long ascending fibers from the upper six thoracic and all the cervical spinal nerves.

The fibers of the fasciculus gracilis and fasciculus cuneatus ascend **ipsilaterally** and terminate by synapsing on the second-order neurons in the **nuclei gracilis** and **cuneatus** of the medulla oblongata (Fig. 4-12). The axons of the second-order neurons, called the **internal arcuate fibers**, sweep anteromedially around the central gray matter and **cross the median plane**, decussating with the corresponding fibers of the opposite side in the **sensory decussation** (Fig. 4-12). The fibers then ascend as a single compact bundle, the **medial lemniscus**, through the medulla oblongata, the pons, and the midbrain (Fig. 4-12). The fibers terminate by synapsing on the third-order neurons in the ventral posterolateral nucleus of the thalamus.

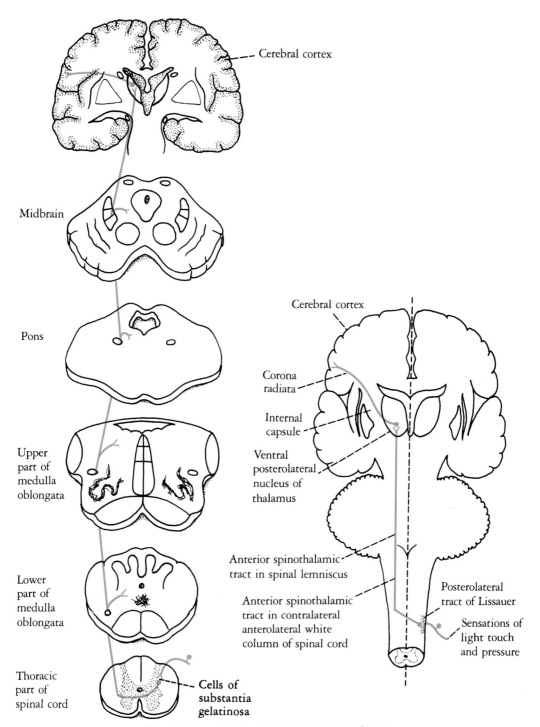

Cerebral cortex

Midbrain

Pons

Upper part of medulla oblongata

Lower part of medulla oblongata

Thoracic part of spinal cord

Cells of substantia gelatinosa

Cerebral cortex

Corona radiata

Internal capsule

Ventral posterolateral nucleus of thalamus

Anterior spinothalamic tract in spinal lemniscus

Anterior spinothalamic tract in contralateral anterolateral white column of spinal cord

Posterolateral tract of Lissauer

Sensations of light touch and pressure

Figure 4–11 Light touch and pressure pathways.

The axons of the third-order neuron leave and pass through the posterior limb of the **internal capsule** and **corona radiata** to reach the somesthetic area in the postcentral gyrus of the cerebral cortex (Fig. 4-12). The contralateral half of the body is represented inverted, with the hand and mouth situated inferiorly, as de-scribed previously. (For details, see p. 288 and 289.) In this manner, the impressions of touch with fine grada-tions of intensity, exact localization, and two-point dis-crimination can be appreciated. Vibratory sense and the position of the different parts of the body can be con-sciously recognized.

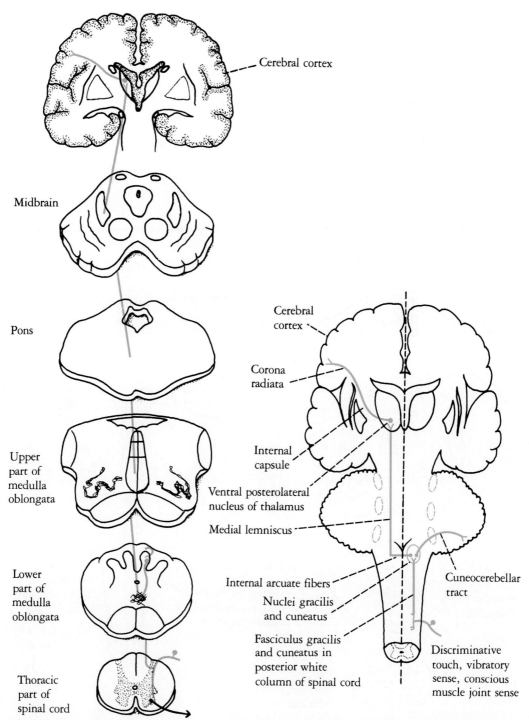

Figure 4–12 Discriminative touch, vibratory sense, and conscious muscle joint sense pathways.

Many fibers in the fasciculus cuneatus from the cervical and upper thoracic segments, having terminated on the second-order neuron of the nucleus cuneatus, are relayed and travel as the axons of the second-order neurons to enter the cerebellum through the inferior cerebellar peduncle of the same side (Fig. 4-12). The pathway is referred to as the **cuneocerebellar tract** and the fibers are known as the **posterior external arcuate fibers**. The function of these fibers is to convey information of muscle joint sense to the cerebellum.

The main somatosensory pathways are summarized in Table 4-2.

Table 4–2 The Main Somatosensory Pathways to Consciousness*

Sensation	Receptor	First-Order Neuron	Second-Order Neuron	Third-Order Neuron	Pathways	Destination
Pain and temperature	Free nerve endings	Posterior root ganglion	Substantia gelatinosa	Ventral posterolateral nucleus of thalamus	Lateral spinothalamic, spinal lemniscus	Post. central gyrus
Light touch and pressure	Free nerve endings	Posterior root ganglion	Substantia gelatinosa	Ventral posterolateral nucleus of thalamus	Anterior spinothalamic, spinal lemniscus	Post. central gyrus
Discriminative touch, vibratory sense, conscious, muscle joint sense	Meissner's corpuscles, pacinian corpuscles, muscle spindles, tendon organs	Posterior root ganglion	Nuclei gracilis and cuneatus	Ventral posterolateral nucleus of thalamus	Fasciculi gracilis and cuneatus, medial lemniscus	Post. central gyrus

*Note that all ascending pathways send branches to the reticular activating system.

Muscle Joint Sense Pathways To The Cerebellum

POSTERIOR SPINOCEREBELLAR TRACT

The axons entering the spinal cord from the posterior root ganglion enter the posterior gray column and terminate by synapsing on the second-order neurons at the base of the posterior gray column (Fig. 4-13). These neurons are known collectively as the **nucleus dorsalis (Clark's column)**. The axons of the second-order neurons enter the posterolateral part of the lateral white column on the **same side** and ascend as the posterior spinocerebellar tract to the medulla oblongata. Here the tract joins the inferior cerebellar peduncle and terminates in the cerebellar cortex (Fig. 4-13). Note that it does not ascend to the cerebral cortex. Because the nucleus dorsalis (Clark's column) extends only from the eighth cervical segment caudally to the third or fourth lumbar segment, axons entering the spinal cord from the posterior roots of the lower lumbar and sacral segments ascend in the posterior white column until they reach the third or fourth lumbar segment, where they enter the nucleus dorsalis.

The posterior spinocerebellar fibers receive muscle joint information, from the muscle spindles, tendon organs, and joint receptors of the trunk and lower limbs. This information concerning tension of muscle tendons and the movements of muscles and joints is used by the cerebellum in the coordination of limb movements and the maintenance of posture.

ANTERIOR SPINOCEREBELLAR TRACT

The axons entering the spinal cord from the posterior root ganglion terminate by synapsing with the second-order neurons in the **nucleus dorsalis** at the base of the posterior gray column (Fig. 4-13). The majority of the axons of the second-order neurons **cross** to the opposite side and ascend as the anterior spinocerebellar tract in the contralateral white column; the minority of the axons ascend as the anterior spinocerebellar tract in the lateral white column of the **same side** (Fig. 4-13). The fibers, having ascended through the medulla oblongata and pons, enter the cerebellum through the superior cerebellar peduncle and terminate in the cerebellar cortex. It is believed that those fibers that crossed over to the opposite side in the spinal cord **cross back** within the cerebellum (Fig. 4-13). The anterior spinocerebellar tract conveys muscle joint information from the muscle spindles, tendon organs, and joint receptors of the trunk and the upper and lower limbs. It is also believed that the cerebellum receives information from the skin and superficial fascia by this tract.

The muscle joint sense pathways to the cerebellum are summarized in Table 4-3.

CUNEOCEREBELLAR TRACT

These fibers have already been described on page 152. They originate in the nucleus cuneatus and enter the cerebellum through the inferior cerebellar peduncle of the **same side** (Fig. 4-12). The fibers are known as the **posterior external arcuate fibers** and their function is to convey information of muscle joint sense to the cerebellum.

Other Ascending Pathways

SPINOTECTAL TRACT

The axons enter the spinal cord from the posterior root ganglion and travel to the gray matter where they synapse on unknown second-order neurons (Fig. 4-14). The axons of the second-order neurons **cross the median plane** and ascend as the spinotectal tract in the anterolateral white column lying close to the lateral spinothalamic tract. After passing through the medulla oblongata and pons, they terminate by synapsing with neurons in the superior colliculus of the

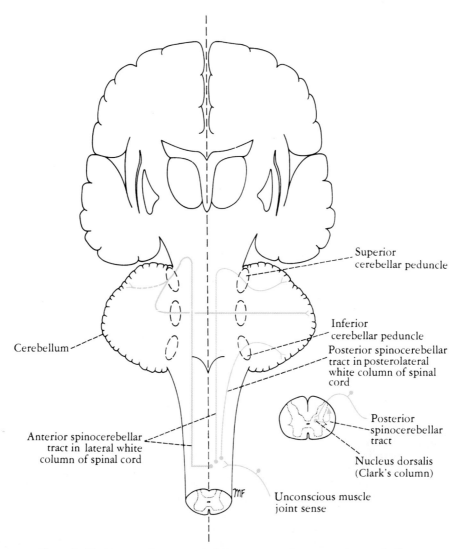

Figure 4–13 Unconscious muscle joint sense pathways to the cerebellum.

		Table 4-3 Muscle Joint Sense Pathways to the Cerebellum			
Sensation	**Receptor**	**First-Order Neuron**	**Second-Order Neuron**	**Pathways**	**Destination**
Unconscious muscle joint sense	Muscle spindles, tendon organs, joint receptors	Posterior root ganglion	Nucleus dorsalis	Anterior and posterior spinocerebellar	Cerebellar cortex

midbrain (Fig. 4-14). This pathway provides afferent information for spinovisual reflexes and brings about movements of the eyes and head toward the source of the stimulation.

SPINORETICULAR TRACT

The axons enter the spinal cord from the posterior root ganglion and terminate on unknown second-order neurons in the gray matter (Fig. 4-14). The axons from these second-order neurons ascend the spinal cord as the spinoreticular tract in the lateral white column mixed with the lateral spinothalamic tract. The majority of the fibers are **uncrossed** and terminate by synapsing with neurons of the reticular formation in the medulla oblongata, pons, and midbrain (Fig. 4-14). The spinoreticular tract provides an afferent pathway for the reticular formation, which plays an important role in influencing levels of consciousness. (For details, see p. 295.)

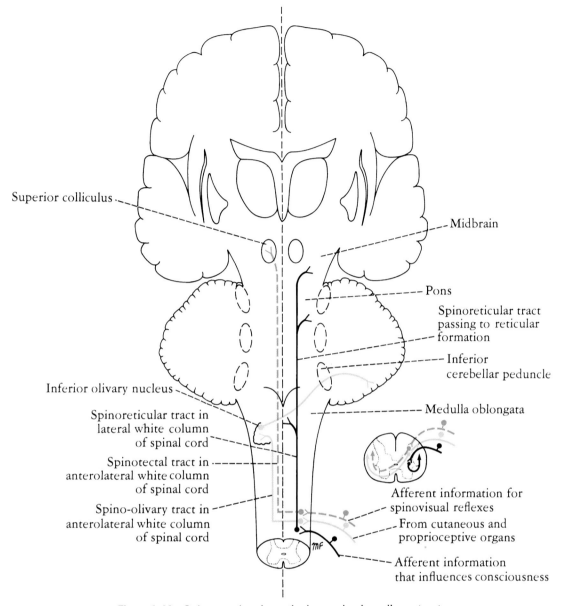

Figure 4–14 Spinotectal, spinoreticular, and spino-olivary tracts.

SPINO-OLIVARY TRACT

The axons enter the spinal cord from the posterior root ganglion and terminate on unknown second-order neurons in the posterior gray column (Fig. 4-14). The axons from the second-order neurons **cross the midline** and ascend as the spino-olivary tract in the white matter at the junction of the anterior and lateral columns. The axons end by synapsing on third-order neurons in the inferior olivary nuclei in the medulla oblongata (Fig. 4-14). The axons of the third-order neurons cross the midline and enter the cerebellum through the inferior cerebellar peduncle. The spinoolivary tract conveys information to the cerebellum from cutaneous and proprioceptive organs.

Visceral Sensory Tracts

Sensations that arise in viscera located in the thorax and abdomen enter the spinal cord through the posterior roots. The cell bodies of the first-order neuron are situated in the posterior root ganglia. The peripheral processes of these cells receive nerve impulses from pain* and stretch receptor endings in the viscera. The central processes, having entered the spinal cord, synapse with second-order neurons

---

*The causes of visceral pain include ischemia, chemical damage, spasm of smooth muscle, and distention.

in the gray matter, probably in the posterior or lateral gray columns.

The axons of the second-order neurons are believed to join the spinothalamic tracts and ascend and terminate on the third-order neurons in the ventral posterolateral nucleus of the thalamus. The final destination of the axons of the third-order neurons is probably in the postcentral gyrus of the cerebral cortex.

Many of the visceral afferent fibers that enter the spinal cord branch participate in reflex activity.

THE DESCENDING TRACTS OF THE SPINAL CORD

The motor neurons situated in the anterior gray columns of the spinal cord send axons to innervate skeletal muscle through the anterior roots of the spinal nerves. These motor neurons are sometimes referred to as the **lower motor neurons** and constitute the final common pathway to the muscles (Fig. 4-15).

The lower motor neurons are constantly bombarded by nervous impulses that descend from the medulla, pons,

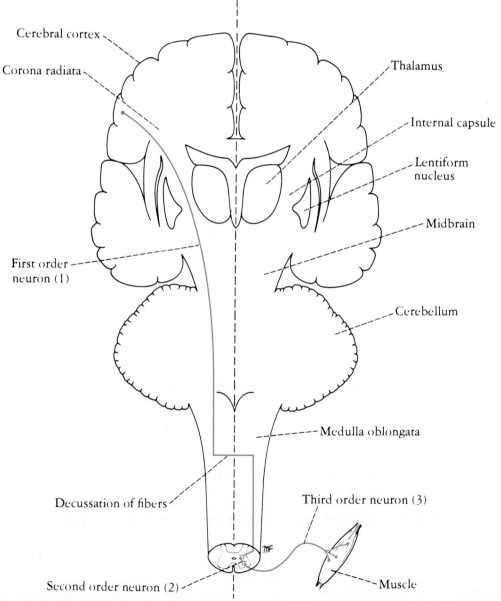

Figure 4–15 Simple form of the descending motor pathway from the cerebral cortex to the skeletal muscle. Note the three neurons involved.

midbrain, and cerebral cortex, as well as those that enter along sensory fibers from the posterior roots. The nerve fibers that descend in the white matter from different supraspinal nerve centers are segregated into nerve bundles called the **descending tracts**. These supraspinal neurons and their tracts are sometimes referred to as the **upper motor neurons** and they provide numerous separate pathways that can influence motor activity.

 ## ANATOMICAL ORGANIZATION

Control of skeletal muscle activity from the cerebral cortex and other higher centers is conducted through the nervous system by a series of neurons (Fig. 4-15). The descending pathway from the cerebral cortex is often made up of three neurons. The first neuron, the **first-order neuron**, has its cell body in the cerebral cortex. Its axon descends to synapse on the **second-order neuron**, an internuncial neuron, situated in the anterior gray column of the spinal cord (Fig. 4-15). The axon of the second-order neuron is short and synapses with the **third-order neuron**, the lower motor neuron, in the anterior gray column (Fig. 4-15). The axon of the third-order neuron innervates the skeletal muscle through the anterior root and spinal nerve. In some instances, the axon of the first-order neuron terminates directly on the third-order neuron (as in reflex arcs).

 ## FUNCTIONS OF THE DESCENDING TRACTS

The **corticospinal tracts** (Fig. 4-16) are the pathways concerned with voluntary, discrete, skilled movements, especially those of the distal parts of the limbs. The **reticulospinal tracts** may facilitate or inhibit the activity of the alpha and gamma motor neurons in the anterior gray columns and may, therefore, facilitate or inhibit voluntary movement or reflex activity. The **tectospinal tract** (Fig. 4-16) is concerned with reflex postural movements in response to visual stimuli. Those fibers that are associated with the sympathetic neurons in the lateral gray column are concerned with the pupillodilation reflex in response to darkness. The **rubrospinal tract** (Fig. 4-16) acts on both the alpha and gamma motor neurons in the anterior gray columns and facilitates the activity of flexor muscles and inhibits the activity of extensor or antigravity muscles. The **vestibulospinal tract** (Fig. 4-16), by acting on the motor neurons in the anterior gray columns, facilitates the activity of the extensor muscles, inhibits the activity of the flexor muscles, and is concerned with the postural activity associated with balance. The **olivospinal tract** (Fig. 4-16) may play a role in muscular activity, but there is doubt that it exists. The **descending autonomic fibers** are concerned with the control of visceral activity.

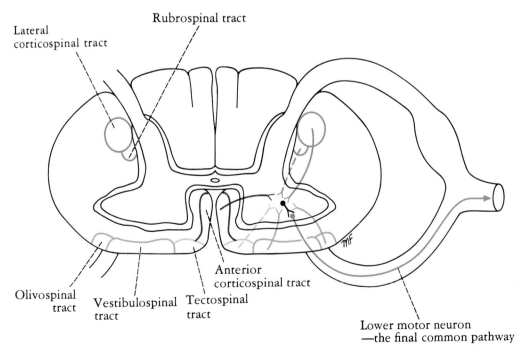

Figure 4–16 Transverse section of the spinal cord, showing the termination of the descending motor tracts. Note that there is now considerable doubt as to the existence of the olivospinal tract as a separate pathway.

CORTICOSPINAL TRACTS

Fibers of the corticospinal tract arise as axons of pyramidal cells situated in the fifth layer of the cerebral cortex (Fig. 4-17). About one-third of the fibers originate from the primary motor cortex (area 4), one-third from the secondary motor cortex (area 6), and one-third from the parietal lobe (areas 3, 1, and 2); thus, two-thirds of the fibers arise from the precentral gyrus and one-third from the postcentral gyrus. *Since electrical stimulation of different parts of the precentral gyrus produces movements of different parts of the

---

*These fibers do not control motor activity but influence sensory input to the nervous system.

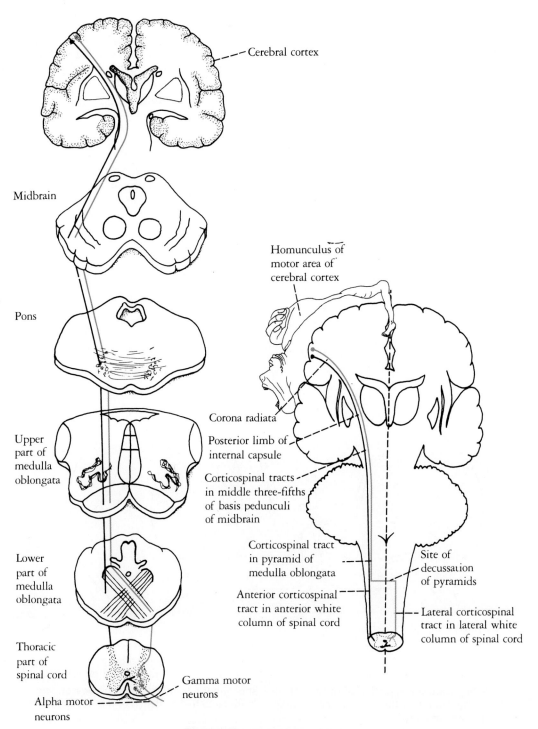

Cerebral cortex

Midbrain

Pons

Homunculus of motor area of cerebral cortex

Corona radiata

Upper part of medulla oblongata

Posterior limb of internal capsule

Corticospinal tracts in middle three-fifths of basis pedunculi of midbrain

Corticospinal tract in pyramid of medulla oblongata

Site of decussation of pyramids

Lower part of medulla oblongata

Anterior corticospinal tract in anterior white column of spinal cord

Lateral corticospinal tract in lateral white column of spinal cord

Thoracic part of spinal cord

Gamma motor neurons

Alpha motor neurons

Figure 4–17   Corticospinal tracts.

opposite side of the body, we can represent the parts of the body in this area of the cortex. Such a homunculus is shown in Figure 4-17. Note that the region controlling the face is situated inferiorly and that controlling the lower limb is situated superiorly and on the medial surface of the hemisphere. The homunculus is a distorted picture of the body, with the various parts having a size proportional to the area of the cerebral cortex devoted to their control. It is interesting to find that the majority of the corticospinal fibers are myelinated and are relatively slow-conducting, small fibers.

The descending fibers converge in the **corona radiata** and then pass through the posterior limb of the **internal capsule** (Fig. 4-17). Here, the fibers are organized so that those closest to the genu are concerned with cervical por-

tions of the body, while those situated more posteriorly are concerned with the lower extremity. The tract then continues through the middle three-fifths of the **basis pedunculi of the midbrain** (Fig. 4-17). Here, the fibers concerned with cervical portions of the body are situated medially, while those concerned with the leg are placed laterally.

On entering the pons, the tract is broken into many bundles by the **transverse pontocerebellar fibers** (see Figs. 5-12, 5-14, and 5-15). In the medulla oblongata, the bundles become grouped together along the anterior border to form a swelling known as the **pyramid** (hence the alternative name, **pyramidal tract**) (see Fig. 5-2). At the junction of the medulla oblongata and the spinal cord, most of the fibers **cross** the midline at the **decussation of the pyra-**

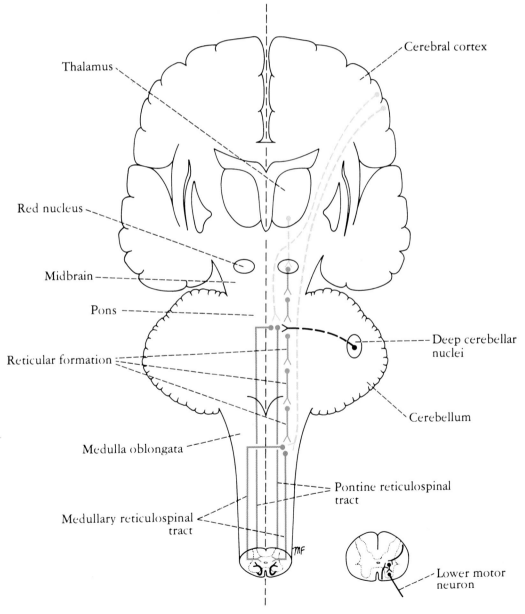

Figure 4–18   Reticulospinal tracts.

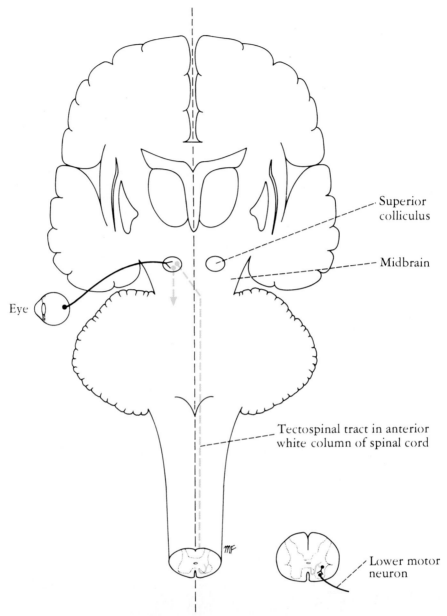

Figure 4–19 Tectospinal tract.

mids (Fig. 4-17) and enter the lateral white column of the spinal cord to form the **lateral corticospinal tract** (Fig. 4-16). The remaining fibers do not cross in the decussation, but descend in the anterior white column of the spinal cord as the **anterior corticospinal tract** (Figs. 4-16 and 4-17). These fibers eventually **cross** the midline and terminate in the anterior gray column of the spinal cord segments in the cervical and upper thoracic regions.

The lateral corticospinal tract descends the length of the spinal cord; its fibers terminate in the anterior gray column of all the spinal cord segments.

Most corticospinal fibers synapse with internuncial neurons, which in turn synapse with alpha motor neurons and some gamma motor neurons. Only the largest corticospinal fibers synapse directly with the motor neurons.

The corticospinal tracts are not the sole pathway for serving voluntary movement. Rather, they form the pathway that confers speed and agility to voluntary movements and is thus used in performing rapid skilled movements. Many of the simple, basic voluntary movements are mediated by other descending tracts.

Branches

1. Branches are given off early in their descent and return to the cerebral cortex to inhibit activity in adjacent regions of the cortex.
2. Branches pass to the caudate and lentiform nuclei, the red nuclei, and the olivary nuclei and the reticular formation. These branches keep the subcortical regions

informed about the cortical motor activity. Once alerted, the subcortical regions may react and send their own nervous impulses to the alpha and gamma motor neurons by other descending pathways.

RETICULOSPINAL TRACTS

Throughout the midbrain, pons, and medulla oblongata, groups of scattered nerve cells and nerve fibers exist that are collectively known as the **reticular formation**. From the pons, these neurons send axons, which are mostly **uncrossed**, down into the spinal cord and form the **pontine reticulospinal tract** (Fig. 4-18). From the medulla, similar neurons send axons, which are crossed and uncrossed, to the spinal cord and form the **medullary reticulospinal tract**.

The reticulospinal fibers from the pons descend through the anterior white column, while those from the medulla oblongata descend in the lateral white column (Fig. 4-18). Both sets of fibers enter the anterior gray columns of the spinal cord and may facilitate or inhibit the activity of the alpha and gamma motor neurons. By this means the reticulospinal tracts influence voluntary movements and reflex activity. The reticulospinal fibers are also now thought to include the descending autonomic fibers. The reticulospinal tracts thus provide a pathway by which the hypothalamus can control the sympathetic outflow and the sacral parasympathetic outflow.

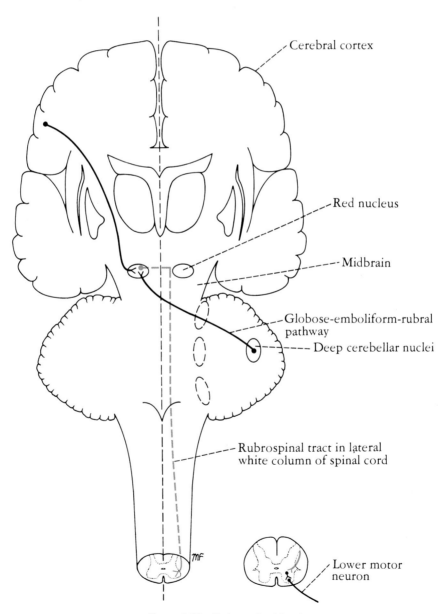

Figure 4–20 Rubrospinal tract.

TECTOSPINAL TRACT

Fibers of this tract arise from nerve cells in the **superior colliculus** of the midbrain (Fig. 4-19). Most of the fibers **cross** the midline soon after their origin and descend through the brainstem close to the **medial longitudinal fasciculus**. The tectospinal tract descends through the anterior white column of the spinal cord close to the anterior median fissure (Figs. 4-16 and 4-19). The majority of the fibers terminate in the anterior gray column in the upper cervical segments of the spinal cord by synapsing with internuncial neurons. These fibers are believed to be concerned with reflex postural movements in response to visual stimuli.

RUBROSPINAL TRACT

The **red nucleus** is situated in the tegmentum of the midbrain at the level of the superior colliculus (Fig. 4-20). The axons of neurons in this nucleus cross the midline at the level of the nucleus and descend as the rubrospinal tract through the pons and medulla oblongata to enter the lateral white column of the spinal cord (Figs. 4-16 and 4-20). The fibers terminate by synapsing with internuncial neurons in the anterior gray column of the cord.

The neurons of the red nucleus receive afferent impulses through connections with the cerebral cortex and the cerebellum. This is believed to be an important indirect pathway by

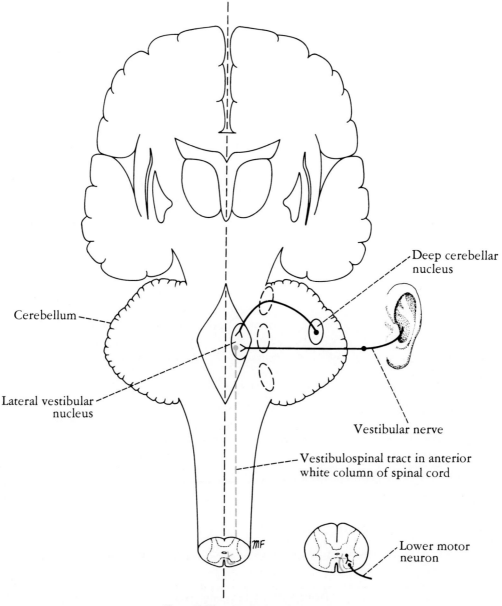

Figure 4–21   Vestibulospinal tract.

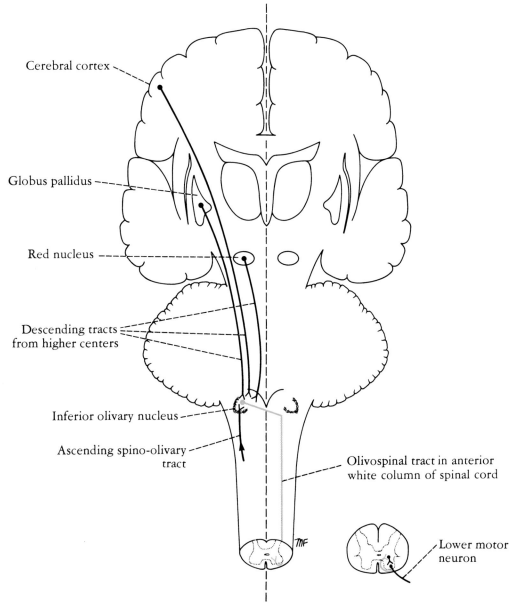

Figure 4–22   Olivospinal tract. There is now considerable doubt as to the existence of this tract as a separate pathway.

which the cerebral cortex and the cerebellum can influence the activity of the alpha and gamma motor neurons of the spinal cord. The tract facilitates the activity of the flexor muscles and inhibits the activity of the extensor or antigravity muscles.

 VESTIBULOSPINAL TRACT

The **vestibular nuclei** are situated in the pons and medulla oblongata beneath the floor of the fourth ventricle (Fig. 4-21). The vestibular nuclei receive afferent fibers from the inner ear through the vestibular nerve and from the cerebellum. The neurons of the lateral vestibular nucleus give rise to the axons that form the vestibulospinal tract. The tract descends **uncrossed** through the medulla and

through the length of the spinal cord in the anterior white column (Figs. 4-16 and 4-21). The fibers terminate by synapsing with internuncial neurons of the anterior gray column of the spinal cord.

The inner ear and the cerebellum, by means of this tract, facilitate the activity of the extensor muscles and inhibit activity of the flexor muscles in association with the maintenance of balance.

OLIVOSPINAL TRACT

The olivospinal tract was thought to arise from the inferior olivary nucleus and to descend in the lateral white column of the spinal cord (Fig. 4-22), to influence the activity of the motor neurons in the anterior gray column. There is now considerable doubt that it exists.

DESCENDING AUTONOMIC FIBERS

The higher centers of the central nervous system associated with the control of autonomic activity are situated in the cerebral cortex, hypothalamus, amygdaloid complex, and reticular formation. Although distinct tracts have not been recognized, investigation of spinal cord lesions has demonstrated that descending autonomic tracts do exist and probably form part of the reticulospinal tract.

The fibers arise from neurons in the higher centers and cross the midline in the brainstem. They are believed to descend in the lateral white column of the spinal cord and to terminate by synapsing on the autonomic motor cells in the lateral gray columns in the thoracic and upper lumbar (sympathetic outflow) and midsacral (parasympathetic) levels of the spinal cord.

A summary of the main descending pathways in the spinal cord is shown in Table 4-4.

INTERSEGMENTAL TRACTS

Short ascending and descending tracts that originate and end within the spinal cord exist in the anterior, lateral, and

Table 4–4   The Main Descending Pathways to the Spinal Cord*

Pathway	Function	Origin	Site of Crossover	Destination	Branches to
Corticospinal tracts	Rapid, skilled, voluntary movements, especially distal ends of limbs	Primary motor cortex (area 4), secondary motor cortex (area 6), parietal lobe (areas 3, 1, and 2)	Most cross at decussation of pyramids and descend as lateral corticospinal tracts; some continue as anterior corticospinal tracts and cross over at level of destination	Internuncial neurons or alpha motor neurons	Cerebral cortex, basal nuclei, red nucleus, olivary nuclei, reticular formation
Reticulospinal tracts	Inhibit or facilitate voluntary movement; hypothalamus controls sympathetic, parasympathetic outflows	Reticular formation	Some cross at various levels	Alpha and gamma motor neurons	Multiple branches as they descend
Tectospinal tract	Reflex postural movements concerning sight	Superior colliculus	Soon after origin	Alpha and gamma motor neurons	?
Rubrospinal tract	Facilitates activity of flexor muscles and inhibits activity of extensor muscles	Red nucleus	Immediately	Alpha and gamma motor neurons	?
Vestibulospinal tract	Facilitates activity of extensor muscles and inhibits flexor muscles	Vestibular nuclei	Uncrossed	Alpha and gamma motor neurons	?
Olivospinal tract	??	Inferior olivary nuclei		? Alpha and gamma motor neurons	—
Descending autonomic fibers	Control sympathetic and parasympathetic systems	Cerebral cortex, hypothalamus, amygdaloid complex, reticular formation	Cross in brainstem	Sympathetic and parasympathetic outflows	—

*Note that the corticospinal tracts are believed to control the prime mover muscles (especially the highly skilled movements), whereas the other descending tracts are important in controlling the simple basic movements.
For simplicity, the internuncial neurons are omitted from this table.

posterior white columns. The function of these pathways is to interconnect the neurons of different segmental levels, and they are particularly important in intersegmental spinal reflexes.

REFLEX ARC

A **reflex** may be defined as an involuntary response to a stimulus. It depends on the integrity of the reflex arc (Fig. 4-23). In its simplest form, a reflex arc consists of the following anatomical structures: (1) a receptor organ, (2) an afferent neuron, (3) an effector neuron, and (4) an effector organ. Such a reflex arc involving only one synapse is referred to as a **mono-**synaptic reflex arc. Interruption of the reflex arc at any point along its course would abolish the response.

In the spinal cord, reflex arcs play an important role in maintaining muscle tone, which is the basis for body posture. The receptor organ is situated in the skin, muscle, or tendon. The cell body of the afferent neuron is located in the posterior root ganglion, and the central axon of this first-order neuron terminates by synapsing on the effector neuron. Since the afferent fibers are of large diameter and are rapidly conducting, and because of the presence of only one synapse, a very quick response is possible.

Physiological study of the electrical activity of the effector neuron shows that following the very quick monosynaptic discharge there is a prolonged asynchro-

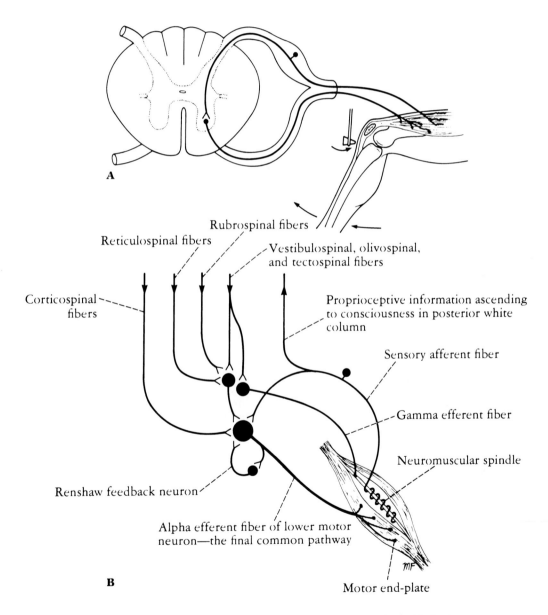

Figure 4–23   A. A monosynaptic reflex arc. B. Multiple neurons synapsing with the lower motor neuron. Note the presence of the Renshaw feedback neuron.

nous discharge. The reason for this later discharge is that the afferent fibers entering the spinal cord frequently branch, and the branches synapse with many internuncial neurons, which ultimately synapse with the effector neuron (Fig. 4-24). These additional neuronal circuits prolong the bombardment of the effector neurons after the initial stimulation by the afferent neuron has ceased. The presence of internuncial neurons also results in the spread of the afferent stimulus to neurons at different segmental levels of the spinal cord.

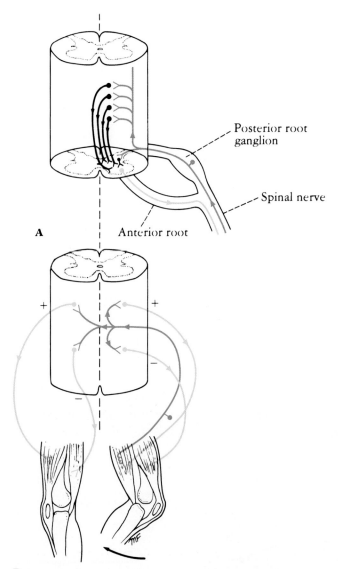

Figure 4–24 A. Multiple branching of afferent fibers entering the spinal cord and the presence of many internuncial neurons that synapse with the effector neuron. B. Law of reciprocal innervation and the crossed extensor reflex.

In considering reflex skeletal muscle activity it is important to understand the **law of reciprocal innervation** (Fig. 4-24). Simply stated, it means that the flexor and extensor reflexes of the same limb cannot be made to contract simultaneously. For this law to work, the afferent nerve fibers responsible for flexor reflex muscle action must have branches that synapse with the extensor motor neurons of the same limb, causing them to be inhibited.

Another interesting property of spinal reflexes should be pointed out. The evocation of a reflex on one side of the body causes opposite effects on the limb of the other side of the body. This **crossed extensor reflex** (Fig. 4-24) may be demonstrated as follows. Afferent stimulation of the reflex arc that causes the ipsilateral limb to flex results in the contralateral limb being extended.

INFLUENCE OF HIGHER NEURONAL CENTERS ON THE ACTIVITIES OF SPINAL REFLEXES

The spinal segmental reflex arc involving motor activity is greatly influenced by higher centers in the brain. These influences are mediated through the corticospinal, reticulospinal, tectospinal, rubrospinal, and vestibulospinal tracts. In the clinical condition known as spinal shock (see p. 172), which follows the sudden removal of these influences by severance of the spinal cord, the segmental spinal reflexes are depressed. When the so-called spinal shock disappears in a few weeks, the segmental spinal reflexes return and the muscle tone is increased. This so-called **decerebrate rigidity** is due to the overactivity of the gamma efferent nerve fibers to the muscle spindles, which results from the release of these neurons from the higher centers (see p. 106 and 107). The next stage may be **paraplegia in extension** with domination of the increased tone of the extensor muscles over the flexor muscles. Some neurologists believe that this condition is due to incomplete severance of all the descending tracts with persistence of the vestibulospinal tract. Should all the descending tracts be severed, the condition of **paraplegia in flexion** occurs. In this condition, the reflex responses are flexor in nature and the tone of the extensor muscles is diminished.

RENSHAW CELLS AND LOWER MOTOR NEURON INHIBITION

Lower motor neuron axons give off collateral branches as they pass through the white matter to reach the anterior roots of the spinal nerve. These collaterals synapse on neurons described by Renshaw, which in turn synapse on the lower motor neurons (Fig. 4-23). These internuncial neurons are believed to provide feedback on the lower motor neurons, inhibiting their activity.

CLINICAL NOTES

GENERAL ANATOMICAL FEATURES OF CLINICAL IMPORTANCE

The spinal cord may be described, for practical purposes, as consisting of columns of motor and sensory nerve cells, the gray matter, surrounded by ascending and descending tracts, the white matter. It lies within the vertebral canal and is protected by three surrounding fibrous membranes, the meninges. It is cushioned against trauma by the cerebrospinal fluid and is held in position by the denticulate ligaments on each side and the filum terminale inferiorly. The spinal cord is segmented, and paired posterior (sensory) and anterior (motor) roots corresponding to each segment of the cord leave the vertebral canal through the intervertebral foramina.

The spinal cord is shorter than the vertebral column and terminates inferiorly in the adult at the level of the lower border of the first lumbar vertebra. The subarachnoid space extends inferiorly beyond the end of the cord and ends at the level of the lower border of the second sacral vertebra.

Because of the shortness of the spinal cord relative to the length of the vertebral column, the nerve roots of the lumbar and sacral segments have to take an oblique course downward to reach their respective intervertebral foramina; the resulting leash of nerve roots forms the cauda equina.

A spinal tap needle may be inserted into the subarachnoid space below the level of the second lumbar vertebra without damaging the spinal cord. (For details, see p. 18.)

LESIONS OF THE ANTERIOR AND POSTERIOR NERVE ROOTS

Each nerve root has a covering of pia, arachnoid, and dura mater. The anterior and posterior roots unite in the intervertebral foramina to form the spinal nerves. Here the meninges fuse with the epineurium of the spinal nerves. Either or both spinal nerve roots may be involved in syphilitic spinal meningitis or pyogenic meningitis. The posterior roots may be involved in tabes dorsalis and herpes zoster. Their anatomical location, both in the vertebral canal and in the intervertebral foramina, exposes them to compression from tumors of the vertebral column and to irritation from abnormal constituents of the cerebrospinal fluid, such as blood following a subarachnoid hemorrhage. A herniated intervertebral disc, a primary or secondary vertebral tumor, vertebral destruction by tumor or infection, or a fracture dislocation can press upon the spinal nerve roots in the intervertebral foramina. Even severe scoliosis may result in compression of the nerve roots.

A lesion of one posterior spinal nerve root will produce pain in the area of skin innervated by that root, and also in the muscles that receive their sensory nerve supply from that root. Movements of the vertebral column in the region of the lesion will heighten the pain, and coughing and sneezing will also make it worse by raising the pressure within the vertebral canal. Before there is actual loss of sensation in the dermatome, there may be evidence of hyperalgesia and hyperesthesia.

A lesion of an anterior root will result in paralysis of any muscle that is supplied exclusively by that root and a partial paralysis of any muscle that is supplied partially by that root. In both cases, fasciculation and muscle atrophy occur.

Clinical Significance of Lamination of The Ascending Tracts

Within the anterolateral white column of the spinal cord, the axons of the spinothalamic tracts from the sacral and lumbar segments of the body are deflected laterally by axons crossing the midline at successively higher levels. Within the posterior white column, the axons from the sacral and lumbar segments of the body are pushed medially by the axons from higher segments of the body. This deflection of the tracts produces lamination, so that in the spinothalamic tracts (anterolateral system) the cervical to sacral segments are located from medial to lateral and in the posterior white column (medial lemniscus system), the sacral to cervical segments are located from medial to lateral. This is shown diagrammatically in Figure 4-25.

This detailed information is of practical value in patients in whom there is external pressure exerted on the spinal cord in the region of the spinothalamic tracts. It explains, for example, why they will first experience a loss of pain and temperature sensations in the sacral dermatomes of the body and, if the pressure increases, the other higher segmental dermatomes of the body will be affected.

INJURY TO THE ASCENDING TRACTS WITHIN THE SPINAL CORD

Lateral Spinothalamic Tract

Destruction of this tract produces contralateral loss of pain and thermal sensibilities below the level of the lesion. The patient will not, therefore, respond to pinprick or recognize hot and cold objects placed in contact with the skin.

Anterior Spinothalamic Tract

Destruction of this tract produces contralateral loss of light touch and pressure sensibilities below the level of the lesion. Remember that discriminative touch will still be present, because this information is conducted through the fasciculus gracilis and fasciculus cuneatus. The patient will not feel the light touch of a piece of cotton placed against the skin or feel pressure from a blunt object placed against the skin.

Fasciculus Gracilis and Fasciculus Cuneatus

Destruction of these tracts cuts off the supply of information from the muscles and joints to consciousness; thus, the individual does not know about the position and move-

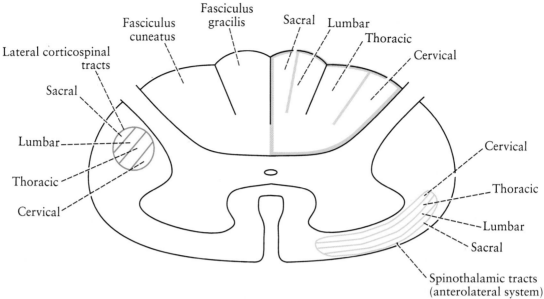

Figure 4–25 Segmental organization of the tracts in the posterior, lateral, and anterior white columns of the spinal cord.

ments of the ipsilateral limbs below the level of the lesion. With the patient's eyes closed, he or she is unable to tell where the limb or part of the limb is in space. For example, if you passively dorsiflex the patient's big toe, he or she is unable to tell you whether the toe is pointing upward or downward. The patient has impaired muscular control and the movements are jerky or ataxic.

The patient also has loss of vibration sense below the level of the lesion on the same side. This is easily tested by applying a vibrating tuning fork to a bony prominence such as the lateral malleolus of the fibula or the styloid process of the radius.

There will also be a loss of tactile discrimination on the side of the lesion. This is tested most easily by gradually separating the two points of a compass until the patient can appreciate them as two separate points, not as one, when they are applied to the skin surface. Tactile discrimination varies from one part of the body to another. In a normal individual, the points have to be separated by about 3 to 4 mm before they are recognized as separate points on the tips of the fingers. On the back, however, the points have to be separated by 65 mm or more before they can be recognized as separate points.

The sense of general light touch would be unaffected, because these impulses ascend in the anterior spinothalamic tracts.

It should be pointed out that it is extremely rare for a lesion of the spinal cord to be so localized as to affect one sensory tract only. It is more usual to have several ascending and descending tracts involved.

SOMATIC AND VISCERAL PAIN

Somatic pain has been considered extensively in this chapter. The sense organs for somatic pain are the naked nerve endings. The initial sharp pain is transmitted by fastconducting fibers and the more prolonged burning pain travels in the slow-conducting nerve fibers (see p. 149).

In the viscera, there are special receptors, chemoreceptors, baroreceptors, osmoreceptors, and stretch receptors that are sensitive to a variety of stimuli including ischemia, stretching, and chemical damage. Afferent fibers from the visceral receptors reach the central nervous system via the sympathetic and parasympathetic parts of the autonomic nervous system. Once within the central nervous system, the pain impulses travel by the same ascending tracts as does the somatic pain and ultimately reach the postcentral gyrus.

Visceral pain is poorly localized and often associated with salivation, nausea, vomiting, tachycardia, and sweating. Visceral pain may be referred from the organ involved to a distant area of the body **(referred pain).**

TREATMENT OF ACUTE PAIN

Drugs such as salicylates can be used to reduce the synthesis of prostaglandin, a substance that sensitizes free nerve endings to painful stimuli. Local anesthetics such as procaine can be used to block nerve conduction in peripheral nerves.

Narcotic analgesics such as morphine and codeine reduce the affective reaction to pain and act on the opiate receptor sites in the cells in the posterior gray column of the spinal cord, as well as other cells in the analgesic system in the brain. It is believed that opiates act by inhibiting the release of glutamate, substance P, and other transmitters from the sensory nerve endings. To minimize the side effects of morphine given by systemic injection, the narcotic can be given by local injection directly into the posterior gray horn of the spinal cord or by injection indirectly into the cerebrospinal fluid in the subarachnoid space. Long term

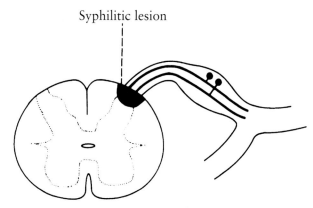

Syphilitic lesion

Figure 4–26 Site of a syphilitic lesion on the spinal cord.

cancer pain has been treated successfully by the continuous infusion of morphine into the spinal cord.

TREATMENT OF CHRONIC PAIN

New techniques, such as acupuncture and electrical stimulation of the skin, are now being used with success. Relief of pain can be achieved by the use of placebos in a few patients. The anticipation of the relief of pain is thought to stimulate the release of endorphins, which inhibit the normal pain pathway.

RELIEF OF PAIN BY RHIZOTOMY OR CORDOTOMY

Surgical relief of pain has been used extensively in patients with terminal cancer. Posterior rhizotomy or division of the posterior root of a spinal nerve effectively severs the conduction of pain into the central nervous system. It is a relatively simple procedure, but, unfortunately, the operation deprives the patient of other sensations besides pain. Moreover, if the pain sensation is entering the spinal cord through more than one spinal nerve, it may be necessary to divide several posterior roots.

Thoracic cordotomy has been performed with success in patients with severe pain originating from the lower abdomen or pelvis. Essentially, the operation consists of dividing the lateral spinothalamic tracts by inserting a knife into the anterolateral quadrant of the spinal cord. It is important to remember that the lateral spinothalamic fibers have originated in cells of the substantia gelatinosa in the opposite posterior gray column, and that they cross the spinal cord obliquely and reach their tract in the white column three or four segments higher than their posterior root of entry. Cervical cordotomy has been performed successfully in patients with intractable pain in the neck or thorax.

TABES DORSALIS

Tabes dorsalis is caused by syphilis. The organism causes a selective destruction of nerve fibers at the point of entrance of the posterior root into the spinal cord, especially in the lower thoracic and lumbosacral regions (Fig. 4-26).

The following symptoms and signs may be present: (1) stabbing pains in the lower limbs, which may be very severe; (2) paresthesia, with numbness in the lower limbs; (3) hypersensitivity of skin to touch, heat, and cold; (4) loss of sensation in the skin of parts of the trunk and lower limbs and loss of awareness that the urinary bladder is full; (5) loss of appreciation of posture or passive movements of the limbs, especially the legs; (6) loss of deep pain sensation, such as when the muscles are forcibly compressed or when the tendo Achillis is compressed between the finger and thumb; (7) loss of pain sensation in the skin in certain areas of the body, such as the side of the nose or the medial border of the forearm, or the thoracic wall between the nipples, or the lateral border of the leg; (8) ataxia of the lower limbs as the result of loss of proprioceptive sensibility (the unsteadiness in gait is compensated to some extent by vision; however, in the dark, or if the eyes are closed, the ataxia becomes worse and the person may fall); (9) hypotonia as the result of loss of proprioceptive information that arises from the muscles and joints; and (10) loss of tendon reflexes, owing to degeneration of the afferent fiber component of the reflex arc (the knee and ankle tendon jerks are lost early in the disease).

MUSCLE ACTIVITY

Muscle Tone

Muscle tone is a state of continuous partial contraction of a muscle and is dependent on the integrity of a monosynaptic reflex arc (see description on p. 106 and 107). The receptor organs are the muscle spindles. The afferent neuron enters the spinal cord through the posterior root and synapses with the effector neuron or lower motor neuron in the anterior gray column. The lower motor neuron supplies the muscle fibers by traveling through the anterior roots, the spinal nerves, and peripheral nerves. Muscle tone is abolished if any part of that simple reflex arc is destroyed. An atonic muscle feels soft and flabby and atrophies rapidly.

Normal muscle tone exhibits a certain resilience or elasticity, and when a muscle is passively stretched by moving a joint, a certain degree of resistance is felt. Normal muscle tone depends on the integrity of the monosynaptic reflex arc described above, and the control superimposed on it by impulses received through the descending tracts from supraspinal levels. Note that muscle spindles are excitatory to muscle tone, whereas neurotendinous receptors are inhibitory to muscle tone.

Voluntary Movement

Voluntary movement is initiated by the individual. A series of different muscles are made to contract for the purpose of reaching a goal. This would suggest that the descending tracts that influence the activity of the lower motor neurons are driven by information received by the sensory systems, the eyes, the ears, and the muscles themselves, and are affected further by past afferent information that has been stored in the memory. Moreover, the whole process may be colored by past and present emotional input. The limbic structures appear to play a role in emotion, motivation, and memory and they may influence the initiation process of voluntary movement by their projections to the cerebral cortex.

The descending pathways from the cerebral cortex and the brainstem, that is, the upper motor neurons, influence the activity of the lower motor neurons either directly or through internuncial neurons. Most of the tracts originating in the brainstem that descend to the spinal cord also are receiving input from the cerebral cortex.

The corticospinal tracts are believed to control the prime mover muscles, especially those responsible for the highly skilled movements of the distal parts of the limbs. The other supraspinal descending tracts play a major role in the simple basic voluntary movements, and in addition bring about an adjustment of the muscle tone, so that easy and rapid movements of the joints can take place.

It is interesting to note that the basal ganglia and the cerebellum do not give rise directly to descending tracts that influence the activities of the lower motor neuron, and yet these parts of the nervous system greatly influence voluntary movements. This influence is accomplished indirectly by fibers that project to the cerebral cortex and brainstem nuclei, which are the sites of origin of the descending tracts.

Pyramidal And Extrapyramidal Tracts

The term **pyramidal tract** is used commonly by clinicians and refers specifically to the corticospinal tracts. The term came into common usage when it was learned that the corticospinal fibers become concentrated on the anterior part of the medulla oblongata in an area referred to as the **pyramids**.

The term **extrapyramidal tracts** refers to all the descending tracts other than the corticospinal tracts.

UPPER MOTOR NEURON LESIONS

Lesions Of The Corticospinal Tracts (Pyramidal Tracts)

Lesions restricted to the corticospinal tracts produce the following clinical signs:

1. The **Babinski sign** is present. The great toe becomes dorsally flexed and the other toes fan outward in response to scratching the skin along the lateral aspect of the sole of the foot. The normal response is plantar flexion of all the toes. Remember that the Babinski sign normally is present during the first year of life, because the corticospinal tract is not myelinated until the end of the first year of life.

The explanation for the Babinski response is thought to be the following. Normally, the corticospinal tracts produce plantar flexion of the toes in response to sensory stimulation of the skin of the sole. When the corticospinal tracts are nonfunctional, the influence of the other descending tracts on the toes becomes apparent, and a kind of withdrawal reflex takes place in response to stimulation of the sole, with the great toe being dorsally flexed and the other toes fanning out.

2. The **superficial abdominal reflexes** are absent. The abdominal muscles fail to contract when the skin of the abdomen is scratched. This reflex is dependent on the integrity of the corticospinal tracts, which exert a tonic excitatory influence on the internuncial neurons.

3. The **cremasteric reflex** is absent. The cremaster muscle fails to contract when the skin on the medial side of the thigh is stroked. This reflex arc passes through the first lumbar segment of the spinal cord. This reflex is dependent on the integrity of the corticospinal tracts, which exert a tonic excitatory influence on the internuncial neurons.

4. There is **loss of performance of fine skilled voluntary movements**. This occurs especially at the distal end of the limbs.

Lesions of the Descending Tracts Other Than the Corticospinal Tracts (Extrapyramidal Tracts)

The following clinical signs are present in lesions restricted to the other descending tracts:

1. **Severe paralysis** with little or no muscle atrophy (except secondary to disuse).
2. **Spasticity** or **hypertonicity** of the muscles. The lower limb is maintained in extension and the upper limb is maintained in flexion.
3. **Exaggerated deep muscle reflexes** and clonus may be present in the flexors of the fingers, the quadriceps femoris, and the calf muscles.
4. **Clasp-knife reaction**. When passive movement of a joint is attempted, there is resistance owing to spasticity of the muscles. The muscles, on stretching, suddenly give way due to neurotendinous organ-mediated inhibition.

It should be pointed out that in clinical practice it is rare to have an organic lesion that is restricted only to the pyramidal tracts, or only to the extrapyramidal tracts. Usually, both sets of tracts are affected to a variable extent, producing both groups of clinical signs. As the pyramidal tracts normally tend to increase muscle tone and the extrapyramidal tracts inhibit muscle tone, the balance between these opposing effects will be altered, producing different degrees of muscle tone.

LOWER MOTOR NEURON LESIONS

Trauma, infection (poliomyelitis), vascular disorders, degenerative diseases, and neoplasms may all produce a lesion of the lower motor neuron by destroying the cell body in the anterior gray column or its axon in the anterior root or spinal nerve. The following clinical signs are present with lower motor neuron lesions:

1. **Flaccid paralysis** of muscles supplied.
2. **Atrophy** of muscles supplied.
3. **Loss of reflexes** of muscles supplied.
4. **Muscular fasciculation**. This is twitching of muscles seen only when there is slow destruction of the lower motor neuron cell.
5. **Muscular contracture**. This is a shortening of the paralyzed muscles. It occurs more often in the antagonist muscles whose action is no longer opposed by the paralyzed muscles.
6. **Reaction of degeneration**. Normally innervated muscles respond to stimulation by the application of faradic (interrupted) current and the contraction continues as long as the current is passing. Galvanic or direct current causes contraction only when the current is turned on or turned off. When the lower motor neuron is cut, a muscle will no longer respond to interrupted electrical stimulation 7 days after nerve section, although it still will respond to direct current. After 10 days, the response to direct current also ceases. This change in muscle response to electrical stimulation is known as the **reaction of degeneration**.

TYPES OF PARALYSIS

Hemiplegia is a paralysis of one side of the body and includes the upper limb, one side of the trunk, and the lower limb.

Monoplegia is a paralysis of one limb only.

Diplegia is a paralysis of two corresponding limbs (i.e., arms or legs).

Paraplegia is a paralysis of the two lower limbs.

Quadriplegia is a paralysis of all four limbs.

RELATIONSHIP OF MUSCULAR SIGNS AND SYMPTOMS TO LESIONS OF THE NERVOUS SYSTEM

Abnormal Muscle Tone

HYPOTONIA

This condition exists when the muscle tone is diminished or absent. It occurs when any part of the monosynaptic stretch reflex arc is interrupted. It also occurs in cerebellar disease as the result of diminished influence on the gamma motor neurons from the cerebellum.

HYPERTONIA (SPASTICITY, RIGIDITY)

This condition exists when the muscle tone is increased. It occurs when lesions exist that involve supraspinal centers or their descending tracts but *not* the corticospinal tract. It also may occur at the local spinal segmental level and be produced by local excitation of the stretch reflex by sensory irritation (e.g., spasm of back muscles secondary to prolapsed intervertebral disc, spasm of abdominal muscles secondary to peritonitis).

TREMORS

Tremors are rhythmic involuntary movements that result from the contraction of opposing muscle groups. These may be slow, as in **parkinsonism**, or fast, as in toxic tremors from thyrotoxicosis. They may occur at rest, as in parkinsonism, or with action, the so-called intention tremor, as seen in cerebellar disease.

SPASMS

Spasms are sudden involuntary contractions of large groups of muscles. Examples of spasms are seen in paraplegia and are due to lesions involving the descending tracts but not the corticospinal tract.

ATHETOSIS

Athetosis means continuous, slow, involuntary, dysrhythmic movements that are always the same in the same patient and disappear during sleep. They impede voluntary movement. Athetosis occurs with lesions of the corpus striatum.

CHOREA

Chorea consists of a series of continuous, rapid, involuntary, jerky, coarse, purposeless movements, which may occur during sleep. Chorea occurs with lesions of the corpus striatum.

DYSTONIA

Dystonia consists of frequent, maintained contractions of hypertonic muscles, leading to bizarre postures. It occurs with lesions of the lentiform nucleus.

MYOCLONUS

Myoclonus is a sudden contraction of an isolated muscle or part of a muscle. It occurs irregularly and commonly involves a muscle of a limb. It may be present with diseases that involve the reticular formation and the cerebellum. Normal myoclonic jerks sometimes occur in individuals as they are falling asleep and are believed to be due to a sudden temporary reactivation of the reticular formation.

HEMIBALLISMUS

Hemiballismus is a rare form of involuntary movement confined to one side of the body. It usually involves the proximal extremity musculature and the limb involved is made to fly about in all directions. The lesion responsible occurs in the opposite subthalamic nucleus.

SPINAL CORD INJURIES

Acute Spinal Cord Injuries

The incidence of acute spinal cord injuries in the United States is about 10,000 per year. The injury is catastrophic, since little or no regeneration of the severed nerve tracts takes place (see p. 114) and the individual is permanently disabled. Treatment has been restricted to anatomical realignment and stabilization of the vertebral column or decompression of the spinal cord. During the recovery process the patient goes through intensive rehabilitation to optimize the remaining neurological function. Apart from improved management of medical complications, very little new therapy has been successful in spite of an enormous amount of research into the problem of neuronal regeneration in the spinal cord. Recently, the use of certain drugs (GM₁ ganglioside and methylprednisolone) administered to the patient soon after injury has resulted in some improvement in the neurological deficit. Animal experiments appear to indicate that these drugs enhance the functional recovery of damaged neurons.

CHRONIC COMPRESSION OF THE SPINAL CORD

If injuries to the spinal cord are excluded (see p. 16), the causes of compression may be divided into extradural and intradural. The intradural causes may be divided into those that arise outside the spinal cord (extramedullary) and those that arise within the cord (intramedullary).

The extradural causes include herniation of an intervertebral disc, infection of the vertebrae with tuberculosis, and primary and secondary tumors of the vertebra; leukemic deposits and extradural abscesses may also compress the spinal cord. The two common extramedullary tumors are meningiomas and nerve fibromas. Intramedullary causes include primary tumors of the spinal cord, such as gliomas.

The clinical signs and symptoms are produced by an interference with the normal anatomical and physiological functions of the spinal cord. Pressure on the spinal arteries causes ischemia of the spinal cord with degeneration of nerve cells and their fibers. Pressure on the spinal veins causes edema of the spinal cord with interference in the function of the neurons. Finally, direct pressure on the white and gray matter of the spinal cord and the spinal nerve roots interferes with nerve conduction. At the same time, the circulation of the cerebrospinal fluid is obstructed, and the composition of the fluid changes below the level of obstruction.

Clinical Signs

One of the earliest signs is pain. This may be local pain in the vertebra involved or pain radiating along the distribution of one or more spinal nerve roots. The pain is made worse by coughing or sneezing and is usually worse at night, when the patient is recumbent.

Interference with motor function occurs early. Involvement of the anterior gray column motor cells at the level of the lesion results in partial or complete paralysis of muscles, with loss of tone and muscle wasting. The early involvement of the corticospinal and other descending tracts produces muscular weakness, increased muscle tone (spasticity), increased tendon reflexes below the level of the lesion, and an extensor plantar response. The degree of sensory loss will depend on the nerve tracts involved. A lesion of the posterior white columns of the spinal cord will cause loss of muscle joint sense (proprioception), vibration sense, and tactile discrimination below the level of the lesion on the same side. Involvement of the lateral spinal thalamic tracts will cause loss of pain and heat and cold sensations on the opposite side of the body below the level of the lesion. A more detailed discussion of the symptoms and signs following injury to the ascending and descending tracts in the spinal cord is given on pp. 167.

Since many spinal tumors are benign and can be successfully removed (provided that irreversible damage to the

spinal cord has not occurred as a result of compression of the blood supply), an early accurate diagnosis is essential. The following investigations should be performed: (1) radiography of the vertebral column, including CT and MRI; (2) spinal tap; and in cases where the making of the diagnosis is difficult(3) myelography.

CLINICAL SYNDROMES AFFECTING THE SPINAL CORD

Spinal Shock Syndrome

This clinical condition follows acute severe damage to the spinal cord. All cord functions below the level of the lesion become depressed or lost and sensory impairment and a flaccid paralysis occur. The segmental spinal reflexes are depressed due to the removal of influences from the higher centers that are mediated through the corticospinal, reticulospinal, tectospinal, rubrospinal, and vestibulospinal tracts. Spinal shock, especially when the lesion is at a high level of the cord, may also cause severe hypotension from loss of sympathetic vasomotor tone.

In most patients the shock persists for less than 24 hours, whereas in others it may persist for as long as 1 to 4 weeks. As the shock diminishes, the neurons regain their excitability and the effects of the upper motor neuron loss on the segments of the cord below the lesion, for example, spasticity and exaggerated reflexes, will make their appearance.

The presence of spinal shock can be determined by testing for the activity of the anal sphincter reflex. The reflex can be initiated by placing a gloved finger in the anal canal and stimulating the anal sphincter to contract by squeezing the glans penis or clitoris, or gently tugging on an inserted Foley catheter. An absent anal reflex would indicate the existence of spinal shock. A cord lesion involving the sacral segments of the cord would nullify this test, since the neurons giving rise to the inferior hemorrhoidal nerve to the anal sphincter (S2-4) would be nonfunctioning.

Destructive Spinal Cord Syndromes

When neurological impairment is identified following the disappearance of spinal shock, it can often be categorized into one of the following syndromes: (1) complete cord transection syndrome, (2) anterior cord syndrome, (3) central cord syndrome, or (4) Brown-Séquard syndrome or hemisection of the cord. The clinical findings often indicate a combination of lower motor neuron injury (at the level of destruction of the cord) and upper motor neuron injury (for those segments below the level of destruction).

COMPLETE CORD TRANSECTION SYNDROME

This transection (Fig.4-27) results in complete loss of all sensibility and voluntary movement below the level of the lesion. It can be caused by fracture dislocation of the vertebral column, by a bullet or stab wound, or by an expanding tumor. The following characteristic clinical features will be seen *after* the period of spinal shock has ended:

1. Bilateral lower motor neuron paralysis and muscular atrophy in the segment of the lesion. This results from

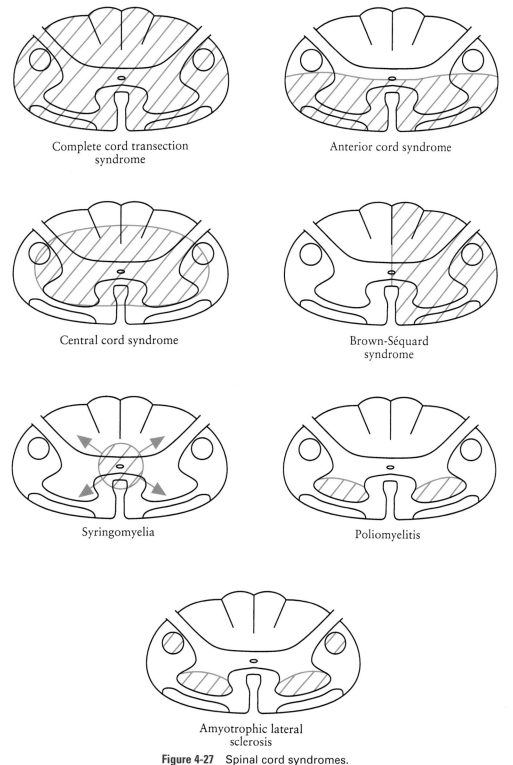

Complete cord transection
syndrome

Anterior cord syndrome

Central cord syndrome

Brown-Séquard
syndrome

Syringomyelia

Poliomyelitis

Amyotrophic lateral
sclerosis

Figure 4-27 Spinal cord syndromes.

damage to the neurons in the anterior gray columns (i.e.,
lower motor neuron) and possibly from damage to the
nerve roots of the same segment.
2. Bilateral spastic paralysis below the level of the lesion. A
bilateral Babinski sign is present and, depending on the
level of the segment of the spinal cord damaged, bilat-

eral loss of the superficial abdominal and cremaster
reflexes occurs. All these signs are caused by an interruption of the corticospinal tracts on both sides of the
cord. The bilateral spastic paralysis is produced by the
cutting of the descending tracts other than the corticospinal tracts.

3. Bilateral loss of all sensations below the level of the lesion. The loss of tactile discrimination and vibratory and proprioceptive sensations is due to bilateral destruction of the ascending tracts in the posterior white columns. The loss of pain, temperature, and light touch sensations is caused by section of the lateral and anterior spinothalamic tracts on both sides. Because these tracts cross obliquely, the loss of thermal and light touch sensations occurs two or three segments below the lesion distally.
4. Bladder and bowel functions are no longer under voluntary control, since all the descending autonomic fibers have been destroyed.

If there is a complete fracture dislocation at the L2-3 vertebral level (i.e., a level below the lower end of the cord in the adult), no cord injury occurs and neural damage is confined to the cauda equina, and lower motor neuron, autonomic, and sensory fibers are involved.

ANTERIOR CORD SYNDROME

The anterior cord syndrome (Fig. 4-27) can be caused by cord contusion during vertebral fracture or dislocation, from injury to the anterior spinal artery or its feeder arteries with resultant ischemia of the cord, or by a herniated intervertebral disc. The following characteristic clinical features are seen *after* the period of spinal shock has ended:

1. Bilateral lower motor neuron paralysis in the segment of the lesion and muscular atrophy. This is caused by damage to the neurons in the anterior gray columns (i.e., lower motor neuron) and possibly by damage to the anterior nerve roots of the same segment.
2. Bilateral spastic paralysis below the level of the lesion, the extent of which depends on the size of the injured area of the cord. The bilateral paralysis is caused by the interruption of the anterior corticospinal tracts on both sides of the cord. The bilateral muscular spasticity is produced by the interruption of tracts other than the corticospinal tracts.
3. Bilateral loss of pain, temperature, and light touch sensations below the level of the lesion. These signs are caused by interruption of the anterior and lateral spinothalamic tracts on both sides.
4. Tactile discrimination and vibratory and proprioceptive sensations are preserved because the posterior white columns on both sides are undamaged.

CENTRAL CORD SYNDROME

This syndrome is most often caused by hyperextension of the cervical region of the spine (see Fig. 4-27). The cord is pressed upon anteriorly by the vertebral bodies and posteriorly by the bulging of the ligamentum flavum, causing damage to the central region of the spinal cord. Radiographs of these injuries often appear normal because no fracture or dislocation has occurred. The following characteristic clinical features are seen *after* the period of spinal shock has ended:

1. Bilateral lower motor neuron paralysis in the segment of the lesion and muscular atrophy. This is caused by damage to the neurons in the anterior gray columns (i.e., lower motor neuron) and possibly by damage to the nerve roots of the same segment.
2. Bilateral spastic paralysis below the level of the lesion with characteristic sacral "sparing." The lower limb fibers are affected less than the upper limb fibers because the descending fibers in the lateral corticospinal tracts are laminated, with the upper limb fibers located medially and the lower limb fibers located laterally (Fig. 4-25).
3. Bilateral loss of pain, temperature, light touch, and pressure sensations below the level of the lesion with characteristic sacral "sparing." Because the ascending fibers in the lateral and anterior spinothalamic tracts are also laminated, with the upper limb fibers located medially and the lower limb fibers located laterally, the upper limb fibers are more susceptible to damage than are those of the lower limb (Fig. 4-25).

It follows from this discussion that the clinical picture of a patient with a history of a hyperextension injury of the neck, presenting with motor and sensory tract injuries involving principally the upper limb, would strongly suggest central cord syndrome. The sparing of the lower part of the body may be evidenced by (1) the presence of perianal sensation, (2) good anal sphincter tone, and (3) the ability to move the toes slightly. In patients whose damage is caused by edema of the spinal cord alone, the prognosis is often very good. A mild central cord syndrome that consists only of paresthesias of the upper part of the arm and some mild arm and hand weakness can occur.

BROWN-SÉQUARD SYNDROME OR HEMISECTION OF THE CORD

Hemisection of the spinal cord can be caused by fracture dislocation of the vertebral column, by a bullet or stab wound, or by an expanding tumor (Fig. 4-27). Incomplete hemisection is common; complete hemisection is rare. The following characteristic clinical features are seen in patients with a complete hemisection of the cord (Fig. 4-28) *after* the period of spinal shock has ended:

1. Ipsilateral lower motor neuron paralysis in the segment of the lesion and muscular atrophy. These signs are caused by damage to the neurons on the anterior gray column and possibly by damage to the nerve roots of the same segment.
2. Ipsilateral spastic paralysis below the level of the lesion. An ipsilateral Babinski sign is present, and depending on the segment of the cord damaged, an ipsilateral loss of the superficial abdominal reflexes and cremasteric reflex occurs. All these signs are due to loss of the corticospinal tracts on the side of the lesion. Spastic paralysis is produced by interruption of the descending tracts other than the corticospinal tracts.
3. Ipsilateral band of cutaneous anesthesia in the segment of the lesion. This results from the destruction of the posterior root and its entrance into the spinal cord at the level of the lesion.
4. Ipsilateral loss of tactile discrimination and of vibratory and proprioceptive sensations below the level of the

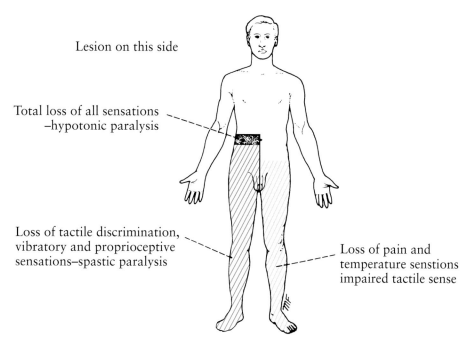

Figure 4–28 Brown-Séquard syndrome with a spinal cord lesion at the right tenth thoracic level.

Lesion on this side

Total loss of all sensations –hypotonic paralysis

Loss of tactile discrimination, vibratory and proprioceptive sensations–spastic paralysis

Loss of pain and temperature senstions impaired tactile sense

lesion. These signs are caused by destruction of the ascending tracts in the posterior white column on the same side of the lesion.

5. Contralateral loss of pain and temperature sensations below the level of the lesion. This is due to destruction of the crossed lateral spinothalamic tracts on the same side of the lesion. Because the tracts cross obliquely, the sensory loss occurs two or three segments below the lesion distally.

6. Contralateral but not complete loss of tactile sensation below the level of the lesion. This condition is brought about by destruction of the crossed anterior spinothalamic tracts on the side of the lesion. Here, again, because the tracts cross obliquely, the sensory impairment occurs two or three segments below the level of the lesion distally. The contralateral loss of tactile sense is incomplete because discriminative touch traveling in the ascending tracts in the contralateral posterior white column remains intact.

Syringomyelia

This condition, which is due to a developmental abnormality in the formation of the central canal, most often affects the brainstem and cervical region of the spinal cord. At the site of the lesion there is cavitation and gliosis in the central region of the neuroaxis (Fig. 4-29). The following characteristic signs and symptoms are found:

1. Loss of pain and temperature sensations in dermatomes on both sides of the body related to the affected segments

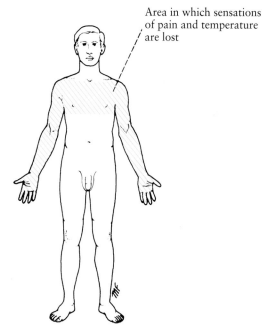

Figure 4–29 Skin area in which the sensations of pain and temperature are lost in syringomyelia.

Area in which sensations of pain and temperature are lost

of the cord. This loss commonly has a shawl-like distribution, caused by the interruption of the lateral spinothalamic tracts as they cross the midline in the anterior gray and white commissures. The patient commonly complains of accidental burning injuries to the fingers.

2. Tactile discrimination, vibratory sense, and proprioceptive sense are normal. The reason is that the ascending tracts in the posterior white column are unaffected.
3. Lower motor neuron weakness is present in the small muscles of the hand. It may be bilateral or one hand may suffer before the other. As the lesion expands in the lower cervical and upper thoracic region, it destroys the anterior horn cells of these segments. Later, the other muscles of the arm and shoulder girdles undergo atrophy.
4. Bilateral spastic paralysis of both legs may occur, with exaggerated deep tendon reflexes and the presence of a positive Babinski response. These signs are produced by the further expansion of the lesion laterally into the white column to involve the descending tracts.
5. A Horner's syndrome may be present. This is caused by the interruption of the descending autonomic fibers in among the reticulospinal tracts in the lateral white column by the expanding lesion.

Poliomyelitis

Poliomyelitis is an acute viral infection of the neurons of the anterior gray columns of the spinal cord (Fig. 4-27) and the motor nuclei of the cranial nerves. Immunization has greatly reduced the incidence of poliomyelitis, once a feared disease. Following death of the motor nerve cells there is paralysis and wasting of the muscles. The muscles of the lower limb are more often affected than are those of the upper limb. In severe poliomyelitis, respiration may be threatened due to the paralysis spreading to the intercostal muscles and diaphragm. The muscles of the face, pharynx, larynx, and tongue may also be paralyzed. Improvement usually begins at the end of the first week as the edema in the affected area subsides and function returns to the neurons that have not been destroyed.

Multiple Sclerosis (MS)

Multiple sclerosis is a common disease confined to the central nervous system and causing demyelination of the ascending and descending tracts. It is a disease of young adults and the cause is unknown. The loss of the myelin sheath results in the breakdown of the insulation around the axons and the velocity of the action potentials is reduced and ultimately becomes blocked.

Although myelin is relatively rich in lipid (70-80%), it also contains proteins which play a role in myelin compaction. It has been found that many of the proteins in the myelin of the central nervous system differ from those in the peripheral nervous system. Experimentally, it has been shown that basic myelin proteins can produce a strong immune response when injected into animals and demyelination in the central nervous system occurs. It is possible that mutations in the structure of myelin protein can occur and be responsible for some inherited forms of demyelination. It is also possible that in MS that autoantigens develop.

The course of multiple sclerosis is chronic with exacerbations and remissions. Because of the widespread involvement of different tracts at different levels of the neuraxis, the signs and symptoms are multiple but remissions do occur.

Weakness of the limbs is the most common sign of the disease. Ataxia due to involvement of the tracts of the cerebellum may occur but spastic paralysis may also be present.

Recent research has suggested that the remissions in multiple sclerosis may in part be explained by the remodelling of the demyelinated axonal plasma membrane so that it acquires a higher than normal number of sodium channels, which permit conduction of action potentials despite the loss of myelin.

In patients who have the progressive form of the disease without remissions, it is has been shown that they have a substantial damage to the axons as well as the myelin. This would suggest that multiple sclerosis is not just a demyelinating disease but one in which there is axonal pathology.

Amyotrophic Lateral Sclerosis (ALS) (Lou Gehrig's Disease)

Amyotrophic lateral sclerosis is a disease confined to the corticospinal tracts and the motor neurons of the anterior gray columns of the spinal cord (Fig. 4-27). It is rarely familial and is inherited in about 10% of patients. Amyotrophic lateral sclerosis is a chronic progressive disease of unknown etiology. Typically it occurs in late middle age and is inevitably fatal in 2 to 6 years. The lower motor neuron signs of progressive muscular atrophy, paresis, and fasciculations are superimposed on the signs and symptoms of upper motor neuron disease with paresis, spasticity, and Babinski response. The motor nuclei of some cranial nerves may also be involved.

Parkinson's Disease

This disease is associated with neuronal degeneration in the substantia nigra and to a lesser extent in the globus pallidus, putamen, and caudate nucleus. The degeneration of the inhibitory nigrostriate fibers results in a reduction in the release of the neurotransmitter dopamine within the corpus striatum. This leads to hypersensitivity of the dopamine receptors in the postsynaptic neurons in the corpus striatum, which become overactive. The characteristic signs of the disease include tremor and cogwheel rigidity (hyperkinetic activity) and difficulty initiating voluntary movements, which are slow (hypokinetic activity).

Pernicious Anemia

This form of megaloblastic anemia is caused by Vitamin B_{12} deficiency. The disease may produce extensive damage to the tracts in the posterior and lateral white columns of the spinal cord as well as peripheral nerve degeneration. Widespread sensory and motor losses may be present due to involvement of the ascending and descending tracts of the spinal cord.

Radiographic Appearances of the Vertebral Column

The views commonly used in radiography are anteroposterior, lateral, and oblique. Vertebral destruction owing to tuberculosis or to primary or secondary tumors of the vertebrae, or fractures owing to trauma usually can be revealed by radiographic examination. Erosion of the pedicles by a tumor within the intervertebral foramina may be seen. Narrowing of the space between the vertebral bodies with bony spurs because of osteoarthritic changes in adjacent vertebral bodies can also be seen.

CT and MRI of the Vertebral Column and Spinal Cord

CT scans of the vertebrae and joints can be obtained (Fig. 4-30). A protrusion of an intervertebral disc can be identified and the presence of narrowing of the vertebral canal (**spinal stenosis**) can be diagnosed.

Sagittal MRI is increasingly being used to replace CT and myelography. The parts of a vertebra, the intervertebral disc, the posterior longitudinal ligament, and meningeal sac (**thecal sac**) can easily be identified(Fig. 4-31).

Myelography

The subarachnoid space can be studied radiographically by the injection of a contrast medium into the subarachnoid space by spinal tap. Iodized oil has been used with success. This technique is referred to as **myelography** (Figs. 4-32 and 4-33).

If the patient is sitting in the upright position, the oil sinks to the lower limit of the subarachnoid space at the level of the lower border of the second sacral vertebra. By placing the patient on a tilting table, the oil can be made to gravitate gradually to higher levels of the vertebral column.

A normal myelogram will show pointed lateral projections at regular intervals at the intervertebral space levels. The reason for this is that the opaque medium fills the lateral extensions of the subarachnoid space around each spinal nerve. The presence of a tumor or a prolapsed intervertebral disc may obstruct the movement of the oil from one region to another when the patient is tilted.

With the recent technological advances in CT scans and MRIs, it is now unusual to require an intrusive procedure such as myelography to make a diagnosis.

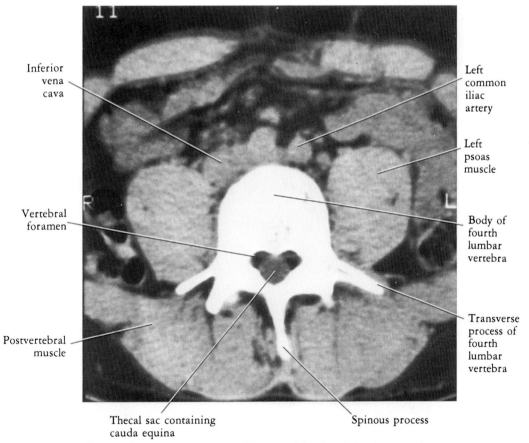

Figure 4–30   Horizontal (axial) CT scan of the fourth lumbar vertebra.

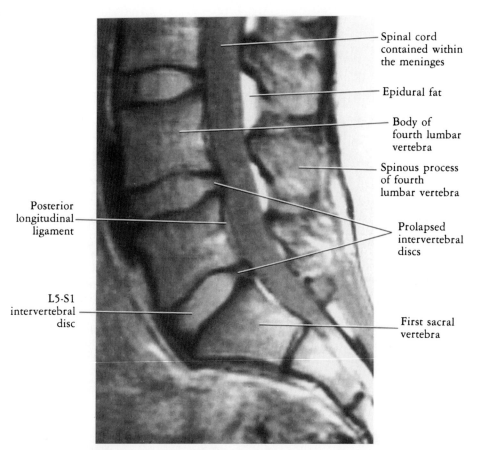

Spinal cord
contained within
the meninges

Epidural fat

Body of
fourth lumbar
vertebra

Spinous process
of fourth
lumbar vertebra

Prolapsed
intervertebral
discs

First sacral
vertebra

Posterior
longitudinal
ligament

L5-S1
intervertebral
disc

Figure 4–31   Sagittal MRI of the lumbosacral part of the vertebral column, showing several prolapsed intervertebral discs. (Courtesy Dr. Pait.)

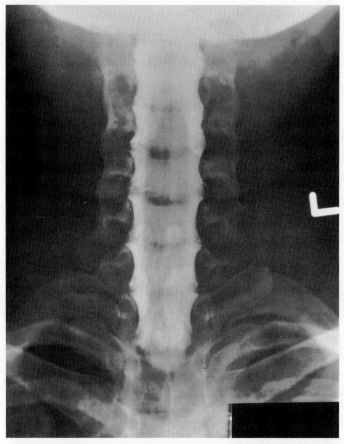

Figure 4–32   Posteroanterior myelogram of the cervical region of a 22-year-old woman.

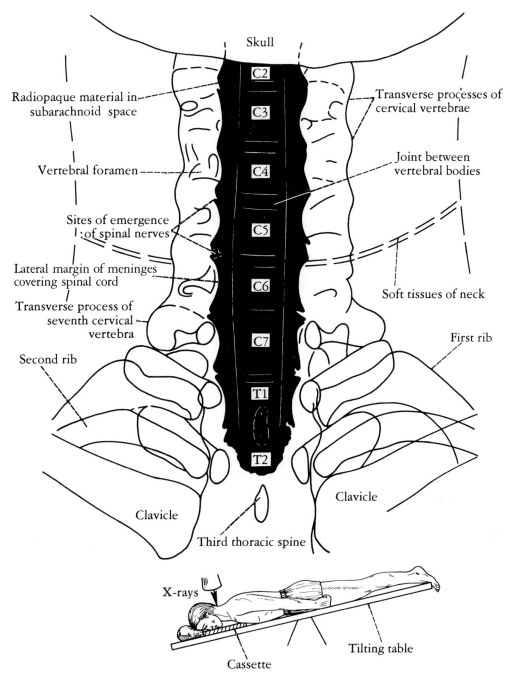

Figure 4–33   Diagrammatic explanation of the myelogram shown in Figure 4–32.

Clinical Problem Solving

1. A 53-year-old widower was admitted to the hospital complaining of a burning pain over his right shoulder region and the upper part of his right arm. The pain had started 3 weeks previously and since that time had progressively worsened. The pain was accentuated by moving his neck and by coughing. Two years previously he had been treated for osteoarthritis of his vertebral column. The patient stated that he had been a football player at college and since that time he continued to take an active part in the game until his forty-second year. Physical examination revealed weakness, wasting, and fasciculation of the right deltoid and biceps brachii muscles. The right biceps tendon reflex was absent. Radiological examination revealed extensive spur formation on the bodies of the fourth, fifth, and sixth cervical vertebrae. The patient demonstrated hyperesthesia and partial analgesia in the skin over the lower part of the right deltoid and down the lateral side of the arm. Using your knowledge of neuroanatomy, make the diagnosis. How is the pain produced? Why is the pain made worse by coughing?

2. A 66-year-old woman was admitted to the hospital because of her increasing difficulty with walking. Two weeks before admission she had been able to walk with the help of a stick. Since that time walking had become increasingly difficult and for the past 2 days she could not walk at all. She had complete control of micturition and defecation. On examination, the handgrip was weak on both sides but power was normal in the proximal segments of the upper extremities. The tendon reflexes of the upper limbs and the sensory function were normal. Both lower limbs showed muscular weakness with increased muscle tone, especially on the left side. The knee jerks and ankle jerks (tendon reflexes) in both lower limbs were grossly exaggerated and there were bilateral extensor plantar responses. The patient had a loss of sensation of pain below the fifth thoracic dermatome on both sides of the body. Postural sense was impaired in both great toes and vibration sense was absent below the fifth thoracic segmental level. Radiological examination, including an MRI, of the vertebral column showed nothing abnormal. A myelogram in the lumbar region revealed a complete block at the lower border of the fourth thoracic vertebra. Using your knowledge of neuroanatomy, suggest a possible diagnosis. How would you treat this patient? Name the tracts in the spinal cord that are responsible for conduction of the sensation of pain. What is the position of these tracts in the spinal cord? Name the tracts responsible for the conduction of postural sense and vibration sense from the spinal cord to the brain. Why did the patient have increasing difficulty in walking? Why were the tendon reflexes in the lower limbs exaggerated, and why did the patient exhibit bilateral extensor plantar responses?

3. A 20-year-old male student celebrated the passing of an examination by drinking several beers at a party. On the way home, he drove his car head-on into a bridge abutment. On examination in the emergency department, he was found to have a fracture dislocation of the ninth thoracic vertebra with signs and symptoms of severe damage to the spinal cord. On physical examination, he had an upper motor neuron paralysis of the left leg. He also had loss of muscle joint sense of the left leg. On testing of cutaneous sensibility, he had a band of cutaneous hyperesthesia extending around the abdominal wall on the left side at the level of the umbilicus. Just below this, he had a narrow band of anesthesia and analgesia. On the right side, there was total analgesia, thermoanesthesia, and partial loss of tactile sense of the skin of the abdominal wall below the level of the umbilicus and involving the whole of the right leg. Using your knowledge of neuroanatomy, state the level at which the spinal cord was damaged. Was the spinal cord completely sectioned? If not, on which side did the hemisection occur? Explain the sensory losses found on examination in this patient.

4. A 35-year-old woman was admitted to the hospital for investigation. She had symptoms of analgesia and thermoanesthesia on the medial side of the left hand of 6 months' duration. Three weeks prior to her admittance, she had severely burned the little finger of her left hand on a hot stove, and was unaware that the burn had occurred until she smelled the burning skin. On physical examination, she was found to have considerably reduced pain and temperature sense involving the eighth cervical and first thoracic dermatomes of the left hand. However, her sense of tactile discrimination was perfectly normal in these areas. Examination of the right arm showed a similar but much less severe dissociated sensory loss involving the same areas. No further abnormal signs were discovered. Using your knowledge of neuroanatomy, state which tract or tracts were involved in this pathological process. Name this disease.

5. A 60-year-old man walked into the neurology clinic and the physician paid particular attention to his gait. The patient raised his feet unnecessarily high and brought them to the ground in a stamping manner. While he was waiting for the physician, it was noticed that he stood with his feet wide apart. On questioning, the patient said that he was finding it increasingly difficult to walk and was starting to use a stick, especially when he went out for walks in the dark. The physician asked the patient to stand with his toes and heels together and to close his eyes. The patient immediately started to sway and the nurse had to steady him to prevent him from falling. On further examination, the patient was found to have loss of muscle joint sense of both legs and was unable to detect any feeling of vibration when a vibrating tuning fork was placed on the medial malleolus of either leg. No other sensory losses were noted. Using your knowledge of neuroanatomy, name the ascending

pathways that are involved, by disease, in this patient. Name a disease that could be responsible for these findings.

6. A 68-year-old man had an advanced inoperable carcinoma of the prostate with multiple metastases in the lumbar vertebrae and hip bones. Apart from the severe intractable pain, the patient was still able to enjoy life among his family. After a full discussion of the prognosis with the patient and his wife, she turned to the physician and said, "Can't you do something to stop this terrible pain, so that my husband can die happy?" What can a physician do to help a patient under these circumstances?

7. A third-year medical student attended a lecture on the effects of trauma on the vertebral column. The orthopedic surgeon described very superficially the different neurological deficits that may follow injury to the spinal cord. At the end of the lecture, the student said he did not understand what was meant by the term *spinal shock*. He could not understand what the underlying mechanism for this condition was. He also asked the surgeon to explain what was meant by paraplegia in extension and paraplegia in flexion. Could the surgeon explain why one condition sometimes passes into the other? These are good questions. Can you answer them?

8. While examining a patient with a right-sided hemiplegia caused by a cerebrovascular accident, the neurologist asked the student which clinical signs could be attributed to an interruption of the corticospinal tracts and which signs could be attributed to damage to other descending tracts. Using your knowledge of neuroanatomy, answer this question.

9. A large civilian aircraft was forced to abort its takeoff because three tires had burst as the plane sped along the runway. The pilot miraculously managed to halt the plane as it veered off the runway and came to an abrupt halt in a ditch. All the passengers escaped injury, but one of the stewardesses was admitted to the emergency department with suspected spinal cord injury. On questioning, the 25-year-old patient said that although she had her seat belt fastened, she was thrown violently forward on impact. She said she could not feel anything in either leg and could not move her legs. On examination, there was complete motor and sensory loss of both legs below the inguinal ligament and absence of all deep tendon reflexes of both legs. Twelve hours later, it was noted that she could move the toes and ankle of her left lower limb and she had a return of sensations to her right leg except for loss of tactile discrimination, vibratory sense, and proprioceptive sense. She had a band of complete anesthesia over her right inguinal ligament. Her left leg showed a total analgesia, thermoanesthesia, and partial loss of tactile sense. Her right leg was totally paralyzed and the muscles were spastic.

There was a right-sided Babinski response, and it was possible to demonstrate right-sided ankle clonus. The right knee jerk was exaggerated. Using your knowledge of neuroanatomy, explain the symptoms and signs found in this patient. Which vertebra was damaged?

10. Why is it dangerous to move a patient who is suspected of having a fracture or dislocation of the vertebral column?

11. An 18-year-old man was admitted to the hospital following a severe automobile accident. After a complete neurological investigation, his family was told that he would be paralyzed from the waist downward for the rest of his life. The neurologist outlined to the medical personnel the importance of preventing complications in these cases. The common complications are the following: (a) urinary infection, (b) bedsores, (c) nutritional deficiency, (d) muscular spasms, and (e) pain. Using your knowledge of neuroanatomy, explain the underlying reasons for these complications. How long after the accident do you think it would be possible to give an accurate prognosis in this patient?

12. A 67-year-old man was brought to the neurology clinic by his daughter because she had noticed that his right arm had a tremor. Apparently this had started about 6 months previously and was becoming steadily worse. When questioned, the patient said he noticed that the muscles of his limbs sometimes felt stiff but he had put this down to old age. While talking, it was noticed, the patient rarely smiled and then only with difficulty. It was also noted that he infrequently blinked his eyes. The patient tended to speak in a low, faint voice. When asked to walk, the patient was seen to have normal posture and gait, although he tended to hold his right arm flexed at the elbow joint. When he was sitting, it was noted that the fingers of the right hand were alternately contracting and relaxing and there was a fine tremor involving the wrist and elbow on the right side. It was particularly noticed that the tremor was worse when the arm was at rest. When he was asked to hold a book in his right hand, the tremor stopped momentarily, but it started again immediately after the book was placed on the table. The daughter said that when her father falls asleep, the tremor stops immediately. On examination, it was found that the passive movements of the right elbow and wrist showed an increase in tone and there was some cogwheel rigidity. There was no sensory loss, either cutaneous or deep sensibility, and the reflexes were normal. Using your knowledge of neuroanatomy, make a diagnosis. Which regions of the brain are diseased?

13. Name a center in the central nervous system that may be responsible for the following clinical signs: (a) intention tremor, (b) athetosis, (c) chorea, (d) dystonia, and (e) hemiballismus.

Answers to Clinical Problem Solving

1. This patient was suffering from spondylosis, which is a general term used for degenerative changes in the vertebral column caused by osteoarthritis. In the cervical region the growth of osteophytes was exerting pressure on the anterior and posterior roots of the fifth and sixth spinal nerves. As the result of repeated trauma and of aging, degenerative changes occurred at the articulating surfaces of the fourth, fifth, and sixth cervical vertebrae. Extensive spur formation resulted in narrowing of the intervertebral foramina with pressure on the nerve roots. The burning pain, hyperesthesia, and partial analgesia were due to pressure on the posterior roots, and weakness, wasting, and fasciculation of the deltoid and biceps brachii muscles were due to pressure on the anterior roots. Movements of the neck presumably intensified the symptoms by exerting further traction or pressure on the nerve roots. Coughing or sneezing raised the pressure within the vertebral canal and resulted in further pressure on the nerve roots.

2. The patient was operated on and a laminectomy of the third, fourth, and fifth thoracic vertebrae was carried out. At the level of the fourth thoracic vertebra a small swelling was seen on the posterior surface of the spinal cord; it was attached to the dura mater. Histological examination showed that it was a meningioma. The tumor was easily removed and the patient successfully recovered from the operation. There was a progressive recovery in the power of the lower limbs, with the patient walking without a stick. This patient emphasizes the importance of making an early, accurate diagnosis, because benign extramedullary spinal tumors are readily treatable. The lateral spinal thalamic tracts are responsible for the conduction of pain impulses up the spinal cord. These tracts are situated in the lateral white columns of the spinal cord (see p. 146). Postural sense and vibration sense are conducted up the spinal cord in the posterior white column through the fasciculus cuneatus from the upper limbs and the upper part of the thorax, and in the fasciculus gracilis from the lower part of the trunk and the leg. The difficulty in walking was due to pressure on the corticospinal tracts in the lateral white column. The exaggeration in the tendon reflexes of the lower limbs and the bilateral extensor plantar responses were due to the pressure on the descending tracts in the spinal cord at the level of the tumor. This also resulted in spastic paralysis of the muscles of the lower limbs.

3. A fracture dislocation of the ninth thoracic vertebra would result in severe damage to the tenth thoracic segment of the spinal cord. The unequal sensory and motor losses on the two sides indicate a left hemisection of the cord. The narrow band of hyperesthesia on the left side was due to the irritation of the cord immediately above the site of the lesion. The band of anesthesia and analgesia was due to the destruction of the cord on the left side at the level of the tenth thoracic segment—that is, all afferent fibers entering the cord at that point were interrupted. The loss of pain and thermal sensibilities and the loss of light touch below the level of the umbilicus on the right side were caused by the interruption of the lateral and anterior spinothalamic tracts on the left side of the cord.

4. This patient has the early signs and symptoms of syringomyelia. The gliosis and cavitation had resulted in interruption of the lateral and anterior spinothalamic tracts as they decussated in the anterior gray and white commissures of the spinal cord at the level of the eighth cervical and first thoracic segments of the spinal cord. Because of uneven growth of the cavitation, the condition was worse on the left than on the right side. Since tactile discrimination was normal in both upper limbs, the fasciculus cuneatus in both posterior white columns was unaffected. This dissociated sensory loss is characteristic of this disease.

5. The peculiar stamping gait and the swaying posture on closing the eyes are the characteristic signs of loss of appreciation of proprioceptive sensation from the lower limbs. These, together with the inability to detect the vibrations of a tuning fork placed on the medial malleoli of both legs, indicated that the patient had a lesion involving the fasciculus gracilis in both posterior white columns. Further questioning of this patient indicated that he had been treated for syphilis. The diagnosis was tabes dorsalis.

6. The treatment of intractable pain in terminal cancer is a difficult problem. The narcotic drugs with their strong analgesic action are generally used. The likelihood that these drugs will be habit-forming is accepted in a dying patient. Alternative treatments include the continuous infusion of morphine directly into the spinal cord (See page 168) or the surgical section of the nerve fibers carrying the sensations of pain into the nervous system. The techniques of posterior rhizotomy and cordotomy are described on page 169.

7. Spinal shock is a temporary interruption of the physiological function of the spinal cord following injury. It may in part be a vascular phenomenon involving the gray matter of the spinal cord; on the other hand, some authorities believe it is due to the sudden interruption of the influence of the higher centers on the local segmental reflexes. Whatever the cause, it usually disappears after 1 to 4 weeks. The condition is characterized by a flaccid paralysis and loss of sensation and reflex activity below the level of the lesion; this includes paralysis of the bladder and rectum.

   Paraplegia in extension and paraplegia in flexion follow severe injury to the spinal cord. Paraplegia in extension indicates an increase in the extensor muscle tone owing to the overactivity of the gamma efferent nerve fibers to the muscle spindles as the result of the release of these neurons from the higher centers. However, some neurologists believe that the vestibulospinal tracts are intact in these cases. Should all the descending tracts be severed, the condition of paraplegia in flexion occurs where the reflex responses are flexor in nature when a noxious stimulus is applied. It should be emphasized that paraplegia in extension and paraplegia in flexion occur only after spinal shock has ceased. Paraplegia in extension may change to paraplegia in flexion if the damage to the spinal cord becomes more extensive and the vestibulospinal tracts are destroyed.

8. If it is assumed that this patient had a lesion in the left internal capsule following a cerebral hemorrhage, the corticospinal fibers would have been interrupted as they descended through the posterior limb of the internal capsule. Since most of these fibers crossed to the right side at the decussation of the pyramids, or lower down at the segmental level of the spinal cord, the muscles of the opposite side would have been affected. Interruption of these corticospinal fibers would have produced the following clinical signs: (a) Babinski sign positive; (b) loss of superficial abdominal and cremasteric reflexes; and (c) loss of performance of fine, skilled voluntary movements, especially at the distal ends of the limbs.

   In patients with severe hemorrhage into the internal capsule, subcortical connections between the cerebral cortex and the caudate nucleus and the globus pallidus and other subcortical nuclei may be damaged. Moreover, some of the nuclei themselves may be destroyed. The interruption of other descending tracts from these subcortical centers would produce the following clinical signs: (a) severe paralysis on the opposite side of the body; (b) spasticity of the paralyzed muscles; (c) exaggerated deep muscle reflexes on the opposite side of the body to the lesion (clonus may be demonstrated); and (d) clasp-knife reaction, which may be felt in the paralyzed muscles.

9. A lateral radiograph of the thoracic part of the vertebral column showed a fracture dislocation involving the tenth thoracic vertebra. The first lumbar segment of the spinal cord is related to this vertebra. The first lumbar dermatome overlies the inguinal ligament and the total anesthesia over the right ligament would suggest a partial lesion of the spinal cord involving the total sensory input at that level. The loss of tactile discrimination and vibratory and proprioceptive senses in the right leg was caused by the interruption of the ascending tracts in the posterior white column on the right side of the spinal cord. The loss of pain and temperature senses in the skin of the left leg was due to destruction of the crossed lateral spinothalamic tracts on the right side at the level of the lesion. The loss of tactile sense in the skin of the left leg was caused by the destruction of the crossed anterior spinothalamic tracts on the right side. The spastic paralysis of the right leg and the right-sided ankle clonus were due to the interruption of the right-sided descending tracts other than the corticospinal tracts. The right-sided Babinski response was brought about

by the interruption of the corticospinal fibers on the right side.

   The complete motor and sensory loss of both legs and the absence of all deep tendon reflexes of both legs during the first 12 hours were due to spinal shock.

10. The spinal cord occupies the vertebral canal of the vertebral column and under normal circumstances, therefore, is well protected. Unfortunately, once the integrity of the bony protection is destroyed by a fracture dislocation, especially in the thoracic region, where the canal is of small diameter, the bone can damage the cord and sever it just as a knife cuts through butter. It is essential that all patients suspected of having an injury to the spine be handled with great care to prevent the bones undergoing further dislocation and causing further injury to the cord. The patient should be carefully lifted by multiple supports under the feet, knees, pelvis, back, shoulders, and head and placed on a rigid stretcher or board for transportation to the nearest medical center.

11. Urinary infection secondary to bladder dysfunction is extremely common in paraplegic patients. The patient not only has lost control of the bladder but also does not know when it is full. An indwelling Foley catheter is placed in the bladder immediately for continuous drainage and antibiotic therapy is instituted.

   Bedsores are very common in patients who have lost all sensory perception over their bony points, such as the ischial tuberosities and the sacrum. Bedsores are best prevented by (a) keeping the skin scrupulously clean, (b) frequently changing the position of the patient, and (c) keeping soft padding beneath the bony points.

   Nutritional deficiency is common in active individuals who are suddenly confined to their beds and who are paralyzed. Loss of appetite must be combated by giving the patients a high-calorie diet that has all the required ingredients, especially vitamins.

   Muscle spasms occur in paraplegia in extension or paraplegia in flexion and may follow only minor stimuli. The cause is unknown, but neuronal irritation at the site of injury may be responsible. Warm baths are helpful but occasionally, in extreme cases, nerve section may be necessary.

   Pain occurs in the anesthetic areas in about one-fourth of patients who have a complete section of the spinal cord. The pain may be burning or shooting and superficial, or deep visceral. Here again, neuronal irritation at the site of injury may be responsible. Analgesics should be tried, but in some individuals rhizotomy or even chordotomy may be necessary.

   An accurate prognosis is not possible until the stage of spinal shock has ended and this may last as long as 4 weeks.

12. The characteristic coarse tremor of the right hand (pill rolling) and right arm, the unsmiling masklike face with unblinking eyes, and the cogwheel rigidity of the involved muscles make the diagnosis of early Parkinson's disease (paralysis agitans) certain. Degen-

erative lesions occur in the substantia nigra and other subcortical nuclei, including the lentiform nucleus. The loss of normal function of these subcortical areas and the absence of their influence on the lower motor neurons are responsible for the increased tone and tremor.

13. (a) Intention tremor occurs in cerebellar disease.
    (b) Athetosis occurs in lesions of the corpus striatum.
    (c) Chorea occurs in lesions of the corpus striatum.
    (d) Dystonia occurs in disease of the lentiform nucleus.
    (e) Hemiballismus occurs in disease of the opposite subthalamic nucleus.

Review Questions

Directions: Each of the numbered items in this section is followed by answers that are positively phrased. Select the ONE lettered answer that is an EXCEPTION.

1. The following statements concerning the spinal cord are correct **except**:
   (a) The anterior and posterior gray columns on the two sides are united by a gray commissure.
   (b) The terminal ventricle is the expanded lower end of the central canal.
   (c) The larger nerve cell bodies in the anterior gray horns give rise to the alpha efferent nerve fibers in the anterior roots.
   (d) The substantia gelatinosa groups of cells are located at the base of each posterior gray column.
   (e) The nucleus dorsalis (Clark's column) is a group of nerve cells found in the posterior gray column and extending from the eighth cervical segment caudally to the third or fourth lumbar segment.
2. The following statements concerning the white columns of the spinal cord are correct **except**:
   (a) The posterior spinocerebellar tract is situated in the lateral white column.
   (b) The anterior spinothalamic tract is found in the anterior white column.
   (c) The lateral spinothalamic tract is found in the lateral white column.
   (d) The fasciculus gracilis is found in the lateral white column.
   (e) The rubrospinal tract is found in the lateral white column.
3. The following statements concerning the spinal cord are correct **except**:
   (a) The spinal cord has a cervical enlargement for the brachial plexus.
   (b) It possesses 34 pairs of spinal nerves.
   (c) In the adult, the spinal cord usually ends inferiorly at the lower border of the first lumbar vertebra.
   (d) The ligamentum denticulatum anchors the spinal cord to the dura mater along each side.
   (e) The central canal communicates with the fourth ventricle of the brain.

Directions: Matching Questions

In Figure 4-34, match the numbers listed on the left with the appropriate lettered structure listed on the right. Each lettered option may be selected once, more than once, or not at all.

4. Number 1   (a) Nucleus proprius
5. Number 2   (b) Preganglionic sympathetic outflow
6. Number 3   (c) Nucleus dorsalis
7. Number 4   (d) Substantia gelatinosa
8. Number 5   (e) None of the above
9. Number 6

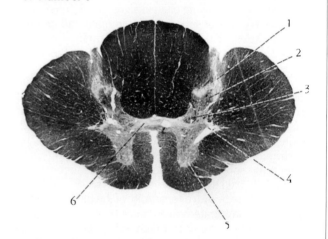

Directions: Each of the numbered items in this section is followed by answers that are positively phrased. Select the ONE lettered answer that is an EXCEPTION.

10. The following statements concerning the cell of origin of the tracts listed below are correct **except**:
    (a) The fasciculus cuneatus arises from the cells in the posterior root ganglion.
    (b) The anterior spinal thalamic arises from the cells in substantia gelatinosa.
    (c) The fasciculus gracilis arises from the cells in the posterior root ganglion.
    (d) The anterior spinocerebellar arises from the cells in Clark's column.
    (e) The lateral spinothalamic arises from the cells in the posterior root ganglion.
11. The following statements concerning the courses taken by the tracts listed below are correct **except**:
    (a) The fasciculus gracilis does not cross to the opposite side of the neural axis.
    (b) The spinotectal tract crosses to the opposite side of the spinal cord.

(c) The lateral spinothalamic tract does not cross to the opposite side of the spinal cord.
(d) The posterior spinocerebellar tract does not cross to the opposite side of the neural axis.
(e) The anterior spinothalamic tract crosses very obliquely to the opposite side of the spinal cord.

12. The following statements concerning the nucleus of termination of the tracts listed below are correct **except**:
(a) The posterior white column tracts terminate in the inferior colliculus.
(b) The anterior spinothalamic tract terminates in the ventral posterolateral nucleus of the thalamus.
(c) The spinotectal tract terminates in the superior colliculus.
(d) The spinoreticular tract terminates on the neurons of the reticular formation in the medulla, pons, and midbrain.
(e) The anterior spinocerebellar tract terminates in the cerebellar cortex.

13. The following statements relating sensations with the appropriate nervous pathways are correct **except**:
(a) Two-point tactile discrimination travel in the fasciculus cuneatus.
(b) Pain travels in the anterior spinothalamic tract.
(c) Unconscious muscle joint sense travels in the anterior spinocerebellar tract.
(d) Pressure travels in the anterior spinothalamic tract.
(e) Vibration travels in the fasciculus gracilis.

14. The following statements are consistent with the gating theory of pain **except**:
(a) Stimulation of large non-pain-conducting fibers in a peripheral nerve may reduce pain sensitivity.
(b) Massage applied to the skin over a painful joint may reduce pain sensitivity.
(c) Stimulation of delta A- and C-type fibers in a posterior root of a spinal nerve may decrease pain sensitivity.
(d) Degeneration of large non-pain-conducting fibers in a peripheral nerve increases pain sensitivity.
(e) Inhibition of pain conduction in the spinal cord could be brought about by means of connector neurons.

15. The following statements concerning the reception of pain are correct **except**:
(a) The slow-conducting C-type fibers are responsible for prolonged, burning pain.
(b) Substance P, a peptide, is thought to be the neurotransmitter at the synapses where the first-order neuron terminates on the cells in the posterior gray column of the spinal cord.
(c) The enkephalins and endorphins may serve to inhibit the release of substance P in the posterior gray column of the spinal cord.

(d) Many of the tracts conducting the initial, sharp, pricking pain terminate in the ventral posterolateral nucleus of the thalamus.
(e) Serotonin is not a transmitter substance in the analgesic system.

16. The following statements concerning the corticospinal tracts are correct **except**:
(a) Those that control the movements of the upper limb originate in the precentral gyrus on the medial side of the cerebral hemisphere.
(b) They are mainly responsible for controlling the voluntary movements in the distal muscles of the limbs.
(c) They arise as axons of the pyramidal cells in the fifth layer of the cerebral cortex.
(d) They occupy the posterior limb of the internal capsule.
(e) Those that are concerned with the movements of the lower limb are located in the lateral area of the middle three-fifths of the basis pedunculi.

17. The following statements concerning the course taken by the tracts listed below are correct **except**:
(a) The rubrospinal tract crosses the midline of the neuroaxis in the midbrain.
(b) The tectospinal tract (most of the nerve fibers) crosses the midline in the midbrain.
(c) The lateral corticospinal tract has crossed the midline in the medulla oblongata.
(d) The vestibulospinal tract crosses the midline in the medulla oblongata.
(e) The anterior corticospinal tract crosses the midline in the spinal cord.

18. The following statements concerning the nerve cells of origin for the tracts listed below are correct **except**:
(a) The vestibulospinal tract originates from cells of the lateral vestibular nucleus situated in the pons.
(b) The tectospinal tract originates from cells in the inferior colliculus.
(c) The lateral corticospinal tract originates from cells in area 4 of the cerebral cortex.
(d) The rubrospinal tract originates from cells in the red nucleus.
(e) The reticulospinal tract originates from cells in the reticular formation in the midbrain, pons, and medulla oblongata.

19. The following statements concerning muscle movement are correct **except**:
(a) Hyperactive ankle-jerk reflexes and ankle clonus indicate a release of the lower motor neurons from supraspinal inhibition.
(b) Muscle spindle afferent nerve fibers send information to the brain as well as to the spinal cord.
(c) In Parkinson's disease there is a degeneration of dopamine-secreting neurons that originate in the substantia nigra.

(d) Brain neuronal activity preceding a voluntary movement is limited to the precentral gyrus (area 4).
(e) Muscular fasciculation is seen only when there is slow destruction of the lower motor neurons.
20. After a hemorrhage into the left internal capsule in a right-handed person, the following signs or symptoms might be present **except**:
(a) Right homonymous hemianopia
(b) Right astereognosis
(c) Left hemiplegia
(d) Aphasia
(e) Right-sided positive Babinski response
21. A patient with a traumatic lesion of the left half of the spinal cord at the level of the eighth cervical segment might present the following signs and symptoms **except:**
(a) Loss of pain and temperature sensations on the left side below the level of the lesion
(b) Loss of position sense of the left leg
(c) Left hemiplegia
(d) Left positive Babinski sign
(e) Left-sided lower motor paralysis in the segment of the lesion and muscular atrophy

Directions: Each of the numbered items in this section is followed by answers. Select the ONE lettered answer that is BEST in each case.

22. Which of the signs and symptoms listed below **are** indicative of a cerebellar lesion?
(a) Cogwheel rigidity
(b) Hemiballismus
(c) Chorea
(d) Intention tremor
(e) Athetosis
23. Which of the following regions of white matter would **not** contain corticospinal fibers?
(a) Pyramid of medulla oblongata
(b) Lateral white column of the spinal cord
(c) Cerebral peduncle of the midbrain
(d) Anterior limb of the internal capsule
(e) Corona radiata

Directions: Read the case histories then answer the questions. You will be required to select ONE BEST lettered answer.

A 59-year-old woman was experiencing pain in the back and showed evidence of loss of pain and temperature sensations down the back of her left leg. Three years previously she underwent a radical mastectomy followed by radiation and chemotherapy for advanced carcinoma of her right breast.
On examination it was found that she was experiencing pain over the lower part of the back, with loss of the skin sensations of pain and temperature down the back of her left leg in the area of the S1, 2, and 3 dermatomes. No other neurological deficits were identified. Radiographic examination of the vertebral column showed evidence of metastases in the bodies of the ninth and tenth thoracic

vertebrae. An MRI revealed an extension of one of the metastases into the vertebral canal, with slight indentation of the spinal cord on the right side.
24. The pain in the back could be explained in this patient by the following facts **except:**
(a) Osteoarthritis of the joints of the vertebral column.
(b) The presence of metastases in the bodies of the ninth and tenth thoracic vertebrae.
(c) The pressure of the tumor on the posterior roots of the spinal nerves.
(d) A prolapsed intervertebral disc pressing on the spinal nerves.
(e) Spasm of the postvertebral muscles following pressure of the tumor on the posterior white columns of the spinal cord.
25. The loss of pain and temperature sensations down the back of the patient's left leg in the area of the S1,2 and 3 dermatomes could be explained by the following facts **except**:
(a) The lateral spinothalamic tracts in the spinal cord conduct the sensations of pain.
(b) The lateral spinothalamic tracts are laminated, with the sacral segments of the body located most laterally.
(c) The sacral segments of the tracts are the most exposed to external cord pressure from a metastasising tumor.
(d) The loss of temperature sensations in the leg could be explained by pressure of the tumor on the anterior spinothalamic tract.
26. The severe intractable pain in the back in this patient could be treated by the following methods **except**:
(a) The prescription of salicylates in large doses.
(b) The intramuscular injection of morphine or even the direct injection of the opiate into the spinal cord.
(c) The operation of posterior rhizotomy.
(d) The operation of cordotomy.
(e) The injection of opiates into the subarachnoid space.

A 33-year-old mailman received a gunshot wound in his back while he was delivering mail. On examination in the emergency department, the patient was conscious and was found to have an entry wound to the right of the midline in the region of the eighth thoracic vertebra; there was no exit wound.
27. A thorough neurological examination revealed the following motor deficits **except**:
(a) A right-sided lower motor neuron paralysis involving the muscles of the anterior abdominal wall below the umbilicus (the body wall bulged forward in that region).
(b) Spastic paralysis of the right leg.
(c) A left-sided Babinski response.
(d) A right-sided loss of the lower superficial abdominal reflexes.
(e) A loss of the cremasteric reflex on the right side.

28. Further neurological examination also revealed the following sensory deficits **except**:
    (a) A band of cutaneous anesthesia on the right side involving the eleventh thoracic dermatome.
    (b) A left-sided partial loss of tactile discrimination below the level of the eleventh thoracic segment.
    (c) A right-sided partial loss of vibratory sense below the level of the eleventh thoracic segment.
    (d) A right-sided loss of proprioceptive sense below the level of the eleventh thoracic segment.
    (e) A left-sided partial loss of pain and temperature senses below the level of the eleventh thoracic segment.
29. Following a complete radiological workup , including an MRI, and based on the clinical signs and symptoms noted above, the **most likely** diagnosis to be considered was:
    (a) A complete cord transection at the level of the eleventh thoracic segment.
    (b) An anterior cord syndrome at the level of the eleventh thoracic segment.
    (c) A central cord syndrome at the level of the eleventh thoracic segment.
    (d) A Brown-Séquard syndrome involving the right side of the spinal cord at the level of the eleventh thoracic segment.
    (e) A Brown-Séquard syndrome involving the left side of the spinal cord at the level of the eleventh thoracic segment.

Answers to Review Questions

1. D
2. D
3. B
4. D
5. A
6. C
7. B
8. E
9. E
10. E
11. C
12. A
13. B
14. C
15. E
16. A
17. D
18. B
19. D
20. C
21. A
22. D
23. D

24. E. Spasm of the postvertebral muscles would not be produced by pressure on the posterior white columns of the spinal cord.
25. D. The sensation of temperature travels in the lateral spinothalamic tract along with the pain impulses.
26. A. Salicylates, such as aspirin, sodium salicylate, and diflunisal are used clinically only for the relief of mild to moderate pain, as found in patients suffering from headache, and dysmenorrhea.
27. C. A lesion of the corticospinal tracts on the right side would produce a right-sided Babinski response.
28. B. Damage to the right posterior white column of the spinal cord would have interrupted the fasciculus gracilis on the right side. This would have prevented the sensations of tactile discrimination, vibration, and proprioception from the right lower part of the body ascending to the brain.
29. D. The radiographic examination showed the bullet to be lodged in the vertebral canal on the right side of the vertebral column at the level of the eighth thoracic vertebra. This produced severe damage to the right side of the spinal cord at the level of the eleventh thoracic segment and caused the signs and symptoms indicative of a right-sided Brown-Séquard syndrome.

ADDITIONAL READING

Austin, G. *The Spinal Cord.* New York: Igaku Shoin, 1981.

Barson, A. J. The vertebral level of termination of the spinal cord during normal and abnormal development. *J. Anat.* 106:489, 1970.

Basbaum, A. I., and Fields, H. L. Endogenous pain control systems: Brainstem spinal pathways and endorphin circuitry. *Annu. Rev. Neurosci.* 7:309, 1984.

Basbaum, A.I., Unlocking pain's secrets. In: *Encyclopedia Britannica.* Medical Health Annual, pp. 74-95. Chicago: Encyclopedia Britannica, 1995.

Bennett, G. J., Abdelmoumine, M., Hayashi, H., and Dubner, R. Physiology and morphology of substantia gelatinosa neurons intracellularly stained with horseradish peroxidase. *J. Comp. Neurol.* 194:809, 1980.

Bonica, J.J. *The Management of Pain,* 2nd ed. Philadelphia: Lea & Febiger, 1990.

Bracken, M. B., Shepard, M. J., Collins, W. F., et al. A randomized, controlled trial of methylprednisolone or naloxone in the treatment of acute spinal-cord injury: Results of the second national acute spinal cord injury study. *N. Engl. J. Med.* 322:1405, 1990.

Bracken, M. B., et al. Methylprednisone or naloxone treatment after acute spinal cord injury: 1-Year follow up data: Results of the Second National Acute Spinal Cord Injury Study. *J. Neurosurg.* 76:23, 1992.

Brazis, P. W., Masden, J. C., and Biller, J. *Localization in Clinical Neurology.* Boston: Little, Brown, 1990.

Cordo, P., et al. Proprioceptive coordination of movement sequences: role of velocity and position information. *J. Neurophysiol.* 71:1848, 1994.

Chiles, B. W., and Cooper, P. R. Acute spinal cord injury. *N. Engl. J. Med.* 334:514, 1996.

Craig, C. R., and Stitzel, R. E. *Modern Pharmacology* (4th ed.). Boston: Little, Brown, 1994.

Dawnay, N. A. H., and Glees, F. P. Mapping the primate corticospinal pathway. *J. Anat.* 133:124, 1981.

Ekerot, C. F., Larson, B., and Oscarsson, O. Information carried by the spinocerebellar tracts. *Prog. Brain Res.* 50:79, 1979.

Fields, H.L., Liebeskind, J.C. (eds). Pharmacological Approaches to the Treatment of Chronic Pain: New Concepts and Critical Issues. The Bristol-Myers Squibb Symposium on Pain Research, Seattle: IASP Press, 1994.

Frymoyer, J. W. Back pain and sciatica. *N. Engl. J. Med.* 318:291, 1988.

Geisler, F. H., Dorsey, F. C., and Coleman, W. P. Recovery of motor function after spinal cord injury: A randomized, placebo-controlled trial with G. M.-1 ganglioside. *N. Engl. J. Med.* 344:1829, 1991.

Guyton, A.C., and Hall, J.E. *Textbook of Medical Physiology*, 9th ed. W.B.Saunders, Philadelphia, London, 1996.

Koehler, P. J., and Endtz, L. J. The Brown-Séquard syndrome—true or false? *Arch. Neurol.* 43:921, 1986.

Scott, S.A. *Sensory Neurons: Diversity, Development, and Plasticity.* New York, Oxford University Press, 1992.

Snell, R. S. *Clinical Anatomy for Medical Students* (6th ed.). Philadelphia: Lippincott Williams and Wilkins, 2000.

Snell, R. S., and Smith, M. S. *Clinical Anatomy for Emergency Medicine.* St. Louis: Mosby, 1993.

Trapp, B. D. et al. Axonal Transection in the Lesions of Multiple Sclerosis. *N. Engl. J. Med.* 338:278-85, 1998.

Wall, P. D., Melzak, R. (eds). *Textbook of Pain,* 3rd ed. Edinburgh: Churchill Livingstone, 1994.

Waxman, S.G. Demyelinating Diseases-New Pathological Insights, New Therapeutic Targets. *N. Engl. J. Med.* 338:323-325, 1998.

Williams, P. L., et al., *Gray's Anatomy* (38th Br. ed.). New York: London: Churchill Livingstone, 1995.

Wolinsky, J. S. Multiple sclerosis. *Curr. Neurol.* 13:167, 1993.

5

The Brainstem

A 58-year-old woman was referred to a neurologist because of recent onset of difficulty with walking. It was noted that she stood and walked with her left arm flexed at the elbow and the left leg extended (left hemiparesis). While walking, the patient had difficulty flexing the left hip and knee and dorsiflexing the ankle; the forward motion was possible by swinging the left leg outward at the hip to avoid dragging the foot on the ground. The left arm remained motionless.

Neurological examination showed no signs of facial paralysis but there was evidence of weakness of the movements of the tongue. On protrusion, the tongue deviated toward the right side (right hypoglossal nerve palsy). Cutaneous sensations were found to be normal but there was evidence of impairment of muscle joint sense, tactile discrimination, and vibratory sense on the left side of the body.

Based on the neurological findings, a diagnosis of right-sided medial medullary syndrome was made. The medial part of the right side of the medulla oblongata receives its arterial supply from the right vertebral artery. Occlusion of this artery or its branch to the medulla results in destruction of the right pyramid (left hemiparesis), destruction of the right hypoglossal nucleus and nerve (right hypoglossal palsy), and destruction of the medial lemniscus on the right side (left-sided loss of muscle joint sense, vibratory sense, and tactile discrimination). The absence of facial palsy showed that the facial nerve nuclei and the facial nerves and the corticobulbar fibers to the facial nuclei were intact. The sparing of the sensations of touch, pain, and temperature showed that the spinal lemniscus was intact.

This diagnosis was possible as the result of carefully sorting out the neurological findings. A clear knowledge of the position and function of the various nerve tracts and nuclei in the medulla oblongata is essential before one can reach a diagnosis in this case.

C H A P T E R   O B J E C T I V E S

The brain stem consists of the medulla oblongata, the pons, and the midbrain. The purpose of this chapter is to develop a three-dimensional picture of the interior of the brainstem. The student will know the positions of several of the cranial nerve nuclei, the olivary nuclear complex, and the paths taken by the various ascending and descending nerve tracts as they ascend to the higher brain centers or descend to the spinal cord. By understanding the internal arrangement of the brainstem, the physician should be able to assess the signs and symptoms presented by the patient and identify the exact location of a structural lesion.

INTRODUCTION

The brainstem is made up of the medulla oblongata, the pons, and the midbrain and occupies the posterior cranial fossa of the skull (See Fig.5-1). It is stalklike in shape and connects the narrow spinal cord with the expanded forebrain.

The brainstem has three broad functions: 1. It serves as a conduit for the ascending tracts and descending tracts connecting the spinal cord to the different parts of the higher centers in the forebrain. 2. It contains important reflex centers associated with the control of respiration and the cardiovascular system; it also is associated with the control of consciousness. 3. It contains the important nuclei of cranial nerves III through XII.

GROSS APPEARANCE OF THE MEDULLA OBLONGATA

The medulla oblongata connects the pons superiorly with the spinal cord inferiorly (Fig. 5-1). The junction of the medulla and spinal cord is at the origin of the anterior and posterior roots of the first cervical spinal nerve, which corresponds approximately to the level of the foramen magnum. The medulla oblongata is conical in shape, its broad extremity being directed superiorly (Fig. 5-2). The **central canal** of the spinal cord continues upward into the lower half of the medulla; in the upper half of the medulla it expands as the **cavity of the fourth ventricle** (Fig. 5-2).

On the anterior surface of the medulla is the anterior median fissure, which is continuous inferiorly with the **anterior median fissure** of the spinal cord (Fig. 5-2). On each side of the median fissure there is a swelling called the **pyramid**. The pyramids are composed of bundles of nerve fibers, corticospinal fibers, which originate in large nerve cells in the precentral gyrus of the cerebral cortex. The pyramids taper inferiorly and it is here that the majority of the descending fibers cross over to the opposite side, forming the **decussation of the pyramids** (Fig. 5-2). The **anterior external arcuate fibers** are a few nerve fibers that emerge from the anterior median fissure above the decussation and pass laterally over the surface of the medulla oblongata to enter the cerebellum. Posterolateral to the pyramids are the

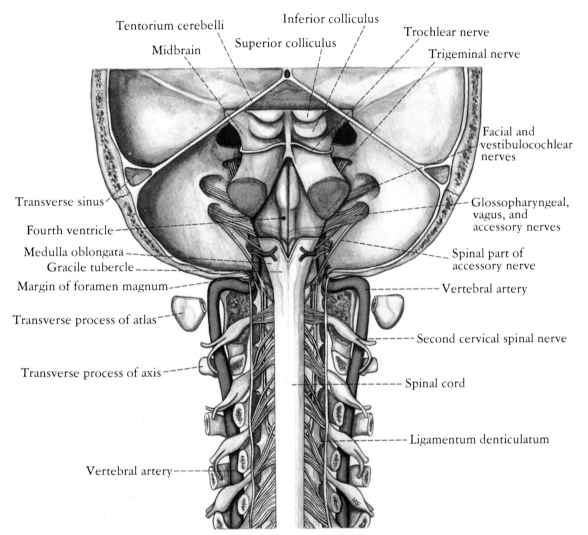

Figure 5–1 Posterior view of the brainstem after removal of the occipital and parietal bones and the cerebrum, the cerebellum, and the roof of the fourth ventricle. Laminae of the upper cervical vertebrae have also been removed.

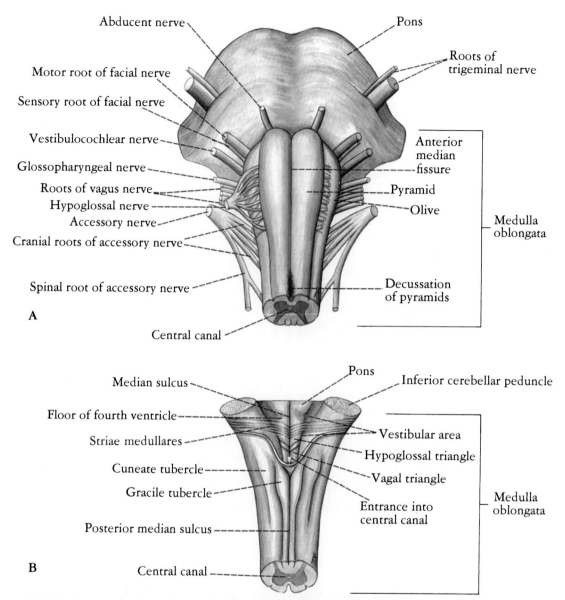

Figure 5–2 Medulla oblongata. **A.** Anterior view. **B.** Posterior view. Note that the roof of the fourth ventricle and the cerebellum have been removed.

olives, which are oval elevations produced by the underlying **inferior olivary nuclei**. In the groove between the pyramid and the olive emerge the rootlets of the hypoglossal nerve. Posterior to the olives are the **inferior cerebellar peduncles** (Fig. 5-2), which connect the medulla to the cerebellum. In the groove between the olive and the inferior cerebellar peduncle emerge the roots of the glossopharyngeal and vagus nerves and the cranial roots of the accessory nerve (see Fig. 5-2).

The posterior surface of the superior half of the medulla oblongata forms the lower part of the **floor of the fourth ventricle** (Fig. 5-2). The posterior surface of the inferior half of the medulla is continuous with the posterior aspect of the spinal cord and possesses a **posterior median sulcus**. On each side of the median sulcus there is an elongated swelling, the gracile tubercle, produced by the underlying **gracile nucleus** (Fig. 5-2). Lateral to the gracile tubercle is a similar swelling, the **cuneate tubercle**, produced by the underlying **cuneate nucleus**.

INTERNAL STRUCTURE

As in the spinal cord, the medulla oblongata consists of white matter and gray matter, but a study of transverse sections of this region shows that they have been extensively rearranged. This rearrangement can be explained embryologically by the expansion of the **neural tube** to form the

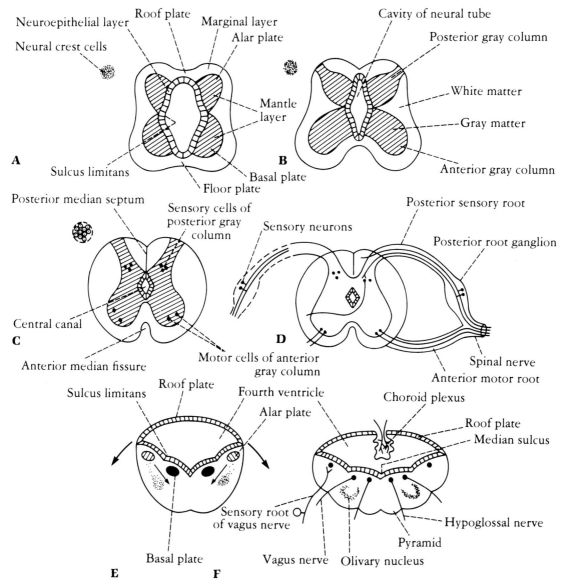

Figure 5-3 Stages in the development of the spinal cord (**A, B, C, D**) and the medulla oblongata (**E, F**). The neural crest cells will form the first afferent sensory neurons in the posterior root ganglia of the spinal nerves and the sensory ganglia of the cranial nerves.

hindbrain vesicle, which becomes the fourth ventricle (Fig. 5-3). The extensive lateral spread of the **fourth ventricle** results in an alteration in the position of the derivatives of the **alar** and **basal plates** of the embryo. To assist in understanding this concept, remember that in the spinal cord the derivatives of the alar and basal plates are situated posterior and anterior to the **sulcus limitans**, respectively, and in the case of the medulla oblongata they are situated lateral and medial to the sulcus limitans, respectively (Fig. 5-3).

The internal structure of the medulla oblongata is considered at four levels: (1) level of decussation of pyramids,

Table 5–1 Comparison of the Different Levels of the Medulla Oblongata, Showing the Major Structures at Each Level*

Level	Cavity	Nuclei	Motor Tracts	Sensory Tracts
Decussation of pyramids	Central canal	Nucleus gracilis, nucleus cuneatus, spinal nucleus of cranial nerve V, accessory nucleus	Decussation of corticospinal tracts, pyramids	Spinal tract of cranial nerve V, posterior spinocerebellar tract, lateral spinothalamic tract, anterior spinocerebellar tract
Decussation of medial lemnisci	Central canal	Nucleus gracilis, nucleus cuneatus, spinal nucleus of cranial nerve V, accessory nucleus, hypoglossal nucleus	Pyramids	Decussation of medial lemnisci, fasciculus gracilis, fasciculus cuneatus, spinal tract of cranial nerve V, posterior spinocerebellar tract, lateral spinothalamic tract, anterior spinocerebellar tract
Olives, inferior cerebellar peduncle	Fourth ventricle	Inferior olivary nucleus, spinal nucleus of cranial nerve V, vestibular nucleus, glossopharyngeal nucleus, vagal nucleus, hypoglossal nucleus, nucleus ambiguus, nucleus of tractus solitarius	Pyramids	Medial longitudinal fasciculus, tectospinal tract, medial lemniscus, spinal tract of cranial nerve V, lateral spinothalamic tract, anterior spinocerebellar tract
Just inferior to pons	Fourth ventricle	Lateral vestibular nucleus, cochlear nuclei	No major changes in distribution of gray and white matter	

*Note that the reticular formation is present at all levels.

(2) level of decussation of lemnisci, (3) level of the olives, and (4) level just inferior to the pons. See Table 5-1 for a comparison of the different levels of the medulla oblongata and the major structures present at each level.

Level of Decussation of Pyramids

A transverse section through the inferior half of the medulla oblongata (Figs. 5-4A and 5-5) passes through the **decussation of the pyramids**, the great motor decussation. In the superior part of the medulla the corticospinal fibers occupy and form the pyramid, but inferiorly about three-fourths of the fibers cross the median plane and continue down the spinal cord in the lateral white column as the **lateral corticospinal tract**. As these fibers cross the midline, they sever the continuity between the anterior column of the gray matter of the spinal cord and the gray matter that surrounds the central canal.

The **fasciculus gracilis** and the **fasciculus cuneatus** continue to ascend superiorly posterior to the central gray matter (Figs. 5-4A and 5-5). The **nucleus gracilis** and the **nucleus cuneatus** appear as posterior extensions of the central gray matter.

The **substantia gelatinosa** in the posterior gray column of the spinal cord becomes continuous with the inferior end

of the **nucleus of the spinal tract of the trigeminal nerve**. The fibers of the tract of the nucleus are situated between the nucleus and the surface of the medulla oblongata.

The lateral and anterior white columns of the spinal cord are easily identified in these sections and their fiber arrangement is unchanged (Figs. 5-4A and 5-5).

Level of Decussation of Lemnisci

A transverse section through the inferior half of the medulla oblongata, a short distance above the level of the decussation of the pyramids, passes through the **decussation of lemnisci**, the great sensory decussation (Figs. 5-4B and 5-6). The decussation of the lemnisci takes place anterior to the central gray matter and posterior to the pyramids. It should be understood that the lemnisci have been formed from the **internal arcuate fibers**, which have emerged from the anterior aspects of the **nucleus gracilis** and **nucleus cuneatus**. The internal arcuate fibers first travel anteriorly and laterally around the central gray matter. They then curve medially toward the midline, where they decussate with the corresponding fibers of the opposite side (Figs. 5-4B and 5-6).

The **nucleus of the spinal tract of the trigeminal nerve** lies lateral to the internal arcuate fibers. The **spinal**

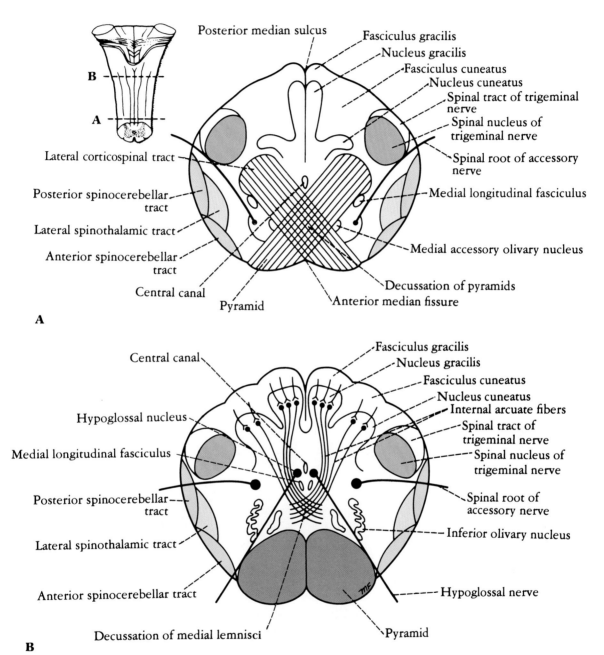

Figure 5–4 Transverse sections of the medulla oblongata. **A**. Level of decussation of the pyramids. **B**. Level of decussation of the medial lemnisci.

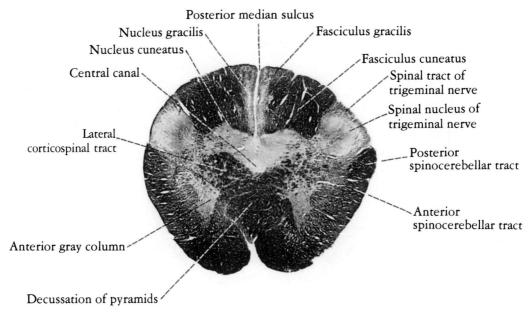

Posterior median sulcus

Nucleus gracilis

Fasciculus gracilis

Nucleus cuneatus

Central canal

Fasciculus cuneatus

Spinal tract of
trigeminal nerve

Spinal nucleus of
trigeminal nerve

Lateral
corticospinal tract

Posterior
spinocerebellar tract

Anterior
spinocerebellar tract

Anterior gray column

Decussation of pyramids

Figure 5–5 Transverse section of the medulla oblongata at the level of decussation of the pyramids. (Weigert stain.)

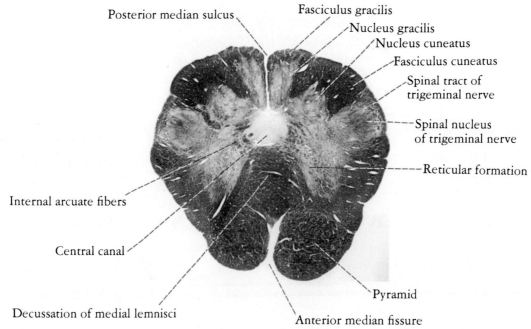

Posterior median sulcus

Fasciculus gracilis

Nucleus gracilis

Nucleus cuneatus

Fasciculus cuneatus

Spinal tract of
trigeminal nerve

Spinal nucleus
of trigeminal nerve

Reticular formation

Internal arcuate fibers

Central canal

Pyramid

Decussation of medial lemnisci

Anterior median fissure

Figure 5–6 Transverse section of the medulla oblongata at the level of decussation of the medial lemnisci. (Weigert stain.)

tract of the **trigeminal nerve** lies lateral to the nucleus (Figs. 5-4B and 5-6).

The **lateral** and **anterior spinothalamic tracts** and the **spinotectal tracts** occupy an area lateral to the decussation of the lemnisci (Fig. 5-4B). They are very close to one another and collectively are known as the **spinal lemniscus**. The **spinocerebellar**, **vestibulospinal**, and the

rubrospinal tracts are situated in the anterolateral region of the medulla oblongata.

Level of the Olives

A transverse section through the olives passes across the inferior part of the fourth ventricle (Figs. 5-7 and 5-8). The

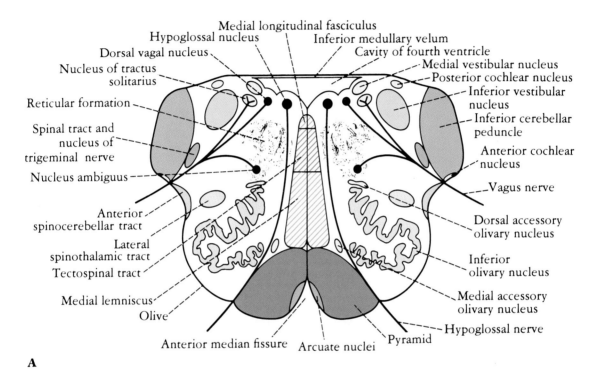

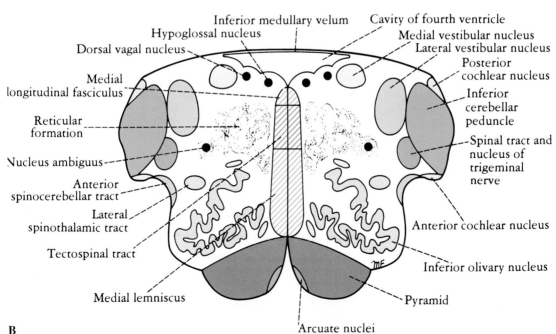

Figure 5–7 Transverse sections of the medulla oblongata at the level of: **A**. The middle of the olivary nuclei. **B**. The superior part of the olivary nuclei just inferior to the pons.

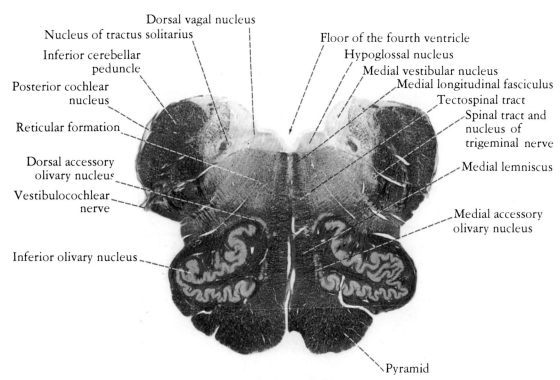

Figure 5–8 Transverse section of the medulla oblongata at the level of the middle of the olivary nuclei. (Weigert stain.)

amount of gray matter has increased at this level owing to the presence of the olivary nuclear complex; the nuclei of the vestibulocochlear, glossopharyngeal, vagus, accessory, and hypoglossal nerves; and the arcuate nuclei.

OLIVARY NUCLEAR COMPLEX

The largest nucleus of this complex is the **inferior olivary nucleus** (Figs. 5-7 and 5-8). The gray matter is shaped like a crumpled bag with its mouth directed medially; it is responsible for the elevation on the surface of the medulla called the **olive**. Smaller **dorsal** and **medial accessory olivary nuclei** also are present. The cells of the inferior olivary nucleus send fibers medially across the midline to enter the cerebellum through the inferior cerebellar peduncle. Afferent fibers reach the inferior olivary nuclei from the spinal cord (the **spino-olivary tracts**) and from the cerebellum and cerebral cortex. The function of the olivary nuclei is associated with voluntary muscle movement.

VESTIBULOCOCHLEAR NUCLEI

The **vestibular nuclear complex** is made up of the following nuclei: (1) **medial vestibular nucleus**, (2) **inferior vestibular nucleus**, (3) **lateral vestibular nucleus**, and (4) **superior vestibular nucleus**. The details of these nuclei and their connections are discussed later. The medial and inferior vestibular nuclei can be seen on section at this level (Figs. 5-7 and 5-8).

The **cochlear nuclei** are two in number. The **anterior cochlear nucleus** is situated on the anterolateral aspect of the inferior cerebellar peduncle and the **posterior cochlear nucleus** is situated on the posterior aspect of the peduncle lateral to the floor of the fourth ventricle (Figs. 5-7 and 5-8). The connections of these nuclei are described later.

THE NUCLEUS AMBIGUUS

The nucleus ambiguus consists of large motor neurons and is situated deep within the reticular formation (Figs. 5-7 and 5-9). The emerging nerve fibers join the glossopharyngeal, vagus, and cranial part of the accessory nerve and are distributed to voluntary skeletal muscle.

CENTRAL GRAY MATTER

The central gray matter lies beneath the floor of the fourth ventricle at this level (Figs. 5-7 and 5-8). Passing from medial to lateral (Fig. 5-9), the following important structures may be recognized: (1) the **hypoglossal nucleus**, (2) the **dorsal nucleus of the vagus**, (3) the **nucleus of the tractus solitarius**, and (4) the **medial** and **inferior vestibular nuclei** (see above). The nucleus ambiguus, referred to above, has become deeply placed within the reticular formation (Fig. 5-7). The connections and functional significance of these nuclei are described in Chapter 11.

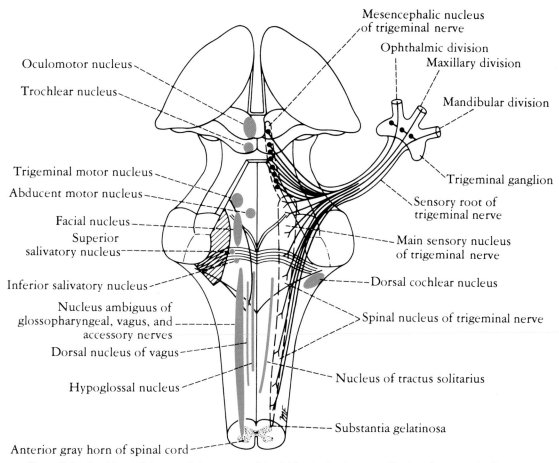

Figure 5–9 Position of the cranial nerve nuclei within the brainstem. The hatched area indicates the position of the vestibular nuclei.

The arcuate nuclei are thought to be inferiorly displaced **pontine nuclei** (see p. 202) and are situated on the anterior surface of the pyramids (Fig. 5-7). They receive nerve fibers from the cerebral cortex and send efferent fibers to the cerebellum through the **anterior external arcuate fibers**.

The **pyramids** containing the corticospinal and some corticonuclear fibers are situated in the anterior part of the medulla separated by the anterior median fissure (Figs. 5-7 and 5-8); the corticospinal fibers descend to the spinal cord and the corticonuclear fibers are distributed to the motor nuclei of the cranial nerves situated within the medulla.

The **medial lemniscus** forms a flattened tract on each side of the midline posterior to the pyramid (Figs. 5-7 and 5-8). These fibers emerge from the decussation of the lemnisci and convey sensory information to the thalamus.

The **medial longitudinal fasciculus** forms a small tract of nerve fibers situated on each side of the midline posterior to the medial lemniscus and anterior to the hypoglossal nucleus (see Figs. 5-7 and 5-8). It consists of ascending and descending fibers, the connections of which are described on page 202.

The **inferior cerebellar peduncle** is situated in the posterolateral corner of the section on the lateral side of the fourth ventricle (Figs. 5-7 and 5-8).

The **spinal tract of the trigeminal nerve** and **its nucleus** are situated on the anteromedial aspect of the inferior cerebellar peduncle (Figs. 5-7 and 5-8).

The **anterior spinocerebellar tract** is situated near the surface in the interval between the inferior olivary nucleus and the nucleus of the spinal tract of the trigeminal nerve (Figs. 5-7 and 5-8). The **spinal lemniscus**, consisting of the **anterior spinothalamic**, the **lateral spinothalamic**, and **spinotectal tracts** is deeply placed.

The **reticular formation**, consisting of a diffuse mixture of nerve fibers and small groups of nerve cells, is deeply placed posterior to the olivary nucleus (Figs. 5-7 and 5-8). The reticular formation represents, at this level, only a small part of this system, which is also present in the pons and midbrain.

The **glossopharyngeal, vagus,** and **cranial part of the accessory nerves** can be seen running forward and laterally through the reticular formation (Fig. 5-7). The nerve fibers emerge between the olives and the inferior cerebellar peduncles. The **hypoglossal nerves** also run anteriorly and laterally through the reticular formation and emerge between the pyramids and the olives (Fig. 5-7).

Level Just Inferior to the Pons

There are no major changes, in comparison to the previous level, in the distribution of the gray and white matter (Figs. 5-7 and 5-9). The lateral vestibular nucleus has replaced the inferior vestibular nucleus, and the cochlear nuclei now are visible on the anterior and posterior surfaces of the inferior cerebellar peduncle.

GROSS APPEARANCE OF THE PONS

The pons is anterior to the cerebellum (Fig. 5-10) and connects the medulla oblongata to the midbrain. It is about 1 inch (2.5 cm) long and owes its name to the appearance presented on the anterior surface, which is that of a bridge connecting the right and left cerebellar hemispheres.

The anterior surface is convex from side to side and shows many transverse fibers that converge on each side to form the **middle cerebellar peduncle** (Fig. 5-10). There is

a shallow groove in the midline, the **basilar groove**, which lodges the basilar artery. On the anterolateral surface of the pons the **trigeminal nerve** emerges on each side. Each nerve consists of a smaller, medial part—the **motor root**—and a larger, lateral part—the **sensory root**. In the groove between the pons and the medulla oblongata there emerge, from medial to lateral, the **abducent, facial,** and **vestibulocochlear nerves** (Fig. 5-10).

The posterior surface of the pons is hidden from view by the cerebellum (Fig. 5-11). It forms the upper half of the floor of the fourth ventricle and is triangular in shape. The posterior surface is limited laterally by the **superior cerebellar peduncles** and is divided into symmetrical halves by a **median sulcus**. Lateral to this sulcus is an elongated elevation, the **medial eminence**, which is bounded laterally by a sulcus, the **sulcus limitans** (Fig. 5-11). The inferior end of the medial eminence is slightly expanded to form the **facial colliculus**, which is produced by the root of the facial nerve winding around the nucleus of the abducent nerve (Fig. 5-12). The floor of the superior part of the **sulcus limitans** is bluish-gray in color and is called the **substantia ferruginea**; it owes its color to a group of deeply pigmented nerve cells. Lateral to the sulcus limitans is the **area vestibuli** produced by the underlying vestibular nuclei (Fig. 5-11).

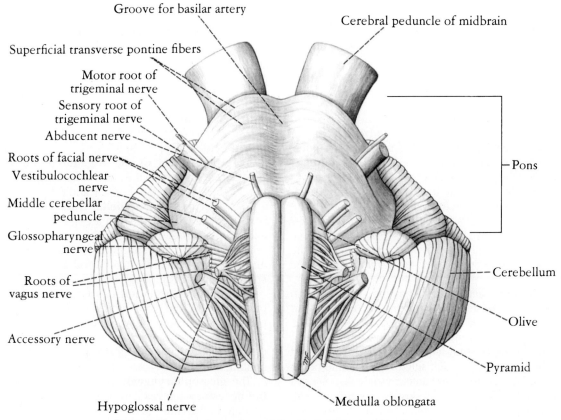

Figure 5–10   Anterior surface of the brainstem showing the pons.

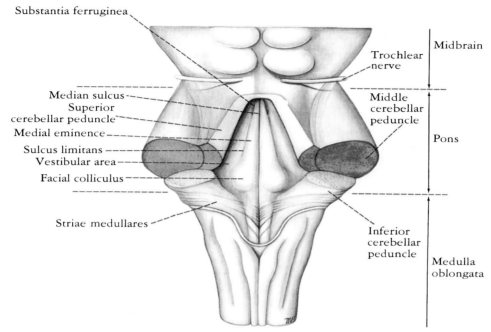

Figure 5–11 Posterior surface of the brainstem showing the pons. The cerebellum has been removed.

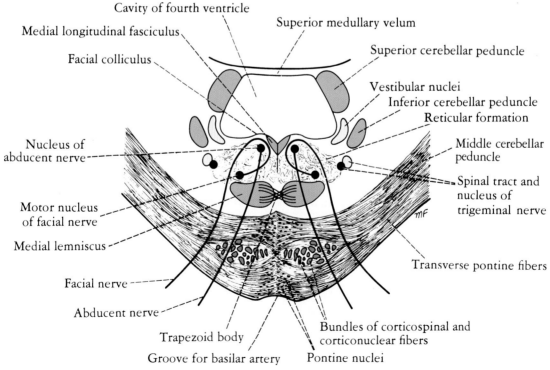

Figure 5–12 Transverse section through the caudal part of the pons at the level of the facial colliculus.

INTERNAL STRUCTURE OF THE PONS

For purposes of description, the pons is commonly divided into a posterior part, the **tegmentum**, and an anterior **basal part** by the transversely running fibers of the **trapezoid body** (Fig. 5-12).

The structure of the pons may be studied at two levels: (1) transverse section through the caudal part, passing through the facial colliculus, and (2) transverse section through the cranial part, passing through the trigeminal nuclei. See Table 5-2 for a comparison of the two levels of the pons and the major structures present at each level.

Transverse Section Through the Caudal Part

The **medial lemniscus** rotates as it passes from the medulla into the pons. It is situated in the most anterior part of the tegmentum with its long axis running transversely (Fig. 5-12). The medial lemniscus is accompanied by the spinal and lateral lemnisci.

The **facial nucleus** lies posterior to the lateral part of the medial lemniscus. The fibers of the facial nerve wind around the **nucleus of the abducent nerve**, producing the **facial colliculus** (Fig. 5-12). The fibers of the facial nerve then pass anteriorly between the facial nucleus and the superior end of the nucleus of the spinal tract of the trigeminal nerve.

The **medial longitudinal fasciculus** is situated beneath the floor of the fourth ventricle on either side of the midline (Fig. 5-12). The medial longitudinal fasciculus is the main pathway that connects the vestibular and cochlear nuclei with the nuclei controlling the extraocular muscles (oculomotor, trochlear, and abducent nuclei).

The **medial vestibular nucleus** is situated lateral to the abducent nucleus (Fig. 5-12) and is in close relationship to the inferior cerebellar peduncle. The superior part of the lat-

eral and the inferior part of the superior vestibular nucleus are found at this level. The **posterior** and **anterior cochlear nuclei** are also found at this level.

The **spinal nucleus of the trigeminal nerve** and its tract lie on the anteromedial aspect of the inferior cerebellar peduncle (Fig. 5-12).

The **trapezoid body** is made up of fibers derived from the cochlear nuclei and the nuclei of the trapezoid body. They run transversely (Fig. 5-12) in the anterior part of the tegmentum (p. 201).

The basilar part of the pons, at this level, contains small masses of nerve cells called **pontine nuclei** (Fig. 5-12). The **corticopontine fibers** of the crus cerebri of the midbrain terminate in the pontine nuclei. The axons of these cells give origin to the **transverse fibers** of the pons, which cross the midline and intersect the corticospinal and corticonuclear tracts, breaking them up into small bundles. The transverse fibers of the pons enter the middle cerebellar peduncle and are distributed to the cerebellar hemisphere. This connection forms the main pathway linking the cerebral cortex to the cerebellum.

Transverse Section Through the Cranial Part

The internal structure of the cranial part of the pons is similar to that seen at the caudal level (Figs. 5-13 through 5-15), but it now contains the motor and principal sensory nuclei of the trigeminal nerve.

The **motor nucleus of the trigeminal nerve** is situated beneath the lateral part of the fourth ventricle within the reticular formation (Figs. 5-13 and 5-14). The emerging motor fibers travel anteriorly through the substance of the pons and exit on its anterior surface.

The **principal sensory nucleus of the trigeminal nerve** is situated on the lateral side of the motor nucleus (Figs. 5-13 and 5-14); it is continuous inferiorly with the nucleus of the spinal tract. The entering sensory fibers travel

Table 5–2   Comparison of the Different Levels of the Pons Showing the Major Structures at Each Level*

Level	Cavity	Nuclei	Motor Tracts	Sensory Tracts
Facial colliculus	Fourth ventricle	Facial nucleus, abducent nucleus, medial vestibular nucleus, spinal nucleus of cranial nerve V, pontine nuclei, trapezoid nuclei	Corticospinal and corticonuclear tracts, transverse pontine fibers, medial longitudinal fasciculus	Spinal tract of cranial nerve V; lateral, spinal, and medial lemnisci
Trigeminal nuclei	Fourth ventricle	Main sensory and motor nucleus of cranial nerve V, pontine nuclei, trapezoid nuclei	Corticospinal and corticonuclear tracts, transverse pontine fibers, medial longitudinal fasciculus	Lateral, spinal, and medial lemnisci

*Note that the reticular formation is present at all levels.

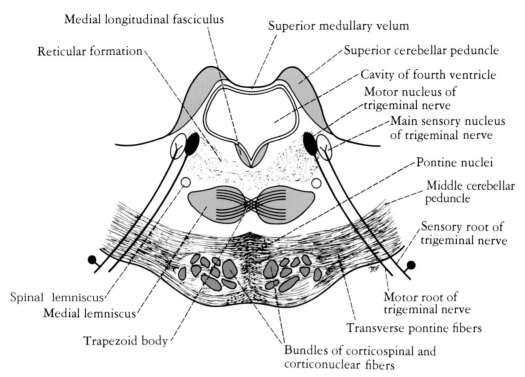

Medial longitudinal fasciculus

Superior medullary velum

Reticular formation

Superior cerebellar peduncle

Cavity of fourth ventricle

Motor nucleus of trigeminal nerve

Main sensory nucleus of trigeminal nerve

Pontine nuclei

Middle cerebellar peduncle

Sensory root of trigeminal nerve

Spinal lemniscus

Medial lemniscus

Motor root of trigeminal nerve

Transverse pontine fibers

Trapezoid body

Bundles of corticospinal and corticonuclear fibers

Figure 5–13   Transverse section through the pons at the level of the trigeminal nuclei.

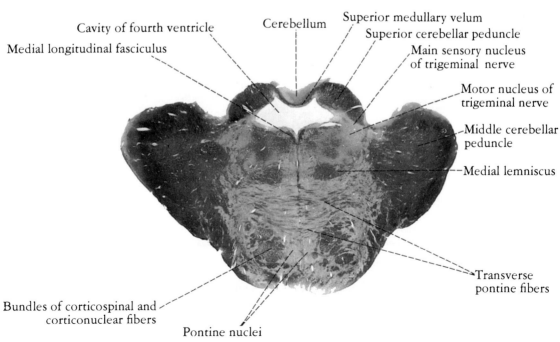

Cavity of fourth ventricle

Cerebellum

Superior medullary velum

Medial longitudinal fasciculus

Superior cerebellar peduncle

Main sensory nucleus of trigeminal nerve

Motor nucleus of trigeminal nerve

Middle cerebellar peduncle

Medial lemniscus

Transverse pontine fibers

Bundles of corticospinal and corticonuclear fibers

Pontine nuclei

Figure 5–14   Photomicrograph of a transverse section of the pons at the level of the trigeminal nuclei.

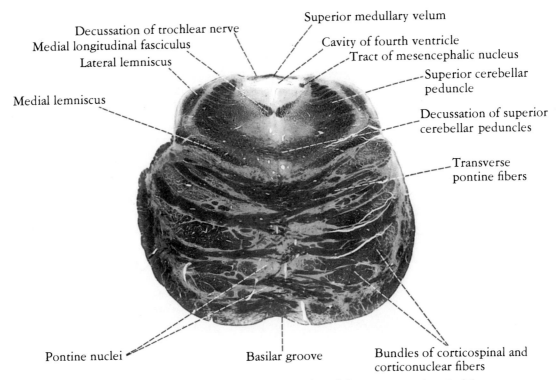

Decussation of trochlear nerve
Medial longitudinal fasciculus
Lateral lemniscus
Medial lemniscus
Superior medullary velum
Cavity of fourth ventricle
Tract of mesencephalic nucleus
Superior cerebellar peduncle
Decussation of superior cerebellar peduncles
Transverse pontine fibers
Pontine nuclei
Basilar groove
Bundles of corticospinal and corticonuclear fibers

Figure 5–15 Photomicrograph of a transverse section of the most rostral part of the pons.

through the substance of the pons and lie lateral to the motor fibers (Fig. 5-13).

The **superior cerebellar peduncle** is situated postero-lateral to the motor nucleus of the trigeminal nerve (Figs. 5-13 and 5-14). It is joined by the **anterior spinocerebellar tract**.

The **trapezoid body** and the **medial lemniscus** are situated in the same position as they were in the previous section (Fig. 5-13). The **lateral** and **spinal lemnisci** lies at the lateral extremity of the medial lemniscus (Figs. 5-13 and 5-15).

GROSS APPEARANCE OF THE MIDBRAIN

The midbrain measures about 0.8 inch (2 cm) in length and connects the pons and cerebellum with the forebrain (Fig. 5-16). Its long axis inclines anteriorly as it ascends through the opening in the tentorium cerebelli. The midbrain is traversed by a narrow channel, the **cerebral aqueduct**, which is filled with cerebrospinal fluid (Figs. 5-17, 5-18 through 5-21).

On the posterior surface are four **colliculi** (corpora quadrigemina). These are rounded eminences that are divided into superior and inferior pairs by a vertical and a transverse groove (Fig. 5-19). The superior colliculi are centers for visual reflexes (p. 208), and the inferior are lower auditory centers. In the midline below the inferior colliculi

the **trochlear** nerves emerge. These are small-diameter nerves that wind around the lateral aspect of the midbrain to enter the lateral wall of the cavernous sinus.

On the lateral aspect of the midbrain, the superior and inferior brachia ascend in an anterolateral direction (Fig. 5-16). The **superior brachium** passes from the superior colliculus to the lateral geniculate body and the optic tract. The **inferior brachium** connects the inferior colliculus to the **medial geniculate body**.

On the anterior aspect of the midbrain (Fig. 5-16) there is a deep depression in the midline, the **interpeduncular fossa**, which is bounded on either side by the **crus cerebri**. Many small blood vessels perforate the floor of the interpeduncular fossa and this region is termed the **posterior perforated substance** (Fig. 5-16). The oculomotor nerve emerges from a groove on the medial side of the crus cerebri and passes forward in the lateral wall of the cavernous sinus.

INTERNAL STRUCTURE OF THE MIDBRAIN

The midbrain comprises two lateral halves, called the **cerebral peduncles**; each of these is divided into an anterior part, the **crus cerebri**, and a posterior part, the **tegmentum**, by a pigmented band of gray matter, the **substantia nigra** (Figs. 5-17 and 5-18). The narrow cavity of the midbrain is the **cerebral aqueduct**, which connects the third

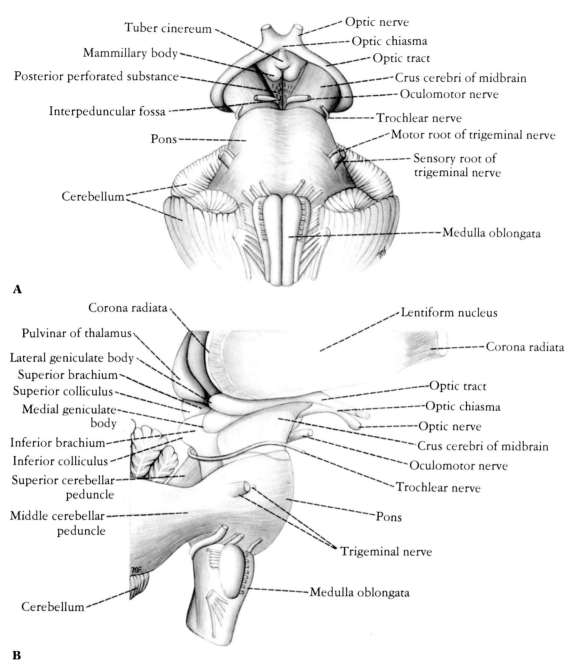

Tuber cinereum

Mammillary body

Posterior perforated substance

Interpeduncular fossa

Pons

Cerebellum

Optic nerve

Optic chiasma

Optic tract

Crus cerebri of midbrain

Oculomotor nerve

Trochlear nerve

Motor root of trigeminal nerve

Sensory root of trigeminal nerve

Medulla oblongata

A

Corona radiata

Pulvinar of thalamus

Lateral geniculate body

Superior brachium

Superior colliculus

Medial geniculate body

Inferior brachium

Inferior colliculus

Superior cerebellar peduncle

Middle cerebellar peduncle

Cerebellum

Lentiform nucleus

Corona radiata

Optic tract

Optic chiasma

Optic nerve

Crus cerebri of midbrain

Oculomotor nerve

Trochlear nerve

Pons

Trigeminal nerve

Medulla oblongata

B

Figure 5–16   The midbrain. **A**. Anterior view. **B**. Lateral view.

and fourth ventricles. The **tectum** is the part of the midbrain posterior to the cerebral aqueduct; it has four small surface swellings referred to previously: the **two superior** and **two inferior colliculi** (Figs. 5-17 and 5-18). The cerebral aqueduct is lined by ependyma and is surrounded by the **central gray matter**. On transverse sections of the midbrain the interpeduncular fossa can be seen to separate the crura cerebri, whereas the tegmentum is continuous across the median plane (see Fig. 5-17).

Transverse Section of the Midbrain at the Level of the Inferior Colliculi

The **inferior colliculus**, consisting of a large nucleus of gray matter, lies beneath the corresponding surface elevation and forms part of the auditory pathway (Figs. 5-18A and 5-20). It receives many of the terminal fibers of the lateral lemniscus. The pathway then continues through the inferior brachium to the medial geniculate body.

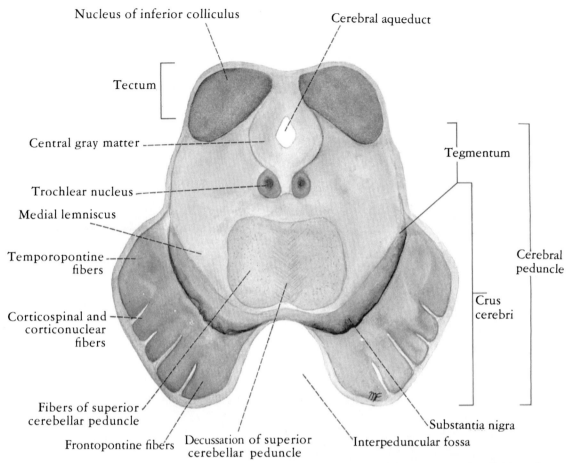

Figure 5–17 Transverse section of the midbrain through the inferior colliculi shows the division of the midbrain into the tectum and the cerebral peduncles. Note that the cerebral peduncles are subdivided by the substantia nigra into the tegmentum and the crus cerebri.

The **trochlear nucleus** is situated in the central gray matter close to the median plane just posterior to the **medial longitudinal fasciculus**. The emerging fibers of the trochlear nucleus pass laterally and posteriorly around the central gray matter and leave the midbrain just below the inferior colliculi. The fibers of the trochlear nerve now **decussate completely** in the superior medullary velum. The **mesencephalic nuclei of the trigeminal nerve** are lateral to the cerebral aqueduct (Figs. 5-18A and 5-20). The **decussation of the superior cerebellar peduncles** occupies the central part of the tegmentum anterior to the cerebral aqueduct. The **reticular formation** is smaller than that of the pons and is situated lateral to the decussation.

The **medial lemniscus** ascends posterior to the substantia nigra; the **spinal** and **trigeminal lemnisci** are situated lateral to the medial lemniscus (Figs. 5-18 and 5-20). The **lateral lemniscus** is located posterior to the trigeminal lemniscus.

The **substantia nigra** (Figs. 5-18 and 5-20) is a large motor nucleus situated between the tegmentum and the crus cerebri and is found throughout the midbrain. The nucleus is composed of medium-size multipolar neurons that possess inclusion granules of melanin pigment within their cytoplasm. The substantia nigra is concerned with muscle tone and is connected to the cerebral cortex, spinal cord, hypothalamus, and basal nuclei.

The **crus cerebri** contains important descending tracts and is separated from the tegmentum by the substantia nigra (Figs. 5-18 and 5-20). The corticospinal and corticonuclear fibers occupy the middle two-thirds of the crus. The frontopontine fibers occupy the medial part of the crus and the temporopontine fibers occupy the lateral part of the crus (Figs. 5-18 and 5-20). These descending tracts connect the cerebral cortex to the anterior gray column cells of the spinal cord, the cranial nerve nuclei, the pons, and the cerebellum (Table 5-3).

Transverse Section of the Midbrain at the Level of the Superior Colliculi

The **superior colliculus** (Figs. 5-18B and 5-21), a large nucleus of gray matter that lies beneath the corresponding surface elevation, forms part of the visual reflexes. It is connected to the lateral geniculate body by the superior

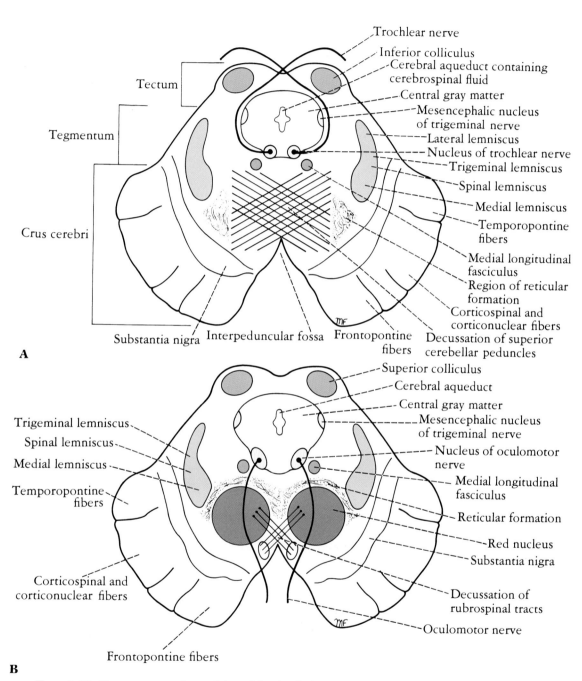

Figure 5–18 Transverse sections of the midbrain. **A.** At the level of the inferior colliculus. **B.** At the level of the superior colliculus. Note that trochlear nerves completely decussate within the superior medullary velum.

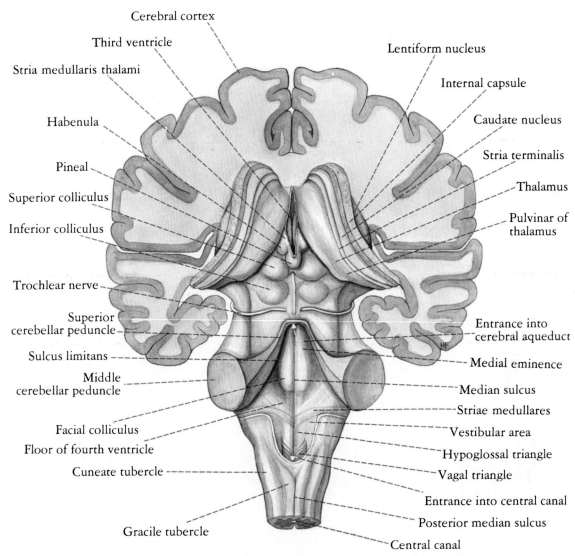

Cerebral cortex

Third ventricle

Stria medullaris thalami

Habenula

Pineal

Superior colliculus

Inferior colliculus

Trochlear nerve

Superior
cerebellar peduncle

Sulcus limitans

Middle
cerebellar peduncle

Facial colliculus

Floor of fourth ventricle

Cuneate tubercle

Gracile tubercle

Lentiform nucleus

Internal capsule

Caudate nucleus

Stria terminalis

Thalamus

Pulvinar of
thalamus

Entrance into
cerebral aqueduct

Medial eminence

Median sulcus

Striae medullares

Vestibular area

Hypoglossal triangle

Vagal triangle

Entrance into central canal

Posterior median sulcus

Central canal

Figure 5–19 Posterior view of the brainstem showing the two superior and the two inferior colliculi of the tectum.

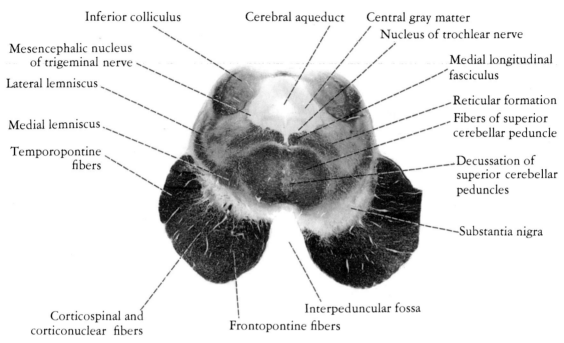

Figure 5–20 Photomicrograph of a transverse section of the midbrain at the level of the inferior colliculus. (Weigert stain.)

Table 5–3		Comparison of Two Levels of the Midbrain, Showing the Major Structures at Each Level*		
Level	**Cavity**	**Nuclei**	**Motor Tract**	**Sensory Tracts**
Inferior colliculi	Cerebral aqueduct	Inferior colliculus, substantia nigra, trochlear nucleus, mesencephalic nuclei of cranial nerve V	Corticospinal and corticonuclear tracts, temporopontine, frontopontine, medial longitudinal fasciculus	Lateral, trigeminal, spinal, and medial lemnisci, decussation of superior cerebellar peduncles
Superior colliculi	Cerebral aqueduct	Superior colliculus, substantia nigra, oculomotor nucleus, Edinger-Westphal nucleus, red nucleus, mesencephalic nucleus of cranial nerve V	Corticospinal and corticonuclear tracts, temporopontine, frontopontine, medial longitudinal fasciculus, decussation of rubrospinal tract	Trigeminal, spinal, and medial lemnisci

*Note that the reticular formation is present at all levels.

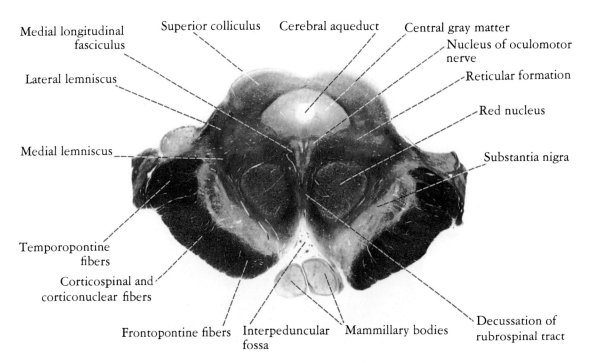

Medial longitudinal fasciculus
Superior colliculus
Cerebral aqueduct
Central gray matter
Nucleus of oculomotor nerve
Lateral lemniscus
Reticular formation
Red nucleus
Medial lemniscus
Substantia nigra
Temporopontine fibers
Corticospinal and corticonuclear fibers
Frontopontine fibers
Interpeduncular fossa
Mammillary bodies
Decussation of rubrospinal tract

Figure 5–21 Photomicrograph of a transverse section of the midbrain at the level of the superior colliculus. (Weigert stain.)

brachium. It receives afferent fibers from the optic nerve, the visual cortex, and the spinotectal tract. The efferent fibers form the tectospinal and tectobulbar tracts, which are probably responsible for the reflex movements of the eyes, head, and neck in response to visual stimuli. The afferent pathway for the **light reflex** ends in the **pretectal nucleus**. This is a small group of neurons situated close to the lateral part of the superior colliculus. After relaying in the pretectal nucleus, the fibers pass to the parasympathetic nucleus of the oculomotor nerve (Edinger-Westphal nucleus). The emerging fibers then pass to the oculomotor nerve. The **oculomotor nucleus** is situated in the central gray matter close to the median plane, just posterior to the **medial longitudinal fasciculus** (Figs. 5-18B and 5-21). The fibers of the oculomotor nucleus pass anteriorly through the red nucleus to emerge on the medial side of the crus cerebri in the interpeduncular fossa. The nucleus of the oculomotor nerve is divisible into a number of cell groups.

The **medial**, **spinal**, and **trigeminal lemnisci** form a curved band posterior to the substantia nigra but the **lateral lemniscus** does not extend superiorly to this level (Figs. 5-18B and 5-21).

The **red nucleus** (Figs. 5-18B and 5-21) is a rounded mass of gray matter situated between the cerebral aqueduct and the substantia nigra. Its reddish hue, seen in fresh specimens, is due to its vascularity and the presence of an iron-containing pigment in the cytoplasm of many of its neurons. Afferent fibers reach the red nucleus from (1) the cerebral cortex through the corticospinal fibers, (2) the cerebellum through the superior cerebellar peduncle, and (3) the lentiform nucleus, subthalamic and hypothalamic nuclei, substantia nigra, and spinal cord. Efferent fibers leave the red nucleus and pass to (1) the spinal cord through the rubrospinal tract (as this tract descends, it decussates), (2) the reticular formation through the rubroreticular tract, (3) the thalamus, and (4) the substantia nigra.

The **reticular formation** is situated in the tegmentum lateral and posterior to the red nucleus (Figs. 5-18B and 5-21).

The **crus cerebri** contains the identical important descending tracts, the **corticospinal**, **corticonuclear**, and **corticopontine fibers**, that are present at the level of the inferior colliculus (see Table 5-3).

The continuity of the various cranial nerve nuclei through the different regions of the brainstem is shown diagrammatically in Figure 5-22.

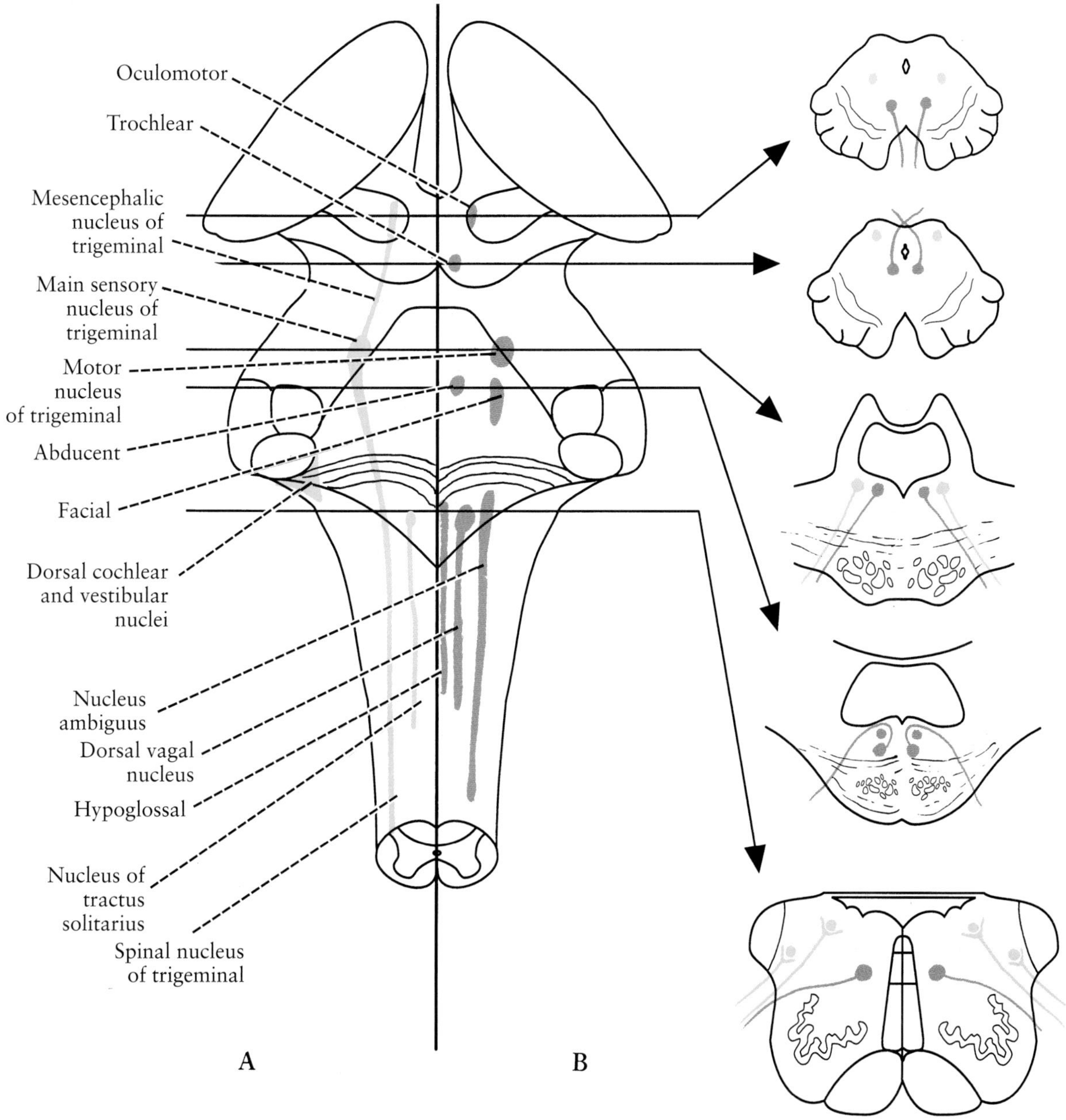
Oculomotor
Trochlear
Mesencephalic nucleus of trigeminal
Main sensory nucleus of trigeminal
Motor nucleus of trigeminal
Abducent
Facial
Dorsal cochlear and vestibular nuclei
Nucleus ambiguus
Dorsal vagal nucleus
Hypoglossal
Nucleus of tractus solitarius
Spinal nucleus of trigeminal
A
B

Figure 5–22 Position of some of the cranial nerve nuclei in the brainstem. **A**. Surface projection on the posterior aspect of the brainstem. **B**. Cross sections. The motor nuclei are in red, and the sensory nuclei in blue.

Clinical Notes

Clinical Significance of the Medulla Oblongata

The medulla oblongata not only contains many cranial nerve nuclei that are concerned with vital functions (e.g., regulation of heart rate and respiration), but also serves as a conduit for the passage of ascending and descending tracts connecting the spinal cord to the higher centers of the nervous system. These tracts may become involved in demyelinating diseases, neoplasms, and vascular disorders.

Raised Pressure in the Posterior Cranial Fossa and Its Effect on the Medulla Oblongata

The medulla oblongata is situated in the posterior cranial fossa, lying beneath the tentorium cerebelli and above the foramen magnum. It is related anteriorly to the basal portion of the occipital bone and the upper part of the odontoid process of the axis and posteriorly to the cerebellum.

In patients with tumors of the posterior cranial fossa, the intracranial pressure is raised and the brain, that is, the cerebellum and the medulla oblongata, tends to be pushed toward the area of least resistance; there is a downward herniation of the medulla and cerebellar tonsils through the foramen magnum. This will produce the symptoms of headache, neck stiffness, and paralysis of the glossopharyngeal, vagus, accessory, and hypoglossal nerves owing to traction. In these circumstances, it is **extremely dangerous to perform a lumbar puncture** because the sudden withdrawal of cerebrospinal fluid may precipitate further herniation of the brain through the foramen magnum and a sudden failure of vital functions, resulting from pressure and ischemia of the cranial nerve nuclei present in the medulla oblongata.

Arnold-Chiari Phenomenon

The **Arnold-Chiari malformation** is a congenital anomaly in which there is a herniation of the tonsils of the cerebellum and the medulla oblongata through the foramen magnum into the vertebral canal (Fig. 5-23). This results in the blockage of the exits in the roof of the fourth ventricle to the cerebrospinal fluid, causing internal hydrocephalus. It is commonly associated with craniovertebral anomalies or various forms of spina bifida. Signs and symptoms related to pressure on the cerebellum and medulla oblongata and involvement of the last four cranial nerves are associated with this condition.

Vascular Disorders of the Medulla Oblongata

LATERAL MEDULLARY SYNDROME OF WALLENBERG

The lateral part of the medulla oblongata is supplied by the posterior inferior cerebellar artery, which is usually a branch of the vertebral artery. Thrombosis of either of these arteries (Fig. 5-24) produces the following signs and symptoms: dysphagia and dysarthria due to paralysis of the ipsilateral palatal and laryngeal muscles (innervated by the nucleus ambiguus); analgesia and thermoanesthesia on the ipsilateral side of the face (nucleus and spinal tract of the trigeminal nerve); vertigo, nausea, vomiting, and nystagmus (vestibular nuclei); ipsilateral Horner's syndrome (descending sympathetic fibers); ipsilateral cerebellar signs—gait and limb ataxia (cerebellum or inferior cerebel-

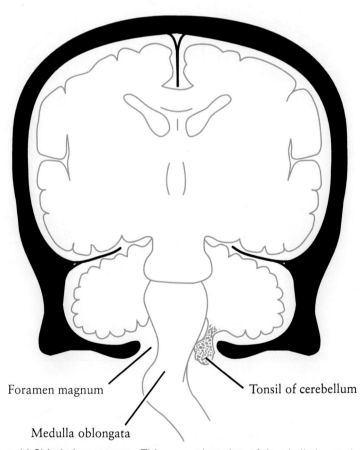

Foramen magnum   Tonsil of cerebellum

Medulla oblongata

Figure 5–23 Arnold-Chiari phenomenon. This coronal section of the skull shows the herniation of the cerebellar tonsil and the medulla oblongata through the foramen magnum into the vertebral canal.

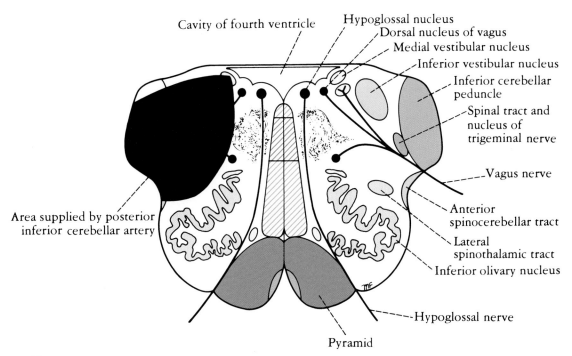

Figure 5–24 Transverse section of the medulla oblongata at the level of the inferior olivary nuclei, showing the extent of the lesion producing the lateral medullary syndrome.

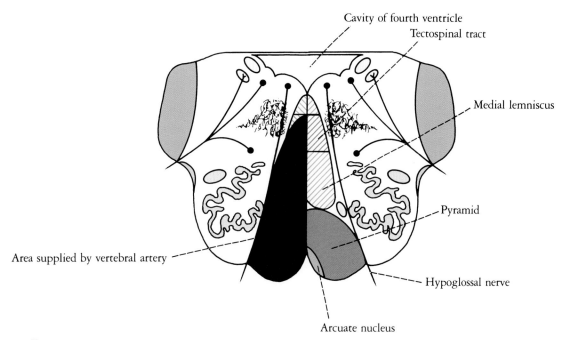

Figure 5–25 Transverse section of the medulla oblongata at the level of the inferior olivary nuclei, showing the extent of the lesion producing the medial medullary syndrome.

lar peduncle); and contralateral loss of sensations of pain and temperature (spinal lemniscus—spinothalamic tract).

MEDIAL MEDULLARY SYNDROME

The medial part of the medulla oblongata is supplied by the vertebral artery. Thrombosis of the medullary branch

(Fig. 5-25) produces the following signs and symptoms: contralateral hemiparesis (pyramidal tract), contralateral impaired sensations of position and movement and tactile discrimination (medial lemniscus), and ipsilateral paralysis of tongue muscles with deviation to the paralyzed side when the tongue is protruded (hypoglossal nerve).

THE CLINICAL SIGNIFICANCE OF THE PONS

The pons, like the medulla oblongata and the cerebellum, is situated in the posterior cranial fossa lying beneath the tentorium cerebelli. It is related anteriorly to the basilar artery, the dorsum sellae of the sphenoid bone, and the basilar part of the occipital bone. In addition to forming the upper half of the floor of the fourth ventricle, it possesses several important cranial nerve nuclei (trigeminal, abducent, facial, and vestibulocochlear) and serves as a conduit for important ascending and descending tracts (corticonuclear, corticopontine, corticospinal, medial longitudinal fasciculus, and medial, spinal, and lateral lemnisci). It is not surprising, therefore, that tumors, hemorrhage, or infarcts in this area of the brain produce a variety of symptoms and signs. For example, involvement of the corticopontocerebellar tracts will produce marked cerebellar ataxia, and voluntary movements are accompanied by a rhythmic tremor that develops and becomes further accentuated as the movements proceed (intention tumor).

Tumors of the Pons

Astrocytoma of the pons occurring in childhood is the most common tumor of the brainstem. The symptoms and signs are those of ipsilateral cranial nerve paralysis and contralateral hemiparesis: weakness of the facial muscles on the same side (facial nerve nucleus), weakness of the lateral rectus muscle on one or both sides (abducent nerve nucleus), nystagmus (vestibular nucleus), weakness of the jaw muscles (trigeminal nerve nucleus), impairment of hearing (cochlear nuclei), contralateral hemiparesis, quadriparesis (corticospinal fibers), anesthesia to light touch with the preservation of appreciation of pain over the skin of the face (principal sensory nucleus of trigeminal nerve involved, leaving spinal nucleus and tract of trigeminal intact), and contralateral sensory defects of the trunk and limbs (medial and spinal lemnisci). Involvement of the corticopontocerebellar tracts may cause ipsilateral cerebellar signs and symptoms. There may be impairment of conjugate deviation of the eyeballs due to involvement of the medial longitudinal fasciculus, which connects the oculomotor, trochlear, and abducent nerve nuclei.

Pontine Hemorrhage

The pons is supplied by the basilar artery and the anterior, inferior, and superior cerebellar arteries. If the hemorrhage occurs from one of those arteries and is unilateral, there will be facial paralysis on the side of the lesion (involvement of the facial nerve nucleus and, therefore, a lower motor neuron palsy) and paralysis of the limbs on the opposite side (involvement of the corticospinal fibers as they pass through the pons). There is often paralysis of conjugate ocular deviation (involvement of the abducent nerve nucleus and the medial longitudinal fasciculus). When the hemorrhage is extensive and bilateral, the pupils may be "pinpoint" (involvement of the ocular sympathetic fibers); there is commonly bilateral paralysis of the face and the limbs. The patient may become poikilothermic because severe damage to the pons has cut off the body from the heat-regulating centers in the hypothalamus.

Infarctions of the Pons

Usually this is due to thrombosis or embolism of the basilar artery or its branches. If it involves the paramedian area of the pons, the corticospinal tracts, the pontine nuclei, and the fibers passing to the cerebellum through the middle cerebellar peduncle may be damaged. A laterally situated infarct will involve the trigeminal nerve, the medial lemniscus, and the middle cerebellar peduncle; the corticospinal fibers to the lower limbs also may be affected.

The clinical conditions mentioned above will be understood more clearly if the ascending and descending tracts of the brain and spinal cord are reviewed (See pages and 145 and 156).

CLINICAL SIGNIFICANCE OF THE MIDBRAIN

The midbrain forms the upper end of the narrow stalk of the brain or brainstem. As it ascends out of the posterior cranial fossa through the relatively small rigid opening in the tentorium cerebelli, it is vulnerable to traumatic injury. It possesses two important cranial nerve nuclei (oculomotor and trochlear), reflex centers (the colliculi), the red nucleus and the substantia nigra, which greatly influence motor function, and it serves as a conduit for many important ascending and descending tracts. As in other parts of the brainstem, it is a site for tumors, hemorrhage or infarcts that will produce a wide variety of symptoms and signs.

Trauma to the Midbrain

Among the mechanisms of injuries to the midbrain, a sudden lateral movement of the head could result in the cerebral peduncles impinging against the sharp rigid free edge of the tentorium cerebelli. Sudden movements of the head resulting from trauma cause different regions of the brain to move at different velocities relative to one another. For example, the large anatomical unit, the forebrain, may move at a different velocity from the remainder of the brain, such as the cerebellum. This will result in the midbrain being bent, stretched, twisted, or torn.

Involvement of the oculomotor nucleus will produce ipsilateral paralysis of the levator palpebrae superioris; the superior, inferior, and medial rectus muscles; and the inferior oblique muscle. Malfunction of the parasympathetic nucleus of the oculomotor nerve produces a dilated pupil that is insensitive to light and does not constrict on accommodation.

Involvement of the trochlear nucleus will produce contralateral paralysis of the superior oblique muscle of the eyeball. Thus it is seen that involvement of one or both of these nuclei, or the corticonuclear fibers that converge upon them, will cause impairment of ocular movements.

Blockage of the Cerebral Aqueduct

The cavity of the midbrain, the cerebral aqueduct, is one of the narrower parts of the ventricular system. Normally, cerebrospinal fluid that has been produced in the lateral and third ventricles passes through this channel to enter the fourth ventricle, and so escapes through the foramina in its roof to enter the subarachnoid space. In congenital hydrocephalus, the cerebral aqueduct may be blocked or replaced by numerous small tubular passages that are insufficient for the normal flow of cerebrospinal fluid. A tumor of the midbrain (Fig. 5-26A) or pressure on the midbrain from a tumor arising outside the midbrain may compress the aqueduct and produce hydrocephalus. When the cerebral aqueduct is blocked, the accumulating cerebrospinal fluid within the third and lateral ventricles produces lesions in the midbrain. The presence of the oculomotor and trochlear nerve nuclei, together with the important descending corticospinal and corticonuclear tracts, will provide symptoms and signs that are helpful in accurately localizing a lesion in the brainstem.

Vascular Lesions of the Midbrain

Weber's Syndrome

Weber's syndrome (Fig. 5-26B), which is commonly produced by occlusion of a branch of the posterior cerebral artery that supplies the midbrain, results in the necrosis of brain tissue involving the oculomotor nerve and the crus cerebri. There is ipsilateral ophthalmoplegia and contralateral paralysis of the lower part of the face, the tongue, and the arm and leg. The eyeball is deviated laterally because of the paralysis of the medial rectus muscle; there is drooping (ptosis) of the upper lid and the pupil is dilated and fixed to light and accommodation.

Benedikt's Syndrome

Benedikt's syndrome (Fig. 5-26C), is similar to Weber's syndrome, but the necrosis involves the medial lemniscus and red nucleus, producing contralateral hemianesthesia and involuntary movements of the limbs of the opposite side.

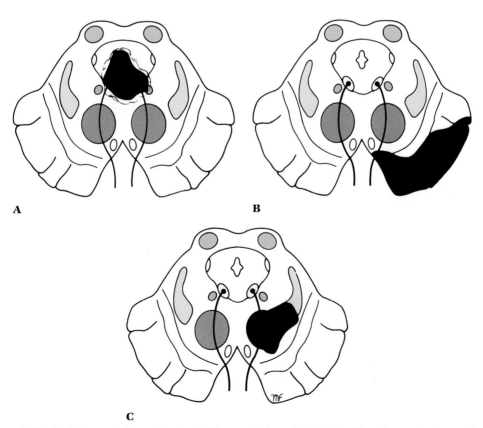

A

B

C

Figure 5–26 Pathology of the midbrain. **A**. Tumor of the midbrain blocking the cerebral aqueduct. **B**. Weber's syndrome, involving the oculomotor nerve and the crus cerebri following occlusion of the blood supply to the midbrain. **C**. Benedikt's syndrome, involving the red nucleus and the medial lemniscus following occlusion of the blood supply to the midbrain.

Clinical Problem Solving

1. While carrying out a physical examination of a patient with an intracranial tumor, the neurologist turned to a medical student and asked, "What signs or symptoms would you look for that would enable you to localize the tumor to the region of the medulla oblongata?" How would you have answered that question?

2. A 6-month-old boy died with hydrocephalus and a myelocele in the lower thoracic region. At autopsy the hindbrain was found to be deformed. The lower part of the medulla oblongata extended inferiorly through the foramen magnum into the vertebral canal as far as the third cervical vertebra. The lower four cranial nerves were longer than normal and the upper cervical nerve roots ascended to reach their exit from the vertebral canal. The cerebellum on the left side extended inferiorly through the foramen magnum to the third cervical vertebra, where it was adherent to the spinal cord. The roof of the fourth ventricle was abnormally low. (a) What is the name of this malformation? (b) Is hydrocephalus common in this condition? (c) Is there a possible association between the thoracic myelocele and the presence of part of the hindbrain in the vertebral canal?

3. A 68-year-old man was admitted to the hospital with the sudden onset of severe dizziness (vertigo), hiccups, and vomiting. He also complained of a hot, painful sensation in the skin of the right side of the face. On physical examination the soft palate was drawn up to the left side when the patient was asked to say "ah," and there was lack of mobility of the right vocal cord as seen on laryngoscopic examination. The patient also showed drooping of the right upper eyelid (ptosis), sunken right eye (enophthalmos), and a constricted right pupil (myosis). When asked to protrude his tongue straight out of his mouth, the patient tried to do so but the tip of the tongue pointed to the right side. There was evidence of impairment of pain and temperature sensation in the trunk and extremities on the left side. Using your knowledge of anatomy, make the diagnosis.

4. The pathologist, while exploring the posterior cranial fossa during an autopsy, was endeavoring to determine where the ninth, tenth, and cranial part of the eleventh cranial nerves emerged from the hindbrain. Describe where these nerves emerge from the hindbrain.

5. A 10-year-old girl was taken to a physician because her mother had noticed that the right half of her face was weak and did not appear to react to emotional changes. It was noted also that her mouth was pulled over slightly to the left, especially when she was tired. On questioning, the patient admitted that food tended to stick inside her right cheek and that the right side of her face "felt funny." The mother had first noticed the facial changes 3 months previously and the condition had progressively worsened. On examination, there was definite weakness of the facial muscles on the right side; the facial muscles on the left side were normal. Skin sensation on stimulation of the face was normal. On testing of the ocular movements there was evidence of slight weakness of the lateral rectus muscle on the right side. Examination of the movements of the arm and leg showed slight weakness on the left side. Using your knowledge of neuroanatomy, relate these symptoms and signs to a lesion in the pons.

6. A 65-year-old man was admitted to the emergency department with a diagnosis of a severe pontine hemorrhage. On examination, he was found to have bilateral "pinpoint" pupils and quadriplegia. How can you explain the presence of the "pinpoint" pupils?

7. A 46-year-old man with symptoms of deafness, vertigo, and double vision (diplopia) visited his physician. On questioning, he said that he also suffered from severe headaches, which were increasing in frequency and severity. The week before, he vomited several times during one of the headache attacks. On examination, he was found to have a slight right internal strabismus and a flattening of the skin furrows on the right side of his forehead and a slight drooping of the right corner of his mouth. There was definite evidence of impairment of hearing on the right side. On testing for sensory loss, there was definite sensory impairment on the right side of the face in the areas supplied by the maxillary and mandibular divisions of the trigeminal nerve. Using your knowledge of anatomy, explain the symptoms and signs.

8. After a severe automobile accident that resulted in the death of the driver of one of the vehicles, an autopsy was performed and the skull was opened. A massive subdural hematoma was found in the middle cranial fossa. The rapid accumulation of blood within the skull had exerted pressure on the brain above the tentorium cerebelli. The uncus of the temporal lobe had been forced inferiorly through the hiatus in the tentorium cerebelli. What effect do you think these intracranial changes had on the midbrain of this patient?

9. A 3-month-old girl was taken to a pediatrician because her mother was concerned about the large size of her head. The child was perfectly normal in every other respect. Examination of the child showed that the diameter of the head was larger than normal for the age; the fontanelles were larger than normal and were moderately tense. The scalp was shiny and the scalp veins were dilated. The eyes were normal and the mental and physical development of the child was within normal limits. CT and MRI of the head revealed gross dilation of the third and lateral ventricles of the brain. What is your diagnosis? What possible treatment would have been suggested to the mother of this child?

10. A 20-year-old man was seen by a neurologist because he had a 3-month history of double vision. On examination of the patient, both eyes at rest were turned downward and laterally. The patient was unable to move the eyes upward or medially. Both upper lids were

drooping (ptosis). Examination of both pupils showed them to be dilated, and they did not constrict when a light was shone into either eye. Facial movements and sensation were normal. Movements of the upper and lower limbs were normal. There was no evidence of loss of or altered skin sensations in the upper or the lower limbs. Using your knowledge of neuroanatomy, make a diagnosis and accurately locate the site of the lesion. Is the lesion unilateral or bilateral?

11. A 57-year-old man with hypertension was admitted to the hospital with a diagnosis of hemorrhage into the midbrain, possibly from a branch of the posterior cerebral artery. He was found, on physical examination, to have paralysis on the right side of the levator palpebrae superioris, the superior rectus, medial rectus, inferior rectus, and inferior oblique muscles. Furthermore, his right pupil was dilated and failed to constrict on exposure to light or on accommodation. The left eye was normal in every respect. He displayed hypersensitivity to touch on the skin of the left side of his face, and loss of skin sensation on the greater part of his left arm and left leg. The left leg also displayed some spontaneous slow writhing movements (athetosis). Using your knowledge of neuroanatomy, explain the signs and symptoms exhibited by this patient.

12. A 41-year-old woman was diagnosed as having a lesion in the midbrain. Physical examination revealed an oculomotor nerve palsy on the left side (paralysis of the left extraocular muscles except the lateral rectus and the superior oblique muscles) and an absence of the light and accommodation reflexes on the left side. There was some weakness but no atrophy of the muscles of the lower part of the face and the tongue on the right side. There was evidence of spastic paralysis of the right arm and leg. There was no evidence of any sensory loss on either side of the head, trunk, or limbs. Using your knowledge of neuroanatomy, precisely place the lesion in the midbrain of this patient.

Answers to Clinical Problem Solving

1. Until involvement of one of the last four cranial nerves occurs, localization of a lesion to the medulla oblongata remains uncertain. For example, involvement of the main ascending sensory pathways or descending pathways may be caused by a lesion in the medulla, the pons, the midbrain, or the spinal cord. Involvement of the glossopharyngeal nerve can be detected by inadequacy of the gag reflex and loss of taste sensation on the posterior third of the tongue. Involvement of the vagus nerve can be assumed if the patient demonstrates some or all of the following symptoms: impairment of pharyngeal sensibility, difficulty in swallowing, nasal regurgitation of fluids with asymmetry of movement of the soft palate, and hoarseness of the voice with paralysis of the laryngeal muscles. The cranial part of the accessory nerve is distributed within the vagus nerve so that it is not possible to test for this nerve alone. The spinal part of the accessory nerve, which supplies the sternocleidomastoid and trapezius muscles, arises from the spinal cord and is therefore unaffected by tumors of the medulla. The hypoglossal nerve involvement may be tested by looking for wasting, fasciculation, and paralysis of one-half of the tongue.

2. (a) The malformation in which the cerebellum and the medulla oblongata are found in the cervical part of the vertebral canal is known as the Arnold-Chiari malformation. (b) Yes, hydrocephalus is common in this condition. The hydrocephalus may be due to distortion or malformation of the openings in the roof of the fourth ventricle, which normally allow the cerebrospinal fluid to escape into the subarachnoid space. (c) Yes, a myelocele is commonly associated with this malformation. The reason for this is not exactly known, although several investigators believe that the myelocele is the primary cause and that it tethers the lower part of the spinal cord to the surrounding tissues at the time when disproportionate growth of the spinal cord and the vertebral column occurs. This would serve to pull the medulla oblongata and the cerebellum inferiorly through the foramen magnum into the vertebral canal.

3. This patient is suffering from a thrombosis of the posterior inferior cerebellar artery or vertebral artery on the right side. The vertigo is caused by the involvement of the cerebellum or the vestibular nuclei, or both. The hot, painful skin sensations are due to the involvement of the spinal tract and nucleus of the trigeminal nerve on the right side. The abnormal movement of the soft palate and the fixation of the right vocal cord are due to involvement of the nucleus of the vagus and accessory nerve on the right side. The ptosis, enophthalmos, and myosis (Horner's syndrome) are due to involvement of the descending fibers of the sympathetic part of the autonomic nervous system. The pointing of the tongue to the right is caused by involvement of the right hypoglossal nucleus (the right genioglossus muscle is paralyzed). The loss of pain and temperature sensations on the opposite side of the body is due to involvement of the ascending lateral spinothalamic tracts. This characteristic clinical syndrome results from cutting off the arterial supply to a wedge-shaped area in the posterolateral part of the medulla oblongata and the inferior surface of the cerebellum.

4. The ninth, tenth, and cranial part of the eleventh cranial nerves emerge from the medulla oblongata in a groove between the olives and the inferior cerebellar peduncles.

5. This 10-year-old girl later was found to have an astrocytoma of the pons. The right unilateral facial weakness, together with weakness of the right lateral rectus muscle of the eye, was due to involvement of the right facial and abducent nuclei by the tumor. The absence of paresthesia of the face indicated that the principal sensory nucleus of the trigeminal nerve was intact on both sides. The weakness in the movements of the left arm and left leg was due to the involvement of the corticospinal fibers in the pons. (Remember that the majority of these fibers cross over to the opposite side at the decussation of the pyramids in the medulla.)

6. "Pinpoint" pupils indicate that the constrictor pupillae muscles are strongly contracted and the dilator pupillae muscles are paralyzed. The dilator pupillae muscles are supplied by the sympathetic fibers, which descend through the pons (position not precisely known) to the lateral gray columns of the thoracic part of the spinal cord. Here the fibers synapse and the thoracolumbar sympathetic outflow occurs.

7. The deafness and vertigo were due to lesions in the cochlear and vestibular nuclei in the upper part of the pons. The double vision (diplopia) was produced by the involvement of the abducent nerve nucleus on the right side of the pons. The history of severe headaches and vomiting was due to a progressive rise in intracranial pressure caused by a tumor of the pons. The right unilateral facial palsy was due to the involvement of the right facial nerve nucleus. The sensory impairment of the skin of the middle and lower part of the right side of the face was due to the tumor involvement of the principal sensory nucleus of the right trigeminal nerve

8. The herniated uncus and the subdural hemorrhage caused pressure of the opposite crus cerebri of the midbrain against the sharp edge of the tentorium. The distortion of the midbrain caused narrowing of the cerebral aqueduct, further raising the supratentorial pressure by blocking the passage of cerebrospinal fluid from the third to the fourth ventricle. Under these circumstances, severe hemorrhage may occur within the midbrain and affect the third and fourth cranial nerve nuclei and various important descending and ascending tracts.

9. This child had hydrocephalus. The physical examination and the special tests showed that the third and lateral ventricles of the brain were grossly dilated owing to the accumulation of cerebrospinal fluid in these cavities. Mechanical obstruction to the flow of cerebrospinal fluid from the third into the fourth ventricle through the cerebral aqueduct was present. After the possibility of the presence of cysts or resectable tumors had been excluded, it was assumed that the cause of the obstruction was a congenital atresia or malformation of the cerebral aqueduct. If the condition were progressing, that is, the block in the aqueduct was complete and the head continued to increase in size at an abnormal rate, some form of neurosurgical procedure should have been performed whereby the cerebrospinal fluid would be shunted from the third or lateral ventricles into the subarachnoid space, or into the venous system of the neck.

10. Two years later the patient died. At autopsy a large astrocytoma that involved the central part of the tegmentum at the level of the superior colliculi was found. The patient had exhibited all signs and symptoms associated with a raised intracranial pressure. The raised pressure was due in part to the expanding tumor, but the problem was compounded by the developing hydrocephalus resulting from blockage of the cerebral aqueduct.

    The symptoms and signs exhibited by the patient when he was first seen by the neurologist could be explained by the presence of the tumor in the central gray matter at the level of the superior colliculi, and involving the third cranial nerve nuclei on both sides. This resulted in bilateral ptosis, bilateral ophthalmoplegia, and bilateral fixed, dilated pupils. The resting position of the eyes in a downward and lateral position was due to the action of the superior oblique muscle (trochlear nerve) and lateral rectus muscle (abducent nerve).

11. The patient had a hemorrhage into the right side of the tegmentum of the midbrain that involved the right third cranial nerve. The ascending tracts of the left trigeminal nerve also were involved. After emerging from the sensory nuclei of the left trigeminal nerve, they cross the midline and ascend through the trigeminal lemniscus on the right side. The loss of sensation seen in the left upper and lower limbs was due to involvement of the right medial and spinal lemnisci. The athetoid movements of the left leg could be explained on the basis of the involvement of the right red nucleus. The absence of spasticity of the left arm and leg would indicate that the lesion did not involve the right descending tracts. For further clarification, consult the descriptions of the various tracts (see p. 170).

12. Autopsy later revealed a vascular lesion involving a branch of the posterior cerebral artery. Considerable brain softening was found in the region of the substantia nigra and crus cerebri on the left side of the midbrain. The left oculomotor nerve was involved as it passed through the infarcted area. The corticonuclear fibers that pass to the facial nerve nucleus and the hypoglossal nucleus were involved as they descended through the left crus cerebri (they cross the midline at the level of the nuclei). The corticospinal fibers on the left side were also involved (they cross in the medulla oblongata), hence the spastic paralysis of the right arm and leg. The left trigeminal and left medial lemnisci were untouched, which explains the absence of sensory changes on the right side of the body. This is a good example of Weber's syndrome.

Review Questions

Directions: Each of the numbered items in this section is followed by answers that are positively phrased. Select the ONE lettered answer that is an EXCEPTION.

1. The following statements concerning the anterior surface of the medulla oblongata are correct **except:**
   (a) The pyramids taper inferiorly and give rise to the decussation of the pyramids.
   (b) On each side of the midline there is an ovoid swelling called the olive, which contains the corticospinal fibers.
   (c) The hypoglossal nerve emerges between the pyramid and the olive.
   (d) The vagus nerve emerges between the olive and the inferior cerebellar peduncle.
   (e) The abducent nerve emerges between the pons and the medulla oblongata.

2. The following general statements concerning the medulla oblongata are correct **except:**
   (a) The caudal half of the floor of the fourth ventricle is formed by the rostral half of the medulla.
   (b) The central canal is limited to the caudal half of the medulla oblongata.
   (c) The nucleus gracilis is situated beneath the gracile tubercle on the anterior surface of the medulla.
   (d) The decussation of the medial lemnisci takes place in the caudal half of the medulla.
   (e) The cerebellum lies posterior to the medulla.

3. The following statements concerning the interior of the lower part of the medulla are true **except:**
   (a) The decussation of the pyramids represents the crossing over from one side of the medulla to the other of three-fourths of the corticospinal fibers.
   (b) The central canal of the spinal cord continues upward into the medulla.
   (c) The substantia gelatinosa becomes continuous with the nucleus of the spinal tract of the trigeminal nerve.
   (d) The medial lemniscus is formed by the anterior spinothalamic tract and the spinotectal tract.
   (e) The internal arcuate fibers emerge from the nucleus gracilis and nucleus cuneatus.

4. The following statements concerning the interior of the upper part of the medulla are true **except:**
   (a) The reticular formation consists of a mixture of nerve fibers and small groups of nerve cells.
   (b) The nucleus ambiguus constitutes the motor nucleus of the vagus, cranial part of the accessory, and hypoglossal nerves.
   (c) Beneath the floor of the fourth ventricle are located the dorsal nucleus of the vagus and the vestibular nuclei.
   (d) The medial longitudinal fasciculus is a bundle of ascending and descending fibers that lie posterior to the medial lemniscus on each side of the midline.
   (e) The inferior cerebellar peduncle connects the medulla to the cerebellum.

5. The following statements concerning the Arnold-Chiari phenomenon are correct **except:**
   (a) It is a congenital anomaly.
   (b) The exits in the roof of the fourth ventricle may be blocked.
   (c) The cerebellum never herniates through the foramen magnum.
   (d) It is commonly associated with various forms of spina bifida.
   (e) It is dangerous to perform a spinal tap in this condition.

6. The following statements concerning the medial medullary syndrome are correct **except:**
   (a) The tongue is paralyzed on the ipsilateral side.
   (b) There is contralateral hemiplegia.
   (c) There are contralateral impaired sensations of position and movement.
   (d) It is commonly caused by thrombosis of a branch of the vertebral artery to the medulla oblongata.
   (e) There is contralateral facial paralysis.

7. The following statements concerning the lateral medullary syndrome are correct **except:**
   (a) The condition may be caused by a thrombosis of the posterior inferior cerebellar artery.
   (b) The nucleus ambiguus of the same side may be damaged.
   (c) There may be analgesia and thermoanesthesia on the ipsilateral side of the face.
   (d) Ipsilateral trunk and extremity hypalgesia and thermoanesthesia may occur.
   (e) There may be nausea and vomiting.

Directions: Matching Questions

In Figure 5-27, match the numbers listed on the left with the appropriate lettered options listed on the right. Each lettered option may be selected once, more than once, or not at all.

8. Number 1   (a) Inferior cerebellar peduncle
9. Number 2   (b) Medial lemniscus
10. Number 3   (c) Hypoglossal nucleus
11. Number 4   (d) Reticular formation
12. Number 5   (e) None of the above
13. Number 6

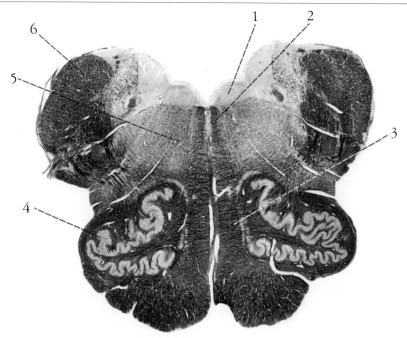

Figure 5–27 Photomicrograph of transverse section of the medulla oblongata. (Weigert Stain.)

Directions: Each of the numbered items in this section is followed by answers that are positively phrased. Select the ONE lettered answer that is an EXCEPTION.

14. The following statements concerning the pons are correct **except:**
    (a) The trigeminal nerve emerges on the anterior aspect of the pons.
    (b) The glossopharyngeal nerve emerges on the anterior aspect of the brainstem in the groove between the pons and the medulla oblongata.
    (c) The basilar artery lies in a centrally placed groove on the anterior aspect of the pons.
    (d) Many nerve fibers present on the anterior aspect of the pons converge laterally to form the middle cerebellar peduncle.
    (e) The pons forms the upper half of the floor of the fourth ventricle.

15. The following important structures are located in the brainstem at the level stated **except:**
    (a) The red nucleus lies within the midbrain.
    (b) The facial colliculus lies in the caudal part of the pons.
    (c) The motor nucleus of the trigeminal nerve lies within the cranial part of the pons.
    (d) The abducent nucleus lies within the cranial part of the pons.
    (e) The trochlear nucleus lies within the midbrain at the level of the inferior colliculus.

16. The following statements concerning the posterior surface of the pons are correct **except:**
    (a) Lateral to the median sulcus is an elongated swelling called the medial eminence.
    (b) The facial colliculus is produced by the root of the abducent nerve winding around the nucleus of the facial nerve.
    (c) The floor of the superior part of the sulcus limitans is pigmented and is called the substantia ferruginea.
    (d) The vestibular area lies lateral to the sulcus limitans.
    (e) The cerebellum lies posterior to the pons.

17. The following statements concerning a transverse section through the caudal part of the pons are correct **except:**
    (a) The medial longitudinal fasciculus lies beneath the floor of the fourth ventricle on either side of the midline.
    (b) The vestibular nuclei lie lateral to the abducent nucleus.
    (c) The trapezoid body is made up of fibers derived from the facial nerve nuclei.
    (d) The tegmentum is the part of the pons lying posterior to the trapezoid body.
    (e) The pontine nuclei lie between the transverse pontine fibers.

18. The following statements concerning a transverse section through the cranial part of the pons are correct **except:**
    (a) The motor nucleus of the trigeminal nerve lies medial to the main sensory nucleus in the tegmentum.
    (b) The medial lemniscus has rotated so that its long axis lies transversely.
    (c) Bundles of corticospinal fibers lie in among the transverse pontine fibers.
    (d) The medial longitudinal fasciculus joins the thalamus to the spinal nucleus of the trigeminal nerve.
    (e) The motor root of the trigeminal nerve is much smaller than the sensory root.
19. The following statements concerning the pons are correct **except:**
    (a) It is related anteriorly to the dorsum sellae of the sphenoid bone.
    (b) It lies in the posterior cranial fossa.
    (c) The corticopontine fibers terminate in the pontine nuclei.
    (d) Glial tumors of the pons are rare.
    (e) The pons receives its blood supply from the basilar artery.

Directions: Matching Questions

In Figure 5-28, match the numbers listed on the left with the appropriate lettered options listed on the right. Each lettered option may be selected once, more than once, or not at all.

20. Number 1   (a) Basilar groove
21. Number 2   (b) Medial longitudinal fasciculus
22. Number 3   (c) Superior cerebellar peduncle
23. Number 4   (d) Superior medullary velum
24. Number 5   (e) None of the above
25. Number 6

Directions: Each of the numbered items in this section is followed by answers that are positively phrased. Select the ONE lettered answer that is an EXCEPTION.

26. The following statements concerning the midbrain are correct **except:**
    (a) It passes superiorly through the opening in the tentorium cerebelli.
    (b) The cavity of the midbrain is called the cerebral aqueduct.
    (c) The oculomotor nerve emerges from the posterior surface below the inferior colliculi.

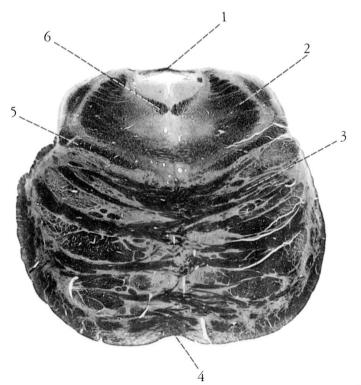

Figure 5–28 Photomicrograph of transverse section of the pons. (Weigert Stain.)

(d) The superior brachium passes from the superior colliculus to the lateral geniculate body.

(e) The interpeduncular fossa is bounded laterally by the crus cerebri.

27. The following statements concerning the midbrain are correct **except:**
    (a) The oculomotor nucleus is found within it at the level of the superior colliculus.
    (b) The trochlear nerve emerges on the posterior surface of the midbrain and decussates completely in the superior medullary velum.
    (c) The trochlear nucleus is situated in the central gray matter at the level of the inferior colliculus.
    (d) The lemnisci are situated lateral to the central gray matter.
    (e) The trigeminal lemniscus lies anterior to the medial lemniscus.

28. The following statements concerning the internal structures of the midbrain are correct **except:**
    (a) The tectum is the part situated posterior to the cerebral aqueduct.
    (b) The crus cerebri on each side lies anterior to the substantia nigra.
    (c) The tegmentum lies posterior to the substantia nigra.
    (d) The central gray matter encircles the red nuclei.
    (e) The reticular formation is present throughout the midbrain.

29. The following statements concerning the colliculi of the midbrain are correct **except:**
    (a) They are located in the tegmentum.
    (b) The superior colliculi are concerned with sight reflexes.
    (c) The inferior colliculi lie at the level of the trochlear nerve nuclei.
    (d) The inferior colliculi are concerned with auditory reflexes.
    (e) The superior colliculi lie at the level of the red nuclei.

30. The following statements concerning the third cranial nerve nuclei are correct **except:**
    (a) The oculomotor nucleus is situated in the central gray matter.
    (b) The parasympathetic part of the oculomotor nucleus is called the Edinger-Westphal nucleus.
    (c) The oculomotor nucleus lies posterior to the cerebral aqueduct.
    (d) The nerve fibers from the oculomotor nucleus pass through the red nucleus.
    (e) The oculomotor nucleus lies close to the medial longitudinal fasciculus.

Directions: Matching Questions

In Figure 5-29, match the numbers listed on the left with the appropriate lettered options listed on the right. Each lettered option may be selected once, more than once, or not at all.

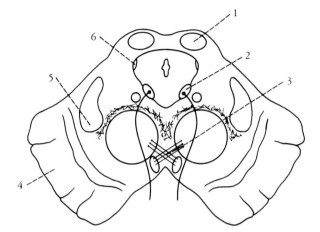

Figure 5–29   Transverse section of the midbrain.

31. Number 1   (a) Medial longitudinal fasciculus
32. Number 2   (b) Inferior colliculus
33. Number 3   (c) Medial lemniscus
34. Number 4   (d) Trochlear nucleus
35. Number 5   (e) None of the above
36. Number 6

Directions: Read the case histories then answer the questions. You will be required to select ONE BEST lettered answer.

A 63-year-old man complaining of difficulty in swallowing, some hoarseness of his voice, and giddiness was seen by a neurologist. All these symptoms started suddenly 4 days previously. On physical examination he was found to have a loss of the pharyngeal gagging reflex on the left side, left-sided facial analgesia, and left-sided paralysis of the vocal cord.

37. Based on the clinical history and the results of the physical examination, select the **most likely** diagnosis.
    (a) A meningeal tumor in the posterior cranial fossa on the right side
    (b) Lateral medullary syndrome on the left side
    (c) Medial medullary syndrome on the left side
    (d) Lateral medullary syndrome on the right side
    (e) Medial medullary syndrome on the right side

A 7-year-old girl was seen by a neurologist because she complained to her mother that she was seeing double. Careful physical examination revealed that the double vision became worse when she looked toward the left. The patient also had evidence of a mild motor paralysis of her right lower limb without spasticity. There was also a slight facial paralysis involving the whole left side of the face.

38. Based on the clinical history and the clinical examination, the following neurological deficits could have been present **except:**
    (a) The double vision caused by weakness of the left lateral rectus muscle.
    (b) The complete left-sided facial paralysis caused by involvement of the left seventh cranial nerve nucleus or its nerve.
    (c) The mild right hemiparesis produced by damage to the corticospinal tract on the right side.
    (d) An MRI revealed the presence of a tumor of the lower part of the pons on the left side.
    (e) There was damage to the left sixth cranial nerve nucleus.

A 42-year-old woman complaining of a severe, persistent headache visited her physician. At first the headache was not continuous and tended to occur during the night. Now, the headache was present all the time and was felt over the whole head. Recently, she has begun to feel nauseous and this has resulted in several episodes of vomiting. Last week, on looking in the mirror, she noted that her right pupil looked much larger than the left. Her right upper lid appeared to droop.

39. The physical examination revealed the following most likely findings **except:**
    (a) Weakness in raising the right eyelid upward.
    (b) There was severe ptosis of the right eye.
    (c) There was obvious dilatation of the right pupil.
    (d) Ophthalmoscopic examination revealed bilateral papilledema.
    (e) There was no evidence of paralysis of either superior oblique muscle.
    (f) Examination of the lower limbs revealed a mild spasticity of the left lower limb muscles.
    (g) Ataxia of the right upper limb was also present.
    (h) Loss of taste sensation on the posterior one third of the tongue on the left side.

40. The combination of the clinical history and the findings in the physical examination enabled the physician to make the following **most likely** diagnosis.
    (a) A tumor involving the left cerebral hemisphere.
    (b) A tumor involving the right side of the midbrain at the level of the superior colliculi.
    (c) Severe migraine.
    (d) A cerebral hemorrhage involving the left cerebral hemisphere.
    (e) A tumor of the left side of the midbrain.

Answers to Review Questions

1. B
2. C
3. D
4. B
5. C
6. E
7. D
8. C
9. E
10. B
11. E
12. D
13. A
14. B
15. D
16. B
17. C
18. D
19. D
20. D
21. C
22. E
23. A
24. E
25. B
26. C
27. E
28. D
29. A
30. C
31. E
32. E
33. E
34. E
35. C
36. E
37. B

38. C. The right sided hemiparesis was caused by damage to the corticospinal tract on the left side of the pons. The corticospinal tract descends through the medulla and crosses to the right side of the midline at the decussation of the pyramids. The patient was later discovered to have a glioma involving the left side of the lower pons.

39. H. The sensation of taste on the posterior one third of the tongue is supplied by the glossopharyngeal nerve which originates in the medulla oblongata.

40. B. The combination of raised intracranial pressure (headache, vomiting, and bilateral papilledema), the involvement of the right third cranial nerve (right-sided ptosis, right pupillary dilatation, and right-sided weakness of ocular deviation upward), spasticity of the left leg (right-sided corticospinal tracts), and ataxia of the right upper limb (cerebellar connections on the right side) led the physician to make a tentative diagnosis of an intracranial tumor in the right side of the midbrain at the level of the superior colliculi. An MRI confirmed the diagnosis.

ADDITIONAL READING

Brazis, P. W., Masdeu, J. C., and Biller, J. *Localization in Clinical Neurology* (2nd ed.). Boston: Little, Brown, 1990.

Brodal, A. *Neurological Anatomy in Relation to Clinical Medicine*, 3rd ed. New York: Oxford Univ. Press,1981.

Crosby, E. C., Humphrey, T., and Lauer, E. W. *Correlative Anatomy of the Nervous System.* New York: Macmillan, 1962.

Martin, J.H. *Neuroanatomy: Text and Atlas*, 2nd ed. Stamford, CT: Appleton & Lange, 1996

Patten, J. P. *Neurological Differential Diagnosis.* London: Harold Stark, 1980.

Paxinos, G. *The Human Nervous System.* San Diego: Academic Press,1990.

Rowland, L. P. (ed.). *Merritt's Textbook of Neurology* (7th ed.). Philadelphia: Lea & Febiger, 1984.

Walton, J. N. *Brain's Diseases of the Nervous System* (9th ed.). New York and London: Oxford University Press, 1984.

Williams, P. L., et al. *Gray's Anatomy* (38th Br. ed.). New York, London, Churchill Livingstone, 1995.

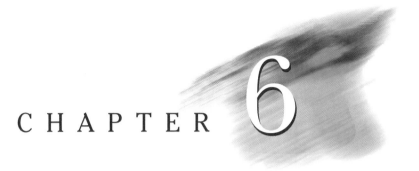

CHAPTER 6

The Cerebellum and Its Connections

A 56-year-old woman was examined by a neurologist for a variety of complaints, including an irregular swaying gait and a tendency to drift to the right when walking. Her family recently noticed that she had difficulty in keeping her balance when standing still and she found that standing with her feet apart helped her keep her balance.

On examination, it was apparent that she had diminished tone of the muscles of her right upper limb as seen when the elbow and wrist joints were passively flexed and extended. Similar evidence was found in the right lower limb. When asked to stretch out her arms in front of her and hold them in position, she demonstrated obvious signs of right-sided tremor. When asked to touch the tip of her nose with the left index finger, she performed the movement without any difficulty, but when she repeated the movement with her right index finger, she either missed her nose or hit it due to the irregularly contracting muscles. When she was asked to quickly pronate and supinate the forearms, the movements were normal on the left side but were jerky and slow on the right side. A mild papilledema of both eyes was found. No other abnormal signs were demonstrated.

The right-sided hypotonia, static tremor, and intention tremor associated with voluntary movements, right-sided dysdiadochokinesia, together with the history, were characteristic of right-sided cerebellar disease. A CT scan revealed a tumor in the right cerebellar hemisphere.

Understanding the structure and the nervous connections of the cerebellum, and in particular, knowing that the right cerebellar hemisphere influences voluntary muscle tone on the same side of the body, enables the neurologist to make an accurate diagnosis and institute treatment.

CHAPTER OUTLINE

CHAPTER OBJECTIVES

The cerebellum is a very important part of the central nervous system. It unconsciously controls the smooth contraction of voluntary muscles and carefully coordinates their actions, together with the relaxation of their antagonists. This chapter considers the structure and functions of the cerebellum.

The connections of the cerebellum to the remainder of the central nervous system are considered in relation to posture and voluntary movement. It is suggested that the reader commit the functions of the connections to memory as this will greatly assist in the retention of the material. Great emphasis is placed on the fact that each cerebellar hemisphere controls muscular movements on the same side of the body and that the cerebellum has no direct pathway to the lower motor neurons but exerts its control via the cerebral cortex and the brainstem.

GROSS APPEARANCE OF THE CEREBELLUM

The cerebellum is situated in the posterior cranial fossa and covered superiorly by the tentorium cerebelli. It is the largest part of the hindbrain and lies posterior to the fourth ventricle, the pons and the medulla oblongata (Fig. 6-1). The cerebellum is somewhat ovoid in shape and constricted in its median part. It consists of two **cerebellar hemispheres** joined by a narrow median **vermis.** The cerebellum is connected to the posterior aspect of the brainstem by three symmetrical bundles of nerve fibers called the **superior, middle,** and **inferior cerebellar peduncles.**

The cerebellum is divided into three main lobes: the **anterior lobe,** the **middle lobe,** and the **flocculonodular lobe.** The **anterior lobe** may be seen on the superior surface of the cerebellum and is separated from the middle lobe by a wide V-shaped fissure called the **primary fissure** (Figs. 6-2 and 6-3). The **middle lobe** (sometimes called the posterior lobe), which is the largest part of the cerebellum, is situated between the primary and **uvulonodular fissures.** The **flocculonodular lobe** is situated posterior to the uvulonodular fissure (Fig. 6-3). A deep **horizontal fissure** that is found along the margin of the cerebellum separates the superior from the inferior surfaces; it is of no morphological or functional significance (Figs. 6-2 and 6-3).

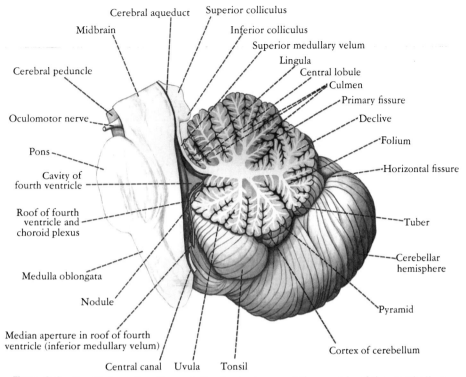

Figure 6–1 Sagittal section through the brainstem and the vermis of the cerebellum.

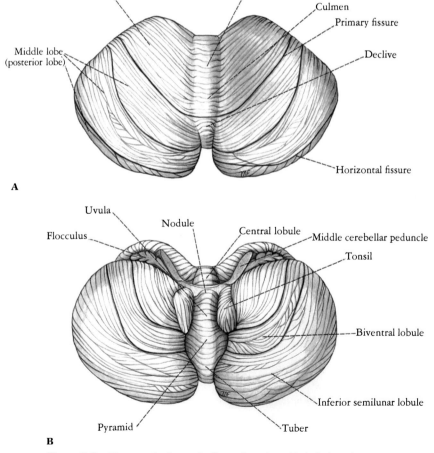

Figure 6–2 The cerebellum. **A.** Superior view. **B.** Inferior view.

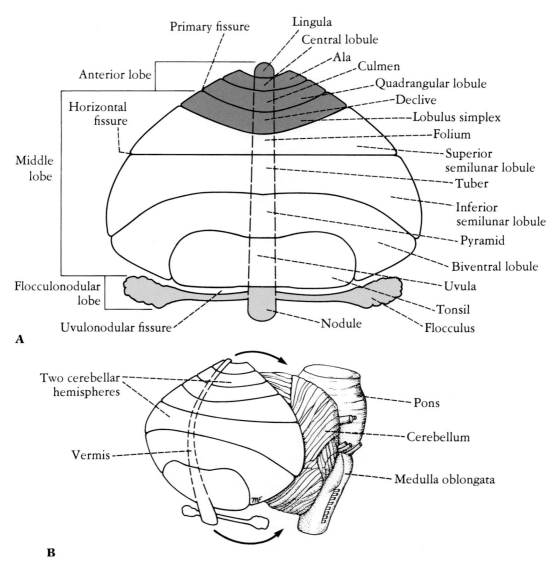

Figure 6–3   A. Flattened view of the cerebellar cortex showing the main cerebellar lobes, lobules, and fissures. **B.** Relationship between the diagram in A and the cerebellum.

STRUCTURE OF THE CEREBELLUM

The cerebellum is composed of an outer covering of gray matter called the **cortex** and inner white matter. Embedded in the white matter of each hemisphere are three masses of gray matter forming the **intracerebellar nuclei.**

Stucture of the Cerebellar Cortex

The cerebellar cortex can be regarded as a large sheet with folds lying in the coronal or transverse plane. Each fold or folium contains a core of white matter covered superficially by gray matter (Fig. 6-1).

A section made through the cerebellum parallel with the median plane divides the folia at right angles, and the cut surface has a branched appearance, called the **arbor vitae** (Fig. 6-1).

The gray matter of the cortex throughout its extent has a uniform structure. It may be divided into three layers: (1) an external layer, the **molecular layer;** (2) a middle layer, the **Purkinje cell layer;** and (3) an internal layer, the **granular layer** (Figs. 6-4 and 6-5).

MOLECULAR LAYER

The molecular layer contains two types of neurons: the outer **stellate cell** and the inner **basket cell** (Fig. 6-4). These neurons are scattered among dendritic arborizations and numerous thin axons that run parallel to the long axis of the folia. Neuroglial cells are found between these structures.

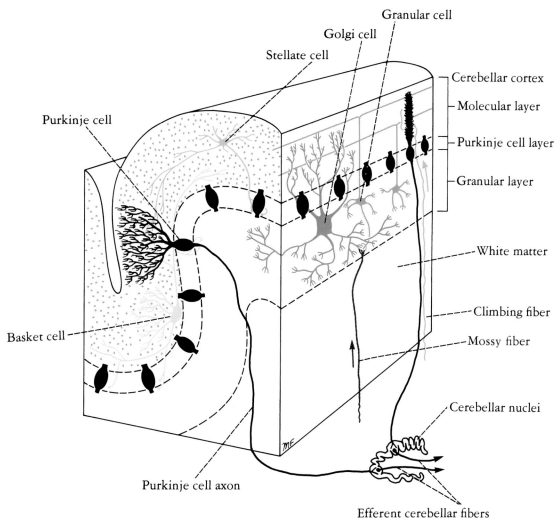

Figure 6–4 Cellular organization of the cerebellar cortex. Note the afferent and efferent fibers.

PURKINJE CELL LAYER

The Purkinje cells are large Golgi type I neurons. They are flask-shaped and are arranged in a single layer (Figs. 6-4 and 6-5). In a plane transverse to the folium, the dendrites of these cells are seen to pass into the molecular layer, where they undergo profuse branching (Figs. 6-4 and 6-5). The primary and secondary branches are smooth and subsequent branches are covered by short, thick **dendritic spines.** It has been shown that the spines form synaptic contacts with the parallel fibers derived from the granule cell axons.

At the base of the Purkinje cell, the axon arises and passes through the granular layer to enter the white matter. On entering the white matter, the axon acquires a myelin sheath and it terminates by synapsing with cells of one of the intracerebellar nuclei. Collateral branches of the Purkinje axon make synaptic contacts with the dendrites of basket and stellate cells of the granular layer in the same

area or in distant folia. A few of the Purkinje cell axons pass directly to end in the vestibular nuclei of the brainstem.

GRANULAR LAYER

The granular layer is packed with small cells with densely staining nuclei and scanty cytoplasm (Figs. 6-4 and 6-5). Each cell gives rise to four or five dendrites, which make clawlike endings and have synaptic contact with mossy fiber input (see pp. 231 and 233). The axon of each granule cell passes into the molecular layer, where it bifurcates at a T junction, the branches running parallel to the long axis of the cerebellar folium (Fig. 6-4). These fibers, known as **parallel fibers,** run at right angles to the dendritic processes of the Purkinje cells. Most of the parallel fibers make synaptic contacts with the spinous processes of the dendrites of the Purkinje cells. Neuroglial cells are found throughout this layer. Scattered throughout the granular layer are Golgi cells

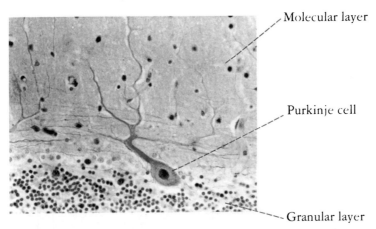

Figure 6–5 Photomicrograph of a cross section of a cerebellar folium, showing the three layers of the cerebellar cortex.

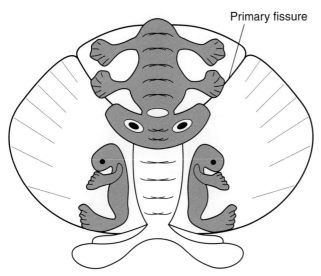

Figure 6–6 Somatosensory projection areas in the cerebellar cortex.

(Fig. 6-4). Their dendrites ramify in the molecular layer and their axons terminate by splitting up into branches that synapse with the dendrites of the granular cells (Fig. 6-5).

Functional Areas of the Cerebellar Cortex

Clinical observations by neurologists and neurosurgeons and the experimental use of the PET scan, have shown that it is possible to divide up the cerebellar cortex into three functional areas.

The cortex of the vermis influences the movements of the long axis of the body, namely the neck, the shoulders, the thorax, the abdomen, and the hips (Fig. 6-6). Immediately lateral to the vermis is a so called intermediate zone of the cerebellar hemisphere. This area has been

shown to control the muscles of the distal parts of the limbs, especially the hands and feet (Fig. 6-6). The lateral zone of each cerebellar hemisphere appears to be concerned with the planning of sequential movements of the entire body and is involved with the conscious assessment of movement errors.

Intracerebellar Nuclei

Four masses of gray matter are embedded in the white matter of the cerebellum on each side of the midline (Fig. 6-7). From lateral to medial these nuclei are the **dentate,** the **emboliform,** the **globose,** and the **fastigial.**

The **dentate nucleus** is the largest of the cerebellar nuclei. It has the shape of a crumpled bag with the opening facing medially (Fig. 6-7). The interior of the bag is filled with white matter made up of efferent fibers that leave the nucleus through the opening to form a large part of the superior cerebellar peduncle.

The **emboliform nucleus** is ovoid and is situated medial to the dentate nucleus, partially covering its hilus (Fig. 6-7).

The **globose nucleus** consists of one or more rounded cell groups that lie medial to the emboliform nucleus (Fig. 6-7).

The **fastigial nucleus** lies near the midline in the vermis and close to the roof of the fourth ventricle; it is larger than the globose nucleus (Fig. 6-7).

The intracerebellar nuclei are composed of large, multipolar neurons with simple branching dendrites. The axons form the cerebellar outflow in the superior and inferior cerebellar peduncles.

White Matter

There is a small amount of white matter in the vermis and it closely resembles the trunk and branches of a tree—the **arbor vitae** (Fig. 6-1). There is a large amount of white matter in each cerebellar hemisphere.

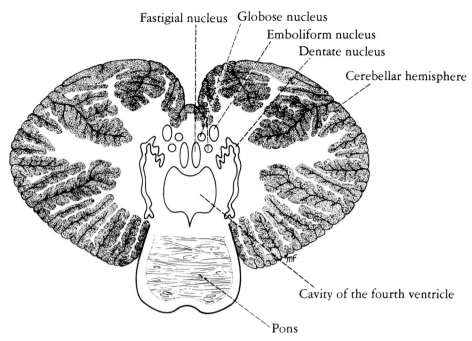

Figure 6–7   Position of the intracerebellar nuclei.

The white matter is made up of three groups of fibers: (1) intrinsic, (2) afferent, and (3) efferent.

The **intrinsic fibers** do not leave the cerebellum but connect different regions of the organ. Some interconnect folia of the cerebellar cortex and vermis on the same side; others connect the two cerebellar hemispheres together.

The **afferent fibers** form the greater part of the white matter and proceed to the cerebellar cortex. They enter the cerebellum mainly through the inferior and middle cerebellar peduncles.

The **efferent fibers** constitute the output of the cerebellum and commence as the axons of the Purkinje cells of the cerebellar cortex. The great majority of the Purkinje cell axons pass to and synapse with the neurons of the cerebellar nuclei (fastigial, globose, emboliform, and dentate). The axons of the neurons then leave the cerebellum. A few Purkinje cell axons in the flocculonodular lobe and in parts of the vermis bypass the cerebellar nuclei and leave the cerebellum without synapsing.

Fibers from the dentate, emboliform, and globose nuclei leave the cerebellum through the superior cerebellar peduncle. Fibers from the fastigial nucleus leave through the inferior cerebellar peduncle.

CEREBELLAR CORTICAL MECHANISMS

As the result of extensive cytological and physiological research, certain basic mechanisms have been attributed to the cerebellar cortex. The climbing and the mossy fibers constitute the two main lines of input to the cortex and are excitatory to the Purkinje cells (Fig. 6-8).

The **climbing fibers** are the terminal fibers of the olivocerebellar tracts (Fig. 6-8). They are so named because they ascend through the layers of the cortex like a vine on a tree. They pass through the granular layer of the cortex and terminate in the molecular layer by dividing repeatedly. Each climbing fiber wraps around and makes a large number of synaptic contacts with the dendrites of a Purkinje cell. A **single** Purkinje neuron makes synaptic contact with only one climbing fiber. However, one climbing fiber makes contact with one to ten Purkinje neurons. A few side branches leave each climbing fiber and synapse with the stellate cells and basket cells.

The **mossy fibers** are the terminal fibers of all other cerebellar afferent tracts. They have multiple branches and exert a much more diffuse excitatory effect. A single mossy fiber may stimulate **thousands** of Purkinje cells through the granule cells (Fig. 6-8). What then is the function of the remaining cells of the cerebellar cortex, namely, the stellate, basket, and Golgi cells? Neurophysiological research, using microelectrodes, would indicate that they serve as inhibitory interneurons. It is believed that they not only limit the area of cortex excited but influence the degree of Purkinje cell excitation produced by the climbing and mossy fiber input. By this means, fluctuating inhibitory impulses are transmitted by the Purkinje cells to the intracerebellar nuclei, which in turn modify muscular activity through the motor control areas of the brainstem and cerebral cortex. It is thus seen that the Purkinje cells form the center of a **functional unit** of the cerebellar cortex.

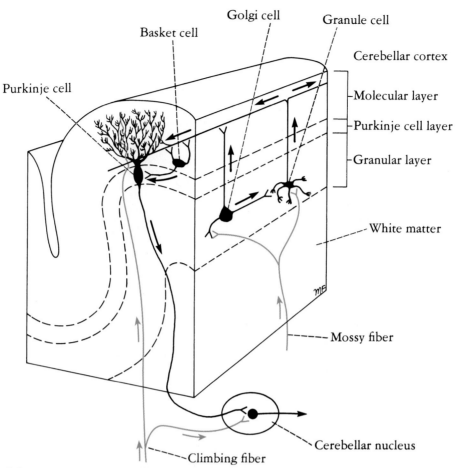

Figure 6–8 Functional organization of the cerebellar cortex. The arrows indicate the direction taken by the nervous impulses.

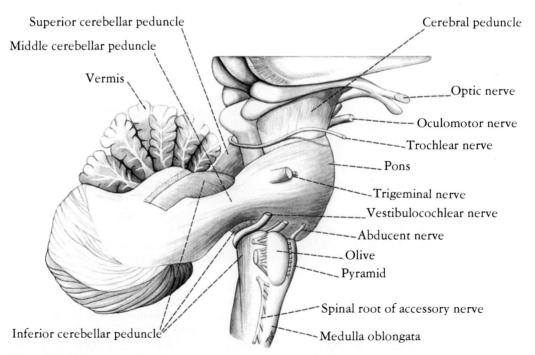

Figure 6–9 Three cerebellar peduncles connecting the cerebellum to the rest of the central nervous system.

Intracerebellar Nuclear Mechanisms

The deep cerebellar nuclei receive afferent nervous information from two sources. 1) The inhibitory axons from the Purkinje cells of the overlying cortex and 2) the excitatory axons that are branches of the afferent climbing and mossy fibers that are passing to the overlying cortex. In this manner a given sensory input to the cerebellum sends excitatory information to the nuclei which a short time later receive cortical processed inhibitory information from the Purkinje cells. Efferent information from the deep cerebellar nuclei leave the cerebellum to be distributed to the remainder of the brain and spinal cord.

Cerebellar Peduncles

The cerebellum is linked to other parts of the central nervous system by numerous efferent and afferent fibers that are grouped together on each side into three large bundles, or peduncles (Fig. 6-9). The superior cerebellar peduncles connect the cerebellum to the midbrain, the middle cerebellar peduncles connect the cerebellum to the pons, and the inferior cerebellar peduncles connect the cerebellum to the medulla oblongata.

 CEREBELLAR AFFERENT FIBERS

Cerebellar Afferent Fibers From The Cerebral Cortex

The cerebral cortex sends information to the cerebellum by three pathways: (1) the corticopontocerebellar pathway, (2) the cerebro-olivocerebellar pathway, and (3) the cerebroreticulocerebellar pathway.

CORTICOPONTOCEREBELLAR PATHWAY

The corticopontine fibers arise from nerve cells in the frontal, parietal, temporal, and occipital lobes of the cerebral cortex and descend through the corona radiata and internal capsule and terminate upon the pontine nuclei (Fig. 6-10). The pontine nuclei give rise to the **transverse fibers of the pons,** which cross the midline and enter the opposite cerebellar hemisphere as the middle cerebellar peduncle (Figs. 5-13, 5-14, and 5-15).

CEREBRO-OLIVOCEREBELLAR PATHWAY

The cortico-olivary fibers arise from nerve cells in the frontal, parietal, temporal, and occipital lobes of the cerebral cortex and descend through the corona radiata and internal capsule to terminate bilaterally upon the inferior olivary nuclei (Fig. 6-10). The inferior olivary nuclei give rise to fibers that cross the midline and enter the opposite cerebellar hemisphere through the inferior cerebellar peduncle. These fibers terminate as the climbing fibers in the cerebellar cortex.

CEREBRORETICULOCEREBELLAR PATHWAY

The corticoreticular fibers arise from nerve cells from many areas of the cerebral cortex, particularly the sensorimotor areas. They descend to terminate in the reticular formation on the same side and on the opposite side in the pons and medulla (Fig. 6-10). The cells in the reticular formation give rise to the reticulocerebellar fibers that enter the cerebellar hemisphere on the same side through the inferior and middle cerebellar peduncles.

This connection between the cerebrum and the cerebellum is important in the control of voluntary movement. Information regarding the initiation of movement in the cerebral cortex is probably transmitted to the cerebellum so that the movement can be monitored and appropriate adjustments in the muscle activity can be made.

Cerebellar Afferent Fibers From The Spinal Cord

The spinal cord sends information to the cerebellum from somatosensory receptors by three pathways: (1) the anterior spinocerebellar tract, (2) the posterior spinocerebellar tract, and (3) the cuneocerebellar tract.

ANTERIOR SPINOCEREBELLAR TRACT

The axons entering the spinal cord from the posterior root ganglion terminate by synapsing with the neurons in the **nucleus dorsalis** (Clark's column) at the base of the posterior gray column. Most of the axons of these neurons cross to the opposite side and ascend as the **anterior spinocerebellar tract** in the contralateral white column; some of the axons ascend as the anterior spinocerebellar tract in the lateral white column of the same side (Fig. 6-11). The fibers enter the cerebellum through the superior cerebellar peduncle and terminate as mossy fibers in the cerebellar cortex. Collateral branches that end in the deep cerebellar nuclei are also given off. It is believed that those fibers that crossed over to the opposite side in the spinal cord cross back within the cerebellum.

The anterior spinocerebellar tract is found at all segments of the spinal cord and its fibers convey muscle joint information from the muscle spindles, tendon organs, and joint receptors of the upper and lower limbs. It is also believed that the cerebellum receives information from the skin and superficial fascia by this tract.

POSTERIOR SPINOCEREBELLAR TRACT

The axons entering the spinal cord from the posterior root ganglion enter the posterior gray column and terminate by synapsing on the neurons at the base of the posterior gray column. These neurons are known collectively as the nucleus dorsalis (Clark's column). The axons of these neurons enter the posterolateral part of the lateral white column on the same side and ascend as the **posterior spinocerebellar tract** to the medulla oblongata (Fig. 6-11). Here the tract enters the cerebellum through the inferior

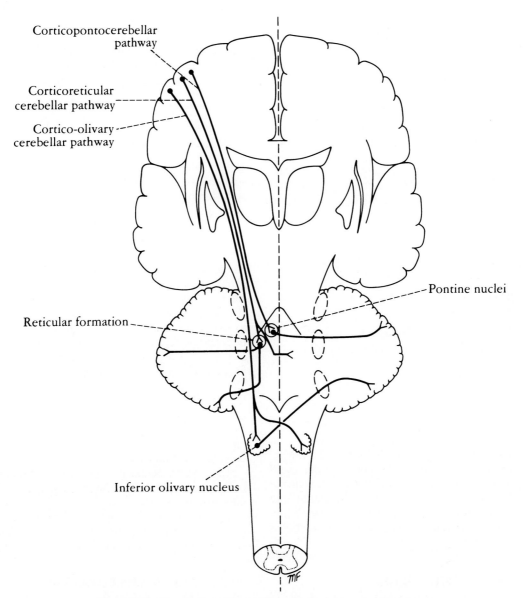

Corticopontocerebellar pathway

Corticoreticular cerebellar pathway

Cortico-olivary cerebellar pathway

Pontine nuclei

Reticular formation

Inferior olivary nucleus

Figure 6–10 Cerebellar afferent fibers from the cerebral cortex.

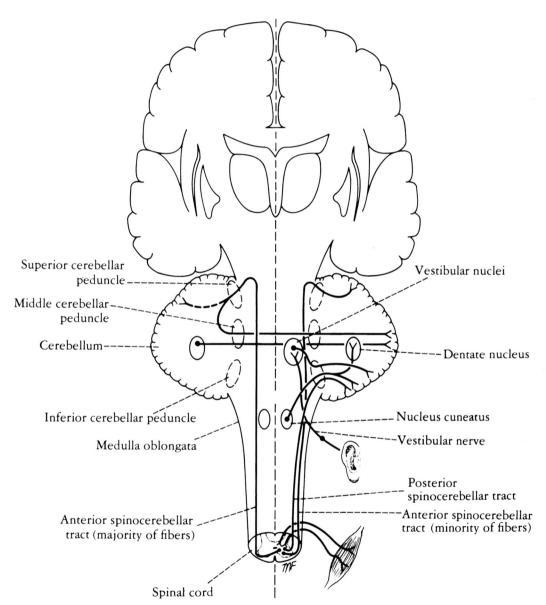

Figure 6–11   Cerebellar afferent fibers from the spinal cord and internal ear.

Table 6-1   The Afferent Cerebellar Pathways

Pathway	Function	Origin	Destination
Corticopontocerebellar	Conveys control from cerebral cortex	Frontal, parietal, temporal, and occipital lobes	Via pontine nuclei and mossy fibers to cerebellar cortex
Cerebro-olivocerebellar	Conveys control from cerebral cortex	Frontal, parietal, temporal, and occipital lobes	Via inferior olivary nuclei and climbing fibers to cerebellar cortex
Cerebroreticulocerebellar	Conveys control from cerebral cortex	Sensorimotor areas	Via reticular formation
Anterior spinocerebellar	Conveys information from muscles and joints	Muscle spindles, tendon organs, and joint receptors	Via mossy fibers to cerebellar cortex
Posterior spinocerebellar	Conveys information from muscles and joints	Muscle spindles, tendon organs, and joint receptors	Via mossy fibers to cerebellar cortex
Cuneocerebellar	Conveys information from muscles and joints of upper limb	Muscle spindles, tendon organs, and joint receptors	Via mossy fibers to cerebellar cortex
Vestibular nerve	Conveys information of head position and movement	Utricle, saccule, and semicircular canals	Via mossy fibers to cortex of flocculonodular lobe
Other afferents	Conveys information from midbrain	Red nucleus, tectum	Cerebellar cortex

cerebellar peduncle and terminates as mossy fibers in the cerebellar cortex. Collateral branches that end in the deep cerebellar nuclei are also given off. The posterior spinocerebellar tract receives muscle joint information from the muscle spindles, tendon organs, and joint receptors of the trunk and lower limbs.

CUNEOCEREBELLAR TRACT

These fibers originate in the nucleus cuneatus of the medulla oblongata and enter the cerebellar hemisphere on the same side through the inferior cerebellar peduncle (Fig. 6-10). The fibers terminate as mossy fibers in the cerebellar cortex. Collateral branches that end in the deep cerebellar nuclei are also given off. The cuneocerebellar tract receives muscle joint information from the muscle spindles, tendon organs, and joint receptors of the upper limb and upper part of the thorax.

Cerebellar Afferent Fibers From The Vestibular Nerve

The vestibular nerve receives information from the inner ear concerning motion from the semicircular canals and position relative to gravity from the utricle and saccule. The vestibular nerve sends many afferent fibers directly to the cerebellum through the inferior cerebellar peduncle on the same side. Other vestibular afferent fibers pass first to the vestibular nuclei in the brainstem, where they synapse and are relayed to the cerebellum (Fig. 6-11). They enter the cerebellum through the inferior cerebellar peduncle on the same side. All the afferent fibers from the inner ear terminate as mossy fibers in the flocculonodular lobe of the cerebellum.

Other Afferent Fibers

In addition, the cerebellum receives small bundles of afferent fibers from the red nucleus and the tectum.

The afferent cerebellar pathways are summarized in Table 6-1.

CEREBELLAR EFFERENT FIBERS

The entire output of the cerebellar cortex is through the axons of the Purkinje cells. Most of the axons of the Purkinje cells end by synapsing on the neurons of the deep cerebellar nuclei (Fig. 6-4). The axons of the neurons that form the cerebellar nuclei constitute the efferent outflow from the cerebellum. A few Purkinje cell axons pass directly out of the cerebellum to the lateral vestibular nucleus. The efferent fibers from the cerebellum connect with the red nucleus, thalamus, vestibular complex, and reticular formation.

Globose-Emboliform-Rubral Pathway

Axons of neurons in the globose and emboliform nuclei travel through the superior cerebellar peduncle and cross the midline to the opposite side in the **decussation of the superior cerebellar peduncles** (Fig. 6-12). The fibers end by synapsing with cells of the contralateral red nucleus, which give rise to axons of the **rubrospinal tract** (Fig. 6-12). Thus it is seen that this pathway crosses twice, once in the decussation of the superior cerebellar peduncle and again in the rubrospinal tract close to its origin. By this means, the globose and emboliform nuclei influence motor activity on the same side of the body.

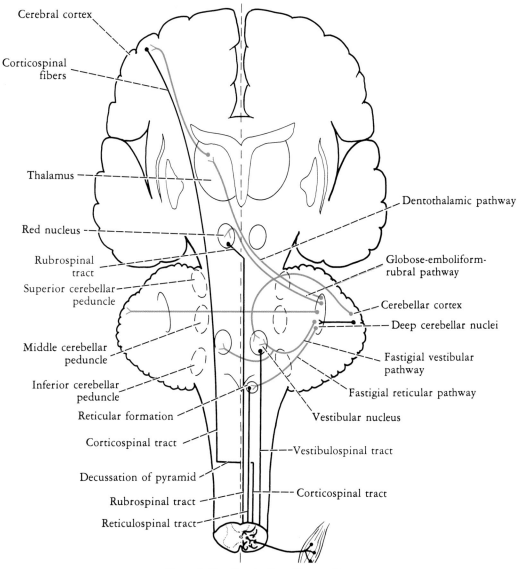

Figure 6–12   Cerebellar efferent fibers.

Dentothalamic Pathway

Axons of neurons in the dentate nucleus travel through the superior cerebellar peduncle and cross the midline to the opposite side in the **decussation of the superior cerebellar peduncle** (Fig. 6-12). The fibers end by synapsing with cells in the contralateral **ventrolateral nucleus of the thalamus.** The axons of the thalamic neurons ascend through the internal capsule and corona radiata and terminate in the primary motor area of the cerebral cortex. By this pathway, the dentate nucleus can influence motor activity by acting upon the motor neurons of the opposite cerebral cortex; impulses from the motor cortex are transmitted to spinal segmental levels through the corticospinal tract. It will be remembered that most of the fibers of the corticospinal tract cross to the opposite side in the decussation

of the pyramids or later at the spinal segmental levels. The dentate nucleus thus is able to coordinate muscle activity on the same side of the body.

Fastigial Vestibular Pathway

The axons of neurons in the fastigial nucleus travel through the inferior cerebellar peduncle and end by projecting on the neurons of the **lateral vestibular nucleus** on both sides (Fig. 6-12). It will be remembered that some Purkinje cell axons project directly to the lateral vestibular nucleus. The neurons of the lateral vestibular nucleus form the **vestibulospinal tract.** The fastigial nucleus exerts a facilitatory influence mainly on the ipsilateral extensor muscle tone.

Table 6–2   The Efferent Cerebellar Pathways*

Pathway	Function	Origin	Destination
Globose-emboliform-rubral	Influences ipsilateral motor activity	Globose and emboliform nuclei	To contralateral red nucleus, then via crossed rubrospinal tract to ipsilateral motor neurons in spinal cord
Dentothalamic	Influences ipsilateral motor activity	Dentate nucleus	To contralateral ventrolateral nucleus of thalamus, then to contralateral motor cerebral cortex; corticospinal tract crosses midline and controls ipsilateral motor neurons in spinal cord
Fastigial vestibular	Influences ipsilateral extensor muscle tone	Fastigial nucleus	Mainly to ipsilateral and to contralateral lateral vestibular nuclei; vestibulospinal tract to ipsilateral motor neurons in spinal cord
Fastigial reticular	Influences ipsilateral muscle tone	Fastigial nucleus	To neurons of reticular formation; reticulospinal tract to ipsilateral motor neurons to spinal cord

*Note that each cerebellar hemisphere influences the voluntary muscle tone on the same side of the body.

Fastigial Reticular Pathway

The axons of neurons in the fastigial nucleus travel through the inferior cerebellar peduncle and end by synapsing with neurons of the reticular formation (Fig. 6-12). Axons of these neurons influence spinal segmental motor activity through the reticulospinal tract. The efferent cerebellar pathways are summarized in Table 6-2.

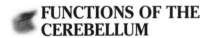

FUNCTIONS OF THE CEREBELLUM

The cerebellum receives afferent information concerning voluntary movement from the cerebral cortex and from the muscles, tendons, and joints. It also receives information concerning balance from the vestibular nerve and possibly concerning sight through the tectocerebellar tract. All this information is fed into the cerebellar cortical circuitry by the mossy fibers and the climbing fibers and converges on the Purkinje cells (Fig.6-8). The axons of the Purkinje cells project with few exceptions on the deep cerebellar nuclei. The output of the vermis projects to the fastigial nucleus, the intermediate regions of the cortex project to the globose and emboliform nuclei, and the output of the lateral part of the cerebellar hemisphere projects to the dentate nucleus. A few Purkinje cell axons pass directly out of the cerebellum and end on the lateral vestibular nucleus in the brainstem. It is now generally believed that the Purkinje axons exert an inhibitory influence on the neurons of the cerebellar nuclei and the lateral vestibular nuclei.

The cerebellar output is conducted to the sites of origin of the descending pathways that influence motor activity at the segmental spinal level. In this respect, the cerebellum has no direct neuronal connections with the lower motor neurons, but exerts its influence indirectly through the cerebral cortex and brainstem.

Physiologists have postulated that the cerebellum functions as a coordinator of precise movements by continually comparing the output of the motor area of the cerebral cortex with the proprioceptive information received from the site of muscle action; it is then able to bring about the necessary adjustments by influencing the activity of the lower motor neurons (Fig. 6-13). This is accomplished by controlling the timing and sequence of firing of the alpha and gamma motor neurons. It is also believed that the cerebellum can send back information to the motor cerebral cortex, to inhibit the agonist muscles and stimulate the antagonist muscles, thus limiting the extent of voluntary movement.

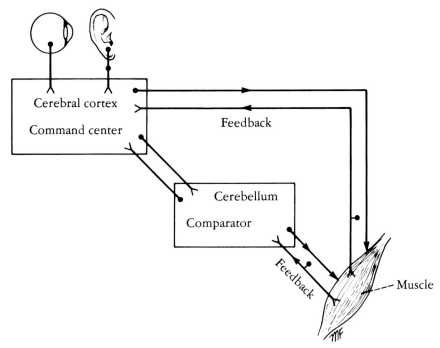

Figure 6–13 Cerebellum serving as a comparator.

CLINICAL NOTES

GENERAL CONSIDERATIONS

Each cerebellar hemisphere is connected by nervous pathways principally with the same side of the body, so that a **lesion in one cerebellar hemisphere gives rise to signs and symptoms that are limited to the same side of the body**. The main connections of the cerebellum are summarized in Figure 6-14.

The essential function of the cerebellum is to coordinate, by synergistic action, all reflex and voluntary muscular activity. It thus graduates and harmonizes muscle tone and maintains normal body posture. It permits voluntary movements such as walking to take place smoothly with precision and economy of effort.

Signs and Symptoms of Cerebellar Disease

While the importance of the cerebellum in the maintenance of muscle tone and the coordination of muscle movement has been emphasized, it should be remembered that the symptoms and signs of acute lesions differ from those produced by chronic lesions. Acute lesions produce sudden, severe symptoms and signs, but there is considerable clinical evidence to show that patients can recover completely from large cerebellar injuries. This suggests that other areas of the central nervous system can compensate for loss of cerebellar function. Chronic lesions, such as slowly enlarging tumors, produce symptoms and signs that are much less severe than those of acute lesions. The reason for this may be that other areas of the central nervous system have time to compensate for loss of cerebellar function. The following symptoms and signs are characteristic of cerebellar dysfunction.

Hypotonia

The muscles lose resilience to palpation. There is diminished resistance to passive movements of joints. Shaking the limb produces excessive movements at the terminal joints. The condition is attributable to loss of cerebellar influence on the simple stretch reflex.

Postural Changes and Alteration of Gait

The head is often rotated and flexed and the shoulder on the side of the lesion is lower than on the normal side. The patient assumes a wide base when he or she stands and is often stiff-legged to compensate for loss of muscle tone. When the individual walks, he or she lurches and staggers toward the affected side.

Disturbances of Voluntary Movement (Ataxia)

The muscles contract irregularly and weakly. **Tremor** occurs when fine movements, such as buttoning clothes, writing, and shaving, are attempted. Muscle groups fail to

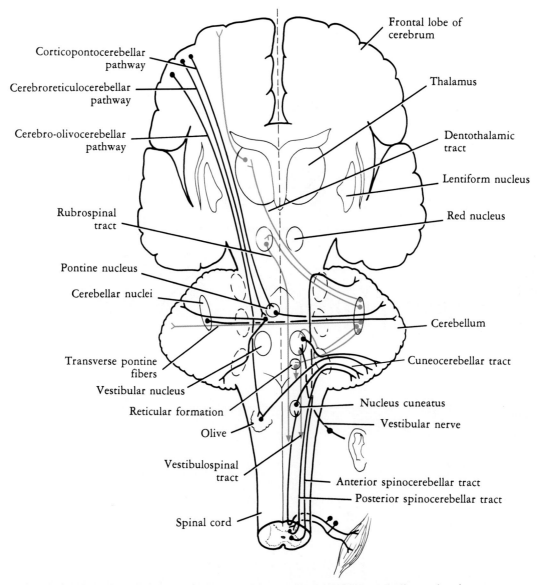

Figure 6–14 Some of the main connections of the cerebellum. The cerebellar peduncles are shown as ovoid dashed lines.

work harmoniously and there is **decomposition of movement.** When the patient is asked to touch the tip of the nose with the index finger, the movements are not properly coordinated and the finger either passes the nose (past-pointing) or hits the nose. A similar test can be performed on the lower limbs by asking the patient to place the heel of one foot on the shin of the opposite leg.

Dysdiadochokinesia

Dysdiadochokinesia is the inability to perform alternating movements regularly and rapidly. Ask the patient to pronate and supinate the forearms rapidly. On the side of the cerebellar lesion the movements are slow, jerky, and incomplete.

Disturbances of Reflexes

Movement produced by tendon reflexes tends to continue for a longer period of time than normal. The **pendular knee jerk,** for example, occurs following tapping of the patellar tendon. Normally the movement occurs and is self-limited by the stretch reflexes of the agonists and antagonists. In cerebellar disease, because of loss of influence on the stretch reflexes, the movement continues as a series of flexion and extension movements at the knee joint; that is, the leg moves like a pendulum.

Disturbances of Ocular Movement

Nystagmus, which is essentially an ataxia of the ocular muscles, is a rhythmical oscillation of the eyes. It is more easily demonstrated when the eyes are deviated in a horizontal direction. This rhythmic oscillation of the eyes may be of the same rate in both directions (**pendular nystagmus**), or quicker in one direction than in the other (**jerk nystagmus**). In the latter situation, the movements are referred to as the slow phase away from the visual object, followed by a quick phase back toward the target. The quick phase is used to describe the form of nystagmus. For example, a patient is said to have a nystagmus to the left if the quick phase is to the left and the slow phase is to the right. The movement of nystagmus may be confined to one plane and may be horizontal or vertical or in many planes, when it is referred to as rotatory nystagmus.

The posture of the eye muscles depends mainly upon the normal functioning of two sets of afferent pathways. The first is the visual pathway whereby the eye views the object of interest, and the second is much more complicated and involves the labyrinths, the vestibular nuclei, and the cerebellum.

Disorders of Speech

Dysarthria occurs in cerebellar disease owing to ataxia of the muscles of the larynx. Articulation is jerky and the syllables often are separated from one another. Speech tends to be explosive and the syllables often are slurred.

In cerebellar lesions, paralysis and sensory changes are not present. Although muscle hypotonia and incoordination may be present, the disorder is not limited to specific muscles or muscle groups; rather, an entire extremity or the entire half of the body is involved, and if both cerebellar hemispheres are involved, then the entire body may show disturbances of muscle action. Even though the muscular contractions may be weak and the patient easily fatigued, there is no atrophy.

CEREBELLAR SYNDROMES

Vermis Syndrome

The most common cause of this syndrome is a **medulloblastoma** of the vermis in children. Involvement of the flocculonodular lobe results in signs and symptoms related to the vestibular system. Since the vermis is unpaired and influences midline structures, muscle incoordination involves the head and trunk and not the limbs. There is a tendency to fall forward or backward. There is difficulty in holding the head steady and in an upright position. There also may be difficulty in holding the trunk erect.

Cerebellar Hemisphere Syndrome

Tumors of one cerebellar hemisphere may be the cause of this syndrome. The symptoms and signs are usually unilateral and involve muscles on the side of the diseased cerebellar hemisphere. Movements of the limbs, especially the arms, are disturbed. Swaying and falling to the side of the lesion often occur. Dysarthria and nystagmus are also common findings. Disorders of the lateral part of the cerebellar hemispheres produces delays in initiating movements and inability to move all limb segments together in a coordinated manner but show a tendency to move one joint at a time.

COMMON DISEASES INVOLVING THE CEREBELLUM

The following frequently involve the cerebellum: congenital agenesis or hypoplasia, trauma, infections, tumors, multiple sclerosis, alcoholism, vascular disorders such as thrombosis of the cerebellar arteries, and poisoning with heavy metals.

The many manifestations of cerebellar disease can be reduced to two basic defects: hypotonia, and loss of influence of the cerebellum on the activities of the cerebral cortex.

Clinical Problem Solving

1. A 10-year-old girl was taken to a neurologist because her parents had noticed that her gait was becoming awkward. Six months previously, the child had complained that she felt her right arm was clumsy and she had inadvertently knocked a teapot off the table. More recently, her family had noticed that her hand movements were becoming jerky and awkward; this was particularly obvious when she was eating with a knife and fork. The mother commented that her daughter had had problems with her right foot since birth and that she had a clubfoot. She also had scoliosis and was attending an orthopedic surgeon for treatment. The mother said she was particularly worried about her daughter because two other members of the family had similar signs and symptoms.

   On physical examination, the child was found to have a lurching gait with a tendency to reel over to the right. Intention tremor was present in the right arm and the right leg. When the strength of the limb muscles was tested, those of the right leg were found to be weaker than those of the left leg. The muscles of the right arm and right lower leg were also hypotonic. She had severe pes cavus of the right foot and a slight pes cavus of the left foot. Kyphoscoliosis of the upper part of the thoracic vertebral column also was present.

   On examination of her sensory system, she was found to have loss of muscle joint sense and vibratory sense of both legs. She also had loss of two-point discrimination of the skin of both legs. Her knee jerks were found to be exaggerated, but her ankle jerks were absent. The biceps and triceps jerks of both arms were normal. She had bilateral Babinski responses. Slight nystagmus was present in both eyes. Using your knowledge of neuroanatomy, explain the symptoms and signs listed above. Did the disease process involve more than one area of the central nervous system? Explain.

2. Two physicians were talking in the street when one turned to the other and said, "Look at that man over there—look at the way he is walking—he is not swinging his right arm at all—it is just hanging down by his side. I wonder if he has a cerebellar lesion." Does a person with a unilateral cerebellar hemisphere tumor tend to hold the arm limply at the side when he walks?

3. A 37-year-old man visited his physician because he had noticed clumsiness of his right arm. The symptoms had started 6 months previously and were getting worse. He also noticed that his right hand had a tremor when he attempted fine movements or tried to insert a key in a lock. When he walks he notices that now and again he tends to reel over to the right, "as if he had too much alcohol to drink." On physical examination, the face was tilted slightly to the left and the right shoulder was held lower than the left. Passive movements of the arms and legs revealed hypotonia and looseness on the right side. When asked to walk heel to toe along a straight line on the floor, the patient swayed over to the right side. When he was asked to touch his nose with his right index finger, the right hand displayed tremor and the finger tended to overshoot the target. Speech was normal and nystagmus was not present. Using your knowledge of neuroanatomy, explain each sign and symptom. Is the lesion of the cerebellum likely to be in the midline or to one side?

4. A 4 1/2-year-old boy was taken to a neurologist because his mother was concerned about his attacks of vomiting on waking in the morning and his tendency to be unsteady on standing up. The mother also noticed that the child walked with an unsteady gait and often fell backward. On physical examination, the child tended to stand with the legs well apart, that is, broad-based. The head was larger than normal for his age and the suture lines of the skull could be easily felt. A retinal examination with an ophthalmoscope showed severe papilledema in both eyes. The muscles of the upper and lower limbs showed some degree of hypotonia. Nystagmus was not present and the child showed no tendency to fall to one side or the other when asked to walk. Using your knowledge of neuroanatomy, explain the symptoms and signs. Is the lesion in the cerebellum likely to be in the midline or to one side?

5. During a ward round, a third-year student was asked to explain the phenomenon of nystagmus. How would you have answered that question? Why do patients with cerebellar disease exhibit nystagmus?

6. What is the essential difference between the symptoms and signs of acute and chronic lesions of the cerebellum? Explain these differences.

Answers to Clinical Problem Solving

1. This 10-year-old girl had the symptoms and signs of Friedreich's ataxia, an inherited degenerative disease of the cerebellum and posterior and lateral parts of the spinal cord.

   Degeneration of the cerebellum was revealed by the altered gait, clumsy movements of the right arm, tendency to fall to the right, intention tremor of the right arm and leg, hypotonicity of the right arm and right leg, and nystagmus of both eyes.

   Involvement of the fasciculus gracilis was evidenced by loss of vibratory sense, loss of two-point discrimination, and loss of muscle joint sense of the lower limbs.

   Corticospinal tract degeneration resulted in weakness of the legs and the presence of the Babinski plantar response. The exaggerated knee jerks were due to involvement of the upper motor neurons other than the corticospinal tract.

   The loss of the ankle jerks was due to the interruption of the reflex arcs at spinal levels S1 and 2 by the degenerative process.

   The clubfoot and scoliosis can be attributed to altered tone of the muscles of the leg and trunk over a period of many years.

2. Yes. A person who has a unilateral lesion involving one cerebellar hemisphere demonstrates absence of coordination between different groups of muscles on the same side of the body. This disturbance affects not only agonists and antagonists in a single joint movement, but also all associated muscle activity. For example, a normal person when walking swings his or her arms at both sides; with cerebellar disease this activity would be lost on the side of the lesion.

3. This man, at operation, was found to have an astrocytoma of the right cerebellar hemisphere. This fact explains the occurrence of unilateral symptoms and signs. The lesion was on the right side and the clumsiness, tremor, muscle incoordination, and hypotonia occurred on the right side of the body. The progressive worsening of the clinical condition could be explained on the basis that more and more of the cerebellum was becoming destroyed as the tumor rapidly expanded. The flaccidity of the muscles of the right arm and leg was due to hypotonia, that is, a removal of the influence of the cerebellum on the simple stretch reflex involving the muscle spindles and tendon organs. The clumsiness, tremor, and overshooting on the finger-nose test were caused by the lack of cerebellar influence on the process of coordination between different groups of muscles. The falling to the right side, the tilting of the head, and the drooping of the right shoulder were due to loss of muscle tone and fatigue.

4. The diagnosis was medulloblastoma of the brain in the region of the roof of the fourth ventricle, with involvement of the vermis of the cerebellum. The child died 9 months

later after extensive deep x-ray therapy. The sudden onset of vomiting, the increased size of the head beyond normal limits, the sutural separation, and the severe bilateral papilledema could all be accounted for by the rapid rise in intracranial pressure owing to the rapid increase in size of the tumor. The broad-based, unsteady gait and the tendency to fall backward (or forward), and not to one side, indicate a tumor involving the vermis. The presence of bilateral hypotonia, especially during the later stages, was due to involvement of both cerebellar hemispheres. At autopsy the tumor was found to have invaded the fourth ventricle extensively, and there was evidence of internal hydrocephalus because the cerebrospinal fluid had been unable to escape through the foramina in the roof of the fourth ventricle.

5. Nystagmus, an involuntary oscillation of the eyeball, may occur physiologically, as when a person watches rapidly moving objects, or by rapid rotation of the body. It commonly occurs in diseases of the nervous system, eye, and inner ear. In cerebellar disease, nystagmus is due to ataxia of the muscles moving the eyeball. There is lack of coordination between the agonists and antagonists involved in the eyeball movement. For full understanding of the different forms of nystagmus, a textbook of neurology should be consulted. See also page 240.

6. Acute lesions, such as those resulting from a thrombosis of a cerebellar artery or a rapidly growing tumor, produce sudden severe symptoms and signs owing to the sudden withdrawal of the influence of the cerebellum on muscular activity. Patients can recover quickly from large cerebellar injuries, and this can be explained on the basis that the cerebellum influences muscular activity not directly, but indirectly, through the vestibular nuclei, reticular formation, red nucleus, tectum, and corpus striatum and the cerebral cortex; it may well be that these other areas of the central nervous system take over this function. In chronic lesions, the symptoms and signs are much less severe and there is enough time to allow the other areas of the central nervous system to compensate for loss of cerebellar function.

Review Questions

Directions: Each of the numbered items in this section is followed by answers that are positively phrased. Select the ONE lettered answer that is an EXCEPTION.

1. The following statements concerning the gross appearance of the cerebellum are correct **except:**
   (a) It is separated from the occipital lobes of the cerebral hemispheres by the tentorium cerebelli.
   (b) It lies posterior to the medulla oblongata and the pons.
   (c) The anterior lobe is separated from the middle (posterior) lobe by the horizontal fissure.
   (d) The flocculonodular lobe is separated from the middle (posterior) lobe by the uvulonodular fissure.
   (e) The fourth ventricle lies anterior to the cerebellum.

2. The following general statements concerning the cerebellum are correct **except:**
   (a) The cerebellum has no influence on the activity of smooth muscle.
   (b) The cerebellum has no influence on the skeletal muscles supplied by the cranial nerves.
   (c) Each cerebellar hemisphere controls the skeletal muscle tone on the same side of the body.
   (d) The important Purkinje cells are Golgi type I neurons.
   (e) The Purkinje cells exert an inhibitory influence on the intracerebellar nuclei.

3. The following statements concerning the structure of the cerebellum are correct **except:**
   (a) The cerebellum consists of two cerebellar hemispheres joined by a narrow median vermis.
   (b) The inferior surface of the cerebellum shows a deep groove, formed by the inferior surface of the vermis.
   (c) The inferior cerebellar peduncles join the cerebellum to the medulla oblongata.
   (d) The gray matter is confined to the cerebellar cortex.
   (e) The white matter and folia of the cortex have a branched appearance on the cut surface, called the arbor vitae.

4. The following statements concerning the structure of the cerebellar cortex are correct **except:**
   (a) The cortex is folded by many transverse fissures into folia.
   (b) The structure of the cortex is identical in different parts of the cerebellum.
   (c) The Purkinje cells are found in the most superficial layer of the cortex.
   (d) The Golgi cells are found in the deepest layer of the cerebellar cortex.
   (e) The axons of the Purkinje cells form the efferent fibers from the cerebellar cortex.

5. The following statements concerning the intracerebellar nuclei are correct **except:**
   (a) The nuclei are found within the substance of the white matter.
   (b) They are located in the roof of the fourth ventricle.
   (c) They are composed of large multipolar neurons.
   (d) Their axons form the main cerebellar outflow.
   (e) The nuclei are named from medial to lateral, dentate, emboliform, globose, and fastigial.

6. The following statements concerning the cerebellar peduncles are correct **except:**
   (a) In the superior cerebellar peduncle most of the fibers are efferent and arise from the neurons of the intracerebellar nuclei.

(b) The cerebellar peduncles are surface structures and can easily be seen by brain dissection.

(c) The inferior cerebellar peduncle is made up exclusively of fibers that pass from the inferior olivary nuclei to the middle lobe of the cerebellar hemisphere.

(d) The middle cerebellar peduncle is formed of fibers that arise from the pontine nuclei.

(e) The anterior spinocerebellar tract enters the cerebellum through the superior cerebellar peduncle.

7. The following statements concerning the afferent fibers entering the cerebellum are correct **except:**

   (a) The mossy fibers end by making synaptic contacts with the dendrites of the Purkinje cells.

   (b) They enter the cerebellum mainly through the inferior and middle cerebellar peduncles.

   (c) The climbing and mossy fibers constitute the two main lines of input to the cerebellar cortex.

   (d) The afferent fibers are excitatory to the Purkinje cells.

   (e) The afferent fibers to the cerebellum are myelinated.

8. The following statements concerning the functions of the cerebellum are correct **except:**

   (a) The cerebellum influences the actions of skeletal muscle.

   (b) The cerebellum controls voluntary movement by coordinating the force and extent of contraction of different muscles.

   (c) The cerebellum inhibits the contraction of antagonistic muscles.

   (d) The cerebellum directly influences skeletal muscle activity without the assistance of the cerebral cortex.

   (e) The cerebellum has no effect on the control of intestinal muscle.

9. The following statements concerning the cerebellum are correct **except:**

   (a) The afferent climbing fibers make multiple synaptic contacts with 1-10 Purkinje cells.

   (b) The afferent mossy fibers may stimulate many Purkinje cells by first stimulating the granular cells.

   (c) The neurons of the intracerebellar nuclei send axons without interruption to the opposite cerebral hemisphere.

   (d) The output of the cerebellar nuclei influences muscle activity so that movements can progress in an orderly sequence from one movement to the next.

   (e) Past pointing is caused by the failure of the cerebellum to inhibit the cerebral cortex after the movement has begun.

10. The following statements concerning the cerebellum are correct **except:**

    (a) The cerebellum has the same uniform microscopic structure in different individuals.

(b) The axons of the Purkinje cells exert a stimulatory influence on the neurons of the deep cerebellar nuclei.

(c) Each cerebellar hemisphere principally influences movement on the same side of the body.

(d) Intention tremor is a sign of cerebellar disease.

(e) The part of the cerebellum that lies in the midline is called the vermis.

Directions: Matching Questions.

Following thrombosis of the posterior inferior cerebellar artery, a patient presents the numbered signs and symptoms listed below; match the signs and symptoms with the appropriate lettered structures involved. Each lettered option may be selected once, more than once, or not at all.

11. Loss of pain and temperature on the left side of the body

12. Nystagmus

13. Hypotonicity of the muscles on the right with a tendency to fall to the right

    (a) Right reticulospinal tract

    (b) Right inferior cerebellar peduncle

    (c) None of the above

Match the numbered nerve tracts listed below with the lettered pathways by which they leave the cerebellum. Each lettered option may be selected once, more than once, or not at all.

14. Corticopontocerebellar

15. Cuneocerebellar

16. Cerebellar reticular

17. Cerebellar rubral

    (a) Superior cerebellar peduncle

    (b) Corpus callosum

    (c) Striae medullaris

    (d) Inferior cerebellar peduncle

    (e) Middle cerebellar peduncle

    (f) None of the above

Directions: Read the following case history then answer the questions. You will be required to select ONE lettered answer.

A 45-year-old man, who was an alcoholic, started to develop a lurching, staggering gait even when he was not intoxicated. The condition became slowly worse over a period of several weeks and then appeared to stabilize. Friends noticed that he had difficulty in walking in tandem with another person and tended to become unsteady on turning quickly.

18. A thorough physical examination of this patient revealed the following findings **except:**

    (a) The patient exhibited instability of trunk movements and incoordination of leg movements.

    (b) While standing still the patient stood with his feet together.

    (c) He had no evidence of polyneuropathy.

(d) The ataxia of the legs was confirmed by performing the heel-to-shin test.
(e) An MRI showed evidence of atrophy of the cerebellar vermis.
19. The following additional abnormal signs might have been observed in this patient **except:**
(a) Nystagmus in both eyes.

(b) Dysarthria.
(c) Tremor of the left hand when reaching for a cup.
(d) Paralysis of the right upper arm muscles.
(e) Dysdiadochokinesia

Answers to Review Questions

1. C.
2. B.
3. D.
4. C.
5. E.
6. C.
7. A.
8. D.
9. C.
10. B.
11. C.
12. B.
13. B.
14. E.
15. D.
16. D.
17. A.
18. B. Patients with cerebellar disease frequently exhibit poor muscle tone and to compensate for this they stand stiff-legged with their feet wide apart.
19. D. Although patients with cerebellar disease display disturbances of voluntary movement none of the muscles are paralysed or show atrophy.

ADDITIONAL READING

Adams, R.D., and Victor, M. Principles of Neurology. Hightstown, NJ, McGraw-Hill,1994.
Angevine, J. B., Mancall, E. L., and Yakovlev, P. I. *The Human Cerebellum.* Boston: Little, Brown, 1961.
Arshavsky, Y. I., Gelfand, I. M., and Olovsky, G. N. The cerebellum and control of rhythmical movements. *Trends Neurosci.* 6:417, 1983.
Bloedel, J. R., and Courville, J. Cerebellar Afferent Systems. In V. B. Brooks (ed.), *Handbook of Physiology.* Sec. 1, Vol. II. Bethesda: American Physiological Society, 1981. P. 735.
Brodal, P. *The Central Nervous System: Structure and Function.* New York, Oxford University Press, 1992.
Chan-Palay, V. *Cerebellar Dentate Nucleus: Organization, Cytology and Transmitters.* Berlin: Springer-Verlag, 1977.
Colin, F., Manil, J., and Desclin, J. C. The olivocerebellar system. 1. Delayed and slow inhibitory effects: An overlooked salient feature of cerebellar climbing fibers. *Brain Res.* 187:3, 1980.
Cordo P., and Harnad. S. *Movement Control.* New York, Cambridge University Press, 1994.
Eccles, J. C., Ito, M., and Szentagothai, J. *The Cerebellum as a Neuronal Machine.* Berlin and Vienna: Springer, 1967.
Fields, W. D., and Willis, W. D., Jr. *The Cerebellum in Health and Disease.* St. Louis: Warren H. Green, 1970.
Forssberg, H., and Hirschfeld, H. *Movement Disorders in Children.* Farmington, CT, S. Karger Publishers. Inc., 1992.
Gilman, S. The mechanisms of cerebellar hypotonia. *Brain* 92:621, 1969.
Gilman, S., Bloedal, J. R., and Lechtenberg, R. *Disorders of the Cerebellum.* Philadelphia: Davis, 1981.
Gilman, S. The Cerebellum: Its Role in Posture and Movement. In M.

Swash and C. Kennard (eds.), *Scientific Basis of Clinical Neurology.* Edinburgh: Churchill Livingstone, 1985. P. 36.
Guyton, A. C., Hall, J.E. *Textbook of Medical Physiology* (9th ed.). Philadelphia: Saunders, 1996.
Ito, M. *The Cerebellum and Neural Control.* New York: Raven, 1984.
Kennedy, P. R., Ross, H. G., and Brooks, V. B. Participation of the principal olivary nucleus in neurocerebellar control. *Exp. Brain Res.* 47:95, 1982.
Leigh, R. J., and Zee, D. S. *The Neurology of Eye Movements* (2nd ed.). Philadelphia: Davis, 1991.
Lewis, A. J. *Mechanisms of Neurological Disease.* Boston: Little, Brown, 1976.
Llinas, R. R. The cortex of the cerebellum. *Sci. Am.* 232:56, 1975.
Llinas, R. R. Electrophysiology of the Cerebellar Networks. In V. B. Brooks (ed.), *Handbook of Physiology.* Sec. 1, Vol. II. Bethesda: American Physiological Society, 1981. P. 831.
Napper, R. M. A., and Harvey, R. J. Number of parallel fiber synapses on an individual Purkinje cell in the cerebellum of the rat. *J. Comp. Neurol.* 274:168, 1988.
Palay, S. L., and Chan-Palay, V. Cortex and Organization. In *Cerebellar Cortex.* Berlin and Vienna: Springer, 1974.
Thach, W.T. On the Specific Role of the Cerebellum in Motor Learning and Cognition: Clues from PET activation and lesion studies in Humans. *Behav. Brain Sci.* 19:411-431,1996.
Thach, W.T., Goodkin, H.G., Keating, J.G. Cerebellum and the Adaptive Coordination of Movement. *Ann. Rev. Neurosci.* 15: 403-442,1992.
Thach, W.T., Perry, J.G., Kane, S.A., Goodkin, H.P. Cerebellar Nuclei: Rapid Alternating Movement, Motor Somatotopy, and a Mechanism for the Control of Muscle Synergy. *Rev. Neurol.* 149: 607-628,1993.
Williams, P. L., et al. *Gray's Anatomy* (Br.38th ed.) New York, Edinburgh,1995.

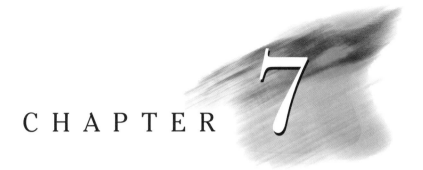

Cerebrum

A 23-year-old man was referred to a neurologist because of intermittent attacks of headaches, dizziness, and weakness and numbness of the left leg. On close questioning, the patient admitted that the headache was made worse by changing the position of his head. A CT scan revealed a small white opaque ball at the anterior end of the third ventricle. A diagnosis of a colloid cyst of the third ventricle was made.

The aggravation of the headache caused by changing the position of the head could be explained by the fact that the cyst was mobile and suspended from the choroid plexus. When the head was moved into certain positions, the ball-like cyst blocked the foramen of Monro on the right side, further raising the intracerebral pressure and increasing the hydrocephalus. The weakness and numbness of the left leg were due to pressure on the right thalamus and the tracts in the right internal capsule, produced by the slowly expanding tumor. The patient made a complete recovery after surgical excision of the tumor.

CHAPTER OBJECTIVES

The objective of this chapter is to introduce the student to the complexities of the forebrain. By studying sagittal, coronal, and horizontal sections of the brain, the student can understand the definition of the diencephalon and accurately localize the thalamus and hypothalamus. It is also important to understand the exact position of the main conduit of the ascending and descending tracts, namely the internal capsule, which is so often the site of pathological lesions.

The cerebral hemispheres are developed from the telencephalon and form the largest part of the brain. Each hemisphere has a covering of gray matter, the cortex and internal masses of gray matter, the basal nuclei, and a lateral ventricle. The basic anatomical structure of this area is described so that the student can be prepared for the complexities associated with functional localization.

SUBDIVISIONS OF THE CEREBRUM

The cerebrum is the largest part of the brain and is situated in the anterior and middle cranial fossae of the skull occupying the whole concavity of the vault of the skull. It may be divided into two parts: the **diencephalon**, which forms the central core, and the **telencephalon**, which forms the **cerebral hemispheres**.

DIENCEPHALON

The diencephalon consists of the third ventricle and the structures that form its boundaries (Fig. 7-1). It extends posteriorly to the point where the third ventricle becomes continuous with the cerebral aqueduct and anteriorly as far as the interventricular foramina (Fig. 7-3). The diencephalon is

thus a midline structure with symmetrical right and left halves. Obviously, these subdivisions of the brain are made for convenience, and from a functional point of view nerve fibers freely cross the boundaries.

Gross Features

The **inferior surface** of the diencephalon is the only area exposed to the surface in the intact brain (Fig. 7-2). It is formed by hypothalamic and other structures, which include, from anterior to posterior, the **optic chiasma**, with the **optic tract** on either side; the **infundibulum**, with **tuber cinereum**; and the **mammillary bodies**.

The **superior surface** of the diencephalon is concealed by the **fornix**, which is a thick bundle of fibers that originates in the **hippocampus** of the temporal lobe and arches posteriorly over the **thalamus** (Fig. 7-3) to join the **mam-**

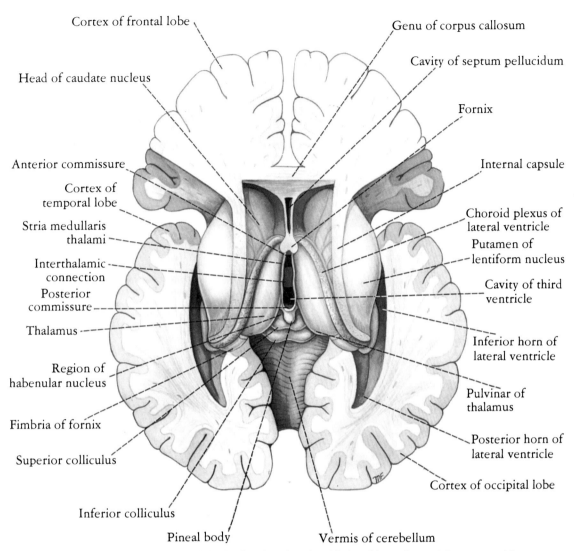

Figure 7–1   Horizontal section of the brain, showing the third and lateral ventricles exposed by dissection from above.

millary body. The actual superior wall of the diencephalon is formed by the **roof of the third ventricle**. This consists of a layer of ependyma, which is continuous with the rest of the ependymal lining of the third ventricle. It is covered superiorly by a vascular fold of pia mater, called the **tela choroidea of the third ventricle**. From the roof of the third ventricle a pair of vascular processes, the **choroid plexuses of the third ventricle**, project downward from the midline into the cavity of the third ventricle.

The **lateral surface** of the diencephalon is bounded by the **internal capsule** of white matter and consists of nerve fibers that connect the cerebral cortex with other parts of the brainstem and spinal cord (Fig. 7-1).

Since the diencephalon is divided into symmetrical halves by the slitlike third ventricle, it also has a **medial surface**. The medial surface of the diencephalon (i.e., the lateral wall of the third ventricle) is formed in its superior part by the medial surface of the **thalamus** and in its inferior

part by the **hypothalamus** (Fig. 7-3). These two areas are separated from one another by a shallow sulcus, the **hypothalamic sulcus**. A bundle of nerve fibers, which are afferent fibers to the habenular nucleus, forms a ridge along the superior margin of the medial surface of the diencephalon and is called the **stria medullaris thalami** (Fig. 7-1).

The diencephalon can be divided into four major parts: (1) the thalamus, (2) the subthalamus, (3) the epithalamus, and (4) the hypothalamus.

Thalamus

The thalamus is a large ovoid mass of gray matter that forms the major part of the diencephalon. It is a region of great functional importance and serves as a cell station to all the main sensory systems (except the olfactory pathway). The thalamus is situated on each side of the third ventricle (Fig. 7-3). The anterior end of the thalamus is narrow and

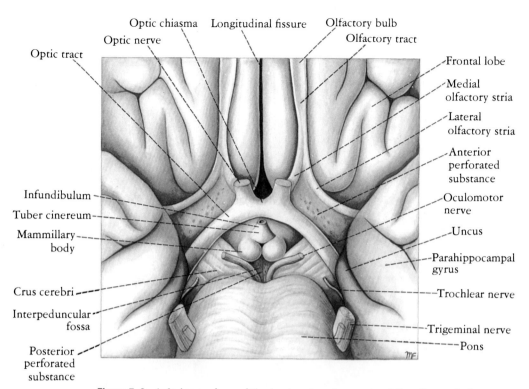

Figure 7–2 Inferior surface of the brain, showing parts of the diencephalon.

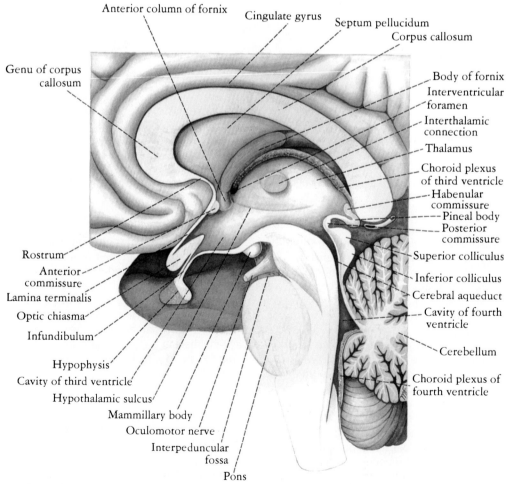

Figure 7–3 Sagittal section of the brain showing the medial surface of the diencephalon.

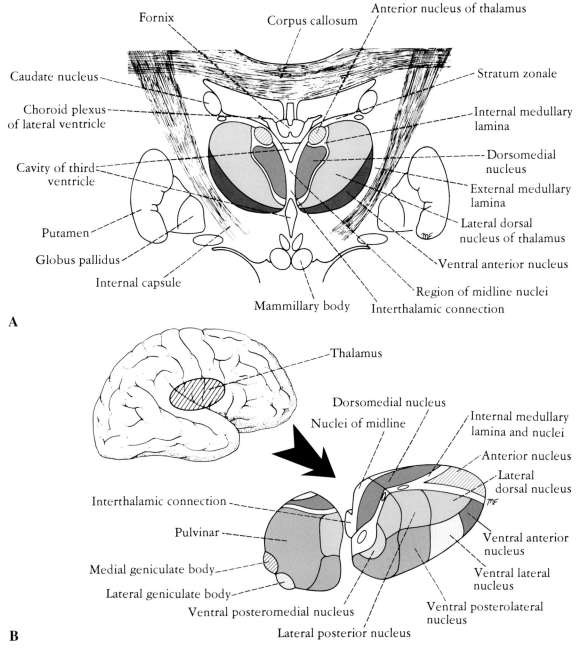

Figure 7–4 Nuclei of the thalamus. **A.** Transverse section through the anterior end of the thalamus. **B.** Diagram showing the position of the thalamus within the right cerebral hemisphere and the relative position of the thalamic nuclei to one another.

rounded and forms the posterior boundary of the interventricular foramen. The posterior end (Fig. 7-4) is expanded to form the **pulvinar**, which overhangs the superior colliculus and the superior brachium. The **lateral geniculate body** forms a small elevation on the under aspect of the lateral portion of the pulvinar.

The superior surface of the thalamus is covered medially by the tela choroidea and the fornix, and laterally it is covered by ependyma and forms part of the floor of the lateral ventricle; the lateral part is partially hidden by the choroid plexus of the lateral ventricle (Fig. 7-1). The inferior surface is continuous with the tegmentum of the midbrain (Fig. 7-3).

The medial surface of the thalamus forms the superior part of the lateral wall of the third ventricle and is usually connected to the opposite thalamus by a band of gray matter, the **interthalamic connection** (interthalamic adhesion) (Fig. 7-3).

The lateral surface of the thalamus is separated from the lentiform nucleus by the very important band of white matter called the **internal capsule** (Fig. 7-1).

Groups of pinealocytes

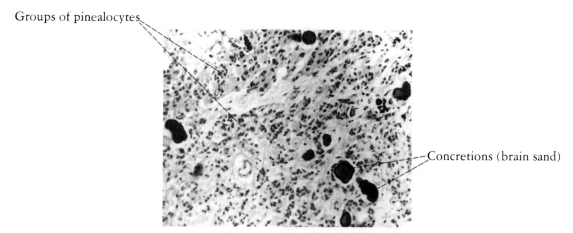

Concretions (brain sand)

Figure 7–5   Photomicrograph of a section of the pineal gland stained with hematoxylin and eosin.

The subdivisions of the thalamus (Fig.7-4) and the detailed description of the thalamic nuclei and their connections are given on page 251.

The thalamus is a very important cell station and receives the main sensory tracts (except the olfactory pathway). It should be regarded as a station where much of the information is integrated and relayed to the cerebral cortex and many other subcortical regions. It also plays a key role in the integration of visceral and somatic functions. For more information on the function of the thalamus see page 249.

Subthalamus

The subthalamus lies inferior to the thalamus and, therefore, is situated between the thalamus and the tegmentum of the midbrain; craniomedially, it is related to the hypothalamus.

The structure of the subthalamus is extremely complex and only a brief description is given here. Among the collections of nerve cells found in the subthalamus are the cranial ends of the **red nuclei** and the **substantia nigra**. The **subthalamic nucleus** has the shape of a biconvex lens. The nucleus has important connections with the corpus striatum (see p. 260); as a result, it is involved in the control of muscle activity.

The subthalamus also contains many important tracts that pass up from the tegmentum to the thalamic nuclei; the cranial ends of the medial, spinal, and trigeminal lemnisci are examples.

Epithalamus

The epithalamus consists of the habenular nuclei and their connections, and the pineal gland.

HABENULAR NUCLEUS

The habenular nucleus is a small group of neurons situated just medial to the posterior surface of the thalamus. Afferent

fibers are received from the amygdaloid nucleus in the temporal lobe (see p. 308) through the stria medullaris thalami; other fibers pass from the hippocampal formation through the fornix. Some of the fibers of the stria medullaris thalami cross the midline and reach the habenular nucleus of the opposite side; these latter fibers form the **habenular commissure** (Fig. 7-3). Axons from the habenular nucleus pass to the interpeduncular nucleus in the roof of the interpeduncular fossa, the tectum of the midbrain, the thalamus, and the reticular formation of the midbrain. The habenular nucleus is believed to be a center for integration of olfactory, visceral, and somatic afferent pathways.

PINEAL GLAND (BODY)

The pineal gland is a small, conical structure that is attached by the pineal stalk to the diencephalon. It projects backward so that it lies posterior to the midbrain (Fig. 7-3). The base of the pineal stalk possesses a recess that is continuous with the cavity of the third ventricle (Fig. 7-3). The superior part of the base of the stalk contains the **habenular commissure**; the inferior part of the base of the stalk contains the **posterior commissure**.

On microscopic section, the pineal gland is seen to be incompletely divided into lobules by connective tissue septa that extend into the substance of the gland from the capsule. Two types of cells are found in the gland, the **pinealocytes** and the **glial cells**. Concretions of calcified material called **brain sand** progressively accumulate within the pineal gland with age (Fig. 7-5).

The pineal gland possesses no nerve cells, but adrenergic sympathetic fibers derived from the superior cervical sympathetic ganglia enter the gland and run in association with the blood vessels and the pinealocytes.

FUNCTIONS OF THE PINEAL GLAND

The pineal gland, once thought to be of little importance, is now recognized as an endocrine gland capable of influencing the activities of the pituitary gland, the islets of Langerhans of the pancreas, the parathyroids, the adrenals, and the gonads. The pineal secretions, produced by the pinealocytes, reach their target organs via the bloodstream or through the cerebrospinal fluid. Their actions are mainly inhibitory and either directly inhibit the production of hormones or indirectly inhibit the secretion of releasing factors by the hypothalamus. It is interesting to note that the pineal gland does not possess a blood-brain barrier.

Animal experiments showed that pineal activity exhibits a circadian rhythm that is influenced by light. The gland has been found to be most active during darkness. The probable nervous pathway from the retina runs to the suprachiasmatic nucleus of the hypothalamus, then to the tegmentum of the midbrain, and then to the pineal gland to stimulate its secretions. The latter part of this pathway may include the reticulospinal tract, the sympathetic outflow of the thoracic part of the spinal cord, the superior cervical sympathetic ganglion and postganglionic nerve fibers that travel to the pineal gland on blood vessels.

Melatonin and enzymes present for its production, are present in high concentrations within the pineal gland. Melatonin and other substances are released into the blood or into the cerebrospinal fluid of the third ventricle where they pass to the anterior lobe of the pituitary gland and inhibit the release of the gonadotrophic hormone. In humans, as in animals, the plasma melatonin level rises in darkness and falls during the day. It would appear that the pineal gland plays an important role in the regulation of reproductive function.

Hypothalamus

The **hypothalamus** is that part of the diencephalon that extends from the region of the optic chiasma to the caudal border of the mammillary bodies (Fig. 7-2). It lies below the hypothalamic sulcus on the lateral wall of the third ventricle. It is thus seen that anatomically the hypothalamus is a relatively small area of the brain that is strategically well placed close to the limbic system, the thalamus, the ascending and descending tracts, and the hypophysis. Microscopically, the hypothalamus is composed of small nerve cells that are arranged in groups or nuclei. The arrangement of these nuclei and their connections are fully described in Chapter 13.

Physiologically, there is hardly any activity in the body that is not influenced by the hypothalamus. The hypothalamus controls and integrates the functions of the autonomic nervous system and the endocrine systems and plays a vital role in maintaining body homeostasis. It is involved in such activities as regulation of body temperature, body fluids, drives to eat and drink, sexual behavior, and emotion.

Relations of the Hypothalamus

Anterior to the hypothalamus is an area that extends forward from the optic chiasma to the lamina terminalis and the anterior commissure; it is referred to as the **preoptic area**. Caudally, the hypothalamus merges into the tegmentum of the midbrain. Superior to the hypothalamus lies the thalamus and inferolaterally is the subthalamic region.

When observed from below, the hypothalamus is seen to be related to the following structures, from anterior to posterior: (1) the optic chiasma, (2) the tuber cinereum and the infundibulum, and (3) the mammillary bodies.

Optic Chiasma

The optic chiasma is a flattened bundle of nerve fibers situated at the junction of the anterior wall and floor of the third ventricle (Figs. 7-2 and 7-3). The superior surface is attached to the **lamina terminalis**, and inferiorly it is related to the **hypophysis cerebri**, from which it is separated by the **diaphragma sellae**. The anterolateral corners of the chiasma are continuous with the **optic nerves**, and the posterolateral corners with the **optic tracts**. A small recess, the **optic recess of the third ventricle**, lies on its superior surface.

It is important to remember that the fibers originating from the nasal half of each retina cross the median plane at the chiasma to enter the optic tract of the opposite side.

Tuber Cinereum

The tuber cinereum is a convex mass of gray matter, as seen from the inferior surface (Figs. 7-2 and 7-3). It is continuous inferiorly with the **infundibulum**. The infundibulum is hollow and becomes continuous with the posterior lobe of the **hypophysis cerebri**. The **median eminence** is a raised part of the tuber cinereum to which is attached the infundibulum. The median eminence, the infundibulum, and the posterior lobe (pars nervosa) of the hypophysis cerebri together form the **neurohypophysis**.

Mammillary Bodies

These are two small hemispherical bodies situated side by side posterior to the tuber cinereum (Figs. 7-2 and 7-3). They possess a central core of gray matter invested by a capsule of myelinated nerve fibers. Posterior to the mammillary bodies lies an area of the brain that is pierced by a number of small apertures and is called the **posterior perforated substance**. These apertures transmit the central branches of the posterior cerebral arteries.

Third Ventricle

The third ventricle, which is derived from the forebrain vesicle, is a slitlike cleft between the two thalami (Figs. 7-1 and 7-3). It communicates anteriorly with the **lateral ventricles** through the **interventricular foramina** (foramina of Monro), and posteriorly with the **fourth ventricle** through the **cerebral aqueduct**. The third ventricle has anterior,

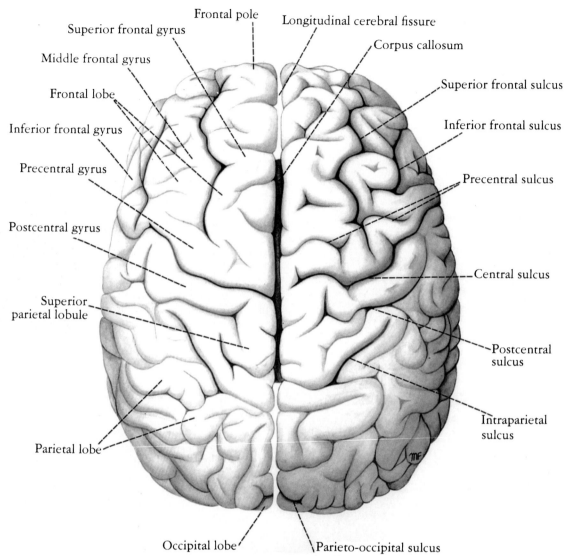

Figure 7–6 Superior view of the cerebral hemispheres.

posterior, lateral, superior, and inferior walls and is lined with ependyma.

The **anterior wall** is formed by a thin sheet of gray matter, the **lamina terminalis**, across which runs the **anterior commissure** (Fig. 7-3). The anterior commissure is a round bundle of nerve fibers that are situated anterior to the **anterior columns of the fornix**; they connect the right and left temporal lobes.

The **posterior wall** is formed by the opening into the cerebral aqueduct (Fig. 7-3). Superior to this opening is the small **posterior commissure**. Superior to the commissure is the **pineal recess**, which projects into the stalk of the **pineal body**. Superior to the pineal recess is the small **habenular commissure**.

The **lateral wall** is formed by the medial surface of the **thalamus** superiorly and the **hypothalamus** inferiorly (Fig. 7-3). These two structures are separated by the **hypothalamic sulcus**. The lateral wall is limited superiorly by the **stria**

medullaris thalami. The lateral walls are joined by the **interthalamic connection**.

The **superior wall** or **roof** is formed by a layer of ependyma that is continuous with the lining of the ventricle. Superior to this layer is a two-layered fold of pia mater called **the tela choroidea of the third ventricle**. The vascular tela choroidea projects downward on each side of the midline, invaginating the ependymal roof to form the **choroid plexuses of the third ventricle**. Within the tela choroidea lie the **internal cerebral veins**. Superiorly, the roof of the ventricle is related to the **fornix** and the **corpus callosum**.

The **inferior wall** or **floor** is formed by the **optic chiasma**, the **tuber cinereum**, the **infundibulum**, with its funnel-shaped recess, and the **mammillary bodies** (Figs. 7-2 and 7-3). The **hypophysis** is attached to the infundibulum. Posterior to these structures lies the **tegmentum of the cerebral peduncles**.

The ventricular system is fully described in Chapter 16.

GENERAL APPEARANCE OF THE CEREBRAL HEMISPHERES

The cerebral hemispheres are the largest part of the brain and are separated by a deep midline sagittal fissure, the **longitudinal cerebral fissure** (Fig. 7-6). The fissure contains the sickle-shaped fold of dura mater, the **falx cerebri**, and the **anterior cerebral arteries**. In the depths of the fissure, the great commissure, the **corpus callosum**, connects the hemispheres across the midline (Fig. 7-6). A second horizontal fold of dura mater separates the cerebral hemispheres from the cerebellum and is called the **tentorium cerebelli**.

To increase the surface area of the cerebral cortex maximally, the surface of each cerebral hemisphere is thrown into **folds** or **gyri**, which are separated from each other by **sulci** or **fissures** (Fig. 7-6). For ease of description, it is customary to divide each hemisphere into **lobes**, which are named according to the cranial bones under which they lie. The **central** and **parieto-occipital sulci** and the **lateral** and **calcarine sulci** are boundaries used for the division of the cerebral hemisphere into **frontal**, **parietal**, **temporal**, and **occipital lobes** (Figs. 7-7 and 7-11).

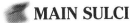

MAIN SULCI

The **central sulcus** (Fig. 7-7) is of great importance because the gyrus that lies anterior to it contains the motor cells that initiate the movements of the opposite side of the body; posterior to it lies the general sensory cortex that receives sensory information from the opposite side of the body. The central sulcus indents the superior medial border of the hemisphere about 0.4 inch (1 cm) behind the midpoint (Fig. 7-8). It runs downward and forward across the lateral aspect of the hemisphere, and its lower end is separated from the posterior ramus of the lateral sulcus by a narrow bridge of cortex. The central sulcus is the only sulcus of any length on this surface of the hemisphere that indents the superomedial border and lies between two parallel gyri.

The **lateral sulcus** (Fig. 7-7) is a deep cleft found mainly on the inferior and lateral surfaces of the cerebral hemisphere. It consists of a short stem that divides into three rami. The stem arises on the inferior surface and on reaching the lateral surface it divides into the **anterior horizontal ramus** and the **anterior ascending ramus**, and continues as the **posterior ramus** (Figs. 7-7 and 7-10). An area of cortex called the **insula** lies at the bottom of the deep lateral sulcus and cannot be seen from the surface unless the lips of the sulcus are separated (Fig. 7-9).

The **parieto-occipital sulcus** begins on the superior medial margin of the hemisphere about 2 inches (5 cm) ante-

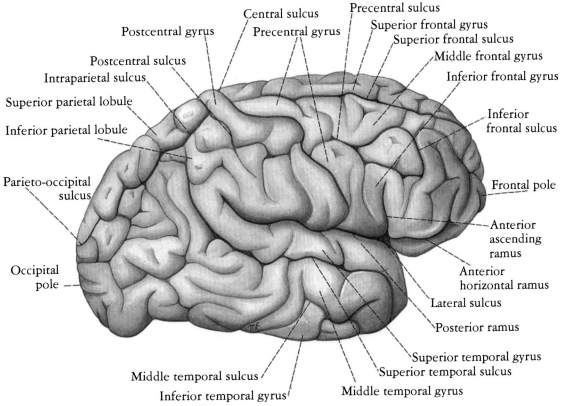

Figure 7-7 Lateral view of the right cerebral hemisphere.

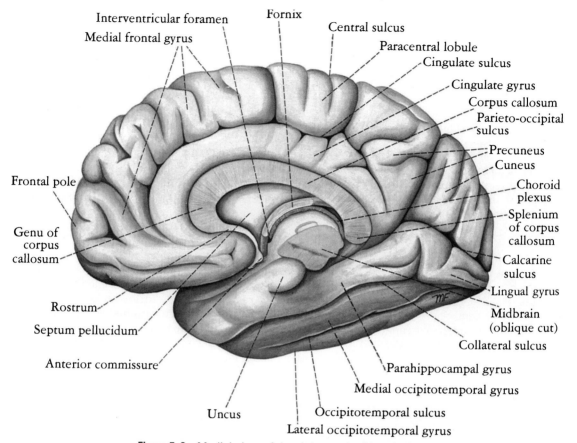

Interventricular foramen
Medial frontal gyrus
Fornix
Central sulcus
Paracentral lobule
Cingulate sulcus
Cingulate gyrus
Corpus callosum
Parieto-occipital sulcus
Precuneus
Cuneus
Choroid plexus
Splenium of corpus callosum
Calcarine sulcus
Lingual gyrus
Midbrain (oblique cut)
Collateral sulcus
Frontal pole
Genu of corpus callosum
Rostrum
Septum pellucidum
Anterior commissure
Uncus
Parahippocampal gyrus
Medial occipitotemporal gyrus
Occipitotemporal sulcus
Lateral occipitotemporal gyrus

Figure 7–8 Medial view of the right cerebral hemisphere.

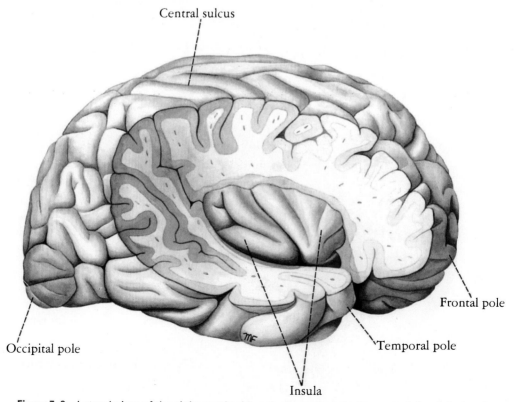

Central sulcus
Frontal pole
Occipital pole
Temporal pole
Insula

Figure 7–9 Lateral view of the right cerebral hemisphere dissected to reveal the right insula.

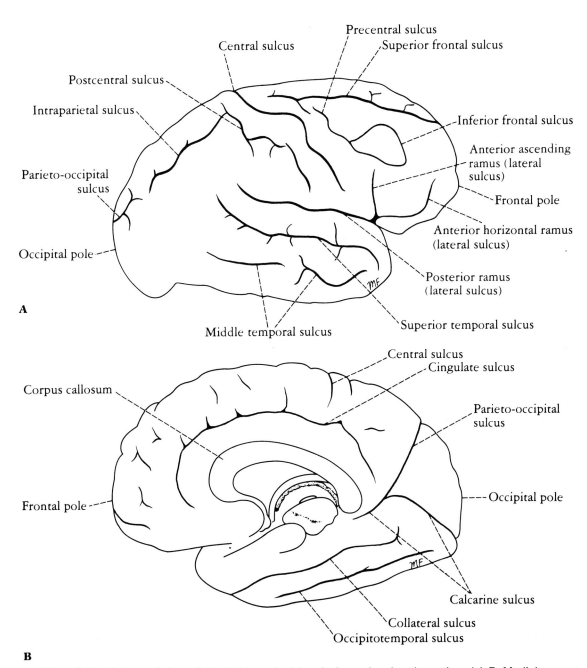

Figure 7–10 A. Lateral view of the right cerebral hemisphere showing the main sulci. **B**. Medial view of the right cerebral hemisphere showing the main sulci.

rior to the occipital pole (Figs. 7-10 and 7-8). It passes downward and anteriorly on the medial surface to meet the calcarine sulcus (Fig. 7-8).

The **calcarine sulcus** is found on the medial surface of the hemisphere (Figs. 7-8 and 7-10). It commences under the posterior end of the corpus callosum and arches upward and backward to reach the occipital pole, where it stops. In some brains, however, it continues for a short distance onto the lateral surface of the hemisphere. The calcarine sulcus is joined at an acute angle by the parietooccipital sulcus about halfway along its length.

LOBES OF THE CEREBRAL HEMISPHERE

Superolateral Surface of the Hemisphere

The **frontal lobe** occupies the area anterior to the central sulcus and superior to the lateral sulcus (Figs. 7-10 and 7-11). The superolateral surface of the frontal lobe is divided by three sulci into four gyri. The **precentral sulcus** runs parallel to the central sulcus and the **precentral gyrus** lies between them

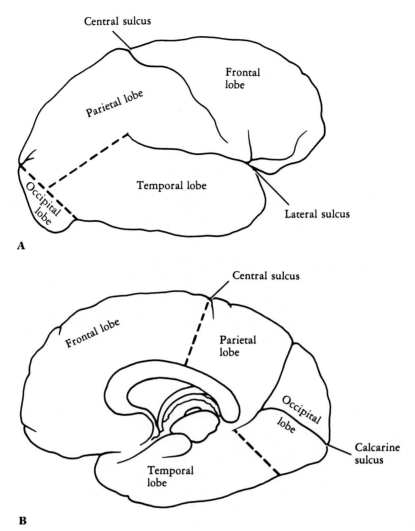

Figure 7–11 **A**. Lateral view of the right cerebral hemisphere showing the lobes. **B**. Medial view of the right cerebral hemisphere showing the lobes. Note that the dashed lines indicate the approximate position of the boundaries where there are no sulci.

(Figs. 7-7 and 7-10). Extending anteriorly from the precentral sulcus are the **superior** and **inferior frontal sulci**. The **superior frontal gyrus** lies superior to the superior frontal sulcus, the **middle frontal gyrus** lies between the superior and inferior frontal sulci, and the **inferior frontal gyrus** lies inferior to the inferior frontal sulcus (Figs. 7-7 and 7-10). The inferior frontal gyrus is invaded by the anterior and ascending rami of the lateral sulcus.

The **parietal lobe** occupies the area posterior to the central sulcus and superior to the lateral sulcus; it extends posteriorly as far as the parieto-occipital sulcus (Figs. 7-7, 7-10, and 7-11). The lateral surface of the parietal lobe is divided by two sulci into three gyri. The postcentral sulcus runs parallel to the central sulcus and the postcentral gyrus lies between them. Running posteriorly from the middle of the postcentral sulcus is the **intraparietal sulcus** (Figs. 7-7 and 7-10). The intraparietal sulcus has superior to it the **superior parietal lobule** (gyrus) and inferior to it the **inferior parietal lobule** (gyrus).

The **temporal lobe** occupies the area inferior to the lateral sulcus (Figs. 7-7, 7-10, and 7-11). The lateral surface of the temporal lobe is divided into three gyri by two sulci. The **superior** and **middle temporal sulci** run parallel to the posterior ramus of the lateral sulcus, and divide the temporal lobe into the **superior**, **middle**, and **inferior temporal gyri**; the inferior temporal gyrus is continued onto the inferior surface of the hemisphere (Figs. 7-7 and 7-10).

The **occipital lobe** occupies the small area behind the parieto-occipital sulcus (Figs. 7-7, 7-10, and 7-11).

Medial and Inferior Surfaces of the Hemisphere

The lobes of the cerebral hemisphere are not clearly defined on the medial and inferior surfaces. However, there are many important areas that should be recognized. The **corpus callosum**, which is the largest commissure of the

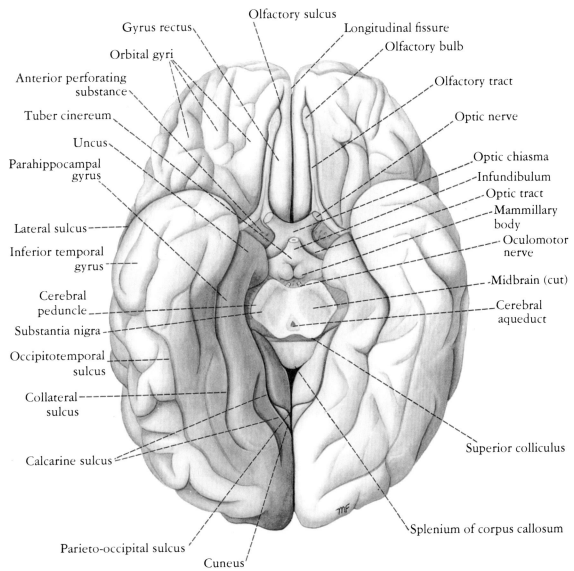

Figure 7–12 Inferior view of the brain; the medulla oblongata, the pons, and the cerebellum have been removed.

brain, forms a striking feature on this surface (Figs. 7-8 and 7-10). The **cingulate gyrus** begins beneath the anterior end of the corpus callosum and continues above the corpus callosum until it reaches its posterior end (Figs. 7-8 and 7-10). The gyrus is separated from the corpus callosum by the **callosal sulcus**. The cingulate gyrus is separated from the superior frontal gyrus by the **cingulate sulcus** (Fig. 7-10).

The **paracentral lobule** is the area of the cerebral cortex that surrounds the indentation produced by the central sulcus on the superior border (Figs. 7-8 and 7-10). The anterior part of this lobule is a continuation of the precentral gyrus on the superior lateral surface, and the posterior part of the lobule is a continuation of the postcentral gyrus.

The **precuneus** (Figs. 7-8 and 7-10) is an area of cortex bounded anteriorly by the upturned posterior end of the cingulate sulcus and posteriorly by the parieto-occipital sulcus.

The **cuneus** (Figs. 7-8 and 7-10) is a triangular area of cortex bounded above by the parieto-occipital sulcus, infe-

riorly by the calcarine sulcus, and posteriorly by the superior medial margin.

The **collateral sulcus** is situated on the inferior surface of the hemisphere (Fig. 7-12 and Fig. 7-8). This runs anteriorly below the calcarine sulcus. Between the collateral sulcus and the **calcarine sulcus** is the **lingual gyrus**. Anterior to the lingual gyrus is the **parahippocampal gyrus**; the latter terminates in front as the hooklike **uncus** (Fig. 7-12).

The **medial occipitotemporal gyrus** extends from the occipital pole to the temporal pole (Fig. 7-12). It is bounded medially by the **collateral** and **rhinal sulci** and laterally by the **occipitotemporal sulcus**. The **occipitotemporal gyrus** lies lateral to the sulcus and is continuous with the inferior temporal gyrus (Fig. 7-12).

On the inferior surface of the frontal lobe, the olfactory bulb and tract overlie a sulcus called the **olfactory sulcus** (Fig. 7-12). Medial to the olfactory sulcus is the **gyrus rectus** and lateral to the sulcus are a number of **orbital gyri**.

INTERNAL STRUCTURE OF THE CEREBRAL HEMISPHERES

The cerebral hemispheres are covered with a layer of gray matter, the cerebral cortex, the structure and function of which are dealt with in Chapter 15. Located in the interior of the cerebral hemispheres are the **lateral ventricles**, masses of gray matter, the **basal nuclei**, and nerve fibers. The nerve fibers are embedded in neuroglia and constitute the **white matter** (Fig. 7-13).

Lateral Ventricles

There are two lateral ventricles and one is present in each cerebral hemisphere (Figs. 7-13 and 7-14). Each ventricle is a roughly C-shaped cavity lined with ependyma and filled with cerebrospinal fluid. The lateral ventricle may be divided into a **body**, which occupies the parietal lobe, and from which **anterior**, **posterior**, and **inferior horns** extend into the frontal, occipital, and temporal lobes, respec-

tively. The lateral ventricle communicates with the cavity of the third ventricle through the **interventricular foramen** (Figs. 7-8 and 7-14). This opening, which lies in the anterior part of the medial wall of the lateral ventricle, is bounded anteriorly by the anterior column of the fornix and posteriorly by the anterior end of the thalamus.

Basal Nuclei (Basal Ganglia)

The term **basal nuclei** is applied to a collection of masses of gray matter situated within each cerebral hemisphere. They are the corpus striatum, the amygdaloid nucleus, and the claustrum.

CORPUS STRIATUM

The corpus striatum is situated lateral to the thalamus. It is almost completely divided by a band of nerve fibers, the **internal capsule**, into the caudate nucleus and the lentiform nucleus (see Figs. 7-13 and 7-18).

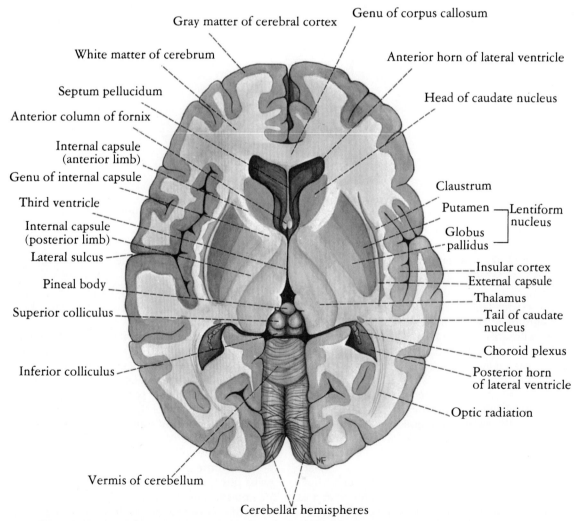

Figure 7–13 Horizontal section of the cerebrum as seen from above, showing the relationship between the lentiform nucleus, the caudate nucleus, the thalamus, and the internal capsule.

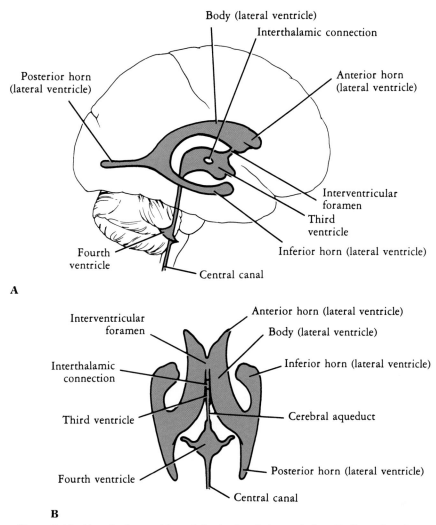

Figure 7–14 Ventricular cavities of the brain. **A**. Lateral view. **B**. Superior view.

The **caudate nucleus**, a large C-shaped mass of gray matter that is closely related to the lateral ventricle, lies lateral to the thalamus (Fig. 7-15). The lateral surface of the nucleus is related to the internal capsule, which separates it from the lentiform nucleus.

The **lentiform nucleus** is a wedge-shaped mass of gray matter whose broad convex base is directed laterally and its blade medially (Figs. 7-13 and 7-15). It is buried deep in the white matter of the cerebral hemisphere and is related medially to the internal capsule, which separates it from the caudate nucleus and the thalamus. The lentiform nucleus is related laterally to a thin sheet of white matter, the **external capsule** (Fig. 7-13), that separates it from a thin sheet of gray matter, called the **claustrum** (Fig. 7-13). The claustrum, in turn, separates the external capsule from the subcortical white matter of the insula. Inferiorly at its anterior end, the lentiform nucleus is continuous with the caudate nucleus.

The detailed structure and connections of the corpus striatum are considered in Chapter 10. Briefly, it may be stated that the corpus striatum receives afferent fibers from different areas of the cerebral cortex, the thalamus, subthalamus, and brainstem. Efferent fibers then travel back to the same areas of the nervous system. The function of the corpus striatum is concerned with muscular movement, which is accomplished by controlling the cerebral cortex rather than through direct descending pathways to the brainstem and spinal cord.

AMYGDALOID NUCLEUS

The amygdaloid nucleus is situated in the temporal lobe close to the uncus (Fig. 7-15). The amygdaloid nucleus is considered part of the limbic system and is described in Chapter 9, p. 308.

CLAUSTRUM

The claustrum is a thin sheet of gray matter that is separated from the lateral surface of the lentiform nucleus by the **external capsule** (Fig. 7-13). Lateral to the claustrum is the

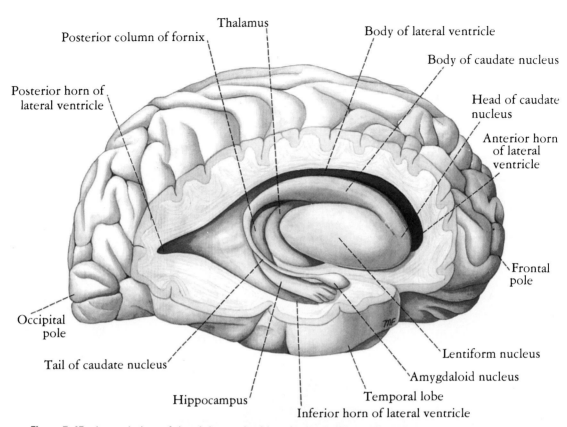

Posterior column of fornix · Thalamus · Body of lateral ventricle

Posterior horn of lateral ventricle · Body of caudate nucleus

Head of caudate nucleus

Anterior horn of lateral ventricle

Frontal pole

Occipital pole

Tail of caudate nucleus

Hippocampus · Inferior horn of lateral ventricle · Temporal lobe · Amygdaloid nucleus · Lentiform nucleus

Figure 7–15 Lateral view of the right cerebral hemisphere dissected to show the position of the lentiform nucleus, the caudate nucleus, the thalamus, and the hippocampus.

subcortical white matter of the insula. The function of the claustrum is unknown.

White Matter of the Cerebral Hemispheres

The white matter is composed of myelinated nerve fibers of different diameters supported by neuroglia. The nerve fibers may be classified into three groups according to their connections: (1) commissural fibers, (2) association fibers, and (3) projection fibers.

COMMISSURE FIBERS

These fibers essentially connect corresponding regions of the two hemispheres. They are as follows: the corpus callosum, the anterior commissure, the posterior commissure, the fornix, and the habenular commissure.

The **corpus callosum**, the largest commissure of the brain, connects the two cerebral hemispheres (Figs. 7-8 and 7-16). It lies at the bottom of the longitudinal fissure. For purposes of description, it is divided into the rostrum, the genu, the body, and the splenium.

The **rostrum** is the thin part of the anterior end of the corpus callosum, which is prolonged posteriorly to be

continuous with the upper end of the lamina terminalis (Fig. 7-8).

The **genu** is the curved anterior end of the corpus callosum that bends inferiorly in front of the septum pellucidum (Figs. 7-8 and 7-16).

The **body** of the corpus callosum arches posteriorly and ends as the thickened posterior portion called the **splenium** (Fig. 7-16).

Traced laterally, the fibers of the genu curve forward into the frontal lobes and form the **forceps minor** (Fig. 7-16). The fibers of the body extend laterally as the **radiation of the corpus callosum** (Fig. 7-16). They intersect with bundles of association and projection fibers as they pass to the cerebral cortex. Some of the fibers form the roof and lateral wall of the posterior horn of the lateral ventricle and the lateral wall of the inferior horn of the lateral ventricle; these fibers are referred to as the **tapetum**. Traced laterally, the fibers in the splenium arch backward into the occipital lobe and form the **forceps major** (Fig. 7-16).

The **anterior commissure** is a small bundle of nerve fibers that cross the midline in the **lamina terminalis** (Fig. 7-8). When traced laterally, a smaller or anterior bundle curves forward on each side toward the anterior perforated substance and the olfactory tract. A larger bundle curves posteriorly on each side and grooves the inferior surface of the lentiform nucleus to reach the temporal lobes.

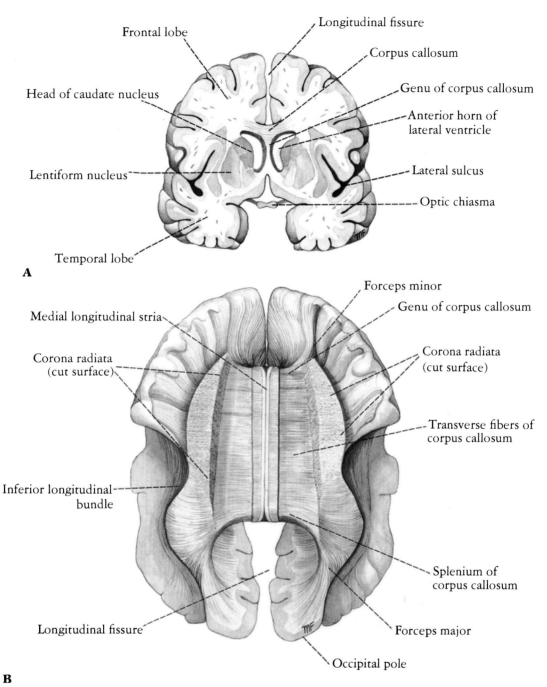

Figure 7–16 **A**. Coronal section of the brain passing through the anterior horn of the lateral ventricle and the optic chiasma. **B**. Superior view of the brain dissected to show the fibers of the corpus callosum and the corona radiata.

The **posterior commissure** is a bundle of nerve fibers that cross the midline immediately above the opening of the cerebral aqueduct into the third ventricle (Fig. 7-3); it is related to the inferior part of the stalk of the pineal gland. Various collections of nerve cells are situated along its length. The destinations and functional significance of many of the nerve fibers are not known. However, the fibers from the pretectal nuclei involved in the pupillary

light reflex are believed to cross in this commissure on their way to the parasympathetic part of the oculomotor nuclei.

The **fornix** is composed of myelinated nerve fibers and constitutes the efferent system of the hippocampus that passes to the mammillary bodies of the hypothalamus. The nerve fibers first form the **alveus** (Fig. 9-5), which is a thin layer of white matter covering the ventricular surface of the

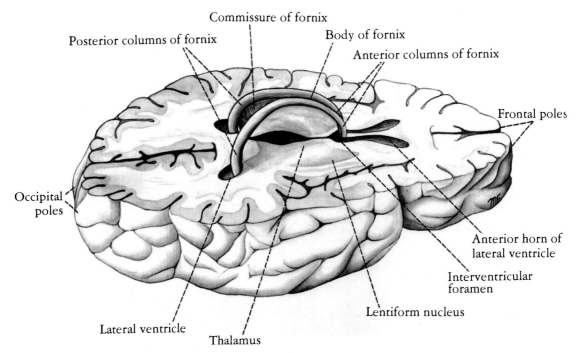

Posterior columns of fornix

Commissure of fornix

Body of fornix

Anterior columns of fornix

Frontal poles

Occipital poles

Anterior horn of lateral ventricle

Interventricular foramen

Lentiform nucleus

Lateral ventricle

Thalamus

Figure 7–17 Horizontal section of the brain leaving the fornix in position.

hippocampus, and then converge to form the **fimbria**. The fimbriae of the two sides increase in thickness and, on reaching the posterior end of the hippocampus, they arch forward above the thalamus and below the corpus callosum to form the **posterior columns of the fornix**. The two columns then come together in the midline to form the **body of the fornix** (Fig. 7-17). A more detailed description of the fornix is given on page 263. The **commissure of the fornix** consists of transverse fibers that cross the midline from one column to another just before the formation of the body of the fornix. The function of the commissure of the fornix is to connect the hippocampal formations of the two sides.

The **habenular commissure** is a small bundle of nerve fibers that cross the midline in the superior part of the root of the pineal stalk (Fig. 7-3). The commissure is associated with the **habenular nuclei**, which are situated on either side of the midline in this region. The habenular nuclei receive many afferents from the amygdaloid nuclei and the hippocampus. These afferent fibers pass to the habenular nuclei in the **stria medullaris thalami**. Some of the fibers cross the midline to reach the contralateral nucleus through the habenular commissure. The function of the habenular nuclei and its connections in humans is unknown.

ASSOCIATION FIBERS

These nerve fibers essentially connect various cortical regions within the same hemisphere and may be divided into short and long groups (Fig. 7-19). The **short association fibers** lie immediately beneath the cortex and connect adjacent gyri; these fibers run transversely to the long axis of

the sulci (Fig. 7-19). The **long association fibers** are collected into named bundles that can be dissected in a formalin-hardened brain. The **uncinate fasciculus** connects the first motor speech area and the gyri on the inferior surface of the frontal lobe with the cortex of the pole of the temporal lobe. The **cingulum** is a long, curved fasciculus lying within the white matter of the cingulate gyrus (Fig. 7-8). It connects the frontal and parietal lobes with parahippocampal and adjacent temporal cortical regions. The **superior longitudinal fasciculus** is the largest bundle of nerve fibers. It connects the anterior part of the frontal lobe to the occipital and temporal lobes. The **inferior longitudinal fasciculus** runs anteriorly from the occipital lobe, passing lateral to the optic radiation, and is distributed to the temporal lobe. The **fronto-occipital fasciculus** connects the frontal lobe to the occipital and temporal lobes. It is situated deep within the cerebral hemisphere and is related to the lateral border of the caudate nucleus.

PROJECTION FIBERS

Afferent and efferent nerve fibers passing to and from the brainstem to the entire cerebral cortex must travel between large nuclear masses of gray matter within the cerebral hemisphere. At the upper part of the brainstem these fibers form a compact band known as the **internal capsule**, which is flanked medially by the caudate nucleus and the thalamus, and laterally by the lentiform nucleus (Fig. 7-13). Because of the wedge shape of the lentiform nucleus, as seen on horizontal section, the internal capsule is bent to form an **anterior limb** and a **posterior limb**, which are continuous with each other at the **genu** (Figs. 7-18 and

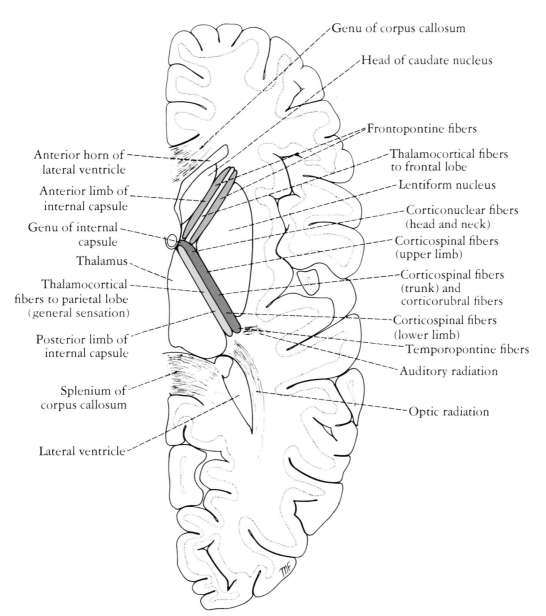

Figure 7–18 Horizontal section of the right cerebral hemisphere showing the relationships and different parts of the internal capsule.

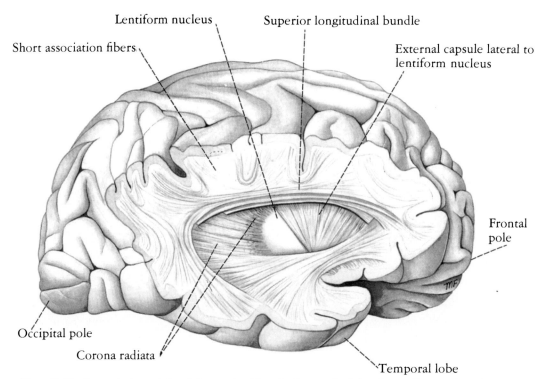

Lentiform nucleus

Superior longitudinal bundle

Short association fibers

External capsule lateral to
lentiform nucleus

Frontal
pole

Occipital pole

Corona radiata

Temporal lobe

Figure 7–19   Lateral view of the right cerebral hemisphere, which has been dissected to show
some of the principal association fibers.

7-20). Once the nerve fibers have emerged superiorly from
between the nuclear masses, they radiate in all directions to
the cerebral cortex. These radiating projection fibers are
known as the **corona radiata** (Fig. 7-20). Most of the projection fibers lie medial to the association fibers, but they intersect the commissural fibers of the corpus callosum and
the anterior commissure. The nerve fibers lying within the
most posterior part of the posterior limb of the internal capsule radiate toward the calcarine sulcus and are known as
the **optic radiation** (Fig. 7-18). The detailed arrangement of
the fibers within the internal capsule is shown in Figure 7-18.

Septum Pellucidum

The septum pellucidum is a thin vertical sheet of nervous
tissue consisting of white and gray matter covered on either
side by ependyma (Figs. 7-8 and 7-13). It stretches between
the fornix and the corpus callosum. Anteriorly, it occupies
the interval between the body of the corpus callosum and
the rostrum. It is essentially a double membrane with a
closed, slitlike cavity between the membranes. The septum
pellucidum forms a partition between the anterior horns of
the lateral ventricles.

Tela Choroidea

The tela choroidea is a two-layered fold of pia mater. It is
situated between the fornix superiorly and the roof of the
third ventricle and the upper surfaces of the two thalami
inferiorly. When seen from above, the anterior end is situated at the interventricular foramina (Fig. 16-6). Its lateral
edges are irregular and project laterally into the body of
the lateral ventricles. Here they are covered by ependyma
and form the choroid plexuses of the lateral ventricle.
Posteriorly, the lateral edges continue into the inferior
horn of the lateral ventricle and are covered with
ependyma so that the choroid plexus projects through the
choroidal fissure.

On either side of the midline the tela choroidea projects
down through the roof of the third ventricle to form the
choroid plexuses of the third ventricle.

The blood supply of the tela choroidea and, therefore,
also the choroid plexuses of the third and lateral ventricles
are derived from the **choroidal branches of the internal
carotid** and **basilar arteries**. The venous blood drains into
the **internal cerebral veins**, which unite to form the **great
cerebral vein**. The great cerebral vein joins the **inferior
sagittal sinus** to form the **straight sinus**.

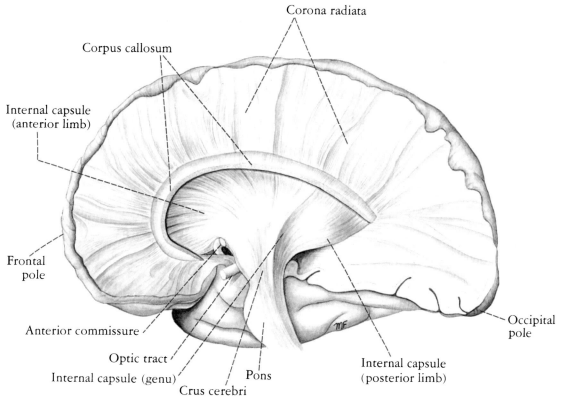

Corona radiata

Corpus callosum

Internal capsule
(anterior limb)

Frontal
pole

Anterior commissure

Optic tract

Internal capsule (genu)

Crus cerebri

Pons

Internal capsule
(posterior limb)

Occipital
pole

Figure 7–20 Medial view of the right cerebral hemisphere, which has been dissected to show the internal capsule and the corona radiata. The thalamus has been removed. Note the interdigitation of the horizontally running fibers of the corpus callosum and the vertical fibers of the corona radiata.

CLINICAL NOTES

LESIONS OF THE THALAMUS

These lesions usually result from thrombosis or hemorrhage of one of the arteries that supply the thalamus. Since the thalamus is concerned with receiving sensory impulses from the opposite side of the body, the disability resulting from a lesion within it will be confined to the contralateral side of the body. There may be a major impairment of all forms of sensation, which could include light touch, tactile localization and discrimination, and loss of appreciation of joint movements.

Subthalamic Lesions

The subthalamus should be regarded as one of the extrapyramidal motor nuclei and has a large connection with the globus pallidus. Lesions of the subthalamus result in sudden, forceful involuntary movements in a contralateral extremity. The movements may be jerky (choreiform) or violent (ballistic).

Pineal Gland

The pineal gland consists essentially of pinealocytes and glial cells supported by a connective tissue framework. As the result of regressive changes that occur with age, calcareous concretions accumulate within the glial cells and connective tissue of the gland. These deposits are useful to the radiologist, since they serve as a landmark and assist in determining whether the pineal gland has been displaced laterally by a space-occupying lesion within the skull.

The functions of the pineal gland are mainly inhibitory and have been shown to influence the pituitary gland, the islets of Langerhans, the parathyroids, the adrenals, and the gonads.

Clinical observation of patients with pineal tumors or tumors of neighboring areas of nervous tissue that may press upon the pineal gland, has shown severe alteration of reproductive function.

Hypothalamus

This is an area of the nervous system that is of great functional importance. Not only does it control emotional states, but it also assists in the regulation of fat, carbohydrate, and water metabolism. Among its many other activities, it influences body temperature, genital functions, sleep, and food intake. The pituitary and the hypothalamus constitute a closely integrated unit and the hypothalamus plays a role in the release of pituitary hormones.

Syndromes of the Hypothalamus

Lesions of the hypothalamus may result from infection, trauma, or vascular disorders. Tumors, such as a **craniopharyngioma** or **chromophobe adenoma of the pituitary** and **pineal tumors**, may interfere with the function of the hypothalamus. The most common abnormalities include **genital hypoplasia** or **atrophy**, **diabetes insipidus**, **obesity**, **disturbances of sleep**, **irregular pyrexia**, and **emaciation**. Some of these disorders may occur together, for example, in the **adiposogenital dystrophy syndrome**.

Cerebral Cortex, Sulci, and Lobes of the Cerebral Hemisphere

The cerebral cortex is composed of gray matter. Only about one-third lies on the exposed convexity of the gyri; the remaining two-thirds form the walls of the sulci. Moreover, different areas of the cortex have different functions, and the anatomical division of the cortex into lobes and gyri by sulci enables the physician to localize loss of function or accurately place a brain lesion. For example, focal lesions of the precentral gyrus will produce contralateral hemiparesis, while lesions of the postcentral gyrus will result in contralateral hemisensory loss. More widespread lesions of the frontal lobe might cause symptoms and signs indicative of loss of attention span or change in social behavior. Widespread degeneration of the cerebral cortex gives rise to symptoms of dementia.

Lateral Ventricles

Each lateral ventricle contains about 7 to 10 ml of cerebrospinal fluid. This fluid is produced in the choroid plexus of the lateral ventricle and normally drains into the third ventricle through the interventricular foramen (foramen of Monro). Blockage of the foramen by a cerebral tumor would result in distention of the ventricle, thus producing a type of **hydrocephalus**.

The choroid plexus of the lateral ventricle is continuous with that of the third ventricle through the interventricular foramen. The choroid plexus is largest where the body and posterior and inferior horns join, and it is here where it may become calcified with age. It is important that this **calcification of the choroid plexus**, as seen on radiographs, is not confused with that of the pineal gland.

In the past, the size and shape of the lateral ventricle were investigated clinically by **pneumoencephalography** (Figs. 7-21 through 7-24). In this procedure, small amounts of air were introduced into the subarachnoid space by lumbar puncture with the patient in the sitting position. If the patient already had a raised intracranial pressure, this method was dangerous (see p. 18), and air or radiopaque fluid was injected directly into the lateral ventricles through a burr hole in the skull (this procedure was referred to as **ventriculography**). This procedure has now been replaced by CT and MRI (Figs. 7-25 through 7-28).

Basal Nuclei

The **basal nuclei**, in this discussion, refers to the masses of gray matter that are deeply placed within the cerebrum. They include the caudate nucleus, the lentiform nucleus, the amygdaloid nucleus, and the claustrum.

Because of the close relationship that exists between these nuclei and the internal capsule, tumors of the caudate or lentiform nuclei may cause severe motor or sensory symptoms on the opposite side of the body. Tumors pressing on the anterior two-thirds of the posterior limb of the internal capsule will cause progressive spastic hemiplegia, while more posteriorly situated tumors will produce impairment of sensation on the opposite side.

Disorders of function of the basal nuclei are considered after the connections of these nuclei are discussed in Chapter 10.

Commissures of the Cerebrum

The major commissure is the large corpus callosum. The majority of the fibers within the corpus callosum interconnect symmetrical areas of the cerebral cortex. Because it transfers information from one hemisphere to another, the corpus callosum is essential for learned discrimination, sensory experience, and memory.

Occasionally the corpus callosum fails to develop and in these individuals no definite signs or symptoms appear. Should the corpus callosum be destroyed by disease in later life, however, each hemisphere becomes isolated and the patient responds as if he or she has two separate brains. The patient's general intelligence and behavior appear normal, since over the years both hemispheres have been trained to respond to different situations. If a pencil is placed in the patient's right hand (with the eyes closed) he or she will recognize the object by touch and be able to describe it. If the pencil is placed in the left hand, the tactile information will pass to the right postcentral gyrus. This information will not be able to travel through the corpus callosum to the speech area in the left hemisphere and, therefore, the patient will be unable to describe the object in his or her left hand.

Section of the corpus callosum has been attempted surgically, with some success, in order to prevent the spread of seizures from one hemisphere to the other.

Lesions of the Internal Capsule

The internal capsule is an important compact band of white matter. It is composed of ascending and descend-

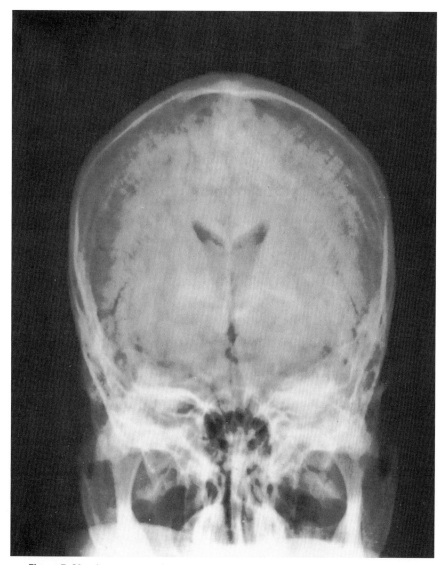

Figure 7–21   Anteroposterior pneumoencephalogram of a 28-year-old man.

ing nerve fibers that connect the cerebral cortex to the brainstem and spinal cord. The internal capsule is flanked medially by the caudate nucleus and thalamus and laterally by the lentiform nucleus. The arrangement of the nerve fibers within the internal capsule is shown in Figure 7-18.

The internal capsule is frequently involved in vascular disorders of the brain. The most common cause of arterial hemorrhage is atheromatous degeneration in an artery in a patient with high blood pressure. Because of the high concentration of important nerve fibers within the internal capsule, even a small hemorrhage can cause widespread effects on the contralateral side of the body. Not only is the immediate neural tissue destroyed by the blood, which later clots, but also neighboring nerve fibers may be compressed or be edematous.

Alzheimer's Disease

Alzheimer's disease is a degenerative disease of the brain occurring in middle to late life, but an early form of the disease is now well recognized. The disease affects more than 4 million people in the United States, resulting in over 100,000 deaths per year. The risk of the disease rises sharply with advancing years.

The cause of Alzheimer's disease is unknown but there is evidence of a genetic predisposition. Several abnormal genes have been found, each of which leads to a similar clinical and pathological syndrome, with only variations in the age of onset and the rate of progression to suggest that there are differences in pathogenetic mechanisms. Some cases of familial Alzheimer's disease, for example, have been shown to have mutations in several genes (App, presenilin 1, presenilin 2).

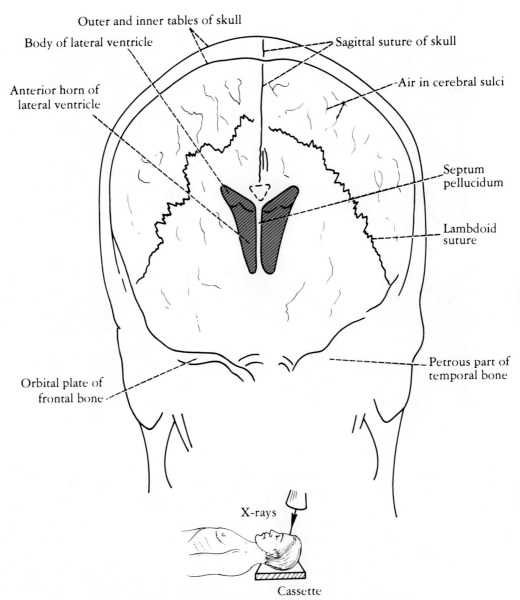

Figure 7–22 Explanation of the radiograph seen in Figure 7-21. Note the position of the x-ray gun relative to the head and the film cassette.

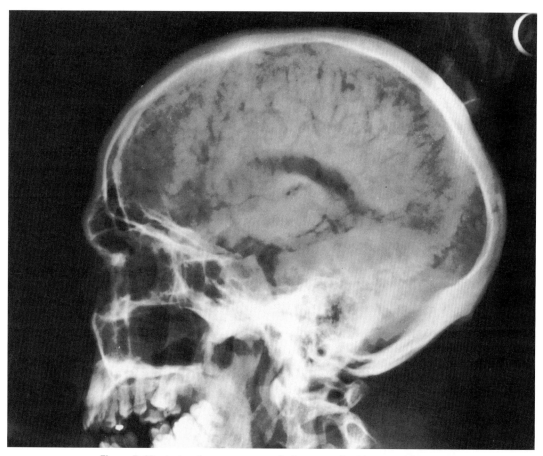

Figure 7–23 Lateral pneumoencephalogram of a 28-year-old man.

Early memory loss, a disintegration of personality, complete disorientation, deterioration in speech, and restlessness are common signs. In the late stages the patient may become mute, incontinent, and bedridden and usually dies of some other disease.

Microscopically, changes eventually occur throughout the cerebral cortex but to begin with certain regions of the brain are selectively involved. The early sites include the hippocampus, the entorrhinal cortex, and the associated areas of the cerebral cortex. Many so-called senile plaques are found in the atrophic cortex. The plaques result from the accumulation of several proteins around deposits of Beta amyloid. In the center of each plaque is an extracellular collection of degenerating nervous tissue; surrounding the core is a rim of large abnormal neuronal processes, probably presynaptic terminals, filled with an excess of intracellular neurofibrils that are tangled and twisted, forming neurofibrillary tangles. The neurofibrillary tangles are aggregations of the microtubular protein tau, which is hyperphosphorylated.

There is a marked loss of choline acetyltransferase, the biosynthetic enzyme for acetylcholine, in the areas of the cortex in which the senile plaques occur. This is thought to be due to loss of the ascending projection fibers rather than a loss of cortical cells. As these cellular changes occur, the affected neurons die.

As yet, there is no clinical test for making the definite diagnosis of Alzheimer's disease. Reliance is placed on taking a careful history, and carrying out numerous neurological, and psychiatric examinations spaced out over time. In this way other causes of dementia can be excluded. Alterations in the levels of amyloid peptides or tau in the serum or cerebrospinal fluid may be helpful. The use of CT scans or MRIs are also used and abnormalities in the medial part of the temporal lobe occur in this disease. In advanced cases, a thin, atrophied cerebral cortex and dilated lateral ventricles may be found. The recent use of positron emission tomography (PET) shows evidence of diminished cortical metabolism (Fig. 7-29).

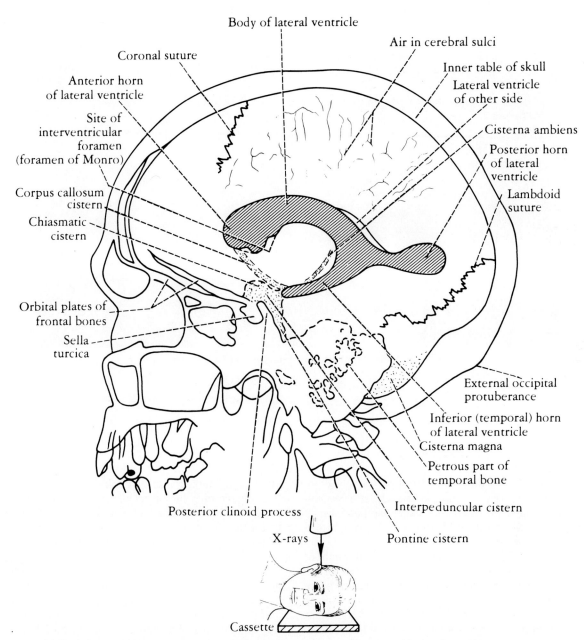

Figure 7–24   Explanation of the radiograph seen in Figure 7-23. Note the position of the x-ray gun relative to the head and the film cassette.

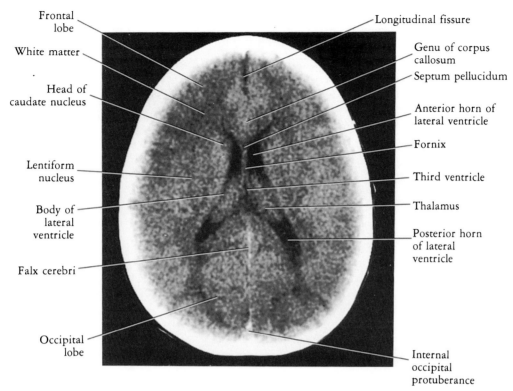

Frontal lobe

White matter

Head of caudate nucleus

Lentiform nucleus

Body of lateral ventricle

Falx cerebri

Occipital lobe

Longitudinal fissure

Genu of corpus callosum

Septum pellucidum

Anterior horn of lateral ventricle

Fornix

Third ventricle

Thalamus

Posterior horn of lateral ventricle

Internal occipital protuberance

Figure 7–25 Horizontal (axial) CT scan of the brain.

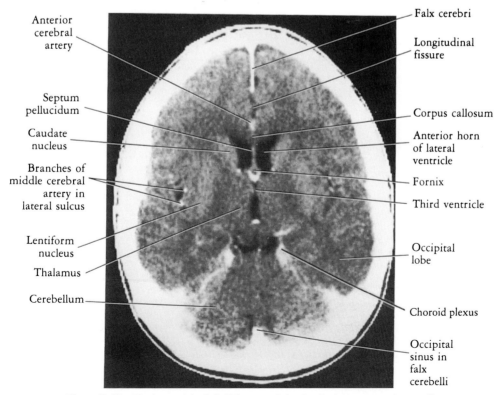

Anterior cerebral artery

Septum pellucidum

Caudate nucleus

Branches of middle cerebral artery in lateral sulcus

Lentiform nucleus

Thalamus

Cerebellum

Falx cerebri

Longitudinal fissure

Corpus callosum

Anterior horn of lateral ventricle

Fornix

Third ventricle

Occipital lobe

Choroid plexus

Occipital sinus in falx cerebelli

Figure 7–26 Horizontal (axial) CT scan of the brain (contrast-enhanced).

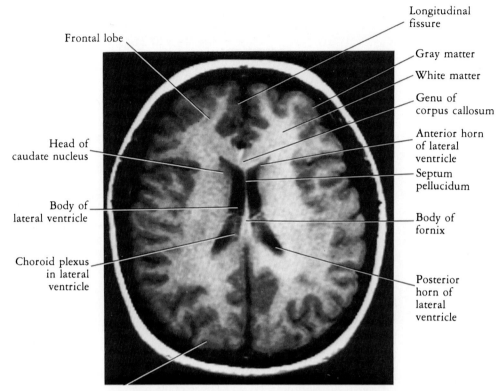

Longitudinal fissure

Gray matter

White matter

Genu of corpus callosum

Anterior horn of lateral ventricle

Septum pellucidum

Body of fornix

Posterior horn of lateral ventricle

Frontal lobe

Head of caudate nucleus

Body of lateral ventricle

Choroid plexus in lateral ventricle

Figure 7–27 Horizontal (axial) MRI of the brain.

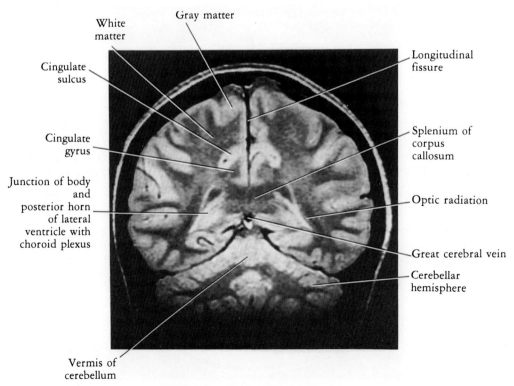

Gray matter

White matter

Cingulate sulcus

Cingulate gyrus

Junction of body and posterior horn of lateral ventricle with choroid plexus

Longitudinal fissure

Splenium of corpus callosum

Optic radiation

Great cerebral vein

Cerebellar hemisphere

Vermis of cerebellum

Figure 7–28 Coronal MRI of the brain.

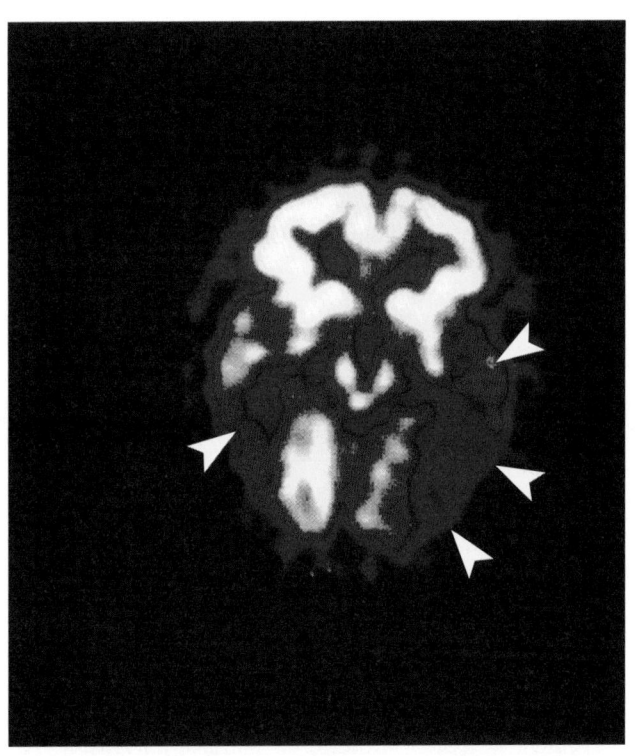

Figure 7–29 Axial (horizontal) PET scan of a male patient with Alzheimer's disease, showing defects (arrowheads) in metabolism in the bitemporoparietal regions of the cerebral cortex, following the injection of 18-fluorodeoxyglucose. The yellow areas indicate regions of high metabolic activity. (Courtesy Dr. Holley Dey.)

Clinical Problem Solving

1. A 53-year-old woman was admitted to an emergency department after she had collapsed in the street. Apart from being confused and disoriented, she exhibited violent, uncoordinated movements of her right arm and right leg and slight spontaneous movements on the right side of her face. The physician was able to ascertain from a friend that the patient had been perfectly fit that morning and had no previous history of this condition. On examination, the involuntary movements of the right limbs were mainly confined to the muscles of the proximal part of the limbs. One week later, the patient died of cardiac failure. What is the medical term used to describe this condition? Which area of the brain is likely to be involved in the production of this condition?

2. A 64-year-old man was admitted to a hospital on the suspicion that he had a cerebral tumor. One of the investigations asked for by the physician was a simple anteroposterior radiograph and lateral radiograph of the head. Using your knowledge of neuroanatomy, name the structure that would assist the radiologist in this case in determining whether lateral displacement of the brain had occurred within the skull.

3. A 12-year-old boy was seen by a pediatrician because his parents were concerned about his excessive weight and lack of development of the external genitalia. On examination, the child was seen to be tall for his age and very obese. The excessive fat was concentrated especially in the lower part of the anterior abdominal wall and the proximal parts of the limbs. His penis and testes were small. Is it possible that disease of the diencephalon might account for this condition?

4. A neurosurgeon explained to her residents that she would attempt to remove the glioma located in the right middle frontal gyrus by turning back a flap of the scalp and removing a rectangular piece of the overlying skull. Where exactly is the right middle frontal gyrus in the brain? What are the names of the sulci that lie above and below this gyrus? Which skull bone overlays this gyrus?

5. While performing an autopsy, a pathologist had great difficulty in finding the central sulcus in each cerebral hemisphere. Since finding this sulcus is the key to localizing many other sulci and gyri, what landmarks would you use to identify the central sulcus? Are the sulci and gyri in the two hemispheres similar in size and shape? Are there individual variations in the arrangement of the sulci and gyri?

6. A fourth-year medical student was shown coronal and horizontal MRIs of the brain and was asked to comment

on his observations. The patient was a 55-year-old man. The student responded by saying that the left lateral ventricle was larger than normal and that there was an area of low signal intensity close to the left interventricular foramen suggesting the presence of a brain tumor. On looking at a standard lateral radiograph of the skull and brain, he noted a small area of "calcification" situated in the region of the posterior part of the left ventricle. Using your knowledge of neuroanatomy, describe the location of the lateral ventricle in the brain. What are the different parts of the lateral ventricle? Where is the cerebrospinal fluid in the lateral ventricle produced and what does it normally drain into? What is responsible for the calcification seen in the left lateral ventricle in this patient?

7. A medical student, while performing an autopsy, found that the patient had no corpus callosum. On consulting the patient's clinical notes she was surprised to find no reference to a neurological disorder. Are you surprised that this patient had no recorded neurological signs and symptoms?

Answers to Clinical Problem Solving

1. This woman exhibited continuous uncoordinated activity of the proximal musculature of the right arm and right leg, resulting in the limbs being flung violently about. The muscles of the right side of the face were also slightly affected. This condition is known as *hemiballismus.* It was caused by hemorrhage into the left subthalamic nucleus.

2. During the third decade of life, calcareous concretions appear in the neuroglia and connective tissue of the pineal gland. This provides a useful midline landmark to the radiologist. A lateral displacement of such a landmark would indicate the presence of an intracranial mass. In this patient, the pineal gland shadow was in the midline and all the other investigations, including CT, showed no evidence of a cerebral tumor.

3. Yes. Adiposity alone or associated with genital dystrophy can occur with disease of the hypothalamus.

4. The right middle frontal gyrus is located on the lateral surface of the frontal lobe of the right cerebral hemisphere. It is bounded superiorly and inferiorly by the superior and inferior frontal sulci, respectively. The right middle frontal gyrus is overlaid by the frontal bone of the skull.

5. The important central sulcus is large and runs downward and forward across the lateral aspect of each hemisphere. Superiorly, it indents the superior medial border of the hemisphere about 1 cm behind the midpoint; it lies between two parallel gyri. It is the only sulcus of any length that indents the superior medial border. The arrangement of the sulci and gyri is very similar on both sides of the brain. There are, however, great individual variations in the details of their arrangement.

6. The lateral ventricle is a C-shaped cavity situated within each cerebral hemisphere. The lateral ventricle wraps itself around the thalamus, the lentiform nucleus, and the caudate nucleus. It is divided into a body that occupies the parietal lobe, an anterior horn that extends into the frontal lobe, a posterior horn that extends into the occipital lobe, and an inferior horn that runs forward and inferiorly into the temporal lobe. The cerebrospinal fluid is produced in the choroid plexus of the lateral ventricle and drains through the small interventricular foramen into the third ventricle. In later life, the choroid plexus, especially in its posterior part, sometimes shows calcified deposits, which are occasionally revealed on radiographs, as in this case. This patient later was found to have a cerebral tumor that was compressing the left interventricular foramen, hence the enlarged left ventricle.

7. No. The corpus callosum occasionally fails to develop and in those patients no definite neurological signs and symptoms appear. If, however, the corpus callosum is divided during a surgical procedure in the adult, the loss of interconnections between the two hemispheres becomes apparent (see p. 268).

Review Questions

Directions: Each of the numbered items in this section is followed by answers that are positively phrased. Select the ONE lettered answer that is an EXCEPTION.

1. The following statements concerning the diencephalon are correct **except:**
   (a) It extends anteriorly as far as the interventricular foramen.
   (b) It is bounded laterally by the internal capsule.
   (c) The thalamus is located in the lateral wall of the third ventricle.
   (d) The epithalamus is formed by the cranial end of the substantia nigra and the red nuclei.
   (e) It extends posteriorly as far as the cerebral aqueduct.

2. The following statements concerning the pineal gland are correct **except:**
   (a) It produces a secretion that is opaque to x-rays.
   (b) It contains high concentrations of melatonin.
   (c) Melatonin inhibits the release of the gonadotrophic hormone from the anterior lobe of the pituitary gland.

(d) There is an increase in the production of secretions of the pineal gland during darkness.

(e) The pinealocytes are stimulated by the sympathetic nerve endings.

3. The following statements concerning the thalamus are correct **except:**

(a) It is the largest part of the diencephalon and serves as a relay station to all the main sensory tracts (except the olfactory pathway).

(b) It is separated from the lentiform nucleus by the internal capsule.

(c) It forms the anterior boundary of the interventricular foramen.

(d) It may be joined to the thalamus on the opposite side.

(e) The thalamus is a large ovoid mass of gray matter.

4. The following statements concerning the hypothalamus are correct **except:**

(a) It is formed by the lower part of the lateral wall and floor of the third ventricle.

(b) Functionally, it plays a role in the release of pituitary hormones.

(c) Caudally the hypothalamus merges with the tectum of the midbrain.

(d) The nuclei are composed of groups of small nerve cells.

(e) The mammillary bodies are part of the hypothalamus.

5. The following statements concerning the hypothalamus are correct **except:**

(a) The hypothalamus controls and integrates the activities of the autonomic and endocrine systems.

(b) It receives many afferent visceral and somatic sensory fibers.

(c) It gives off efferent fibers that pass to the sympathetic and parasympathetic outflows in the brain and spinal cord.

(d) It does not assist in the regulation of water metabolism.

(e) The hypothalamus plays a role in controlling emotional states.

6. The following statements concerning the third ventricle are correct **except:**

(a) The posterior wall is formed by the opening into the cerebral aqueduct and the pineal recess.

(b) It does not communicate directly with the lateral ventricles.

(c) The vascular tela choroidea projects from the roof to form the choroid plexus.

(d) Lying in the floor of the ventricle, from anterior to posterior, are the optic chiasma, the tuber cinereum, and the mammillary bodies.

(e) The wall of the ventricle is lined with ependyma.

Directions: Matching Questions

In Figure 7-30, match the numbers listed on the left with the appropriate lettered options listed on the right. Each lettered option may be selected once, more than once, or not at all.

7. Number 1   (a) Genu of corpus callosum
8. Number 2   (b) Interventricular foramen
9. Number 3   (c) Body of fornix
10. Number 4   (d) Anterior commissure
11. Number 5   (e) None of the above
12. Number 6
13. Number 7

Directions: Each of the numbered items in this section is followed by answers that are positively phrased. Select the ONE lettered answer that is an EXCEPTION.

14. The following statements concerning the longitudinal cerebral fissure are correct **except:**

(a) The fissure contains the sickle-shaped fold of dura mater, the falx cerebri.

(b) In the depths of the fissure the corpus callosum crosses the midline.

(c) The fissure contains the middle cerebral arteries.

(d) The superior sagittal sinus lies above it.

(e) The inferior sagittal sinus lies within it.

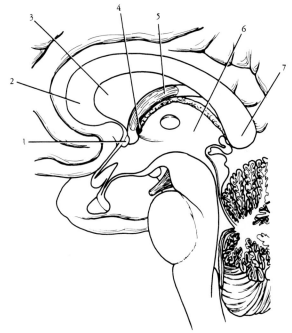

Figure 7–30   Sagittal section of the brain showing the medial surface of the diencephalon.

15. The following statements concerning the central sulcus are correct **except:**
    (a) The frontal lobe lies anterior to it.
    (b) The central sulcus extends onto the medial surface of the cerebral hemisphere.
    (c) The parietal lobe lies behind it.
    (d) The central sulcus is continuous inferiorly with the lateral sulcus.
    (e) The arachnoid mater does not extend into the central sulcus.
16. The following statements concerning the lateral ventricle are correct **except:**
    (a) Each ventricle is C-shaped and filled with cerebrospinal fluid.
    (b) It communicates with the third ventricle through the interventricular foramen.
    (c) The body of the ventricle occupies the parietal lobe.
    (d) The lateral ventricle does not possess a choroid plexus.
    (e) The anterior horn occupies the frontal lobe.
17. The following statements concerning the corpus callosum are correct **except:**
    (a) It is connected to the fornix by the septum pellucidum.
    (b) The rostrum connects the genu to the lamina terminalis.
    (c) Most of the fibers within the corpus callosum interconnect symmetrical areas of the cerebral cortex.
    (d) The fibers of the genu curve forward into the frontal lobes as the forceps major.
    (e) The corpus callosum is related superiorly to the falx cerebri.
18. The following statements concerning the anterior commissure are correct **except:**
    (a) It is embedded in the superior part of the lamina terminalis.
    (b) Some of the fibers are concerned with the sensations of smell.
    (c) It forms the anterior boundary of the interventricular foramen.
    (d) It is formed by a small bundle of nerve fibers.
    (e) When traced laterally, an anterior bundle of fibers curves forward to join the olfactory tract.
19. The following statements concerning the internal capsule are correct **except:**
    (a) It has an anterior limb, a genu, and a posterior limb.
    (b) It is continuous below with the tectum of the midbrain.
    (c) The genu and the anterior part of the posterior limb contain the corticobulbar and corticospinal fibers.
    (d) It is related laterally to the lentiform nucleus.
    (e) It is continuous above with the corona radiata.

20. The following statements concerning the basal ganglia are correct **except:**
    (a) The caudate nucleus is fused with the lentiform nucleus.
    (b) The corpus striatum is concerned with muscular movement.
    (c) The lentiform nucleus is related medially to the external capsule.
    (d) The lentiform nucleus is wedge-shaped as seen on horizontal section.
    (e) The amygdaloid nucleus forms one of the basal ganglia.

Directions: Matching Questions

In Figure 7-31, match the numbers listed on the left with the appropriate lettered options listed on the right. Each lettered option may be selected once, more than once, or not at all.

21. Number 1	(a)	Optic radiation
22. Number 2	(b)	Lateral sulcus
23. Number 3	(c)	Lentiform nucleus
24. Number 4	(d)	Anterior horn of lateral ventricle
25. Number 5	(e)	None of the above

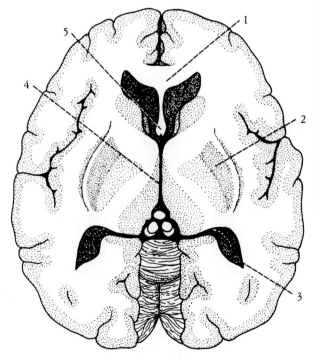

Figure 7–31 Horizontal section of the cerebrum as seen from above.

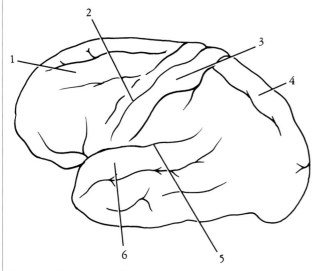

Figure 7–32 Lateral view of the left cerebral hemisphere.

In Figure 7-32, match the numbers listed on the left with the appropriate lettered options listed on the right. Each lettered option may be selected once, more than once, or not at all.

26. Number 1   (a) Central sulcus
27. Number 2   (b) Postcentral gyrus
28. Number 3   (c) Superior temporal gyrus
29. Number 4   (d) Superior parietal lobule
30. Number 5   (e) None of the above
31. Number 6

Directions: Read the case histories then answer the questions. You will be required to select ONE BEST lettered answer.

A 70-year-old man with hypertension was admitted to an emergency department, having suddenly developed hemiparesis on the right side and numbness of the right leg. Axial CT and MRI were undertaken. MRI revealed a small hemorrhage in the left thalamus, which passed horizontally through the lateral ventricles. After careful observation, 2 days later the paresis was much improved and the patient reported that his numbness had disappeared. The patient was discharged from the hospital 1 week later and made an uneventful recovery. His hypertension was brought under control with suitable medication.

32. Using your knowledge of the relationships of the left thalamus, **select** the statement that explains the transient right hemiparesis and numbness.
    (a) The hemorrhage occurred into the third ventricle.
    (b) The hemorrhage into the thalamus extended laterally into the posterior limb of the left internal capsule.
    (c) The hemorrhage was small and confined to the thalamus on the left side.
    (d) The hemorrhage was small and occurred in the lateral part of the left thalamus, producing transient edema in the left internal capsule.
    (e) The hemorrhage extended laterally into the left lateral ventricle.
33. This hypertensive patient had a small thalamic hemorrhage. Select the **most likely** cause for the hemorrhage:
    (a) One of the small diseased thalamic arteries may have ruptured.
    (b) One of the small veins draining the thalamus may have ruptured.
    (c) Vasoconstriction of the thalamic arteries could have occurred.
    (d) Softening of the neuronal tissue around the thalamic arteries might have taken place.
    (e) There is no relation between hypertension and the thalamic hemorrhage in this patient.

An 8-year-old boy with a severe earache on the right side was taken to a pediatrician. The symptoms had started 7 days ago and the pain had progressively worsened. On examination, the boy was found to have severe right-sided otitis media with acute mastoiditis. On being questioned, the boy admitted that his head hurt badly all over and that he felt sick. While he was being examined, he vomited. His body temperature was slightly elevated. In view of the severity of the headache, and the presence of nausea and vomiting, the pediatrician decided to have an MRI performed. The result showed a small, well-defined, right cerebral abscess.

34. The cerebral abscess in this patient was most likely located at which site in the right cerebral hemisphere:
    (a) Frontal lobe
    (b) Thalamus
    (c) Occipital lobe
    (d) Temporal lobe
    (e) Cuneus

Answers to Review Questions

1. D	18. C
2. A	19. B
3. C	20. C
4. C	21. E
5. D	22. C
6. B	23. E
7. D	24. E
8. A	25. E
9. E	26. E
10. B	27. A
11. C	28. B
12. E	29. D
13. E	30. E
14. C	31. C
15. D	32. D
16. D	33. A
17. D	34. D

ADDITIONAL READING

Axelrod, J. The pineal gland. *Endeavour* 29:144, 1970.

Clark, C.M., Ewbank, D., Lee. V.M.Y., and, Trojanowski, J.Q. Molecular Pathology of Alzheimer's Disease: Neuronal Cytoskeletal Abnormalities. In: Growdon, J. H., Rossor, M.N.,eds. *The Dementias.* Vol.19 of Blue Books of Practical Neurology; Boston: Butterworth-Heinemann, 285-304,1998.

Crosby, E. C., Humphrey, T., and Lauer, E. W. *Correlative Anatomy of the Nervous System.* New York: Macmillan, 1962.

Guyton, A. C., and Hall, J.E. *Textbook of Medical Physiology,* 9th ed, Philadelphia, London, W.B. Saunders Co. 1996.

Jacobs, E. R. *Medical Imaging:A Concise Textbook.* New York and Tokyo: Igaku-Shoin, 1987.

Kappers, J. A. Short History of Pineal Discovery and Research. In J. A. Kappers and P. Peret (eds.), *The Pineal Gland of Vertebrates Including Man. Proceedings of the First Colloquium of the European Study Group (EPSG), Amsterdam, 1978* (Progress in Brain Research. Vol. 52). Amsterdam: Biomedical Press, 1978. P. 3.

Kehoe, P., Wavrant-De Vrieze, F., Crook, R., et al. A Full Genome Scan for Late Onset Alzheimer's Disease. *Hum. Mol. Genet.* 8:237-245,1999.

Martin, J.B. Mechanisms of Disease: Molecular Basis of the Neurodegenerative Disorders. *N. Engl. J. Med.* 340:1970-1980,1999.

Marx, J. New Gene Tied to Common Form of Alzheimer's Disease. *Science* 281:507-509,1998.

Neve, R.L., Robakis, N.K. Alzheimer's Disease: A Re-examination of the Amyloid Hypothesis. *Trends Neurosci.* 21:15-29,1998.

Reiman, E. M., et al. Preclinical evidence of Alzheimer's disease in persons homozygous for the ge 4 allele for apolipo-protein E. *N. Engl. J. Med.* 334:752, 1996.

Rhoades, R. A., and Tanner, G. A. *Medical Physiology.* Boston: Little, Brown, 1995.

Selkoe, D. J. Molecular Pathology of Alzheimer's Disease: The Role Amyloid. In: Growdon, J. H., Rossor, M.N., eds. *The Dementias.* Vol.19 of Blue Books of Practical Neurology. Boston: Butterworth-Heinemann, 257-283,1998.

Snell, R. S. Effect of melatonin on mammalian epidermal melanocytes. *J. Invest. Dermatol.* 44:273, 1965.

Swanson, L. W., and Sawchenko, P. E. Hypothalamic integration: Organization of the paraventricular and supraoptic nuclei. *Annu. Rev. Neurosci.* 6:269, 1983.

Walton, J. N. *Brain's Diseases of the Nervous System* (9th ed.). New York and London: Oxford University Press, 1984.

Williams, P. L. et al. *Gray's Anatomy* (38th Br. ed.). New York, Edinburgh, 1995.

CHAPTER 8

The Structure and Functional Localization of the Cerebral Cortex

A 19-year-old woman was involved in an automobile accident. She was not wearing a seat belt and was thrown from the car and suffered severe head injuries. On being examined by the emergency medical technicians, she was found to be unconscious and was admitted to the emergency department. After 5 hours she recovered consciousness and over the next 2 weeks made a remarkable recovery. She left the hospital 1 month after the accident, with very slight weakness of her right leg. Nothing else abnormal was noted. Four months later she was seen by a neurologist because she was experiencing sudden attacks of jerking movements of her right leg and foot. The attacks lasted only a few minutes. One week later the patient had a very severe attack, which involved her right leg and then spread to her right arm. On this occasion, she lost consciousness during the attack.

The neurologist diagnosed Jacksonian epileptic seizures, caused by cerebral scarring secondary to the automobile injury. The weakness of the right leg immediately after the accident was due to damage to the superior part of the left precentral gyrus. Her initial attacks of epilepsy were of the partial variety and were caused by irritation of the area of the left precentral gyrus corresponding to the leg. In her last attack, the epileptiform seizure spread to other areas of the left precentral gyrus, thus involving most of the right side of her body, and she lost consciousness.

Knowledge of the functional localization of the cerebral cortex enabled the physician to make an accurate diagnosis and advise suitable treatment. The cerebral scar tissue was cleanly excised by a neurosurgeon and apart from a small residual weakness of the right leg, the patient had no further epileptiform seizures.

CHAPTER OBJECTIVES

The cerebral cortex is the highest level of the central nervous system and always functions in association with the lower centers. It receives vast amounts of information and responds in a precise manner by bringing about appropriate changes. Many of the responses are influenced by inherited programs, whereas others are colored by programs learned during the individual's life and stored in the cerebral cortex.

The purpose of this chapter is to describe the basic structure and functional localization of the highly complex cerebral cortex. The physician can then use this information to locate hemispheric lesions based on clinical symptoms and signs.

STRUCTURE OF THE CEREBRAL CORTEX

The cerebral cortex forms a complete covering of the cerebral hemisphere. It is composed of gray matter and has been estimated to contain approximately 10 billion neurons. The surface area of the cortex has been increased by throwing it into convolutions, or gyri, separated by fissures or sulci. The thickness of the cortex varies from 1.5 to 4.5 mm. The cortex is thickest over the crest of a gyrus and thinnest in the depth of a sulcus. The cerebral cortex, like gray matter elsewhere in the central nervous system, consists of a mixture of nerve cells, nerve fibers, neuroglia, and blood vessels. The following types of nerve cells are present in the cerebral cortex: (1) pyramidal cells, (2) stellate cells, (3) fusiform cells, (4) horizontal cells of Cajal, and (5) cells of Martinotti (Fig. 8-1).

Nerve Cells of the Cerebral Cortex

The **pyramidal cells** are named from the shape of their cell bodies (Fig. 8-1). Most of the cell bodies measure 10 to 50 μm

long. However, there are giant pyramidal cells, also known as **Betz cells**, whose cell bodies measure as much as 120 μm; these are found in the motor precentral gyrus of the frontal lobe.

The apices of the pyramidal cells are oriented toward the pial surface of the cortex. From the apex of each cell a thick apical dendrite extends upward toward the pia, giving off collateral branches. From the basal angles, several basal dendrites pass laterally into the surrounding neuropil. Each dendrite possesses numerous **dendritic spines** for synaptic junctions with axons of other neurons (Fig. 8-1). The axon arises from the base of the cell body and either terminates in the deeper cortical layers or, more commonly, enters the white matter of the cerebral hemisphere as a projection, association, or commissural fiber.

The **stellate cells**, sometimes called granule cells because of their small size, are polygonal in shape and their cell bodies measure about 8 μm in diameter (Fig. 8-1). These cells have multiple branching dendrites and a relatively short axon, which terminates on a nearby neuron.

The **fusiform cells** have their long axis vertical to the surface and are concentrated mainly in the deepest cortical

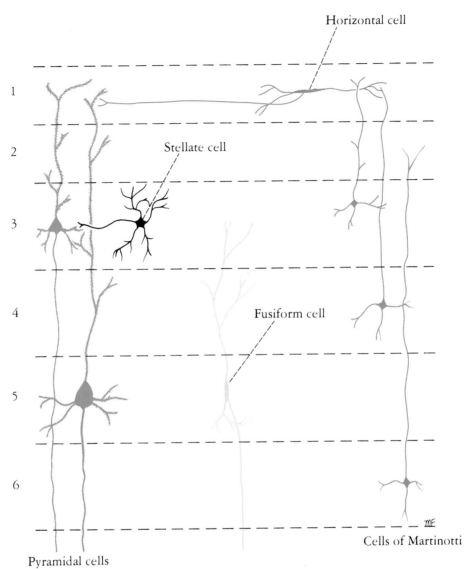

Figure 8–1 Main types of neurons found in the cerebral cortex.

layers (see Fig. 8-1). Dendrites arise from each pole of the cell body. The inferior dendrite branches within the same cellular layer, while the superficial dendrite ascends toward the surface of the cortex and branches in the superficial layers. The axon arises from the inferior part of the cell body and enters the white matter as a projection, association, or commissural fiber.

The **horizontal cells of Cajal** are small, fusiform, horizontally oriented cells found in the most superficial layers of the cortex (Fig. 8-1). A dendrite emerges from each end of the cell and an axon runs parallel to the surface of the cortex, making contact with the dendrites of pyramidal cells.

The **cells of Martinotti** are small, multipolar cells that are present throughout the levels of the cortex (Fig. 8-1). The cell has short dendrites, but the axon is directed toward the pial surface of the cortex, where it ends in a more superficial layer, commonly the most superficial layer. The axon gives origin to a few short collateral branches en route.

Nerve Fibers of the Cerebral Cortex

The nerve fibers of the cerebral cortex are arranged both radially and tangentially (Figs. 8-2 and 8-3). The **radial fibers** run at right angles to the cortical surface. They include the afferent entering projection, association, and commissural fibers that terminate within the cortex, and the axons of pyramidal, stellate, and fusiform cells, which leave the cortex to become projection, association, and commissural fibers of the white matter of the cerebral hemisphere.

The **tangential fibers** run parallel to the cortical surface and are, for the most part, collateral and terminal branches of afferent fibers. They include also the axons of horizontal and stellate cells, and collateral branches of pyramidal and

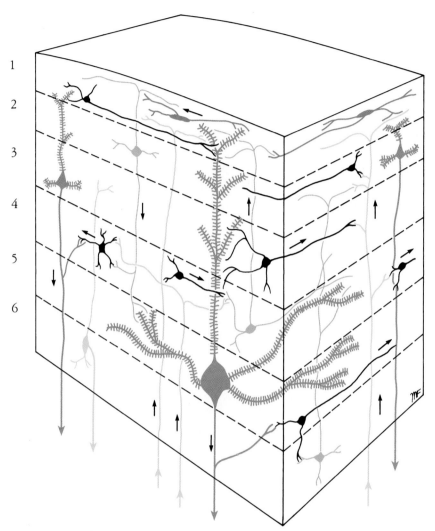

Figure 8–2 Neuronal connections of the cerebral cortex. Note the presence of the afferent and efferent fibers.

fusiform cells. The tangential fibers are most concentrated in layers 4 and 5, where they are referred to as the outer and inner **bands of Baillarger**, respectively (Figs. 8-2 and 8-3). The bands of Baillarger are particularly well developed in the sensory areas due to the high concentration of the terminal parts of the thalamocortical fibers. In the visual cortex, the outer **band of Baillarger**, which is so thick it can be seen with the naked eye, is known as the **stria of Gennari**. Because of this obvious band, or stria, the visual cortex in the walls of the calcarine sulcus is sometimes called the **striate cortex**.

Layers of the Cerebral Cortex

It is convenient, for descriptive purposes, to divide the cerebral cortex into layers that may be distinguished by the types, density, and arrangement of their cells (Figs. 8-1 and 8-3). The names and characteristic features of the layers are described here; regional differences are discussed later.

1. **Molecular layer (plexiform layer).** This is the most superficial layer; it consists mainly of a dense network of tangentially oriented nerve fibers (Figs. 8-1 and 8-3). These fibers are derived from the apical dendrites of the pyramidal cells and fusiform cells, the axons of the stellate cells, and the cells of Martinotti. Afferent fibers originating in the thalamus and in association with commissural fibers also are present. Scattered among these nerve fibers are occasional horizontal cells of Cajal. This most superficial layer of the cortex clearly is where large numbers of synapses between different neurons occur.
2. **External granular layer.** This layer contains large numbers of small pyramidal cells and stellate cells (Figs. 8-1 and 8-3). The dendrites of these cells terminate in the molecular layer, and the axons enter deeper layers, where they terminate or pass on to enter the white matter of the cerebral hemisphere.
3. **External pyramidal layer.** This layer is composed of pyramidal cells, whose cell body size increases from the

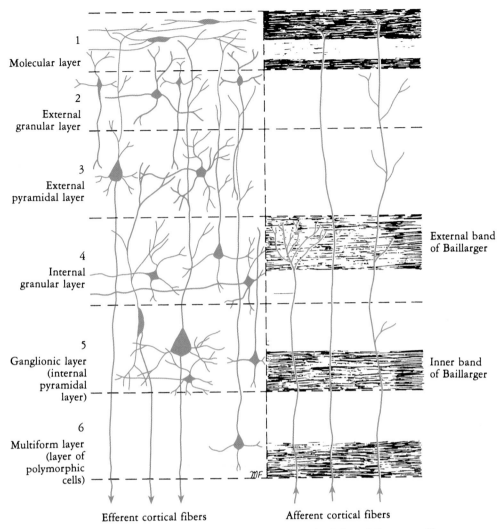

1
Molecular layer

2
External
granular layer

3
External
pyramidal layer

4
Internal
granular layer

External band
of Baillarger

5
Ganglionic layer
(internal
pyramidal
layer)

Inner band
of Baillarger

6
Multiform layer
(layer of
polymorphic
cells)

Efferent cortical fibers   Afferent cortical fibers

Figure 8–3 Layers of the cerebral cortex, showing the neurons on the left and the nerve fibers on the right.

superficial to the deeper borders of the layer (Figs. 8-1 and 8-3). The apical dendrites pass into the molecular layer and the axons enter the white matter as projection, association, or commissural fibers.

4. **Internal granular layer.** This layer is composed of closely packed stellate cells (Figs. 8-1 and 8-3). There is a high concentration of horizontally arranged fibers known collectively as the **external band of Baillarger**.

5. **Ganglionic layer (internal pyramidal layer).** This layer contains very large and medium-size pyramidal cells (Figs. 8-1 and 8-3). Scattered among the pyramidal cells are stellate cells and cells of Martinotti. In addition, there are a large number of horizontally arranged fibers that form the **inner band of Baillarger** (Fig. 8-3). In the motor cortex of the precentral gyrus, the pyramidal cells of this layer are very large and are known as Betz cells. These cells account for about 3 percent of the projection fibers of the **corticospinal** or **pyramidal tract**.

6. **Multiform layer (layer of polymorphic cells).** Although the majority of the cells are fusiform, many of the cells are modified pyramidal cells, whose cell bodies are triangular or ovoid (Figs. 8-1 and 8-3). The cells of Martinotti also are conspicuous in this layer. Many nerve fibers are present that are entering or are leaving the underlying white matter.

Variations In Cortical Structure

The system of numbering and nomenclature of the cortical layers used above is similar to that distinguished by Brodmann (1909). It is important, however, to realize that not all areas of the cerebral cortex possess six layers (Fig. 8-3). Those areas of the cortex in which the basic six layers cannot be recognized are referred to as **heterotypical**, as opposed to the majority, which are **homotypical** and possess six layers. Two heterotypical areas are described: the granular and the agranular type.

In the **granular type**, the granular layers are well developed and contain densely packed stellate cells (Fig. 8-3). Thus, layers 2 and 4 are well developed, and layers 3 and 5 are poorly developed, so that layers 2 through 5 merge into a single layer of predominantly granular cells. It is these cells that receive thalamocortical fibers. The granular type of cortex is found in the postcentral gyrus, in the superior temporal gyrus, and in parts of the hippocampal gyrus.

In the **agranular type** of cortex, the granular layers are poorly developed, so that layers 2 and 4 are practically absent (Fig. 8-3). The pyramidal cells in layers 3 and 5 are densely packed and are very large. The agranular type of cortex is found in the precentral gyrus and other areas in the frontal lobe. These areas give rise to large numbers of efferent fibers that are associated with motor function.

 ## MECHANISMS OF THE CEREBRAL CORTEX

Extensive research in recent years involving electrophysiology, histochemistry, immunocytochemistry, and other microscopic techniques, has resulted in a vast increase in our knowledge of the connections of the neurons of the cerebral cortex. This information combined with new methods of studying the functions of the human cerebral cortex in the living using electroencephalograms (EEG), positron emission tomography (PET) and magnetic resonance imaging (MRI) have led to a new understanding of the functions of the different areas and the different layers of the cerebral cortex. Much of the new information, however, is still merely factual data and cannot be used in the clinical setting.

The cerebral cortex is organized into vertical units or columns of functional activity (Fig. 8-2) measuring about 300-600μm wide. Such a functional unit extends through all six layers from the cortical surface to the white matter. Each unit possesses afferent fibers, internuncial neurons, and efferent fibers. An afferent fiber may synapse directly with an efferent neuron or may involve vertical chains of internuncial neurons. A single vertical chain of neurons may be involved or the wave of excitation may spread to adjacent vertical chains through short axon granular cells. The horizontal cells of Cajal permit activation of vertical units that lie some distance away from the incoming afferent fiber (Fig. 8-2).

 ## CORTICAL AREAS

Clinicopathological studies in humans and electrophysiological and ablation studies in animals have, over the past century, produced evidence that different areas of the cerebral cortex are functionally specialized. However, the precise division of the cortex into different areas of specialization, as described by Brodmann, oversimplifies and misleads the reader. The simple division of cortical areas

into motor and sensory is erroneous, for many of the sensory areas are far more extensive than originally described, and it is known that motor responses can be obtained by stimulation of sensory areas. Until a satisfactory terminology has been devised to describe the various cortical areas, the main cortical areas will be named by their anatomical location.

Some of the main anatomical connections of the cerebral cortex are summarized in Table 8-1.

Frontal Lobe

The **precentral area** is situated in the precentral gyrus and includes the anterior wall of the central sulcus and the posterior parts of the superior, middle, and inferior frontal gyri; it extends over the superomedial border of the hemisphere into the paracentral lobule (Fig. 8-4). Histologically, the characteristic feature of this area is the almost complete absence of the granular layers and the prominence of the pyramidal nerve cells. The giant pyramidal cells of Betz, which can measure as much as 120 μm long and 60 μm wide, are concentrated most highly in the superior part of the precentral gyrus and the paracentral lobule; their numbers diminish as one passes anteriorly in the precentral gyrus or inferiorly toward the lateral fissure. The great majority of the corticospinal and corticobulbar fibers originate from the small pyramidal cells in this area. It has been estimated that the number of Betz cells present is between 25,000 and 30,000 and accounts for only about 3 percent of the corticospinal fibers. It is interesting to note that the postcentral gyrus and the second somatosensory areas, as well as the occipital and temporal lobes, give origin to descending tracts also; they are involved in controlling the sensory input to the nervous system and are not involved in muscular movement.

The precentral area may be divided into posterior and anterior regions. The posterior region—referred to as the **motor area**, **primary motor area**, or Brodmann's area 4—occupies the precentral gyrus extending over the superior border into the paracentral lobule (Fig. 8-4). The anterior region is known as the **premotor area**, **secondary motor area**, or Brodmann's area 6 and parts of areas 8, 44, and 45. It occupies the anterior part of the precentral gyrus and the posterior parts of the superior, middle, and inferior frontal gyri.

The primary motor area, if electrically stimulated, produces isolated movements on the opposite side of the body as well as contraction of muscle groups concerned with the performance of a specific movement. Although isolated ipsilateral movements do not occur, bilateral movements of the extraocular muscles, the muscles of the upper part of the face, the tongue and the mandible, and the larynx and the pharynx do occur.

The movement areas of the body are represented in inverted form in the precentral gyrus (Fig. 8-5). Starting from below and passing superiorly are structures involved in swallowing, tongue, jaw, lips, larynx, eyelid, and brow. The next area is an extensive region for movements of the fingers, especially the thumb, hand, wrist, elbow, shoulder, and trunk.

Table 8–1   Some of the Main Anatomical Connections of the Cerebral Cortex

Function	Origin	Cortical Area	Destination
Sensory			
Somatosensory (most to contralateral side of body; oral to same side; pharynx, larynx, and perineum bilateral)	Ventral posterior lateral and ventral posterior medial nucleus of thalamus	Primary somesthetic area (B3, 1, and 2), posterior central gyrus	Secondary somesthetic area; primary motor area
Vision	Lateral geniculate body	Primary visual area (B17)	Secondary visual area (B18 and 19)
Auditory	Medial geniculate body	Primary auditory area (B41 and 42)	Secondary auditory area (B22)
Taste	Nucleus solitarius	Posterior central gyrus (B43)	
Smell	Olfactory bulb	Primary olfactory area; periamygdaloid and prepiriform areas	Secondary olfactory area (B28)
Motor			
Fine movements (most to contralateral side of body; extraocular muscles, upper face, tongue, mandible, larynx, bilateral)	Thalamus from cerebellum, basal ganglia; somatosensory area; premotor area	Primary motor area (B4)	Motor nuclei of brainstem and anterior horn cells of spinal cord; corpus striatum

B = Brodmann's area.

The movements of the hip, knee, and ankle are represented in the highest areas of the precentral gyrus; the toes are situated on the medial surface of the cerebral hemisphere in the paracentral lobule. The anal and vesical sphincters are also located in the paracentral lobule. The area of cortex controlling a particular movement is proportional to the skill involved in performing the movement and is unrelated to the mass of muscle participating in the movement.

The function of the primary motor area is thus to carry out the individual movements of different parts of the body. To assist in this function, it receives numerous afferent fibers from the premotor area, the sensory cortex, the thalamus, the cerebellum, and the basal ganglia. The primary motor cortex is not responsible for the design of the pattern of movement but is the final station for conversion of the design into execution of the movement.

The premotor area, which is wider superiorly than below and narrows down to be confined to the anterior part of the precentral gyrus, has no giant pyramidal cells of Betz. Electrical stimulation of the premotor area produces muscular movements similar to those obtained by stimulation of the primary motor area; however, stronger stimulation is necessary to produce the same degree of movement.

The premotor area receives numerous inputs from the sensory cortex, the thalamus, and the basal ganglia. The function of the premotor area is to store programs of motor activity assembled as the result of past experience. The premotor area thus programs the activity of the primary motor area. It is particularly involved in controlling coarse postural movements through its connections with the basal ganglia.

The **supplementary motor area** is situated in the medial frontal gyrus on the medial surface of the hemisphere and anterior to the paracentral lobule. Stimulation of this area results in movements of the contralateral limbs, but a stronger stimulus is necessary than when the primary motor area is stimulated. Removal of the supplementary motor area produces no permanent loss of movement.

The **frontal eye field** (Fig. 8-4) extends forward from the facial area of the precentral gyrus into the middle frontal gyrus (parts of Brodmann's areas 6, 8, and 9). Electrical stimulation of this region causes conjugate movements of the eyes, especially toward the opposite side. The exact pathway taken by nerve fibers from this area is not known, but they are thought to pass to the superior colliculus of the midbrain. The superior colliculus is connected to the nuclei of the extraocular muscles by the reticular formation. The frontal eye field is considered to control voluntary scanning movements of the eye and is independent of visual stimuli. The involuntary following of moving objects by the eyes involves the visual area of the occipital cortex to which the frontal eye field is connected by association fibers.

The **motor speech area of Broca** (Fig. 8-4) is located in the inferior frontal gyrus between the anterior and ascending rami and the ascending and posterior rami of the lateral fissure (Brodmann's areas 44 and 45). In the majority of individuals, this area is important on the left or dominant hemisphere and ablation will result in paralysis of speech. In those individuals in whom the right hemisphere is dominant, the area on the right side is of importance. The abla-

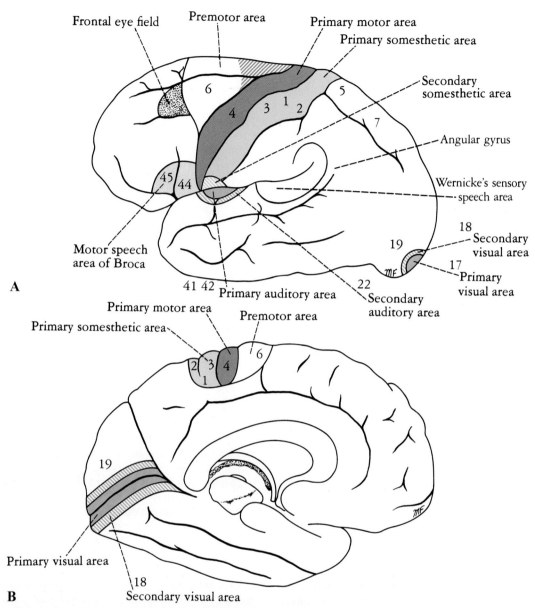

Figure 8–4 Functional localization of the cerebral cortex. **A**. Lateral view of the left cerebral hemisphere. **B**. Medial view of the left cerebral hemisphere.

tion of this region in the nondominant hemisphere has no effect on speech.

Broca's speech area brings about the formation of words by its connections with the adjacent primary motor areas; the muscles of the larynx, mouth, tongue, soft palate, and the respiratory muscles are appropriately stimulated.

The **prefrontal cortex** is an extensive area that lies anterior to the precentral area. It includes the greater parts of the superior, middle, and inferior frontal gyri; the orbital gyri; most of the medial frontal gyrus; and the anterior half of the cingulate gyrus (Brodmann's areas 9, 10, 11, and 12). Large numbers of afferent and efferent pathways connect the prefrontal area with other areas of the cerebral cortex, the thalamus, the hypothalamus, and the corpus striatum. The frontopontine fibers also connect this area to the cerebellum

through the pontine nuclei. The commissural fibers of the forceps minor and genu of the corpus callosum unite these areas in both cerebral hemispheres.

The prefrontal area is concerned with the makeup of the individual's personality. As the result of the input from many cortical and subcortical sources, this area plays a role as a regulator of the person's depth of feeling. It also exerts its influence in determining the initiative and judgment of an individual.

Parietal Lobe

The **primary somesthetic area** (Primary Somatic Sensory Cortex S1) occupies the postcentral gyrus (Fig. 8-4) on the lateral surface of the hemisphere and the posterior part of

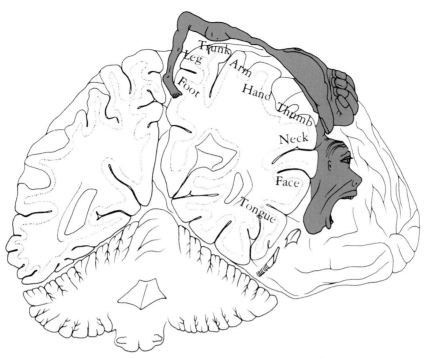

Figure 8–5   Motor homunculus on the precentral gyrus.

the paracentral lobule on the medial surface (Brodmann's areas 3, 1, and 2). Histologically, the anterior part of the postcentral gyrus is the area that borders the central sulcus (area 3), is granular in type, and contains only scattered pyramidal cells. The **outer layer of Baillarger** is broad and very obvious. The posterior part of the postcentral gyrus (areas 1 and 2) possesses fewer granular cells. The primary somesthetic areas of the cerebral cortex receive projection fibers from the ventral posterior lateral and ventral posterior medial nuclei of the thalamus. The opposite half of the body is represented as inverted. The pharyngeal region, tongue, and jaws are represented in the most inferior part of the postcentral gyrus; this is followed by the face, fingers, hand, arm, trunk, and thigh. The leg and the foot areas are found on the medial surface of the hemisphere in the posterior part of the paracentral lobule. The anal and genital regions are also found in this latter area. The apportioning of the cortex for a particular part of the body is related to its functional importance rather than to its size. The face, lips, thumb, and index finger have particularly large areas assigned to them.

Although most sensations reach the cortex from the contralateral side of the body, some from the oral region go to the same side, and those from the pharynx, larynx, and perineum go to both sides. On entering the cortex, the afferent fibers excite the neurons in layer IV and then the signals spread towards the surface of the cerebral unit and toward the deeper layers. From layer VI large numbers of axons leave the cortex and pass to the thalamus providing feedback.

The **secondary somesthetic area** (Secondary Somatic Sensory Cortex, S2) is in the superior lip of the posterior limb of the lateral fissure (Fig. 8-4). The secondary sensory area is much smaller and less important than the primary sensory area. The face area lies most anterior and the leg area is posterior. The body is bilaterally represented with the contralateral side dominant. The detailed connections of this area are unknown. Many sensory impulses come from the primary area and many signals are transmitted from the brain stem. The functional significance of this area is not understood. It has been shown that the neurons respond particularly to transient cutaneous stimuli, such as brush strokes or tapping of the skin.

The **somesthetic association area** (Fig. 8-4) occupies the superior parietal lobule extending onto the medial surface of the hemisphere (Brodmann's areas 5 and 7). This area has many connections with other sensory areas of the cortex. It is believed that its main function is to receive and integrate different sensory modalities. For example, it enables one to recognize objects placed in the hand without the help of vision. In other words, it not only receives information concerning the size and shape of an object but also relates this to past sensory experiences, so that the information may be interpreted and recognition occurs. A quarter placed in the hand can be distinguished from a dime or a nickel by the size, shape, and feel of the coin without having to use one's eyes.

Occipital Lobe

The **primary visual area** (Brodmann's area 17) is situated in the walls of the posterior part of the calcarine sulcus and occasionally extends around the occipital pole onto the lateral surface of the hemisphere (Fig. 8-4). Macroscopically, this area can be recognized by the thinness of the cortex and the visual stria, and microscopically, it is seen to be a granular type of cortex with only a few pyramidal cells present.

The visual cortex receives afferent fibers from the lateral geniculate body. The fibers first pass forward in the white matter of the temporal lobe and then turn back to the primary visual cortex in the occipital lobe. The visual cortex receives fibers from the temporal half of the ipsilateral retina and the nasal half of the contralateral retina. The right half of the field of vision, therefore, is represented in the visual cortex of the left cerebral hemisphere and vice versa. It is also important to note that the superior retinal quadrants (inferior field of vision) pass to the superior wall of the calcarine sulcus, while the inferior retinal quadrants (superior field of vision) pass to the inferior wall of the calcarine sulcus.

The macula lutea, which is the central area of the retina and the area for most perfect vision, is represented on the cortex in the posterior part of area 17 and accounts for one-third of the visual cortex. The visual impulses from the peripheral parts of the retina terminate in concentric circles anterior to the occipital pole in the anterior part of area 17.

The **secondary visual area** (Brodmann's areas 18 and 19) surrounds the primary visual area on the medial and lateral surfaces of the hemisphere (Fig. 8-4). This area receives afferent fibers from area 17 and other cortical areas, as well as from the thalamus. The function of the secondary visual area is to relate the visual information received by the primary visual area to past visual experiences, thus enabling the individual to recognize and appreciate what he or she is seeing.

The **occipital eye field** is thought to exist in the secondary visual area in humans (Fig. 8-4). Stimulation produces conjugate deviation of the eyes, especially to the opposite side. The function of this eye field is believed to be reflex and associated with movements of the eye when it is following an object. The occipital eye fields of both hemispheres are connected by nervous pathways, and also are thought to be connected to the superior colliculus. By contrast, the frontal eye field controls voluntary scanning movements of the eye and is independent of visual stimuli.

Temporal Lobe

The **primary auditory area** (Brodmann's areas 41 and 42) includes the gyrus of Heschl and is situated in the inferior wall of the lateral sulcus (Fig. 8-4). Area 41 is a granular type of cortex; area 42 is homotypical and is mainly an auditory association area.

Projection fibers to the auditory area arise principally in the medial geniculate body and form the **auditory radiation of the internal capsule**. The anterior part of the primary auditory area is concerned with the reception of sounds of low frequency and the posterior part of the area with the sounds of high frequency. A unilateral lesion of the auditory area produces partial deafness in both ears, the greater loss being in the contralateral ear. This can be explained on the basis that the medial geniculate body receives fibers mainly from the organ of Corti of the opposite side as well as some fibers from the same side.

The **secondary auditory area** (auditory association cortex) is situated posterior to the primary auditory area (Fig. 8-4) in the lateral sulcus and in the superior temporal gyrus (Brodmann's area 22). It receives impulses from the primary auditory area and from the thalamus. The secondary auditory area is thought to be necessary for the interpretation of sounds and for the association of the auditory input with other sensory information.

The **sensory speech area of Wernicke** (Fig. 8-4) is localized in the left dominant hemisphere, mainly in the superior temporal gyrus, with extensions around the posterior end of the lateral sulcus into the parietal region. Wernicke's area is connected to Broca's area by a bundle of nerve fibers called the **arcuate fasciculus**. It receives fibers from the visual cortex in the occipital lobe and the auditory cortex in the superior temporal gyrus. Wernicke's area permits the understanding of the written and spoken language and enables a person to read a sentence, understand it, and say it out loud (Figs. 8-6 and 8-7).

Since Wernicke's area represents the site on the cerebral cortex where somatic, visual, and auditory associations areas all come together, it should be regarded as an area of very great importance.

Other Cortical Areas

The **taste area** is situated at the lower end of the postcentral gyrus in the superior wall of the lateral sulcus and in the adjoining area of the insula (Brodmann's area 43). Ascending fibers from the nucleus solitarius probably ascend to the ventral posteromedial nucleus of the thalamus, where they synapse on neurons that send fibers to the cortex.

The **vestibular area** is believed to be situated near the part of the postcentral gyrus concerned with sensations of the face. Its location lies opposite the auditory area in the superior temporal gyrus. The vestibular area and the vestibular part of the inner ear are concerned with appreciation of the positions and movements of the head in space. Through its nerve connections, the movements of the eyes and the muscles of the trunk and limbs are influenced in the maintenance of posture.

The **insula** is an area of the cortex that is buried within the lateral sulcus and forms its floor (Fig. 7-9). It can be examined only when the lips of the lateral sulcus are separated widely. Histologically, the posterior part is granular and the anterior part is agranular, thus resembling the adjoining cortical areas. Its fiber connections are incompletely known. It is believed that this area is important for planning or coordinating the articulatory movements necessary for speech.

Association Cortex

The primary sensory areas with their granular cortex and the primary motor areas with their agranular cortex form only a small part of the total cortical surface area. The remaining areas have all six cellular layers and therefore are referred to as homotypical cortex. Classically, these large remaining areas were known as association areas, though precisely what they associate is not known. The original concept, that

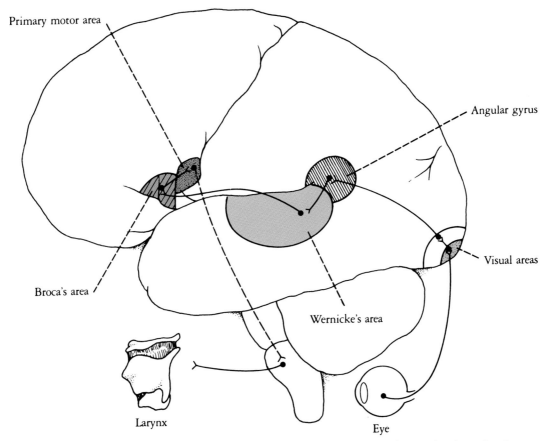

Figure 8–6 Probable nerve pathways involved in reading a sentence and repeating it out loud.

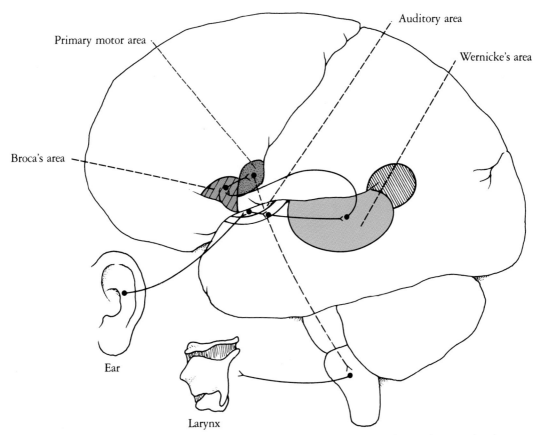

Figure 8–7 Probable nerve pathways involved with hearing a question and answering it.

they receive information from the primary sensory areas that is to be integrated and analyzed in the association cortex and then fed to the motor areas, has not been established. It has now become apparent, as the result of clinical studies and animal experimentation, that these areas of the cortex have multiple inputs and outputs and are very much concerned with behavior, discrimination, and interpretation of sensory experiences. Three main association areas are recognized: prefrontal, anterior temporal, and posterior parietal. The prefrontal cortex is discussed on page 294.

The anterior temporal cortex is thought to play a role in the storage of previous sensory experiences. Stimulation may cause the individual to recall objects seen or music heard in the past.

In the posterior parietal cortex, the visual information from the posterior occipital cortex and the sensory input of touch and pressure and proprioception from the anterior parietal cortex is integrated into concepts of size, form, and texture. This ability is known as **stereognosis**. An appreciation of the body image is also assembled in the posterior parietal cortex. A person is able to develop a body scheme that he or she is able to appreciate consciously. The brain knows at all times where each part of the body is located in relation to its environment. This information is so important when performing body movements. The right side of the body is represented in the left hemisphere and the left side of the body in the right hemisphere.

 CEREBRAL DOMINANCE

An anatomical examination of the two cerebral hemispheres shows that the cortical gyri and fissures are almost identical. Moreover, nervous pathways projecting to the cortex do so largely contralaterally and equally to identical cortical areas. In addition, the cerebral commissures, especially the corpus callosum and the anterior commissure, provide a pathway for information that is received in one hemisphere to be transferred to the other. Nevertheless, certain nervous activity is predominantly performed by one of the two cerebral hemispheres. Handedness, perception of language, and speech are functional areas of behavior that in most individuals are controlled by the dominant hemisphere. By contrast, spatial perception, recognition of faces, and music are interpreted by the nondominant hemisphere (Fig. 8-8).

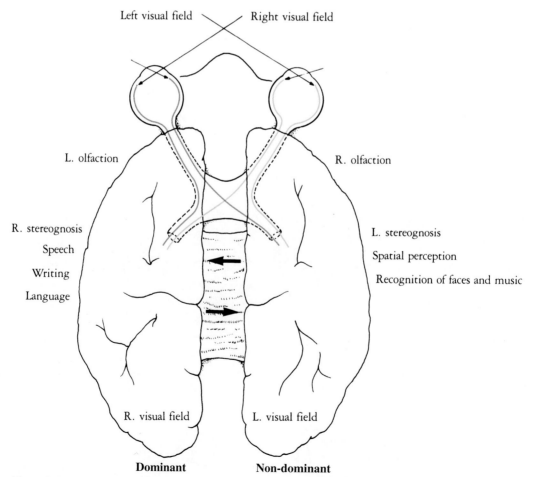

Figure 8–8   Nervous activities performed predominantly by dominant and nondominant hemispheres.

More than 90 percent of the adult population are right-handed and are therefore left hemisphere-dominant. About 96 percent of the adult population are left hemisphere-dominant for speech.

Yakolev and Rakic, in their work on human fetuses and neonates, have shown that more descending fibers in the left pyramid cross over the midline in the decussation than vice versa. This would suggest that in most individuals the anterior horn cells on the right side of the spinal cord have a greater corticospinal innervation than those on the left side, which might explain the dominance of the right hand.

Other workers have shown that the speech area of the adult cortex is larger on the left than on the right. It is believed that the two hemispheres of the newborn have equipotential capabilities. During childhood, one hemisphere slowly comes to dominate the other, and it is only after the first decade that the dominance becomes fixed. This would explain why a 5-year-old child with damage to the dominant hemisphere can easily learn to become left-handed and speak well, whereas in the adult this is almost impossible.

Clinical Notes

General Considerations

The cerebral cortex should be regarded as the last receiving station involved along a line of stations receiving information from the eyes and ears and organs of general sensation. The function of the cortex is, in simple terms, to discriminate, and it relates the received information to past memories. The enriched sensory input is then presumably discarded, stored, or translated into action. In this whole process, there is interplay between the cortex and basal nuclei provided by the many cortical and subcortical nervous connections.

Lesions of the Cerebral Cortex

In humans, the effect of destruction of different areas of the cerebral cortex has been studied by examining patients with lesions resulting from cerebral tumors, vascular accidents, surgery, or head injuries. Moreover, it has been possible to take electrical recordings from different areas of the cortex during surgical exposure of the cerebral cortex, or when stimulating different parts of the cortex in the conscious patient. One thing that has emerged from these studies is that the human cerebral cortex possesses, in a remarkable degree, the ability to reorganize the remaining intact cortex so that a certain amount of cerebral recovery is possible after brain lesions.

The Motor Cortex

Lesions of the primary **motor cortex** in one hemisphere result in paralysis of the contralateral extremities, the finer and more skilled movements suffering most. Destruction of the **primary motor area** (area 4) produces more severe paralysis than destruction of the **secondary motor area** (area 6). Destruction of both areas produces the most complete form of contralateral paralysis.

Lesions of the **secondary motor area** alone produce difficulty in the performance of skilled movements, with little loss of strength.

The **Jacksonian epileptic seizure** is due to an irritative lesion of the primary motor area (area 4). The convulsion

begins in the part of the body represented in the primary motor area that is being irritated. The convulsive movement may be restricted to one part of the body, such as the face or the foot, or it may spread to involve many regions, depending on the spread of irritation of the primary motor area.

Muscle Spasticity

A discrete lesion of the primary motor cortex (area 4) results in little change in the muscle tone. However, larger lesions involving the primary and secondary motor areas (areas 4 and 6), which are the most common, result in muscle spasm. The explanation for this is that the primary motor cortex gives origin to corticospinal and corticonuclear tracts and the secondary motor cortex gives origin to extrapyramidal tracts that pass to the basal ganglia and the reticular formation. The corticospinal and corticonuclear tracts tend to increase muscle tone, but the extrapyramidal fibers transmit inhibitory impulses that lower muscle tone (see p. 170). Destruction of the secondary motor area removes the inhibitory influence and, consequently, the muscles are spastic.

The Frontal Eye Field

Destructive lesions of the frontal eye field of one hemisphere cause the two eyes to deviate to the side of the lesion and an inability to turn the eyes to the opposite side. The involuntary tracking movement of the eyes when following moving objects is unaffected, because the lesion does not involve the visual cortex in the occipital lobe.

Irritative lesions of the frontal eye field of one hemisphere cause the two eyes to periodically deviate to the opposite side of the lesion.

The Motor Speech Area of Broca

Destructive lesions in the left inferior frontal gyrus result in the loss of ability to produce speech, that is, **expressive aphasia**. The patients, however, retain the ability to think the words they wish to say, they can write the words, and they can understand their meaning when they see or hear them.

The Sensory Speech Area of Wernicke

Destructive lesions restricted to Wernicke's speech area in the dominant hemisphere produce a loss of ability to understand the spoken and written word, that is, **receptive aphasia**. Since Broca's area is unaffected, speech is unimpaired, and the patient can produce fluent speech. However, the patient is unaware of the meaning of the words he or she uses, and uses incorrect words or even nonexistent words. The patient is also unaware of any mistakes.

The Motor and Sensory Speech Areas

Destructive lesions involving both Broca's and Wernicke's speech areas result in loss of the production of speech and the understanding of the spoken and written word, that is, **global aphasia**.

Patients who have lesions involving the **insula** have difficulty in pronouncing phonemes in their proper order and usually produce sounds that are close to the target word but are not exactly correct.

The Dominant Angular Gyrus

Destructive lesions in the angular gyrus in the posterior parietal lobe (often considered a part of Wernicke's area) divide the pathway between the visual association area and the anterior part of Wernicke's area. This results in the patient being unable to read (**alexia**) or write (**agraphia**).

The Prefrontal Cortex

It is now generally agreed that destruction of the prefrontal region does not produce any marked loss of intelligence. It is an area of the cortex that is capable of associating experiences that are necessary for the production of abstract ideas, judgment, emotional feeling, and personality. Tumors or traumatic destruction of the prefrontal cortex result in the person's losing initiative and judgment. Emotional changes that occur include a tendency to euphoria. The patient no longer conforms to the accepted mode of social behavior and becomes careless of dress and appearance.

Prefrontal Cortex and Schizophrenia

The prefrontal cortex has a rich dopaminergic innervation. A failure of this innervation may be responsible for some of the symptoms of schizophrenia which include important disorders of thought. It has been shown with PET scans that the blood flow in the prefrontal cortex in schizophrenic patients challenged with executive type functions is much less than in normal individuals.

Frontal Leukotomy and Frontal Lobectomy

Frontal leukotomy (cutting the fiber tracts of the frontal lobe) and frontal lobectomy (removal of the frontal lobe) are surgical procedures that have been used to reduce the emotional responsiveness of patients with obsessive emotional states and intractable pain. The surgical technique was developed to remove the frontal association activity, so that past experience is not recalled and the possibilities of the future are not considered; thus introspection is lessened.

A patient suffering severe pain, such as may be experienced in the terminal stages of cancer, will still feel the pain following frontal lobectomy, but he or she will no longer worry about the pain and therefore will not suffer. It should be pointed out that the introduction of effective tranquilizing and mood-elevating drugs has made these operative procedures largely obsolete.

The Sensory Cortex

The lower centers of the brain, principally the thalamus, relay a large part of the sensory signals to the cerebral cortex for analysis. The sensory cortex is necessary for the appreciation of spatial recognition, recognition of relative intensity, and recognition of similarity and difference.

Lesions of the **primary somesthetic area** of the cortex result in contralateral sensory disturbances, which are most severe in the distal parts of the limbs. Crude painful, tactile, and thermal stimuli often return, but this is believed to be due to the function of the thalamus. The patient remains unable to judge degrees of warmth, unable to localize tactile stimuli accurately, and unable to judge weights of objects. Loss of muscle tone may also be a symptom of lesions of the sensory cortex.

Lesions of the secondary somesthetic area of the cortex do not cause recognizable sensory defects.

The Somesthetic Association Area

Lesions of the superior parietal lobule interfere with the patient's ability to combine touch, pressure, and proprioceptive impulses, so he or she is unable to appreciate texture, size, and form. This loss of integration of sensory impulses is called **astereognosis**. For example, with the eyes closed, the individual would be unable to recognize a key placed in the hand.

Destruction of the posterior part of the parietal lobe, which integrates somatic and visual sensations, will interfere with the appreciation of body image on the opposite side of the body. The individual may fail to recognize the opposite side of the body as his or her own. The patient may fail to wash it or dress it, or to shave that side of the face or legs.

The Primary Visual Area

Lesions involving the walls of the posterior part of one calcarine sulcus result in a loss of sight in the opposite visual field, that is, **crossed homonymous hemianopia**. It is interesting to note that the central part of the visual field, when tested, apparently is normal. This so-called macular sparing is probably due to the patient's shifting the eyes very slightly while the visual fields are being examined. The following clinical defects should be understood. Lesions of the upper half of one primary visual area, that is, the area above the calcarine sulcus, result in **inferior quadrantic hemianopia**, whereas lesions involving one visual area below the calcarine sulcus result in **superior quadrantic hemianopia**. Lesions of the occipital pole produce central scotomas. The most common causes of these lesions are vascular disorders, tumors, and injuries from gunshot wounds.

The Secondary Visual Area

Lesions of the secondary visual area result in a loss of ability to recognize objects seen in the opposite field of vision. The reason for this is that the area of cortex that stores past visual experiences has been lost.

The Primary Auditory Area

Because the primary auditory area in the inferior wall of the lateral sulcus receives nerve fibers from both cochleae, a lesion of one cortical area will produce slight bilateral loss of hearing, but the loss will be greater in the opposite ear. The main defect noted is a loss of ability to locate the source of the sound. Bilateral destruction of the primary auditory areas causes complete deafness.

The Secondary Auditory Area

Lesions of the cortex posterior to the primary auditory area in the lateral sulcus and in the superior temporal gyrus result in an inability to interpret sounds. The patient may experience **word deafness (acoustic verbal agnosia)**.

CEREBRAL DOMINANCE AND CEREBRAL DAMAGE

Although both hemispheres are almost identical in structure, in the majority of the adult population, handedness, perception of language, speech, spatial judgment, and areas of behavior are controlled by one hemisphere and not the other. About 90 percent of people are right-handed, and the control resides in the left hemisphere. The remainder is left-handed, and a few individuals are ambidextrous. In 90 percent of individuals, speech and understanding of spoken and written language are controlled by the left hemisphere. Thus, in most adults, the left cerebral hemisphere is dominant.

From a clinical point of view, the age at which cerebral dominance comes into effect is important. For example, when cerebral damage occurs before the child has learned to speak, speech usually develops and is maintained in the remaining intact hemisphere. This transference of speech control is much more difficult in older persons.

CEREBRAL CORTICAL POTENTIALS

Electrical recordings taken from inside neurons of the cerebral cortex show a negative resting potential of about 60 mV. The action potentials overshoot the zero potential. It is interesting to know that the resting potential shows marked fluctuation, which is probably due to the continuous but variable reception of afferent impulses from other neurons. Spontaneous electrical activity can be recorded from the cortical surface rather than intracellularly; such recordings are known as **electrocorticograms**. Similar recordings can be made by placing the electrodes on the scalp. The result of this latter procedure is referred to as the **electroencephalogram** (EEG). The changes of electrical potential recorded usually are very small and in the order of 50 µV. Characteristically, three frequency bands may be recognized in the normal individual; they are referred to as **alpha**, **beta**, and **delta rhythms**. Abnormalities of the electroencephalogram may be of great value clinically in helping to diagnose cerebral tumors, epilepsy, and cerebral abscess. An electrically silent cortex indicates cerebral death.

CONSCIOUSNESS

A conscious person is awake and aware of himself or herself and the surroundings. For normal consciousness, active functioning of two main parts of the nervous system—the reticular formation (in the brainstem) and the cerebral cortex—is necessary. The reticular formation is responsible for the state of wakefulness. The cerebral cortex is necessary for the state of awareness, that is, the state in which the individual can respond to stimuli and interact with the environment. Eye opening is a brainstem function; speech is a cerebral cortex function. Drugs that produce unconsciousness, such as anesthetics, selectively depress the **reticular alerting mechanism**, while those that cause wakefulness have a stimulating effect on this mechanism.

A physician should be able to recognize the different signs and symptoms associated with different stages of consciousness, namely, **lethargy**, **stupor**, and **coma** (unconsciousness). In a lethargic individual, the speech is slow, and voluntary movement is diminished and slow. The movement of the eyes is slow. A stupored patient will speak only if stimulated with painful stimuli. The voluntary movements are nearly absent, the eyes are closed, and there is very little spontaneous eye movement. A deeply stupored patient will not speak; there will be mass movements of different parts of the body in response to severe pain. The eyes will show even less spontaneous movement.

An unconscious patient will not speak and will respond only reflexly to painful stimuli, or not at all; the eyes are closed and do not move.

Clinically, it is not uncommon to observe a patient with, for example, intracranial bleeding pass progressively from consciousness to lethargy, stupor, and coma, and then, if recovery occurs, pass in the reverse direction. For these altered states of unconsciousness to occur, the thalamocortical system and the reticular formation must be either directly involved bilaterally or indirectly affected by distortion or pressure.

PERSISTENT VEGETATIVE STATE

A person can have an intact reticular formation but a nonfunctioning cerebral cortex. That person is awake (i.e., the eyes are open and move around) and has sleep-awake cycles; however, the person has no awareness and therefore cannot respond to stimuli such as a verbal command or pain. This condition, known as a **persistent vegetative state**, is usually seen following severe head injuries or an anoxic cerebral insult. Unfortunately, the lay observer thinks the patient is "conscious."

It is possible to have wakefulness without awareness; however, it is not possible to have awareness without wakefulness. The cerebral cortex requires the input from the reticular formation in order to function.

SLEEP

Sleep is a changed state of consciousness. The pulse rate, respiratory rate, and blood pressure fall; the eyes deviate upward; the pupils contract but react to light; the tendon reflexes are lost; and the plantar reflex may become extensor. A sleeping person is not, however, unconscious, because he or she may be awakened quickly by the cry of a child, for example, even though he or she has slept through the background noise of an air-conditioner.

Sleep is facilitated by reducing the sensory input and by fatigue. This results in decreased activity of the reticular formation and the thalamocortical activating mechanism. Whether this decreased activity is a passive phenomenon, or whether the reticular formation is actively inhibited, is not known.

EPILEPSY

Epilepsy is a symptom in which there is a sudden transitory disturbance of the normal physiology of the brain, usually the cerebral cortex, that ceases spontaneously and tends to recur. The condition is usually associated with a disturbance of normal electrical activity and in its most typical form is accompanied by seizures. In partial seizures, the abnormality occurs in only one part of the brain and the patient does not lose consciousness. In generalized seizures, the abnormal activity involves large areas of the brain bilaterally and the individual loses consciousness.

In some patients with generalized seizures, there may be nonconvulsive attacks, in which the patient suddenly stares blankly into space. This syndrome is referred to as **petit mal**. In the majority of patients with generalized seizures, there is a sudden loss of consciousness and there are tonic spasm and clonic contractions of the muscles. There are transient apnea and often loss of bowel and bladder control. The convulsions usually last from a few seconds to a few minutes.

In most patients with epilepsy the cause is unknown; in some there appears to be a hereditary predisposition; in a few, a local lesion, such as a cerebral tumor or scarring of the cortex following trauma, is the cause.

Clinical Problem Solving

1. During a practical class in pathology, a student was shown a slide illustrating a particular form of cerebral tumor. At the edge of the section there was a small area of the cerebral cortex. The instructor asked the student whether the tissue had been removed from a motor or sensory area of the cortex. What is the main difference in structure between the motor and sensory areas of the cerebral cortex?

2. A 43-year-old man was examined by a neurologist for a suspected brain tumor. The patient was tested for stereognosis, that is, the appreciation of form in three dimensions. With the patient's eyes closed, a hairbrush was placed in his right hand and he was asked to recognize the object. He was unable to recognize the brush even after the neurologist moved the brush about in the patient's hand. On opening his eyes, the patient immediately recognized the brush. (a) Name the area of the cerebral cortex likely to be diseased in this patient. (b) Do you think that it is necessary for the object to be moved around in the patient's hand?

3. A 65-year-old man attended his physician because he noticed that for the past 3 weeks he had been dragging his right foot when walking. On physical examination, he was found to have an increase in tone of the flexor muscles of the right arm, and when he walked he

tended to hold his right arm adducted and flexed. He also held his right fist tightly clenched. On study of the patient's gait, he was seen to have difficulty in flexing his right hip and knee. There was slight but definite weakness and increased tone of the muscles of the right leg. As the patient walked, he was noted to move his right leg in a semicircle and to place the forefoot on the ground before the heel. Examination of the right shoe showed evidence of increased wear beneath the right toes. Given that this patient had a cerebrovascular lesion involving the cerebral cortex, which area of the cortex was involved to cause these symptoms?

4. While examining an unconscious patient, a physician noted that when the patient's head was gently rotated to the right the two eyes deviated to the left. On rotation of the patient's head to the left, the patient's eyes still looked to the left. Which area of the cortex is likely to be damaged in this patient?

5. A 25-year-old soldier was wounded by an antipersonnel bomb in Vietnam. A small piece of shrapnel entered the right side of his skull over the precentral gyrus. Five years later, he was examined by a physician during a routine physical checkup and was found to have weakness of the left leg. The physician could not detect any increase in muscle tone in his left leg. Explain why it is

that most patients with damage to the motor area of the cerebral cortex have spastic muscle paralysis while in a few the muscle tone remains normal.

6. A distinguished neurobiologist gave a lecture on the physiology of the cerebral cortex to the freshman medical student class. Having reviewed the structure of the different areas of the cerebral cortex and the functional localization of the cerebral cortex, he stated that our knowledge of the cytoarchitecture of the human cerebral cortex has contributed very little to our understanding of the normal functional activity of the cerebral cortex. Do you agree with his statement? What do you understand by the term "the vertical chain theory"?

7. An 18-year-old boy received a gunshot wound that severely damaged his left precentral gyrus. On recovering from the incident, he left the hospital with a spastic paralysis of the right arm and leg. The patient, however, still possessed some coarse voluntary movements of the right shoulder, hip, and knee. Explain the presence of these residual movements on the right side.

8. A 53-year-old professor and chairman of a department of anatomy received a severe head injury while rock climbing. During the ascent of a crevasse, his companion's ice axe fell from his belt and struck the professor's head, causing a depressed fracture of the frontal bone. After convalescing from his accident, the professor

returned to his position in the medical school. It quickly became obvious to the faculty and the student body that the professor's social behavior had changed dramatically. His lectures, although amusing, no longer had direction. Although previously a smartly dressed man, he now had an unkempt appearance. The organization of the department started to deteriorate rapidly. Finally, he was removed from office after being found one morning urinating into the trash basket in one of the classrooms. Use your knowledge of neuroanatomy to explain the professor's altered behavior.

9. A 50-year-old woman with a cerebrovascular lesion, on questioning, was found to experience difficulty in understanding spoken speech, although she fully understood written speech. Which area of the cerebral cortex was damaged?

10. A 62-year-old man, on recovering from a stroke, was found to have difficulty in understanding written speech (alexia) but could easily understand spoken speech and written symbols. Which area of the cerebral cortex is damaged in this patient?

11. What is understood by the following terms: (a) *coma*, (b) *sleep*, and (c) *electroencephalogram?* Name three neurological conditions in which the diagnosis may be assisted by the use of an electroencephalogram.

Answers to Clinical Problem Solving

1. The cerebral cortex is made up of six identifiable layers. In the motor cortex in the precentral gyrus, there is a lack of granular cells in the second and fourth layers, and in the somesthetic cortex in the postcentral gyrus, there is a lack of pyramidal cells in the third and fifth layers. The motor cortex is thicker than the sensory cortex.

2. (a) The area likely to be diseased is the left parietal lobe with advanced destruction of the superior parietal lobule. This is the somesthetic association area, where the sensations of touch, pressure, and proprioception are integrated. (b) Yes. It is essential that the patient be allowed to finger the object so that these different sensations can be appreciated.

3. This patient had a cerebrovascular lesion involving the left precentral gyrus. The damage to the pyramidal cells that give origin to the corticospinal fibers was responsible for the right-sided paralysis. The increased tone of the paralyzed muscles was due to the loss of inhibition caused by involvement of the extrapyramidal fibers (see p. 293).

4. Destructive lesions of the frontal eye field of the left cerebral hemisphere caused the two eyes to deviate to the side of the lesion and an inability to turn the eyes to the opposite side. The frontal eye field is thought to control voluntary scanning movements of the eye and is independent of visual stimuli.

5. A small discrete lesion of the primary motor cortex results in little change in muscle tone. Larger lesions involving the primary and secondary motor areas, which are the most common, result in muscle spasm. The explanation for this is given on page 293.

6. As the result of the patient and extensive histological research of Brodmann, Campbell, Economo, and the Vogts, it has been possible to divide the cerebral cortex into areas that have a different microscopic arrangement and different types of cells. These cortical maps are fundamentally similar and the one proposed by Brodmann is used widely. Because the functional significance of many areas of the human cerebral cortex is not known, it has not been possible to closely correlate structure with function. In general, it can be said that the motor cortices are thicker than the sensory cortices, and that the motor cortex has less prominent second and fourth granular layers and has large pyramidal cells in the fifth layer. Other areas with a different structure may have similar functional roles. More recent studies using electrophysiological techniques have indicated that it is more accurate to divide the cerebral cortex according to its thalamocortical projections. The vertical chain mechanism of the cerebral cortex is fully described on page 286.

7. In this patient, the persistence of coarse voluntary movements of the right shoulder, hip, and knee joints

can be explained on the basis that coarse postural movements are controlled by the premotor area of the cortex and the basal ganglia and these areas were spared in this patient.

8. The professor's altered behavior was due to a severe lesion involving both frontal lobes of the cerebrum secondary to the depressed fracture of the frontal bone. While destruction of the prefrontal cortex does not cause a marked loss of intelligence, it does result in the individual losing initiative and drive, and often the patient no longer conforms to the accepted modes of social behavior.

9. The understanding of spoken speech requires the normal functioning of the secondary auditory area, which is situated posterior to the primary auditory area in the lateral sulcus and in the superior temporal gyrus. This area is believed to be necessary for the interpretation of sounds, and the information is passed on to the sensory speech area of Wernicke.

10. The understanding of written speech requires the normal functioning of the secondary visual area of the cerebral cortex, which is situated in the walls of the posterior part of the calcarine sulcus on the medial and lateral surfaces of the cerebral hemisphere. The function of the secondary visual area is to relate visual information received by the primary visual area to past visual experiences. This information is then passed on to the dominant angular gyrus and relayed to the anterior part of Wernicke's speech area (see p. 290).

11. (a) *Coma* is the term applied to an unconscious patient. The patient will not speak and will respond only reflexly to painful stimuli. In deeply comatose individuals, there will be no response. The eyes are closed and do not move. (b) *Sleep* is a changed state of consciousness; it is discussed on page 296. (c) An *electroencephalogram* (EEG) is a recording of the electrical activity of the cerebral cortex made by placing electrodes on the scalp. Detection of abnormalities of the alpha, beta, and delta rhythms may assist in the diagnosis of cerebral tumors, epilepsy, and cerebral abscesses.

Review Questions

Directions: Each of the numbered items in this section is followed by answers that are positively phrased. Select the ONE lettered answer that is an EXCEPTION.

1. The following statements concerning the cerebral cortex are correct **except:**
   (a) The cerebral cortex is thickest over the crest of a gyrus and thinnest in the depth of a sulcus.
   (b) The largest giant pyramidal cells are found in the precentral gyrus.
   (c) In the visual cortex, the outer band of Baillarger is so thick it can be seen with the naked eye.
   (d) The molecular layer is the most superficial layer of the cerebral cortex and is composed of the small cell bodies of the granular cells.
   (e) From a functional point of view the cerebral cortex is organized into vertical units of activity.

2. The following statements concerning the precentral area of the frontal lobe of the cerebral cortex are true **except:**
   (a) The posterior region is known as the primary motor area.
   (b) The primary motor area is responsible for skilled movements on the opposite side of the body.
   (c) The function of the premotor area is to store programs of motor activity which are conveyed to the primary motor area for the execution of movements.
   (d) Individual muscles are represented in the primary motor area.
   (e) The area of cortex controlling a particular movement is proportional to the skill involved.

3. The following statements concerning the motor speech area of Broca are true **except:**
   (a) In most individuals this area is important on the left or dominant hemisphere.
   (b) Broca's speech area brings about the formation of words by its connections with the primary motor area.
   (c) It is not connected to the sensory speech area of Wernicke.
   (d) It is located in the inferior frontal gyrus between the anterior and ascending rami and the ascending and posterior rami of the lateral fissure.
   (e) Brodmann's areas 44 and 45 represent the motor speech area.

4. The following statements concerning the primary somesthetic area are true **except:**
   (a) It occupies the postcentral gyrus.
   (b) Histologically, it contains large numbers of granular cells and few pyramidal cells.
   (c) The opposite half of the body is represented inverted.
   (d) Although most sensations reach the cortex from the contralateral side of the body, sensations from the hand and mouth go to both sides.
   (e) The area extends onto the posterior part of the paracentral lobule.

5. The following statements concerning the visual areas of the cortex are true **except:**
   (a) The primary visual area is located in the walls of the parieto-occipital sulcus.
   (b) The visual cortex receives afferent fibers from the lateral geniculate body.

(c) The right half of the visual field is represented in the visual cortex of the left cerebral hemisphere.
(d) The superior retinal quadrants pass to the inferior portion of the visual cortex.
(e) The secondary visual area (Brodmann's areas 18 and 19) surrounds the primary visual area on the medial and lateral surfaces of the hemisphere.

6. The following statements concerning the superior temporal gyrus are correct **except:**
 (a) The primary auditory area is situated in the inferior wall of the lateral sulcus.
 (b) The main projection fibers to the primary auditory area arise from the thalamus.
 (c) The sensory speech area of Wernicke is localized in the superior temporal gyrus in the dominant hemisphere.
 (d) A unilateral lesion of the auditory area produces partial deafness in both ears.
 (e) The primary auditory area is sometimes referred to as Brodmann's areas 41 and 42.

7. The following statements concerning the association areas of the cerebral cortex are correct **except:**
 (a) They form a large area of the cortical surface.
 (b) The prefrontal area is concerned with the makeup of the individual's personality.
 (c) They are concerned with the interpretation of sensory experiences.
 (d) An appreciation of the body image is assembled in the posterior parietal cortex and the right side of the body is represented in the left hemisphere.
 (e) The association areas have only four layers of cortex.

8. The following statements concerning cerebral dominance are correct **except:**
 (a) The cortical gyri of the dominant and nondominant hemispheres are arranged differently.
 (b) More than 90 percent of the adult population is right-handed and therefore is left hemisphere-dominant.
 (c) About 96 percent of the adult population is left hemisphere-dominant for speech.
 (d) The nondominant hemisphere interprets spatial perception, recognition of faces, and music.
 (e) After the first decade of life the dominance of the cerebral hemispheres becomes fixed.

Directions: Matching Questions

In Figure 8-9, match the numbers listed on the left with the most likely lettered functional areas of the cerebral cortex listed on the right. Each lettered option may be selected once, more than once, or not at all.
 9. Number 1 (a) Primary motor area
10. Number 2 (b) Secondary auditory area
11. Number 3 (c) Frontal eye field
12. Number 4 (d) Primary somesthetic area
        (e) None of the above

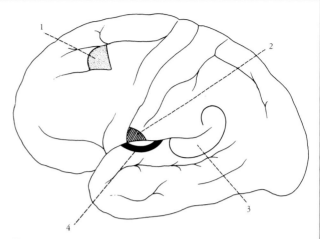

Figure 8–9 Lateral view of the left cerebral hemisphere.

In Figure 8-10, match the numbers listed on the left with the most likely lettered functional areas of the cerebral cortex listed on the right. Each lettered option may be selected once, more than once, or not at all.
13. Number 1 (a) Premotor area
14. Number 2 (b) Primary somesthetic area
15. Number 3 (c) Primary visual area
16. Number 4 (d) Primary motor area
        (e) None of the above

Directions: Read the case histories then answer the questions. You will be required to select ONE BEST lettered answer.

A 54-year-old woman was seen by a neurologist because her sister had noticed a sudden change in her behavior. On questioning, the patient stated that after waking up from a deep sleep about a week ago, she noticed that the left side of her body did not feel as if it belonged to her. Later, the feeling worsened and she became unaware of the existence of her left side. Her sister told the neurologist that the patient now neglects to wash the left side of her body.

17. The neurologist examined the patient and found the following most likely signs **except:**
 (a) It was noted that the patient did not look toward her left side.
 (b) She readily reacted to sensory stimulation of her skin on the left side.
 (c) On being asked to move her left leg, she promptly did so.
 (d) There was definite evidence of muscular weakness of the upper and lower limbs on the left side.

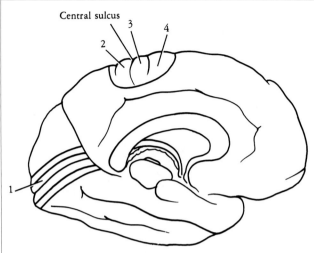

Central sulcus

Figure 8–10 Medial view of the left cerebral hemisphere.

(e) On being asked to walk across the examining room, she tended not to use her left leg as much as her right leg.
18. The neurologist made the following likely conclusions **except:**
    (a) The diagnosis of left hemiasomatognosia (loss of appreciation of the left side of the body) was made.
    (b) This condition probably resulted from a lesion of the left parietal lobe.
    (c) In addition, the patient exhibited left hemiakinesia (unilateral motor neglect).
    (d) There was probably a lesion in areas 6 and 8 of the medial and lateral premotor regions of the right frontal lobe.
    (e) The failure to look toward the left side (visual extinction) suggested a lesion existed in the right parieto-occipital lobes.

 Answers to Review Questions

1. D
2. D
3. C
4. D
5. A
6. B
7. E
8. A
9. C
10. E
11. E

12. B
13. C
14. B
15. D
16. A
17. D. The patient exhibited no weakness of her muscles on the left side in spite of the fact that her sister stated that she tended not to use her left leg.
18. B. An MRI revealed a tumor in the right parieto-occipital lobes; a further lesion was present in the right frontal lobe.

ADDITIONAL READING

Adams, J.H., and Duchen, L.W. *Greenfield's Neuropathology.* New York, Oxford University Press, 1992.

Bates, D. The management of medical coma. *J. Neurol. Neurosurg. Psychiatry* 56:589, 1993.

Benson, D.F. *The Neurology of Thinking.* New York, Oxford University Press,1994.

Bloodstein, O. *Speech Pathology: An Introduction.* Boston: Houghton Mifflin, 1979.

Brodmann, K. *Vergleichende Lokalisationslebre der Grossbirnrinde.* Leipzig: Barth, 1909.

Campbell, A. W. *Histological Studies on the Localization of Cerebral Function.* Cambridge, Massachusetts: Harvard University Press, 1905.

Cowan, N. *Attention and Memory: An Integrated Framework.* New York, Oxford University Press, 1995.

De Gelder, B., and Morais, J. *Speech and Reading.* Hillsdale, NJ, Lawrence Erlbaum Assoc. Inc., 1995.

Easton, J. D. Coma and Related Disorders. In J. H. Stein (ed.), *Internal Medicine* (4th ed.). St. Louis: Mosby, 1993.

Guyton, A. C. and Hall, J.E. *Textbook of Medical Physiology* (9th ed.). Philadelphia: Saunders, 1996.

Iaccino, J, F. *Left Brain-Right Brain Differences: Inquiries, Evidence, and New Approaches.* Hillsdale, NJ , Lawrence Erlbaum Assoc., 1993.

Jackson, J. H. Selected Writings of John Hughlings Jackson. In J. Taylor (ed.), *On Epilepsy and Epileptiform Convulsions.* Vol. 1. London: Hodder & Stoughton, 1931.

Jasper, H. H., Ward, A. A., and Pope, A. (eds.), *Basic Mechanisms of the Epilepsies.* Boston: Little, Brown, 1969.

Kandel, E.R., Schwartz, J.H., and Jessell, T.M. *Principles of Neural Science,* 4ed. McGraw-Hill, New York, 2000.

Kapur, N. *Memory Disorders in Clinical Practice.* Hillsdale, NJ, Lawrence Erlbaum Assoc., 1994.

Levin, H.S., et al. *Frontal Lobe Function and Dysfunction.* New York, Oxford University Press,1991.

Penfield, W., and Boldrey, E. Somatic motor and sensory representation in the cerebral cortex of man as studied by electrical stimulation. *Brain* 60:389, 1937.

Penfield, W., and Rasmussen, T. *The Cerebral Cortex of Man: A Clinical Study of Localization of Function.* New York and London: Macmillan, 1950.

Penfield, W., and Roberts, L. *Speech and Brain Mechanisms.* Princeton, New Jersey: Princeton University Press, 1959.

Porter, R. The Cerebral Cortex and Control of Movement Performance. In M. Swash and C. Kennard (eds.), *Scientific Basis of Clinical Neurology.* Edinburgh: Churchill Livingstone, 1985. P. 19.

Rhoades, R. A., and Tanner, G. A. *Medical Physiology.* Boston: Little, Brown, 1995.

Seeman, P., Gaun, H.C., Van Tol, H.H.M. Dopamine D4 Receptors Elevated in Schizophrenia. *Nature* 365:441-445,1993.

Sholl, D. A. *Organization of the Cerebral Cortex.* London: Methuen, 1956.

Snell, R. S., and Smith, M. S. *Clinical Anatomy for Emergency Medicine.* St. Louis: Mosby, 1993.

Sperry, R. W. Lateral Specialization in the Surgically Separated Hemispheres. In *The Neurosciences, Third Study Program.* Cambridge, Massachusetts: MIT Press, 1974. P. 5.

Williams, P. L., et al. *Gray's Anatomy* (38th Br. ed.). New York and Edinburgh: Churchill Livingstone, 1995.

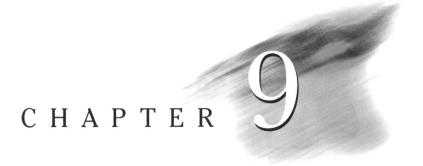

CHAPTER 9

The Reticular Formation and the Limbic System

A 24-year-old medical student was rushed by ambulance to the emergency department after an accident on his motorcycle. On examination he was found to be unconscious and showed evidence of severe injury to the right side of his head. He failed to respond to the spoken word and he did not make any response to deep painful pressure applied over his supraorbital nerve. The plantar reflexes were extensor and the corneal, tendon, and pupillary reflexes were absent. It was clear that the patient was in a deep coma. Further neurological examination revealed nothing that might add to the diagnosis. A CT scan showed a large depressed fracture of the right parietal bone of the skull.

After a week in the intensive care unit, the patient's condition changed. He suddenly showed signs of being awake but not aware of his environment or inner needs. To the delight of his family he followed them with his eyes and responded in a limited manner to primitive postural and reflex movements; he did not, however, speak and did not respond to commands. Although he had sleep-awake cycles, he did not respond appropriately to pain. The patient's neurological condition was unchanged 6 months later.

The neurologist determined that the patient was awake but not aware of his surroundings. He explained to the relatives that the part of the brain referred to as the reticular formation in the brainstem had survived the accident and was responsible for the patient apparently being awake and able to breathe without assistance. However, the tragedy was that his cerebral cortex was dead and the patient would remain in this vegetative state.

CHAPTER OBJECTIVES

Not so very long ago, the reticular system was believed to be a vague network of nerve cells and fibers occupying the central core of the brainstem with no particular function. Today it is known to play a key role in many important activities of the nervous system.

The limbic system was a term loosely used to describe the part of the brain between the cerebral cortex and the hypothalamus, a little understood area of the brain. Today it is known to play a vital role in emotion, behavior, drive, and memory. This chapter provides a brief overview of the structure and function of the reticular formation and presents in the simplest terms the parts of the limbic system and its functions.

RETICULAR FORMATION

The reticular formation, as its name would suggest, resembles a net (reticular) that is made up of nerve cells and nerve fibers. The net extends up through the axis of the central nervous system from the spinal cord to the cerebrum. It is strategically placed among the important nerve tracts and nuclei. It receives input from most of the sensory systems and has efferent fibers that descend and influence nerve cells at all levels of the central nervous system. The exceptionally long dendrites of the neurons of the reticular formation permit input from widely placed ascending and descending pathways. Through its many connections it can influence skeletal muscle activity, somatic and visceral sensations, the autonomic and endocrine systems, and even the level of consciousness.

General Arrangement

The reticular formation consists of a deeply placed continuous network of nerve cells and fibers that extend from the spinal cord, through the medulla, the pons, the midbrain, the subthalamus, the hypothalamus, and the thalamus. The diffuse network may be divided into three longitudinal columns, the first occupying the median plane, called the **median column,** and consisting of intermediate-size neurons, the second called the **medial column** containing large neurons, and the third or **lateral column** containing mainly small neurons (Fig. 9-1).

With the classic neuronal staining techniques, the groups of neurons are poorly defined and it is difficult to trace an anatomical pathway through the network. However, with the new techniques of neurochemistry and cytochemical localization, the reticular formation is shown to contain highly organized groups of transmitter-specific cells that can influence functions in specific areas of the central nervous system. The monoaminergic groups of cells, for example, are located in well-defined areas throughout the reticular formation.

Polysynaptic pathways exist and both crossed and uncrossed ascending and descending pathways are present, involving many neurons that serve both somatic and visceral functions.

Inferiorly, the reticular formation is continuous with the interneurons of the gray matter of the spinal cord, while superiorly impulses are relayed to the cerebral cortex; a substantial projection of fibers also leaves the reticular formation to enter the cerebellum.

Afferent Projections

Many different afferent pathways project onto the reticular formation from most parts of the central nervous system (Fig. 9-2). From the spinal cord there are the spinoreticular tracts, the spinothalamic tracts, and the medial lemniscus. From the cranial nerve nuclei there are ascending afferent tracts which include the vestibular, acoustic, and visual

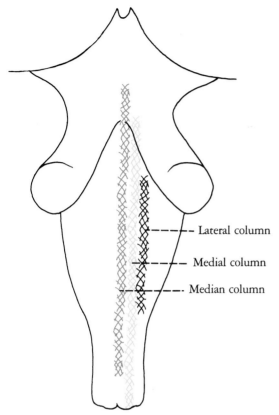

Figure 9–1 Diagram showing the approximate positions of the median, medial, and lateral columns of the reticular formation in the brainstem.

pathways. From the cerebellum, there is the cerebelloreticular pathway. From the subthalamic, hypothalamic, and thalamic nuclei and from the corpus striatum and the limbic system there are further afferent tracts. Other important afferent fibers arise in the primary motor cortex of the frontal lobe and from the somesthetic cortex of the parietal lobe.

Efferent Projections

Multiple efferent pathways extend down to the brainstem and spinal cord through the reticulobulbar and reticulospinal tracts to neurons in the motor nuclei of the cranial nerves and the anterior horn cells of the spinal cord. Other descending pathways extend to the sympathetic outflow and the craniosacral parasympathetic outflow of the autonomic nervous system. Additional pathways extend to the corpus striatum, the cerebellum, the red nucleus, the substantia nigra, the tectum, and the nuclei of the thalamus, subthalamus, and hypothalamus. Most regions of the cerebral cortex receive efferent fibers as well.

Functions of the Reticular Formation

From the previous description of the vast number of connections of the reticular formation to all parts of the nervous system, it is not surprising to find that the functions are many. A few of the more important functions are considered here.

1. **Control of skeletal muscle.** Through the reticulospinal and reticulobulbar tracts, the reticular formation can influence the activity of the alpha and gamma motor neurons. Thus the reticular formation can modulate muscle tone and reflex activity. It can also bring about reciprocal inhibition; for example, when the flexor muscles contract, the antagonistic extensors relax. The reticular formation, assisted by the vestibular apparatus of the inner ear and the vestibular spinal tract, plays an important role in maintaining the tone of the antigravity muscles when standing. The so-called respiratory centers of the brainstem, described by neurophysiologists as being in the control of the respiratory muscles, are now considered part of the reticular formation.

   The reticular formation is important in controlling the muscles of facial expression when associated with emotion. For example, when a person smiles or laughs in response to a joke the motor control is provided by the reticular formation on both sides of the brain. The descending tracts are separate from the corticobulbar fibers. This means that a person who has suffered a stroke that involves the corticobulbar fibers and exhibits facial paralysis on the lower part of the face is still able to smile symmetrically (See page 360).

2. **Control of somatic and visceral sensations.** By virtue of its central location in the cerebrospinal axis, the reticular formation can influence all ascending pathways that pass to supraspinal levels. The influence may be facilitative or inhibitory. In particular, the reticular formation may have a key role in the "gating mechanism" for the control of pain perception (see p. 149).

3. **Control of the autonomic nervous system.** Higher control of the autonomic nervous system, from the cerebral cortex, hypothalamus, and other subcortical nuclei, can be exerted by the reticulobulbar and reticulospinal tracts, which descend to the sympathetic outflow and the parasympathetic craniosacral outflow.

4. **Control of the endocrine nervous system.** Either directly or indirectly through the hypothalamic nuclei, the reticular formation can influence the synthesis or release of releasing or release-inhibiting factors and thereby control the activity of the hypophysis cerebri.

5. **Influence on the biological clocks.** By means of its multiple afferent and efferent pathways to the hypothalamus, the reticular formation probably influences the biological rhythms.

6. **The reticular activating system.** Arousal and the level of consciousness are controlled by the reticular formation. Multiple ascending pathways carrying sensory information to higher centers are channeled through the reticular formation, which in turn projects this information to different parts of the cerebral cortex, causing a sleeping person to awaken. In fact, it is now believed that the state of consciousness is dependent on the continuous projection of sensory information to the cortex.

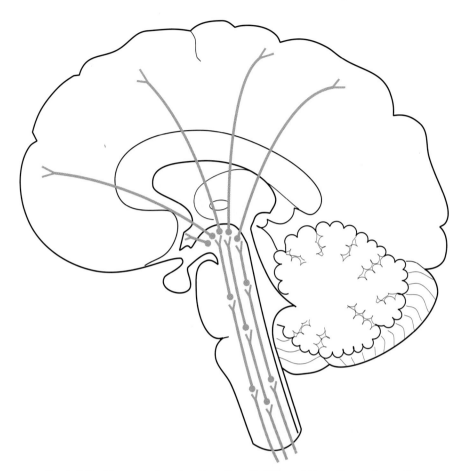

Figure 9–2 Diagram showing the afferent fibers of the reticular formation.

Different degrees of wakefulness seem to depend on the degree of activity of the reticular formation.

From the above description it must be apparent that in the network of neurons in the cerebrospinal axis, almost totally ignored in the past, is now being shown to influence practically all activities of the body.

 LIMBIC SYSTEM
....

The word *limbic* means border or margin and the term *limbic system* was loosely used to include a group of structures that lie in the border zone between the cerebral cortex and the hypothalamus. Now it is recognized, as the result of research, that the limbic system is involved with many other structures beyond the border zone in the control of emotion, behavior, and drive; it also appears to be important to memory.

Anatomically, the limbic structures include the subcallosal, the cingulate, and the parahippocampal gyri, the hippocampal formation, the amygdaloid nucleus, the mammillary bodies, and the anterior thalamic nucleus (Fig. 9-3). The alveus, the fimbria, the fornix, the mammillothalamic tract, and the stria terminalis constitute the connecting pathways of this system.

Hippocampal Formation

The hippocampal formation consists of the hippocampus, the dentate gyrus, and the parahippocampal gyrus.

The **hippocampus** is a curved elevation of gray matter that extends throughout the entire length of the floor of the inferior horn of the lateral ventricle (Fig. 9-4). Its anterior end is expanded to form the **pes hippocampus.** It is named hippocampus because it resembles a sea horse in coronal section. The convex ventricular surface is covered with ependyma, beneath which lies a thin layer of white matter called the **alveus** (Fig. 9-5). The alveus consists of nerve fibers that have originated in the hippocampus and these converge medially to form a bundle called the **fimbria** (Figs. 9-4 and 9-5). The fimbria in turn becomes continuous with the crus of the fornix (Fig. 9-4). The hippocampus terminates posteriorly beneath the splenium of the corpus callosum.

The **dentate gyrus** is a narrow, notched band of gray matter that lies between the fimbria of the hippocampus and the parahippocampal gyrus (Fig. 9-4). Posteriorly, the gyrus accompanies the fimbria almost to the splenium of the corpus callosum and becomes continuous with the **indusium griseum.** The indusium griseum is a thin, vestigial layer of gray matter that covers the superior surface of the corpus callosum (Fig. 9-6). Embedded in the superior

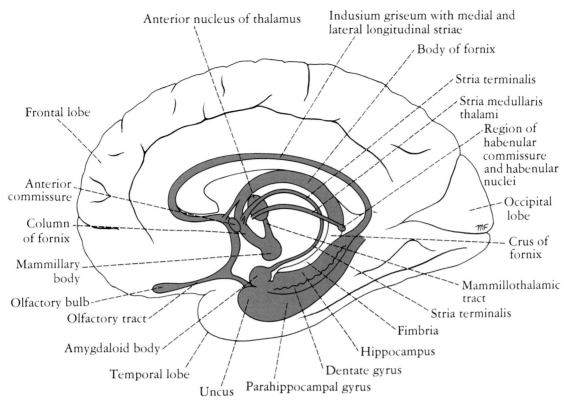

Figure 9–3 Medial aspect of the right cerebral hemisphere, showing structures that form the limbic system.

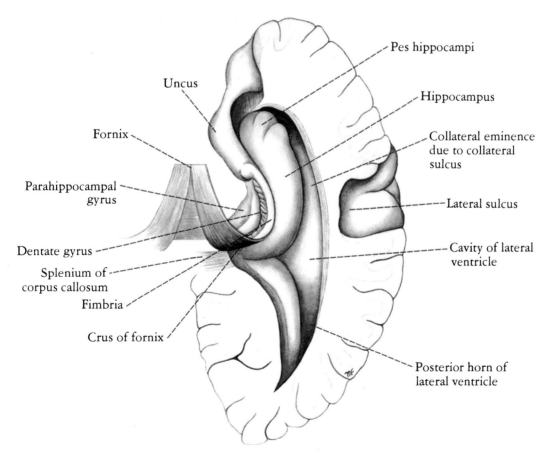

Figure 9–4 Dissection of the right cerebral hemisphere exposing the cavity of the lateral ventricle, showing the hippocampus, the dentate gyrus, and the fornix.

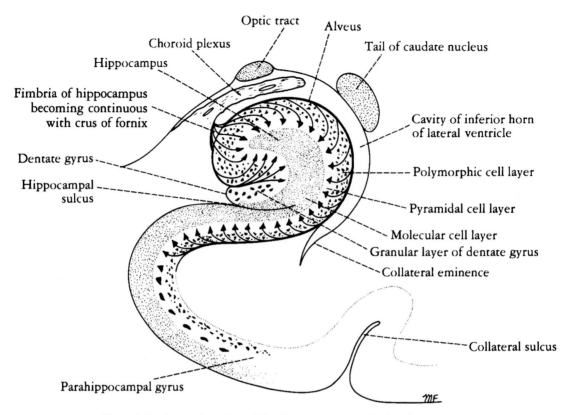

Figure 9–5 Coronal section of the hippocampus and related structures.

surface of the indusium griseum are two slender bundles of white fibers on each side called the **medial** and **lateral longitudinal striae.** The striae are the remains of the white matter of the vestigial indusium griseum. Anteriorly, the dentate gyrus is continued into the **uncus.**

The **parahippocampal gyrus** lies between the hippocampal fissure and the collateral sulcus and is continuous with the hippocampus along the medial edge of the temporal lobe (Figs. 9-4 and 9-5).

Amygdaloid Nucleus

The amygdaloid nucleus is so named because it resembles an almond. It is situated partly anterior and partly superior to the tip of the inferior horn of the lateral ventricle (Fig. 7-15). It is fused with the tip of the tail of the caudate nucleus, which has passed anteriorly in the roof of the inferior horn of the lateral ventricle. The stria terminalis emerges from its posterior aspect. The mammillary bodies and the anterior nucleus of the thalamus are considered elsewhere in this text.

Connecting Pathways of the Limbic System

These pathways are the alveus, the fimbria, the fornix, the mammillothalamic tract, and the stria terminalis.

The **alveus** consists of a thin layer of white matter that lies on the superior or ventricular surface of the hippocam-

pus (Fig. 9-5). It is composed of nerve fibers that originate in the hippocampal cortex. The fibers converge on the medial border of the hippocampus to form a bundle called the **fimbria.**

The fimbria now leaves the posterior end of the hippocampus as the **crus of the fornix** (Fig. 9-4). The crus from each side curves posteriorly and superiorly beneath the splenium of the corpus callosum and around the posterior surface of the thalamus. The two crura now converge to form the **body of the fornix,** which is applied closely to the undersurface of the corpus callosum (Fig. 9-3). As the two crura come together, they are connected by transverse fibers called the **commissure of the fornix** (Fig. 7-17). These fibers decussate and join the hippocampi of the two sides.

Anteriorly, the body of the fornix is connected to the undersurface of the corpus callosum by the **septum pellucidum.** Inferiorly, the body of the fornix is related to the tela choroidea and the ependymal roof of the third ventricle.

The body of the fornix splits anteriorly into two anterior **columns of the fornix,** each of which curves anteriorly and inferiorly over the interventricular foramen (foramen of Monro). Then each column disappears into the lateral wall of the third ventricle to reach the **mammillary body** (Fig. 9-3).

The **mammillothalamic tract** provides important connections between the mammillary body and the anterior nuclear group of the thalamus.

The **stria terminalis** emerges from the posterior aspect of the amygdaloid nucleus and runs as a bundle of nerve

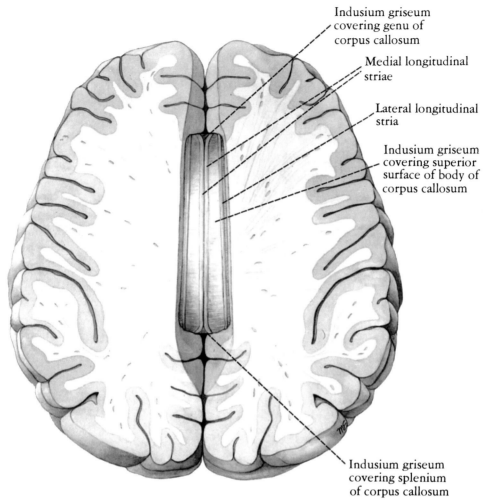

Indusium griseum
covering genu of
corpus callosum

Medial longitudinal
striae

Lateral longitudinal
stria

Indusium griseum
covering superior
surface of body of
corpus callosum

Indusium griseum
covering splenium
of corpus callosum

Figure 9–6   Dissection of both cerebral hemispheres, showing the superior surface of the corpus callosum.

fibers posteriorly in the roof of the inferior horn of the lateral ventricle on the medial side of the tail of the caudate nucleus (Fig. 9-3). It follows the curve of the caudate nucleus and comes to lie in the floor of the body of the lateral ventricle.

Structure of the Hippocampus and the Dentate Gyrus

The cortical structure of the parahippocampal gyrus is six-layered (Fig. 9-5). As the cortex is traced into the hippocampus, there is a gradual transition from a six- to a three-layered arrangement. These three layers are the superficial **molecular layer,** consisting of nerve fibers and scattered small neurons; the **pyramidal layer,** consisting of many large pyramid-shaped neurons; and the inner **polymorphic layer,** which is similar in structure to the polymorphic layer of the cortex seen elsewhere.

The dentate gyrus also has three layers but the pyramidal layer is replaced by the granular layer (Fig. 9-5). The granular layer is composed of densely arranged rounded or oval

neurons that give rise to axons that terminate upon the dendrites of the pyramidal cells in the hippocampus. A few of the axons join the fimbria and enter the fornix.

Afferent Connections of the Hippocampus

Afferent connections of the hippocampus may be divided into six groups (Fig. 9-7):

1. Fibers arising in the cingulate gyrus pass to the hippocampus.
2. Fibers arising from the septal nuclei (nuclei lying within the midline close to the anterior commissure) pass posterior in the fornix to the hippocampus.
3. Fibers arising from one hippocampus pass across the midline to the opposite hippocampus in the commissure of the fornix.
4. Fibers from the indusium griseum pass posteriorly in the longitudinal striae to the hippocampus.

5. Fibers from the entorhinal area or olfactory associated cortex pass to the hippocampus.
6. Fibers arising from the dentate and parahippocampal gyri travel to the hippocampus.

Efferent Connections of the Hippocampus

Axons of the large pyramidal cells of the hippocampus emerge to form the alveus and the fimbria. The fimbria continues as the crus of the fornix. The two crura converge to form the body of the fornix. The body of the fornix splits into the two columns of the fornix, which curve downward and forward in front of the interventricular foramina. The fibers within the fornix are distributed to the following regions (Fig. 9-7):

1. Fibers pass posterior to the anterior commissure to enter the mammillary body, where they end in the medial nucleus.
2. Fibers pass posterior to the anterior commissure to end in the anterior nuclei of the thalamus.
3. Fibers pass posterior to the anterior commissure to enter the tegmentum of the midbrain.
4. Fibers pass anterior to the anterior commissure to end in the septal nuclei, the lateral preoptic area, and the anterior part of the hypothalamus.
5. Fibers join the stria medullaris thalami to reach the habenular nuclei.

Consideration of the above complex anatomical pathways indicates that the structures comprising the limbic system not only are interconnected, but also send projection fibers to many different parts of the nervous system. Physiologists now recognize the importance of the hypothalamus as being the major output pathway of the limbic system.

Functions of the Limbic System

The limbic system, via the hypothalamus and its connections with the outflow of the autonomic nervous system and its control of the endocrine system, is able to influence many aspects of emotional behavior. These include particularly the reactions of fear and anger and the emotions associated with sexual behavior.

There is also evidence that the hippocampus is concerned with converting recent memory to long term memory. A lesion of the hippocampus results in the individual being unable to store long term memory. Memory for remote past events before the lesion developed is unaffected. This condition is called **anterograde amnesia.**

There is no evidence that the limbic system has an olfactory function. The various afferent and efferent connections of the limbic system provide pathways for the integration and effective homeostatic responses to a wide variety of environmental stimuli.

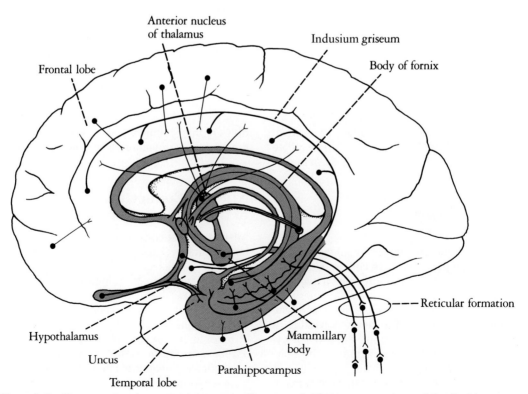

Figure 9–7 Diagram showing some important afferent and efferent connections of the limbic system.

CLINICAL NOTES

RETICULAR FORMATION

The reticular formation is a continuous network of nerve cells and fibers that extend through the neuroaxis from the spinal cord to the cerebral cortex. The reticular formation not only modulates the control of motor systems but influences sensory systems as well. By means of its multiple ascending pathways, which project to different parts of the cerebral cortex, it is believed to influence the state of consciousness.

Loss Of Consciousness

In experimental animals, damage to the reticular formation, which spares the ascending sensory pathways, causes persistent unconsciousness. Pathological lesions of the reticular formation in humans can result in loss of consciousness and even coma. It has been suggested that loss of consciousness that occurs in epilepsy may be due to inhibition of the activity of the reticular formation in the upper part of the diencephalon.

LIMBIC SYSTEM

The anatomical connections of the limbic system are extremely complex and, since their significance is not fully understood, it is unnecessary for a student of medicine to commit all of them to memory. The results of neurophysiological experiments, which have included stimulation and ablation of different parts of the limbic system in animals, are not entirely clear. Nevertheless, certain important roles have been inferred: (1) The limbic structures are involved in the development of sensations of emotion and with the visceral responses accompanying those emotions, and (2) the hippocampus is concerned with recent memory.

Schizophrenia

The symptoms of schizophrenia include chronically disordered thinking, blunted affect, and emotional withdrawal. Paranoid delusions and auditory hallucinations may also be present. Clinical research has shown that if the limbic receptors to dopamine are blocked by a pharmacological agent, the worst symptoms of schizophrenia are lessened. Phenothiazine administration, for example, blocks the dopamine receptors in the limbic system. Unfortunately, this drug, as well as most other antipsychotic drugs, has major motor side effects on the dopaminergic receptors within the extrapyramidal system, producing abnormal involuntary movements. Research is now concentrating on finding a drug that will block the limbic dopamine receptors but without effect on the receptors of the extrapyramidal system (substantia nigra-corpus striatum).

It is clear, however, that there is still no direct evidence that excessive production of dopamine by certain neurons actually contributes to schizophrenia.

Destruction of the Amygdaloid Complex

Unilateral or bilateral destruction of the amygdaloid nucleus and the paraamygdaloid area in patients suffering from aggressive behavior in many cases results in a decrease in aggressiveness, emotional instability, and restlessness; increased interest in food; and hypersexuality. There is no disturbance in memory. Monkeys that have been subjected to bilateral removal of the temporal lobes demonstrate what is known as the **Klüver-Bucy syndrome.** They become docile and show no evidence of fear or anger and are unable to appreciate objects visually. They have an increased appetite and increased sexual activity. Moreover, the animals indiscriminately seek partnerships with male and female animals.

Precise stereotactic lesions in the amygdaloid complex in humans reduce emotional excitability and bring about normalization of behavior in patients with severe disturbances. No loss of memory occurs.

Temporal Lobe Dysfunction

Temporal lobe epilepsy may be preceded by an aura of acoustic or olfactory experience. The olfactory aura is usually an unpleasant odor. The patient is often confused, anxious, and docile and may perform automatic and complicated movements, such as undressing in public or driving a car, and then, following the seizure, may have no memory of what occurred previously.

Clinical Problem Solving

1. While discussing the neurological basis of emotions during a ward round, a neurologist asked a third-year medical student what she knew about the Klüver-Bucy syndrome. What would your answer to that question be? Does it ever occur in humans?
2. A 23-year-old woman with a 4-year history of epileptic attacks visited her neurologist. A friend of hers vividly described one of her attacks. For a few seconds before the convulsions began, the patient would complain of an unpleasant odor, similar to that encountered in a cow shed. This was followed by a shrill cry as she fell to the floor unconscious. Her whole body immediately became involved in generalized tonic and clonic movements. Clearly, this patient had a generalized form of

epileptic seizure. Using your knowledge of neuroanatomy, suggest which lobe of the brain was initially involved in the epileptic discharge.

3. A 54-year-old man died in the hospital with a cerebral tumor. He had always been intellectually very bright and could easily recall events in his childhood. For the past 6 months his family had noticed that he had difficulty in recalling where he had placed things, such as his pipe. He also had difficulty in recalling recent news events and, just before he died, he could not remember that his brother had visited him the day before. Using your knowledge of neuroanatomy, suggest which part of the brain was being affected by the expanding and highly invasive tumor.

Answers to Clinical Problem Solving

1. The Klüver-Bucy syndrome consists of the signs and symptoms found in monkeys following bilateral removal of the temporal lobe. The monkeys become docile and unresponsive and display no signs of fear or anger. They have an increased appetite and increased sexual activity, which is often perverse. They are unable to recognize objects seen. Humans in whom the amygdaloid area is destroyed do not usually demonstrate this syndrome. It has, however, been described in humans following the bilateral removal of large areas of the temporal lobes.

2. The olfactory aura that preceded the general convulsions of the epileptic attack would indicate that the temporal lobe of the cerebral cortex was initially involved.

3. An autopsy study revealed extensive invasion of the hippocampus, fornix, and mammillary bodies in both cerebral hemispheres. It appears that the hippocampus is involved in the storage and categorizing of afferent information related to recent memory.

Review Questions

Directions: Each of the numbered items in this section is followed by answers that are positively phrased. Select the ONE lettered answer that is an EXCEPTION.

1. The following statements concerning the reticular formation are correct **except:**
   (a) Reticulobulbar and reticulospinal tracts form the efferent pathways from the reticular formation to the motor nuclei of the cranial nerves and the anterior horn cells of the spinal cord, respectively.
   (b) The reticular formation extends through the neuroaxis from the spinal cord to the thalamus.
   (c) The main pathways through the reticular formation may easily be traced from one part of the central nervous system to another using silver stains.
   (d) Superiorly the reticular formation is relayed to the cerebral cortex.
   (e) Afferent pathways project into the reticular formation from most parts of the central nervous system.
2. The following statements concerning the functions of the reticular formation are correct **except:**
   (a) It influences the activity of the alpha and gamma motor neurons.
   (b) It opposes the actions of the vestibular spinal tract.

   (c) It brings about reciprocal inhibition during contraction of the prime mover muscles.
   (d) It helps maintain the tone of the antigravity muscles.
   (e) It can modulate reflex activity.
3. The following statements concerning the functions of the reticular formation are correct **except:**
   (a) It does not affect the reception of pain.
   (b) It can influence all ascending pathways to the supraspinal levels.
   (c) By means of its reticulobulbar and reticulospinal tracts it can control the parasympathetic and sympathetic outflows.
   (d) It can affect the biological rhythms.
   (e) It can influence the degree of wakefulness of an individual.
4. The following structures collectively form the limbic system **except:**
   (a) The amygdaloid nucleus
   (b) The pulvinar of the thalamus
   (c) The hippocampal formation
   (d) The cingulate gyrus
   (e) The mammillary bodies
5. The following statements concerning the efferent connections of the hippocampus are correct **except:**
   (a) They arise from the large pyramidal cells of the cortex.

(b) They travel through the fornix.
(c) Some of the fibers enter the mammillary body.
(d) The fibers within the fornix pass posterior to the interventricular foramen.
(e) Some of the fibers end in the anterior nuclei of the thalamus.

6. The following statements concerning the functions of the limbic system are correct **except:**
(a) It is concerned with the reactions of fear and anger.
(b) It is not concerned with visual experiences.
(c) The hippocampus is concerned with recent memory.
(d) The limbic system plays an important role in olfactory function.
(e) It indirectly influences the activity of the endocrine system.

Directions: Matching Questions

In Figure 9-8, match the numbers listed on the left with the appropriate lettered options listed on the right. Each lettered option may be selected once, more than once, or not at all.

7. Number 1   (a) Uncus
8. Number 2   (b) Body of fornix
9. Number 3   (c) Parahippocampal gyrus
10. Number 4   (d) Dentate gyrus
                (e) None of the above

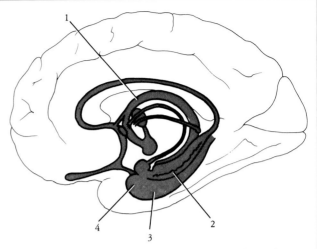

Figure 9–8   Medial aspect of the right cerebral hemisphere, showing structures that form the limbic system.

Answers to Review Questions

1. C
2. B
3. A
4. B
5. D

6. D
7. B
8. D
9. C
10. A

ADDITIONAL READING

Aggleton, J.P. (ed) *The Amygdala: Neurobiological Aspects of Emotion, Memory, and Mental Dysfunction*. Wiley-Liss. 1993

Goldman-Rakic, P. S. Working memory and the mind. *Sci. Am.* 267(3):110, 1992.

Jasper, H.H., Descarries, L., Castelluci, V.F, and, Rossignol, S. (Eds) *Consciousness: At the Frontiers of Neuroscience*. Lippincott-Raven, 1998.

Klemm, W. R. Ascending and descending excitatory influences in the brain stem reticulum: A re-examination. *Brain Res.* 36:444, 1972.

Rowland, L.P. Merritt's *Textbook of Neurology*. Baltimore, Williams & Wilkins, 1995.

Ryan, P. M. Epidemiology, Etiology, Diagnosis and Treatment of Schizophrenia. *Am. J. Hosp. Pharm.* 48:1271, 1991.

Seeman, P., Guan, H.C. and, Van Tol, H.H.M. Dopamine D4 Receptors Elevated in Schizophrenia. *Nature* 365:441-445,1993.

Williams, P. L. et al., eds. *Gray's Anatomy* (Br. 38th ed.). New York and Edinburgh: Churchill Livingstone,1995.

CHAPTER 10

The Basal Nuclei (Basal Ganglia) and Their Connections

A 58-year-old man was seen by a neurologist because he had noticed the development of a slight tremor of his left hand. The tremors involved all of the fingers and the thumb and were present at rest but ceased during voluntary movement.

On examination, the patient tended to perform all his movements slowly and his face had very little expression and was almost masklike. On passively moving the patient's arms, the neurologist found that the muscles showed increased tone and there was a slight jerky resistance to the movements. When asked to stand up straight, the patient did so but with a stooped posture, and when he walked, he did so by shuffling across the examining room.

The neurologist made the diagnosis of Parkinson's disease, based on her knowledge of the structure and function of the basal ganglia and their connections to the substantia nigra of the midbrain. She was able to prescribe appropriate drug therapy, which resulted in a great improvement in the hand tremors.

CHAPTER OUTLINE

CHAPTER OBJECTIVES

The basal nuclei play an important role in the control of posture and voluntary movement. Unlike many other parts of the nervous system concerned with motor control, they have no direct input or output connections with the spinal cord. The purpose of this chapter is to describe the basal nuclei, their connections, and their functions and relate them to diseases commonly affecting this area of the nervous system.

TERMINOLOGY

The term **basal nuclei** is applied to a collection of masses of gray matter situated within each cerebral hemisphere. They are the corpus striatum, the amygdaloid nucleus, and the claustrum.

Clinicians and neuroscientists use a variety of different terminologies to describe the basal nuclei. A summary of the terminologies commonly used is shown in Table 10-1. The subthalamic nuclei, the substantia nigra, and the red nucleus are functionally closely related to the basal nuclei but they should not be included with them.

The interconnections of the basal nuclei are complex, but in this account only the more important pathways are considered. The basal nuclei play an important role in the control of posture and voluntary movement.

Table 10–1 The Terminology Commonly Used to Describe the Basal Nuclei

Neurological Structure	Basal Nucleus (Nuclei)
Caudate nucleus	Caudate nucleus
Lentiform nucleus	Globus pallidus plus putamen
Claustrum	Claustrum
Corpus striatum	Caudate nucleus plus lentiform nucleus
Neostriatum (striatum)	Caudate nucleus plus putamen
Amygdaloid body	Amygdaloid nucleus

The term basal has been used in the past to denote the position of the nuclei at the base of the forebrain.

CORPUS STRIATUM

The corpus striatum (Fig.10-1) is situated lateral to the thalamus and is almost completely divided by a band of nerve fibers, the **internal capsule,** into the caudate nucleus and the lentiform nucleus. The term striatum is used here because of the striated appearance produced by the strands of gray matter passing through the internal capsule and connecting the caudate nucleus to the putamen of the lentiform nucleus (See below).

Caudate Nucleus

The caudate nucleus is a large C-shaped mass of gray matter that is closely related to the lateral ventricle and lies lateral to the thalamus (Fig. 10-1). The lateral surface of the nucleus is related to the internal capsule, which separates it from the lentiform nucleus (Fig. 10-2). For purposes of description, it can be divided into a head, a body, and a tail.

The **head** of the caudate nucleus is large and rounded and forms the lateral wall of the anterior horn of the lateral ventricle (Fig. 10-2). The head is continuous inferiorly with the putamen of the lentiform nucleus (the caudate nucleus and the putamen are sometimes referred to as the **neostriatum** or **striatum**). Just superior to this point of union, strands of gray matter pass through the internal capsule, giving the region a striated appearance, hence the term **corpus striatum.**

The **body** of the caudate nucleus is long and narrow and is continuous with the head in the region of the interven-

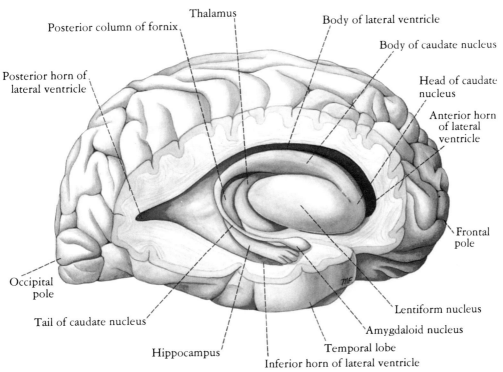

Figure 10–1 Lateral view of the right cerebral hemisphere dissected to show the position of the different basal nuclei.

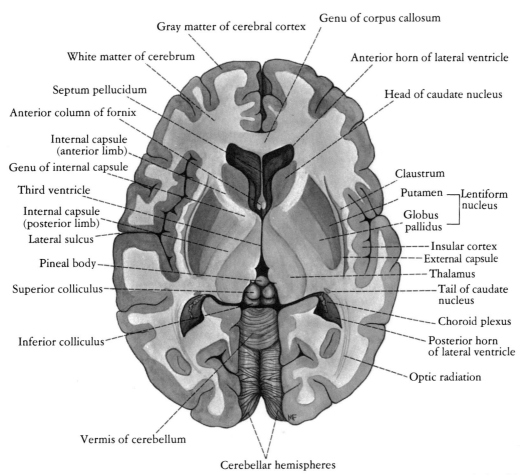

Figure 10–2 Horizontal section of the cerebrum as seen from above, showing the relationships of the different basal nuclei.

tricular foramen. The body of the caudate nucleus forms part of the floor of the body of the lateral ventricle.

The **tail** of the caudate nucleus is long and slender and is continuous with the body in the region of the posterior end of the thalamus. It follows the contour of the lateral ventricle and continues forward in the roof of the inferior horn of the lateral ventricle. It terminates anteriorly in the **amygdaloid nucleus** (Fig. 10-1).

Lentiform Nucleus

The lentiform nucleus is a wedge-shaped mass of gray matter whose broad convex base is directed laterally and its blade medially (Fig. 10-2). It is buried deep in the white matter of the cerebral hemisphere and is related medially to the internal capsule, which separates it from the caudate nucleus and the thalamus. The lentiform nucleus is related lat-

erally to a thin sheet of white matter, the **external capsule** (Fig. 10-2), which separates it from a thin sheet of gray matter, called the **claustrum.** The claustrum, in turn, separates the external capsule from the subcortical white matter of the insula. A vertical plate of white matter divides the nucleus into a larger, darker lateral portion, the **putamen,** and an inner lighter portion, the **globus pallidus** (Fig. 10-2). The paleness of the globus pallidus is due to the presence of a high concentration of myelinated nerve fibers. Inferiorly at its anterior end, the putamen is continuous with the head of the caudate nucleus (Fig. 10-1).

 AMYGDALOID NUCLEUS

The amygdaloid nucleus is situated in the temporal lobe close to the uncus (Fig. 10-1). The amygdaloid nucleus is

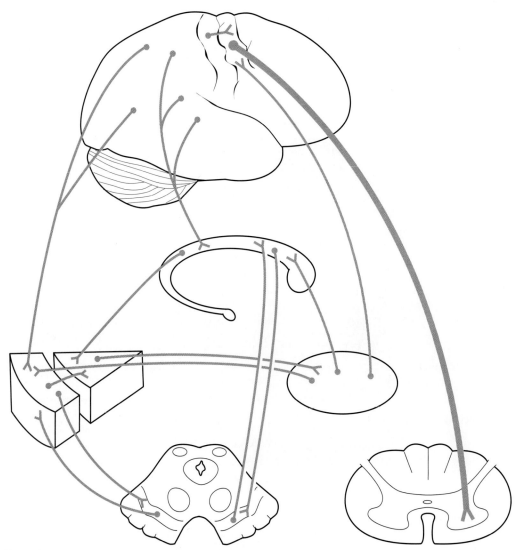

Figure 10–3 Some of the main connections between the cerebral cortex, the basal nuclei, the thalamic nuclei, the brainstem, and the spinal cord.

considered to be part of the limbic system and is described in Chapter 9. Through its connections it can influence the body's response to environmental changes. In the sense of fear, for example, it can change the heart rate, blood pressure, skin color, and rate of respiration.

SUBSTANTIA NIGRA AND SUBTHALAMIC NUCLEI

The substantia nigra of the midbrain and the subthalamic nuclei of the diencephalon are functionally closely related to the activities of the basal nuclei and are described elsewhere (See pp 206 and 252). The neurons of the substantia nigra are dopaminergic and inhibitory and have many connections to the corpus striatum. The neurons of the subthalamic nuclei are glutaminergic and excitatory and have many connections to the globus pallidus and substantia nigra.

CLAUSTRUM

The claustrum is a thin sheet of gray matter that is separated from the lateral surface of the lentiform nucleus by the external capsule (Fig. 10-2). Lateral to the claustrum is the subcortical white matter of the insula. The function of the claustrum is unknown.

CONNECTIONS OF THE CORPUS STRIATUM AND GLOBUS PALLIDUS

The caudate nucleus and the putamen form the main sites for receiving input to the basal nuclei. The globus pallidus forms the major site from which the output leaves the basal nuclei.

They receive no direct input from or output to the spinal cord.

CONNECTIONS OF THE CORPUS STRIATUM

Afferent Fibers

CORTICOSTRIATE FIBERS

All parts of the cerebral cortex send axons to the caudate nucleus and the putamen (Fig. 10-3). Each part of the cerebral cortex projects to a specific part of the caudate-putamen complex. Most of the projections are from the cortex of the same side. The largest input is from the sensory-motor cortex. Glutamate is the neurotransmitter of the corticostriate fibers (Fig. 10-4).

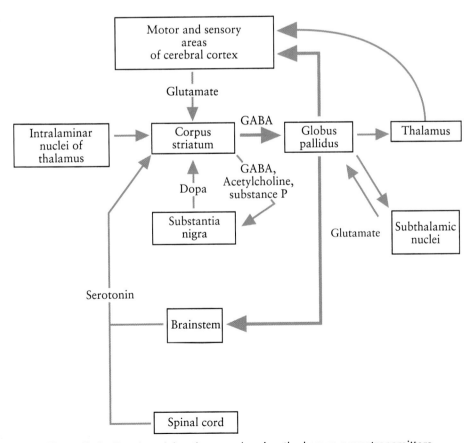

Figure 10–4 Basal nuclei pathways, showing the known neurotransmitters.

THALAMOSTRIATE FIBERS

The intralaminar nuclei of the thalamus send large numbers of axons to the caudate nucleus and the putamen (Fig. 10-3).

NIGROSTRIATE FIBERS

Neurons in the substantia nigra send axons to the caudate nucleus and the putamen (Figs. 10-3 and 10-4) and liberate dopamine at their terminals as the neurotransmitter. It is believed that these fibers are inhibitory in function.

BRAINSTEM STRIATAL FIBERS

Ascending fibers from the brainstem end in the caudate nucleus and putamen (Figs. 10-3 and 10-4) and liberate serotonin at their terminals as the neurotransmitter. It is thought that these fibers are inhibitory in function.

Efferent Fibers

STRIATOPALLIDAL FIBERS

These fibers pass from the caudate nucleus and putamen to the globus pallidus (Fig. 10-3). They have gamma-aminobutyric acid (GABA) as their neurotransmitter (Fig. 10-4).

STRIATONIGRAL FIBERS

Fibers pass from the caudate nucleus and putamen to the substantia nigra (Fig. 10-3). Some of the fibers use GABA or acetylcholine as the neurotransmitter while others use substance P (Fig. 10-4).

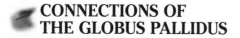

CONNECTIONS OF THE GLOBUS PALLIDUS

Afferent Fibers

STRIATOPALLIDAL FIBERS

These fibers pass from the caudate nucleus and putamen to the globus pallidus. As noted previously, these fibers have GABA as their neurotransmitter (Fig. 10-4).

Efferent Fibers

PALLIDOFUGAL FIBERS

These complicated fibers can be divided into groups: (1) the **ansa lenticularis,** which pass to the thalamic nuclei; (2) the **fasciculus lenticularis,** which pass to the subthal-amus; (3) the **pallidotegmental** fibers, which terminate in the caudal tegmentum of the midbrain; and (4) the **pallidosubthalamic fibers,** which pass to the subthalamic nuclei.

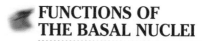

FUNCTIONS OF THE BASAL NUCLEI

The basal nuclei (Fig. 10-5) are joined together and connected with many different regions of the nervous system by a very complex number of neurons.

Basically, the corpus striatum receives afferent information from most of the cerebral cortex, the thalamus, the subthalamus, and the brainstem, including the substantia nigra. The information is integrated within the corpus striatum and the outflow passes back to the areas listed above. This circular pathway is believed to function as follows.

The activity of the basal nuclei is initiated by information received from the premotor and supplemental areas of the motor cortex, the primary sensory cortex, the thalamus, and the brainstem. The outflow from the basal nuclei is channeled through the globus pallidus, which then influences the activities of the motor areas of the cerebral cortex or other motor centers in the brainstem. Thus the basal nuclei control muscular movements by influencing the cerebral cortex and have no direct control through descending pathways to the brainstem and spinal cord. In this way the basal nuclei assist in the regulation of voluntary movement and the learning of motor skills.

Destruction of the primary motor cerebral cortex prevents the individual from performing fine discrete movements of the hands and feet on the opposite side of the body (see pp. 293 and 170). However, the individual is still capable of performing gross crude movements of the opposite limbs. If destruction of the corpus striatum then takes place, paralysis of the remaining movements of the opposite side of the body occurs.

The basal nuclei not only influence the execution of a particular movement of say the limbs, but also help prepare for the movements. This may be achieved by controlling the axial and girdle movements of the body and the positioning of the proximal parts of the limbs. The activity in certain neurons of the globus pallidus increases before active movements take place in the distal limb muscles. This important preparatory function enables the trunk and limbs to be placed in appropriate positions before the primary motor part of the cerebral cortex activates discrete movements in the hands and feet.

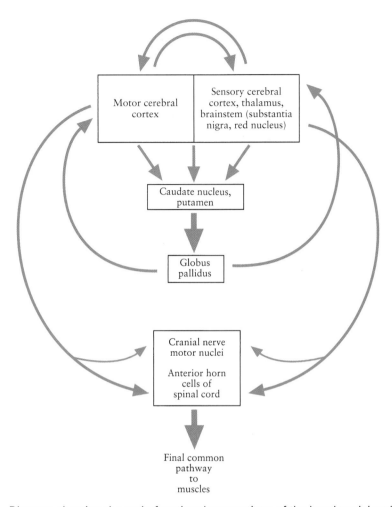

Figure 10–5 Diagram showing the main functional connections of the basal nuclei and how they can influence muscle activity.

CLINICAL NOTES

Disorders of the basal nuclei are of two general types. **Hyperkinetic disorders** are those in which there are excessive and abnormal movements, such as seen with chorea, athetosis, and ballism. **Hypokinetic disorders** include those in which there is a lack or slowness of movement. Parkinson's disease includes both types of motor disturbances.

CHOREA

In this syndrome the patient exhibits involuntary, quick, jerky, irregular movements that are nonrepetitive. Swift grimaces and sudden movements of the head or limbs are good examples.

Huntington's Disease

Huntington's disease is an autosomal dominant inherited disease with the onset occurring most often in adult life. Death occurs 15-20 years after onset. The disease has been traced to a single gene defect on chromosome 4. This gene encodes a protein, **huntingtin**, the function of which is not known. The codon (CAG) that encodes glutamine is repeated many more times than normal. The disease affects men and women with equal frequency and unfortunately often reveals itself only after they have had children.

Patients have the following characteristic signs and symptoms:

1. **Choreiform movements** first appear as involuntary movements of the extremities and twitching of the face (facial grimacing). Later, more muscle groups are involved so that the patient becomes immobile and unable to speak or swallow.
2. **Progressive dementia** occurs with loss of memory and intellectual capacity.

In this disease there is a degeneration of the GABA-secreting, substance P-secreting, and acetylcholine-secreting neurons of the striatonigral inhibiting pathway. This results in the dopa-secreting neurons of the substantia nigra becoming overactive so that the nigrostriatal pathway inhibits the caudate nucleus and the putamen (Fig. 10-6). This inhibition produces the abnormal movements seen in this disease. CT scans show enlarged lateral ventricles due to degeneration of the caudate nuclei. Medical treatment of Huntington's chorea has been disappointing.

Sydenham's Chorea

Sydenham's chorea (St. Vitus' dance) is a disease of childhood in which there are rapid, irregular, involuntary movements of the limbs, face, and trunk. The condition is associated with rheumatic fever. The antigens of the strep-

tococcal bacteria are similar in structure to the proteins present in the membranes of striatal neurons. The host's antibodies not only combine with the bacterial antigens but also attack the membranes of the neurons of the basal ganglia. This results in the production of choreiform movements, which are fortunately transient, and there is full recovery.

HEMIBALLISMUS

This is a form of involuntary movement confined to one side of the body. It usually involves the proximal extremity musculature and the limb suddenly flies about out of control in all directions. The lesion, which is usually a small stroke, occurs in the opposite subthalamic nucleus or its

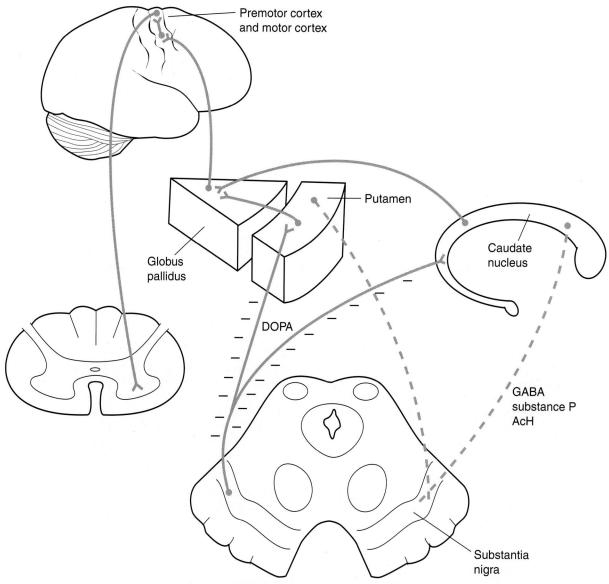

Figure 10–6 Diagram showing the degeneration of the inhibitory pathway between the corpus striatum and the substantia nigra seen in Huntington's disease and the consequent reduction in the liberation of GABA, substance P, and acetylcholine in the substantia nigra.

connections; it is in the subthalamic nucleus that smooth movements of different parts of the body are integrated.

PARKINSON'S DISEASE

This progressive disease of unknown cause commences between the ages of 45 and 55. It is associated with neuronal degeneration in the **substantia nigra** and to a lesser extent in the **globus pallidus, putamen,** and **caudate nucleus.** The disease affects about one million people in the United States.

The degeneration of the neurons of the substantia nigra that send their axons to the corpus striatum results in a reduction in the release of the neurotransmitter dopamine within the corpus striatum (Fig. 10-7 and 10-8). This leads to hypersensitivity of the dopamine receptors in the postsynaptic neurons in the striatum.

Patients have the following characteristic signs and symptoms:

1. **Tremor.** This is the result of the alternating contraction of agonists and antagonists. The tremor is slow and occurs most obviously when the limbs are at rest. It disappears during sleep. It should be distinguished from the intention tremor seen in cerebellar disease, which only occurs when purposeful active movement is attempted.
2. **Rigidity.** This differs from the rigidity caused by lesions of the upper motor neurons in that it is present to an equal extent in opposing muscle groups. If the tremor is absent, the rigidity is felt as resistance to passive movement and is sometimes referred to as **plastic rigidity.** If the tremor is present, the muscle resistance is overcome as a series of jerks, called **cogwheel rigidity.**
3. **Bradykinesis.** There is a difficulty in initiating (**akinesia**) and performing new movements. The movements are slow, the face is expressionless, and the voice is slurred and unmodulated. Swinging of the arms in walking is lost.
4. **Postural disturbances.** The patient stands with a stoop and his or her arms are flexed. The patient walks by taking short steps and often is unable to stop. In fact, he or she may break into a shuffling run to maintain his balance.
5. There is no loss of muscle power and no loss of sensibility. Since the corticospinal tracts are normal, the superficial abdominal reflexes are normal and there is no Babinski response. The deep tendon reflexes are normal.

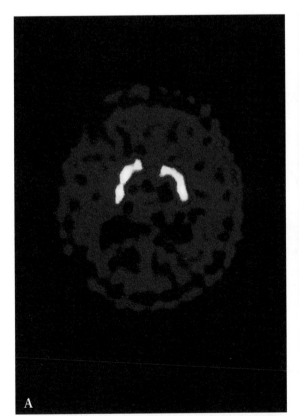
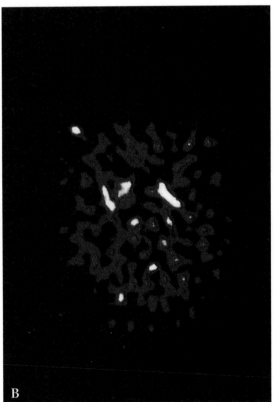

Figure 10–7 Axial (horizontal) PET scans of (A) a normal brain and (B) the brain of a patient with early Parkinson's disease, following the injection of 18-fluoro-6-L-dopa. The normal-brain image shows large amounts of the compound (yellow areas) distributed throughout the corpus striatum in both cerebral hemispheres. In the patient with Parkinson's disease the brain image shows that the total amount of the compound is low and it is unevenly distributed in the corpus striatum. (Courtesy Dr. Holley Dey.)

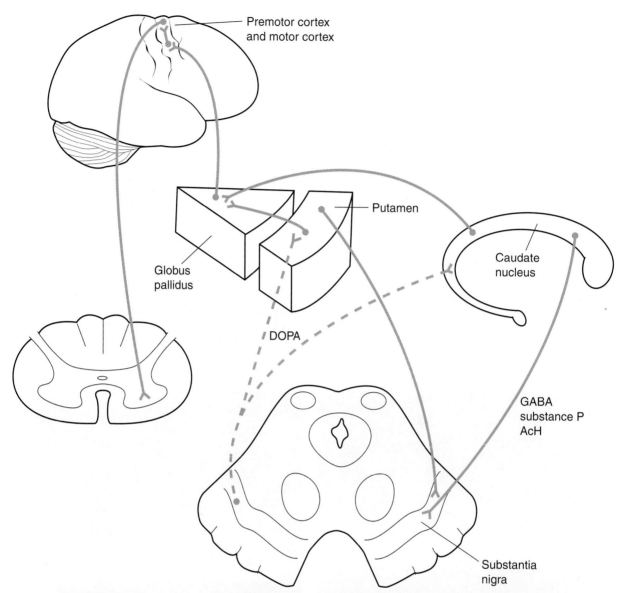

Figure 10–8 Diagram showing the degeneration of the inhibitory pathway between the substantia nigra and the corpus striatum in Parkinson's disease and the consequent reduction in the release of the neurotransmitter dopamine in the striatum.

There are a few types of Parkinson's Disease for which the cause is known. **Postencephalitic Parkinsonism** developed following the viral encephalitis in 1916-1917 in which damage occurred to the basal nuclei. **Iatrogenic Parkinsonism** can be a side effect of antipsychotic drugs (eg.,phenothiazines). Meperidine analogues (used by drug addicts), and poisoning from carbon monoxide and manganese, can also produce the symptoms of Parkinsonism. **Atherosclerotic Parkinsonism** can occur in elderly hypertensive patients.

Parkinson's disease may be treated by elevating the brain dopamine level. Unfortunately dopamine cannot cross the blood-brain barrier but its immediate precursor L-dopa can and is used in its place. L-dopa is taken up by the dopaminergic neurons in the basal nuclei and converted to dopamine. Selegiline, a drug that inhibits monoamine oxi-

dase, which is responsible for destroying dopamine, is also of benefit in the treatment of the disease. There is evidence that selegiline can slow the process of degeneration of the dopa secreting neurons in the substantia nigra.

Transplantation of human embryonic dopamine producing neurons into the caudate nucleus and putamen has been shown to lead to improvement in motor function in Parkinson's disease. There is evidence that the grafts can survive and synaptic contacts are made. Unfortunately many of the grafted neurons do not survive and in many cases the clinical improvement is counteracted by the continuing degeneration of the patient's own dopa producing neurons. Autotransplantation of suprarenal medullary cells can be a source of dopa producing cells but genetically engineered cells could be in the future another source of dopa.

Since most of the symptoms of Parkinson's disease are caused by an increased inhibitory output from the basal nuclei to the thalamus and the precentral motor cortex, surgical lesions in the globus pallidus (**pallidotomy)** have been shown to be effective in alleviating parkinsonian signs. At the present time such procedures are restricted to patients who are no longer responding to medical treatment.

ATHETOSIS

This consists of slow, sinuous, writhing movements that most commonly involve the distal segments of the limbs. Degeneration of the globus pallidus occurs with a breakdown of the circuitry involving the basal nuclei and the cerebral cortex.

Clinical Problem Solving

1. A 10-year-old girl was seen by a neurologist because of the gradual development of involuntary movements. To begin with, the movements were regarded by her parents as general restlessness, but later abnormal facial grimacing and jerking movements of the arms and legs began to occur. The child was now having difficulty in performing normal movements of the arms and walking was becoming increasingly difficult. The abnormal movements appeared to be worse in the upper limbs and were more exaggerated on the right side of the body. The movements were made worse when the child became excited but disappeared completely when she slept. The child was recently treated for rheumatic fever. Is there any possible connection between this child's symptoms and the basal nuclei in the cerebral hemispheres?
2. A 40-year-old man complaining of rapid and jerky involuntary movements involving the upper and lower limbs was seen by his physician. The condition started about

6 months ago and was getting progressively worse. He said that he was extremely worried about his health because his father had developed similar symptoms 20 years ago and had died in a mental institution. His wife told the physician that he also suffered from episodes of extreme depression and that she had noticed that he had periods of irritability and impulsive behavior. The physician made the diagnosis of Huntington's chorea. Using your knowledge of neuroanatomy, explain how this disease involves the basal nuclei.
3. A 61-year-old man suddenly developed uncoordinated movements of the trunk and right arm. The right upper limb would suddenly, vigorously, and aimlessly be thrown about, knocking over anything in its path. The patient was recovering from a right-sided hemiplegia, secondary to a cerebral hemorrhage. What is the name given to this clinical sign? Does this condition involve the basal nuclei?

Answers to Clinical Problem Solving

1. This child is suffering from Sydenham's chorea (see p. 322). This condition occurs, in the majority of cases, in female children between the ages of 5 and 15. It is characterized by the presence of rapid, irregular, involuntary movements that are purposeless. The disease is associated with rheumatic fever and complete recovery is the rule. For details, see page 322.
2. Huntington's chorea is a progressive inherited disease that usually appears between the ages of 30 and 45. The involuntary movements are usually more rapid and jerky than those seen in patients with Sydenham's chorea. Progressive mental changes lead to dementia and death. There is a progressive degeneration of the GABA-secreting, substance P-secreting, and the acetylcholine-secret-

ing neurons of the striatonigral pathway. This results in the dopamine-secreting neurons of the substantia nigra becoming overactive so that the nigrostriatal pathway inhibits the caudate nucleus and the putamen. This causes the involuntary movements. Atrophy of the caudate nucleus and putamen occurs.
3. The clinical sign is known as hemiballismus. The sudden onset is usually caused by vascular impairment due to hemorrhage or occlusion. Yes, hemiballismus does involve the basal nuclei; it is the result of destruction of the contralateral subthalamic nucleus or its neuronal connections, causing the violent, uncoordinated movements of the axial and proximal limb muscles.

Review Questions

Directions: Each of the numbered items in this section is followed by answers that are positively phrased. Select the ONE lettered answer that is an EXCEPTION.

1. The following statements concerning the basal nuclei (ganglia) are correct **except:**
   (a) The caudate nucleus and the putamen form the neostriatum (striatum).
   (b) The head of the caudate nucleus is connected to the putamen.
   (c) The tegmentum of the midbrain forms part of the basal nuclei.
   (d) The internal capsule lies medial to the globus pallidus.
   (e) The basal nuclei are formed of gray matter.

2. The following statements concerning the basal nuclei (ganglia) are correct **except:**
   (a) The amygdaloid nucleus is connected to the caudate nucleus.
   (b) The lentiform nucleus is completely divided by the external capsule into the globus pallidus and the putamen.
   (c) The claustrum forms part of the basal nuclei.
   (d) The corpus striatum lies lateral to the thalamus.
   (e) The function of the claustrum is unknown.

3. The following statements concerning the basal nuclei (ganglia) are correct **except:**
   (a) The corpus striatum is made up of the caudate nucleus and the lentiform nucleus.
   (b) The head of the caudate nucleus lies medial to the internal capsule.
   (c) The insula does not form part of the basal nuclei.
   (d) The tail of the caudate nucleus lies in the floor of the lateral ventricle.
   (e) The subthalamic nuclei are functionally closely related to the basal nuclei but are not considered to be part of them.

4. The following statements concerning the caudate nucleus are correct **except:**
   (a) It is divided into a head, body, and tail.
   (b) It is a C-shaped mass of gray matter.
   (c) The body of the caudate nucleus forms part of the floor of the body of the lateral ventricle.
   (d) The head lies medial to the anterior horn of the lateral ventricle.
   (e) The tail terminates anteriorly in the amygdaloid nucleus.

5. The following statements concerning the afferent corticostriate fibers to the corpus striatum are correct **except:**
   (a) Each part of the cerebral cortex is randomly projected to different parts of the corpus striatum.
   (b) Glutamate is the neurotransmitter.
   (c) All parts of the cerebral cortex send fibers to the caudate nucleus and putamen.
   (d) The largest input is from the sensory-motor part of the cerebral cortex.
   (e) Most of the projections are from the cortex of the same side.

6. The following statements concerning the nigrostriate fibers are correct **except:**
   (a) The neurons in the substantia nigra send axons to the putamen.
   (b) Dopamine is the neurotransmitter.
   (c) The nigrostriate fibers are stimulatory in function.
   (d) The caudate nucleus receives axons from the substantia nigra.
   (e) Parkinson's disease is caused by a reduction in the release of dopamine within the corpus striatum.

7. The following statements concerning the efferent fibers of the corpus striatum are correct **except:**
   (a) None of the efferent fibers descend directly to the motor nuclei of the cranial nerves.
   (b) Some of the striatopallidal fibers have GABA as the neurotransmitter.
   (c) The striatonigral fibers pass from the caudate nucleus to the substantia nigra.
   (d) Many of the efferent fibers pass directly to the cerebellum.
   (e) The anterior horn cells of the spinal cord are not influenced directly by the efferent fibers from the corpus striatum.

8. The following statements concerning the functions of the basal nuclei (ganglia) are correct **except:**
   (a) The corpus striatum does not integrate information received directly from the cerebellar cortex.
   (b) The outflow of the basal nuclei is channeled through the globus pallidus to the motor areas of the cerebral cortex, thus influencing muscular activities.
   (c) The globus pallidus only influences the movements of the axial part of the body.
   (d) The activities of the globus pallidus precede the activities of the motor cortex concerned with discrete movements of the hands and feet.
   (e) The activities of the basal nuclei are initiated by information received from the sensory cortex, the thalamus, and the brainstem.

Directions: Matching Questions

In Figure 10-9, match the numbers listed below on the left with the appropriate lettered options listed on the right. Each lettered option may be selected once, more than once, or not at all.

9. Structure 1	(a) Anterior horn of lateral ventricle
10. Structure 2	(b) Internal capsule
11. Structure 3	(c) Claustrum
12. Structure 4	(d) Putamen
13. Structure 5	(e) External capsule
14. Structure 6	(f) Globus pallidus
	(g) None of the above

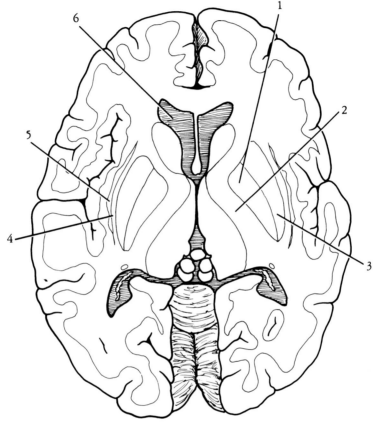

Figure 10–9 Horizontal section of the cerebrum.

Answers to Review Questions

1. C
2. B
3. D
4. D
5. A
6. C
7. D

8. C
9. F
10. B
11. D
12. E
13. C
14. A

ADDITIONAL READING

Albin, R.L., Young, A.B., and Penney, J.B. The Functional Anatomy of Disorders of the Basal Ganglia. *Trends Neurosci.* 200:63, 1995.

Aron, A. M., Freeman, J. M., and Carter, S. The Natural History of Sydenham's Chorea. *Am. J. Med.* 38:83, 1965.

Brooks, D.J., The Role of the Basal Ganglia in Motor Control:Contributions from PET. *J. Neurosci.* 128:1-13, 1995.

Collier, D.S., Berg, M.J., and Fincham, R.W. Parkinsonism Treatment: Part III,-Update. *Ann. Pharmacother.* 26:227,1992.

Craig, C. R., and Stitzel, R. E. *Modern Pharmacology* (4th ed.). Boston: Little, Brown, 1994.

Guyton, A.C. and Hall, J.E. *Textbook of Medical Physiology*, 9th ed. Philadelphia, London, W.B. Saunders,1996.

Kordower, J.H., et al. Neuropathological Evidence of Graft Survival and Striatal Reinervation after the Transplantation of Fetal Mesencephalic Tissue in a Patient with Parkinson's Disease. *N. Engl. J. Med.* 332:1118-1124,1995.

Narabayashi, H., et al. *Parkinson's Disease. From Basic Research to Treatment*. New York, Raven Press, 1993.

Westmoreland, B. F., Benarroch, E. E., Daube, J. R., Reagan, T. J., and Sandok, B. A. *Medical Neurosciences*. Boston: Little, Brown, 1994.

Young, A.B. Huntington's Disease: Lessons from and for Molecular Neuroscience. *The Neuroscientist* 1:51,1990.

CHAPTER 11

The Cranial Nerve Nuclei and Their Central Connections and Distribution

A 49-year-old man woke up one morning to find the right side of his face paralyzed. When examined by his local medical practitioner, he was found to have complete paralysis of the entire right side of the face. He was also found to have severe hypertension. The patient talked with slightly slurred speech. The physician told the patient that he had suffered a mild stroke and he was admitted to the hospital.

The patient was later seen by a neurologist who disagreed with the diagnosis. The original physician had grouped together the facial paralysis, the slurred speech, and the hypertension, and in the absence of other findings made the incorrect diagnosis of cerebral hemorrhage. A lesion of the corticonuclear fibers on one side of the brain will cause paralysis only of the muscles of the lower part of the opposite side of the face. This patient had complete paralysis of the entire right side of the face, which could only be caused by a lesion of the lower motor neuron. The correct diagnosis was Bell's palsy, an inflammation of the connective tissue sheath of the facial nerve, which temporarily interfered with the functions of the axons of the right facial nerve. This case provides a good example of how knowledge of the central connections of a cranial nerve enables a physician to make the correct diagnosis.

CHAPTER OBJECTIVES

The cranial nerves are commonly damaged by trauma or disease, and testing for their integrity forms part of every physical examination. It is important that all physicians know the basic information regarding the motor and sensory nuclei of the cranial nerves, including their locations and central connections. The objective of this chapter is to provide this information.

THE 12 CRANIAL NERVES

There are 12 pairs of cranial nerves, which leave the brain and pass through foramina and fissures in the skull. All the nerves are distributed in the head and neck, except the tenth, which also supplies structures in the thorax and abdomen. The cranial nerves are named as follows:

1. Olfactory
2. Optic
3. Oculomotor
4. Trochlear
5. Trigeminal
6. Abducent
7. Facial
8. Vestibulocochlear
9. Glossopharyngeal
10. Vagus
11. Accessory
12. Hypoglossal

ORGANIZATION OF THE CRANIAL NERVES

The olfactory, optic, and vestibulocochlear nerves are entirely sensory. The oculomotor, trochlear, abducent, accessory, and hypoglossal nerves are entirely motor. The trigeminal, facial, glossopharyngeal, and vagus nerves are both sensory and motor nerves. The letter symbols commonly used to indicate the functional components of each cranial nerve are shown in Table 11-1. The cranial nerves have central motor and/or sensory nuclei within the brain and peripheral nerve fibers that emerge from the brain and exit from the skull to reach their effector or sensory organs.

The different components of the cranial nerves, their functions, and the openings in the skull through which the nerves leave the cranial cavity are summarized in Table 11-2.

Table 11–1 The Letter Symbols Commonly Used to Indicate the Functional Components of Each Cranial Nerve

Component	Function	Letter Symbols
Afferent Fibers	*Sensory*	
General somatic afferent	General sensations	GSA
Special somatic afferent	Hearing, balance, vision	SSA
General visceral afferent	Viscera	GVA
Special visceral afferent	Smell, taste	SVA
Efferent Fibers		
General somatic efferent	Somatic striated muscles	GSE
General visceral efferent	Glands and smooth muscles (parasympathetic innervation)	GVE
Special visceral efferent	Branchial arch striated muscles	SVE

Table 11–2   Cranial Nerves

Number	Name	Components[a]	Function	Opening in Skull
I	Olfactory	Sensory (SVA)	Smell	Openings in cribriform plate of ethmoid
II	Optic	Sensory (SSA)	Vision	Optic canal
III	Oculomotor	Motor (GSE, GVE)	Raises upper eyelid, turns eyeball upward, downward, and medially; constricts pupil; accommodates eye.	Superior orbital fissure
IV	Trochlear	Motor (GSE)	Assists in turning eyeball downward and laterally	Superior orbital fissure
V	Trigeminal[b]			
	Ophthalmic division	Sensory (GSA)	Cornea, skin of forehead, scalp, eyelids, and nose; also mucous membrane of paranasal sinuses and nasal cavity	Superior orbital fissure
	Maxillary division	Sensory (GSA)	Skin of face over maxilla; teeth of upper jaw; mucous membrane of nose, the maxillary sinus, and palate	Foramen rotundum
	Mandibular division	Motor (SVE)	Muscles of mastication, mylohyoid, anterior belly of digastric, tensor veli palatini, and tensor tympani	Foramen ovale
		Sensory (GSA)	Skin of cheek, skin over mandible and side of head, teeth of lower jaw and temporomandibular joint; mucous membrane of mouth and anterior part of tongue	
VI	Abducent	Motor (GSE)	Lateral rectus muscle turns eyeball laterally	Superior orbital fissure
VII	Facial	Motor (SVE)	Muscles of face and scalp, stapedius muscle, posterior belly of digastric and stylohyoid muscles	Internal acoustic meatus, facial canal, stylomastoid foramen
		Sensory (SVA)	Taste from anterior two-thirds of tongue, from floor of mouth and palate	
		Secretomotor (GVE) parasympathetic	Submandibular and sublingual salivary glands, the lacrimal gland, and glands of nose and palate	
VIII	Vestibulocochlear			Internal acoustic meatus
	Vestibular	Sensory (SSA)	From utricle and saccule and semicircular canals—position and movement of head	
	Cochlear	Sensory (SSA)	Organ of Corti—hearing	
IX	Glossopharyngeal	Motor (SVE)	Stylopharyngeus muscle—assists swallowing	Jugular foramen
		Secretomotor (GVE) parasympathetic	Parotid salivary gland	
		Sensory (GVA, SVA, GSA)	General sensation and taste from posterior one-third of tongue and pharynx; carotid sinus (baroreceptor); and carotid body (chemoreceptor)	
X	Vagus	Motor (GVE, SVE) Sensory (GVA, SVA, GSA)	Heart and great thoracic blood vessels; larynx, trachea, bronchi, and lungs; alimentary tract from pharynx to splenic flexure of colon; liver, kidneys, and pancreas	Jugular foramen
XI	Accessory			
	Cranial root	Motor (SVE)	Muscles of soft palate (except tensor veli palatini), pharynx (except stylopharyngeus), and larynx (except cricothyroid) in branches of vagus	Jugular foramen
	Spinal root	Motor (SVE)	Sternocleidomastoid and trapezius muscles	
XII	Hypoglossal	Motor (GSE)	Muscles of tongue (except palatoglossus) controlling its shape and movement	Hypoglossal canal

[a]The letter symbols are explained in Table 11-1.
[b]The trigeminal nerve also carries proprioceptive impulses from the muscles of mastication and the facial and extraocular muscles.

Motor Nuclei of the Cranial Nerves

SOMATIC MOTOR AND BRANCHIOMOTOR NUCLEI

The somatic motor and branchiomotor nerve fibers of a cranial nerve are the axons of nerve cells situated within the brain. These nerve cell groups form motor nuclei and they innervate striated muscle. Each nerve cell with its processes is referred to as a **lower motor neuron**. Such a nerve cell is, therefore, equivalent to the motor cells in the anterior gray columns of the spinal cord.

The motor nuclei of the cranial nerves receive impulses from the cerebral cortex through the corticonuclear (corticobulbar) fibers. These fibers originate from the pyramidal cells in the inferior part of the precentral gyrus (area 4) and from the adjacent part of the postcentral gyrus. The corticonuclear fibers descend through the **corona radiata** and the **genu of the internal capsule**. They pass through the midbrain just medial to the corticospinal fibers in the **basis pedunculi** and end by synapsing either directly with the lower motor neurons within the cranial nerve nuclei or indirectly through the **internuncial neurons**. The corticonuclear fibers thus constitute the **first-order neuron** of the descending pathway, the internuncial neuron constitutes the **second-order neuron**, and the lower motor neuron constitutes the **third-order neuron**.

The majority of the corticonuclear fibers to the motor cranial nerve nuclei cross the median plane before reaching the nuclei. Bilateral connections are present for all the cranial motor nuclei except for part of the facial nucleus that supplies the muscles of the lower part of the face and a part of the hypoglossal nucleus that supplies the genioglossus muscle.

GENERAL VISCERAL MOTOR NUCLEI

The general visceral motor nuclei form the cranial outflow of the parasympathetic portion of the autonomic nervous system. They are the **Edinger-Westphal nucleus** of the oculomotor nerve, the **superior salivatory** and **lacrimal nuclei** of the facial nerve, the **inferior salivatory nucleus** of the glossopharyngeal nerve, and the **dorsal motor nucleus** of the vagus. These nuclei receive numerous afferent fibers including descending pathways from the hypothalamus.

Sensory Nuclei of the Cranial Nerves

These include somatic and visceral afferent nuclei. The sensory or afferent parts of a cranial nerve are the axons of nerve cells outside the brain and are situated in ganglia on the nerve trunks (equivalent to posterior root ganglion of a spinal nerve) or may be situated in a sensory organ, such as the nose, eye, or ear. These cells and their processes form the **first-order neuron**. The central processes of these cells enter the brain and terminate by synapsing with cells forming the sensory nuclei. These cells and their processes form the **second-order neuron**. Axons from these nuclear cells now cross the midline and ascend to other sensory nuclei, such as the thalamus, where they synapse. The nerve cells

of these nuclei form the **third-order neuron** and their axons terminate in the cerebral cortex.

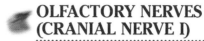

OLFACTORY NERVES (CRANIAL NERVE I)

The olfactory nerves arise from the olfactory receptor nerve cells in the olfactory mucous membrane located in the upper part of the nasal cavity above the level of the superior concha (Fig. 11-1). The **olfactory receptor cells** are scattered among supporting cells. Each receptor cell consists of a small bipolar nerve cell with a coarse peripheral process that passes to the surface of the membrane and a fine central process. From the coarse peripheral process a number of short cilia arise, the **olfactory hairs**, which project into the mucus covering the surface of the mucous membrane. These projecting hairs react to odors in the air and stimulate the olfactory cells.

The fine central processes form the **olfactory nerve fibers** (see Fig. 11-1). Bundles of these nerve fibers pass through the openings of the cribriform plate of the ethmoid bone to enter the olfactory bulb. The olfactory nerve fibers are unmyelinated and are covered with Schwann cells.

Olfactory Bulb

This ovoid structure possesses several types of nerve cells, the largest of which is the **mitral cell** (Fig. 11-1). The incoming olfactory nerve fibers synapse with the dendrites of the mitral cells and form rounded areas known as **synaptic glomeruli**. Smaller nerve cells called **tufted cells** and **granular cells** also synapse with the mitral cells. The olfactory bulb, in addition, receives axons from the contralateral olfactory bulb through the olfactory tract.

Olfactory Tract

This narrow band of white matter runs from the posterior end of the olfactory bulb beneath the inferior surface of the frontal lobe of the brain (Fig. 11-1). It consists of the central axons of the mitral and tufted cells of the bulb and some centrifugal fibers from the opposite olfactory bulb.

As the olfactory tract reaches the **anterior perforated substance**, it divides into **medial** and **lateral olfactory striae**. The lateral stria carries the axons to the **olfactory area of the cerebral cortex**, namely, the **periamygdaloid** and **prepiriform areas** (see Fig. 11-1). The medial olfactory stria carries the fibers that cross the median plane in the anterior commissure to pass to the olfactory bulb of the opposite side.

The periamygdaloid and prepiriform areas of the cerebral cortex are often known as the **primary olfactory cortex**. The **entorhinal area (area 28)** of the parahippocampal gyrus, which receives numerous connections from the primary olfactory cortex, is called the **secondary olfactory cortex**. These areas of the cortex are responsible for the appreciation of olfactory sensations (see Fig. 11-1). Note that, in contrast to all other sensory pathways, the ol-

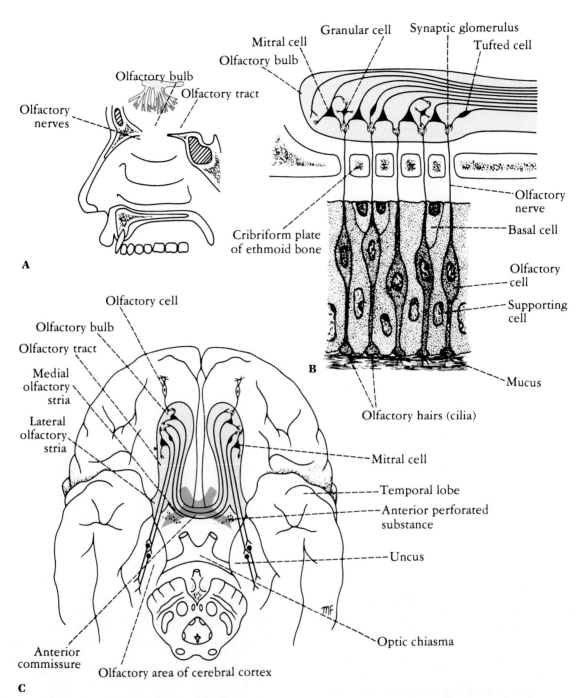

Figure 11–1   A. Distribution of olfactory nerves on the lateral wall of the nose. **B.** Connections between the olfactory cells and the neurons of the olfactory bulb. **C.** Connections between the olfactory cell and the rest of the olfactory system.

factory afferent pathway has only two neurons and reaches the cerebral cortex without synapsing in one of the thalamic nuclei.

The primary olfactory cortex sends nerve fibers to many other centers within the brain to establish connections for emotional and autonomic responses to olfactory sensations.

OPTIC NERVE (CRANIAL NERVE II)

Origin Of The Optic Nerve

The fibers of the optic nerve are the axons of the cells in the **ganglionic layer** of the retina. They converge on the **optic disc** and exit from the eye, about 3 or 4 mm to the nasal side of its center, as the optic nerve (Fig. 11-2). The fibers of the optic nerve are myelinated, but the sheaths are formed from oligodendrocytes rather than Schwann cells, since the optic nerve is comparable to a tract within the central nervous system.

The optic nerve leaves the orbital cavity through the optic canal and unites with the optic nerve of the opposite side to form the **optic chiasma**.

Optic Chiasma

The optic chiasma is situated at the junction of the anterior wall and floor of the third ventricle. Its anterolateral angles are continuous with the optic nerves and the posterolateral angles are continuous with the optic tracts (Fig. 11-2). In the chiasma, the fibers from the nasal (medial) half of each retina, including the nasal half of the **macula,*** cross the midline and enter the optic tract of the opposite side, while the fibers from the temporal (lateral) half of each retina, including the temporal half of the **macula,** pass posteriorly in the optic tract of the same side.

Optic Tract

The optic tract (Fig. 11-2) emerges from the optic chiasma and passes posterolaterally around the cerebral peduncle. Most of the fibers now terminate by synapsing with nerve cells in the **lateral geniculate body**, which is a small projection from the posterior part of the thalamus. A few of the fibers pass to the **pretectal nucleus** and the **superior colliculus** of the midbrain and are concerned with light reflexes (Fig. 11-3).

Lateral Geniculate Body

The lateral geniculate body is a small, oval swelling projecting from the **pulvinar of the thalamus**. It consists of six layers of cells upon which synapse the axons of the optic tract. The axons of the nerve cells within the geniculate body leave it to form the **optic radiation** (Fig. 11-2).

---

*The macula or macula lutea, found at the posterior pole of the eye, is the area of the retina for the most distinct vision. Here the retina is thinned, so that light has greater access to the cones.

Optic Radiation

The fibers of the optic radiation are the axons of the nerve cells of the lateral geniculate body. The tract passes posteriorly through the retrolenticular part of the **internal capsule** and terminates in the **visual cortex (area 17)**, which occupies the upper and lower lips of the calcarine sulcus on the medial surface of the cerebral hemisphere (Fig. 11-2). The visual association cortex (areas 18 and 19) is responsible for recognition of objects and perception of color.

Neurons of the Visual Pathway and Binocular Vision

Four neurons conduct visual impulses to the visual cortex: (1) **rods** and **cones**, which are specialized receptor neurons in the retina; (2) **bipolar neurons**, which connect the rods and cones to the ganglion cells; (3) **ganglion cells**, whose axons pass to the lateral geniculate body; and (4) **neurons of the lateral geniculate body,** whose axons pass to the cerebral cortex.

In binocular vision, the right and left fields of vision are projected on portions of both retinae (Fig. 11-2). The image of an object in the right field of vision is projected on the nasal half of the right retina and the temporal half of the left retina. In the optic chiasma, the axons from these two retinal halves are combined to form the left optic tract. The lateral geniculate body neurons now project the complete right field of vision upon the visual cortex of the left hemisphere, and the left visual field on the visual cortex of the right hemisphere (Fig. 11-2). The lower retinal quadrants (upper field of vision) project on the lower wall of the calcarine sulcus, while the upper retinal quadrants (lower field of vision) project on the upper wall of the sulcus. Note also that the **macula lutea** is represented on the posterior part of area 17, and the periphery of the retina is represented anteriorly.

Visual Reflexes

DIRECT AND CONSENSUAL LIGHT REFLEXES

If a light is shone into one eye, the pupils of both eyes normally constrict. The constriction of the pupil upon which the light is shone is called the **direct light reflex**; the constriction of the opposite pupil even though no light fell upon that eye is called the **consensual light reflex** (Fig. 11-3).

The afferent impulses travel through the optic nerve, optic chiasma, and optic tract (Fig. 11-3). Here a small number of fibers leave the optic tract and synapse on nerve cells in the **pretectal nucleus**, which lies close to the superior colliculus. The impulses are passed by axons of the pretectal nerve cells to the parasympathetic nuclei (**Edinger-Westphal nuclei**) of the third cranial nerve on **both sides**. Here the fibers synapse and the parasympathetic nerves travel through the third cranial nerve to the **ciliary ganglion** in the orbit (Fig. 11-3). Finally, postganglionic parasympathetic fibers pass through the **short ciliary**

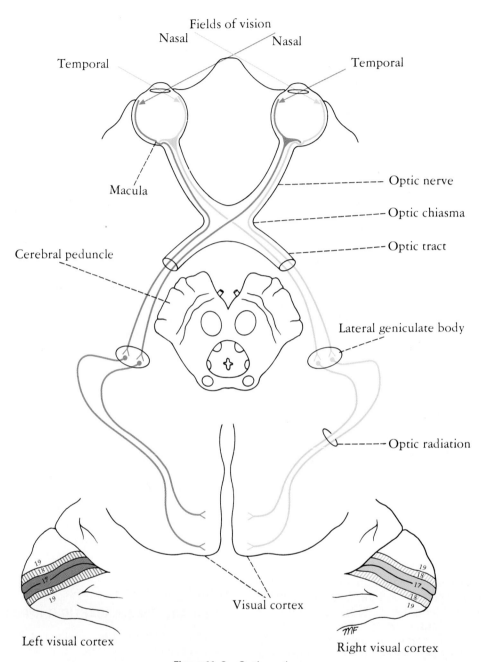

Figure 11–2 Optic pathway.

nerves to the eyeball and the **constrictor pupillae muscle** of the iris. Both pupils constrict in the consensual light reflex because the pretectal nucleus sends fibers to the parasympathetic nuclei on both sides of the midbrain (Fig. 11-3). The fibers that cross the median plane do so close to the cerebral aqueduct in the posterior commissure.

ACCOMMODATION REFLEX

When the eyes are directed from a distant to a near object, contraction of the medial recti brings about convergence of the ocular axes; the lens thicken to increase its refractive power by contraction of the ciliary muscle; and the pupils constrict to restrict the light waves to the thickest central part of the lens. The afferent impulses travel through the optic nerve, the optic chiasma, the optic tract, the lateral geniculate body, and the optic radiation to the visual cortex. The visual cortex is connected to the eye field of the frontal cortex (Fig. 11-3). From here, cortical fibers descend through the internal capsule to the oculomotor nuclei in the midbrain. The oculomotor nerve travels to the medial recti muscles. Some of the descending cortical fibers synapse with the parasympathetic nuclei (Edinger-Westphal nuclei) of the third cranial nerve on **both sides**. Here the fibers

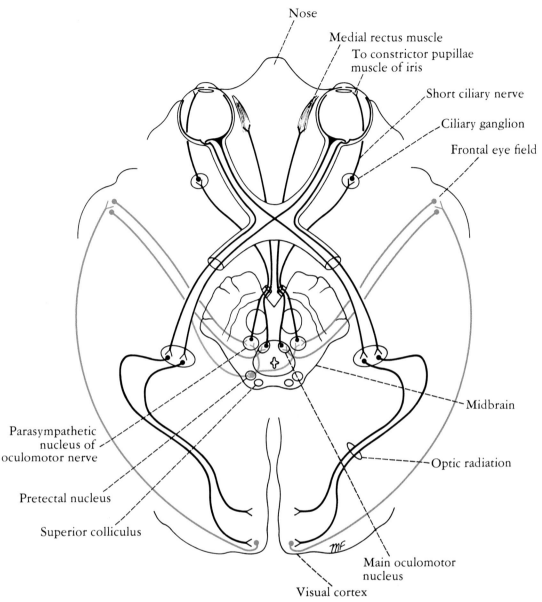

Figure 11–3   Optic pathway and the visual reflexes.

synapse and the parasympathetic nerves travel through the third cranial nerve to the ciliary ganglion in the orbit. Finally, postganglionic parasympathetic fibers pass through the short ciliary nerves to the **ciliary muscle** and the **constrictor pupillae muscle** of the iris (Fig. 11-3).

CORNEAL REFLEX

Light touching of the cornea or conjunctiva results in blinking of the eyelids. Afferent impulses from the cornea or conjunctiva travel through the ophthalmic division of the trigeminal nerve to the sensory nucleus of the trigeminal nerve (Fig. 11-4A). Internuncial neurons connect with the motor nucleus of the facial nerve on both sides through the medial longitudinal fasciculus. The facial nerve and its branches supply the orbicularis oculi muscle, which causes closure of the eyelids.

VISUAL BODY REFLEXES

The automatic scanning movements of the eyes and head made when reading, the automatic movement of the eyes, head, and neck toward the source of the visual stimulus, and the protective closing of the eyes and even the raising of the arm for protection are reflex actions that involve the following reflex arcs (Fig. 11-4B). The visual impulses follow the optic nerves, optic chiasma, and optic tracts to the superior colliculi. Here the impulses are relayed to the tec-

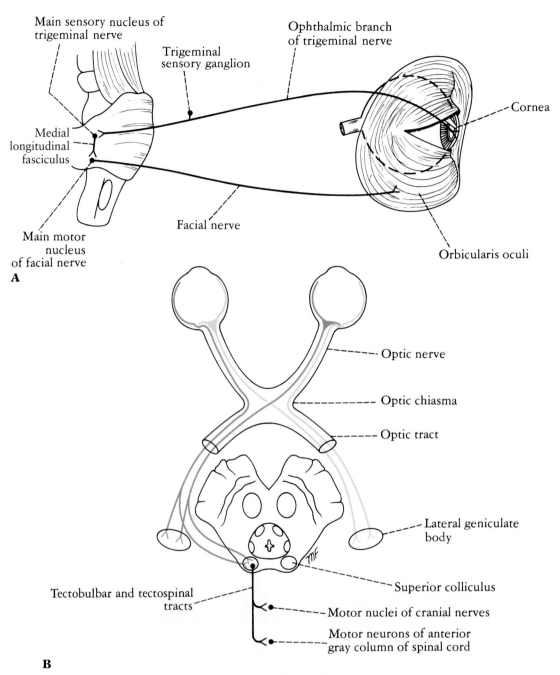

Figure 11–4 **A.** Corneal reflex. **B.** Visual body reflex.

tospinal and tectobulbar (tectonuclear) tracts and to the neurons of the anterior gray columns of the spinal cord and cranial motor nuclei.

PUPILLARY SKIN REFLEX

The pupil will dilate if the skin is painfully stimulated by pinching. The afferent sensory fibers are believed to have connections with the efferent preganglionic sympathetic neurons in the lateral gray columns of the first and second thoracic segments of the spinal cord. The **white rami communicantes** of these segments pass to the sympathetic trunk and the preganglionic fibers ascend to the superior **cervical sympathetic ganglion**. The postganglionic fibers pass through the **internal carotid plexus** and the **long ciliary nerves** to the dilator pupillae muscle of the iris.

OCULOMOTOR NERVE (CRANIAL NERVE III)

The oculomotor nerve is entirely motor in function.

Oculomotor Nerve Nuclei

The oculomotor nerve has two motor nuclei: (1) the main motor nucleus and (2) the accessory parasympathetic nucleus.

The **main oculomotor nucleus** is situated in the anterior part of the gray matter that surrounds the **cerebral aqueduct of the midbrain** (Fig. 11-5). It lies at the level of the **superior colliculus**. The nucleus consists of groups of

nerve cells that supply all the extrinsic muscles of the eye except the superior oblique and the lateral rectus. The outgoing nerve fibers pass anteriorly through the red nucleus and emerge on the anterior surface of the midbrain in the **interpeduncular fossa**. The main oculomotor nucleus receives corticonuclear fibers from both cerebral hemispheres. It receives tectobulbar fibers from the superior colliculus and through this route receives information from the visual cortex. It also receives fibers from the medial longitudinal fasciculus, by which it is connected to the nuclei of the fourth, sixth, and eighth cranial nerves.

The **accessory parasympathetic nucleus (Edinger-Westphal nucleus)** is situated posterior to the main oculo-

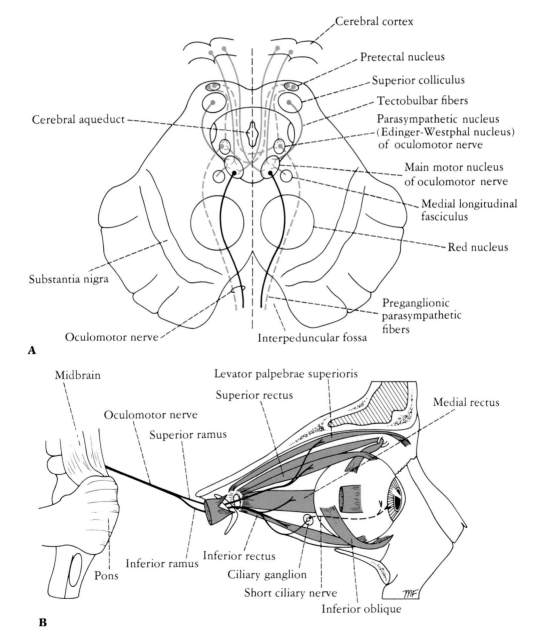

Figure 11–5   A. Oculomotor nerve nuclei and their central connections. **B.** The distribution of the oculomotor nerve.

motor nucleus (Fig. 11-5). The axons of the nerve cells, which are preganglionic, accompany the other oculomotor fibers to the orbit. Here they synapse in the **ciliary ganglion** and postganglionic fibers pass through the **short ciliary nerves** to the constrictor pupillae of the iris and the ciliary muscles. The accessory parasympathetic nucleus receives corticonuclear fibers for the accommodation reflex and fibers from the pretectal nucleus for the direct and consensual light reflexes (Fig. 11-3).

Course of the Oculomotor Nerve

The oculomotor nerve emerges on the anterior surface of the midbrain (Fig. 11-5). It passes forward between the posterior cerebral and the superior cerebellar arteries. It then continues into the middle cranial fossa in the lateral wall of the cavernous sinus. Here, it divides into a superior and an inferior ramus, which enter the orbital cavity through the superior orbital fissure.

The oculomotor nerve supplies the following extrinsic muscles of the eye: the levator palpebrae superioris, superior rectus, medial rectus, inferior rectus, and inferior oblique. It also supplies through its branch to the ciliary ganglion and the short ciliary nerves parasympathetic nerve fibers to the following intrinsic muscles: the constrictor pupillae of the iris and ciliary muscles.

The oculomotor nerve is therefore entirely motor and is responsible for lifting the upper eyelid; turning the eye upward, downward, and medially; constricting the pupil; and accommodating the eye.

TROCHLEAR NERVE (CRANIAL NERVE IV)

The trochlear nerve is entirely motor in function.

Trochlear Nerve Nucleus

The trochlear nucleus is situated in the anterior part of the gray matter that surrounds the **cerebral aqueduct of the midbrain** (Fig. 11-6). It lies inferior to the oculomotor

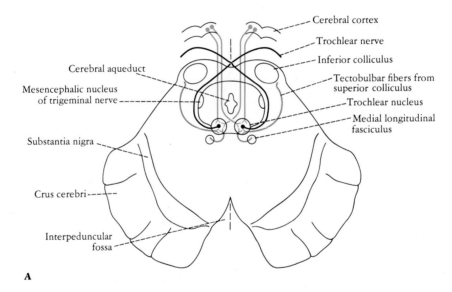

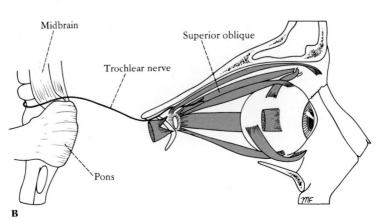

Figure 11–6   A. Trochlear nerve nucleus and its central connections. **B**. Distribution of the trochlear nerve.

nucleus at the level of the **inferior colliculus**. The nerve fibers, after leaving the nucleus, pass posteriorly around the central gray matter to reach the posterior surface of the midbrain.

The trochlear nucleus receives corticonuclear fibers from both cerebral hemispheres. It receives the tectobulbar fibers, which connect it to the visual cortex through the superior colliculus (Fig. 11-6). It also receives fibers from the **medial longitudinal fasciculus**, by which it is connected to the nuclei of the third, sixth, and eighth cranial nerves.

Course of the Trochlear Nerve

The trochlear nerve, the most slender of the cranial nerves, and the only one to leave the posterior surface of the brainstem, emerges from the midbrain and **immediately decussates with the nerve of the opposite side**. The trochlear nerve passes forward through the middle cranial fossa in the lateral wall of the cavernous sinus and enters the orbit through the superior orbital fissure. The nerve supplies the superior oblique muscle of the eyeball. The trochlear nerve is entirely motor and assists in turning the eye downward and laterally.

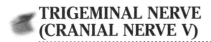

TRIGEMINAL NERVE (CRANIAL NERVE V)

The trigeminal nerve is the largest cranial nerve and contains both sensory and motor fibers. It is the sensory nerve to the greater part of the head and the motor nerve to several muscles, including the muscles of mastication (Fig. 11-8).

Trigeminal Nerve Nuclei

The trigeminal nerve has four nuclei: (1) the main sensory nucleus, (2) the spinal nucleus, (3) the mesencephalic nucleus, and (4) the motor nucleus.

MAIN SENSORY NUCLEUS

This nucleus lies in the posterior part of the pons, lateral to the motor nucleus (Fig. 11-7A). It is continuous below with the spinal nucleus.

SPINAL NUCLEUS

This nucleus is continuous superiorly with the main sensory nucleus in the pons and extends inferiorly through the whole length of the medulla oblongata and into the upper part of the spinal cord as far as the second cervical segment (Fig. 11-7B).

MESENCEPHALIC NUCLEUS

This nucleus is composed of a column of unipolar nerve cells situated in the lateral part of the gray matter around the cerebral aqueduct. It extends inferiorly into the pons as far as the main sensory nucleus (Fig. 11-7).

MOTOR NUCLEUS

This nucleus is situated in the pons medial to the main sensory nucleus (Fig. 11-7).

Sensory Components of the Trigeminal Nerve

The sensations of pain and temperature and touch and pressure from the skin of the face and mucous membranes travel along axons whose cell bodies are situated in the **semilunar** or **trigeminal sensory ganglion** (Fig. 11-7B). The central processes of these cells form the large sensory root of the trigeminal nerve. About half the fibers divide into ascending and descending branches when they enter the pons; the remainder ascend or descend without division (Fig. 11-7B). The ascending branches terminate in the main sensory nucleus and the descending branches terminate in the spinal nucleus. The sensations of touch and pressure are conveyed by nerve fibers that terminate in the main sensory nucleus. The sensations of pain and temperature pass to the spinal nucleus (Fig. 11-7B). The sensory fibers from the ophthalmic division of the trigeminal nerve terminate in the inferior part of the spinal nucleus; fibers from the maxillary division terminate in the middle of the spinal nucleus; and fibers from the mandibular division end in the superior part of the spinal nucleus.

Proprioceptive impulses from the muscles of mastication and from the facial and extraocular muscles are carried by fibers in the sensory root of the trigeminal nerve that have bypassed the semilunar or trigeminal ganglion (Fig. 11-7B). The fibers' cells of origin are the unipolar cells of the mesencephalic nucleus (Fig. 11-7).

The axons of the neurons in the main sensory and spinal nuclei, and the central processes of the cells in the mesencephalic nucleus, now cross the median plane and ascend as the trigeminal lemniscus to terminate on the nerve cells of the ventral posteromedial nucleus of the thalamus. The axons of these cells now travel through the internal capsule to the postcentral gyrus (areas 3, 1, and 2) of the cerebral cortex.

Motor Component of the Trigeminal Nerve

The motor nucleus receives corticonuclear fibers from both cerebral hemispheres (Fig. 11-7). It also receives fibers from the reticular formation, the red nucleus, the tectum, and the medial longitudinal fasciculus. In addition, it receives fibers from the mesencephalic nucleus, thereby forming a monosynaptic reflex arc.

The cells of the motor nucleus give rise to the axons that form the motor root. The motor nucleus supplies the **muscles of mastication**, the **tensor tympani**, the **tensor veli palatini**, and the **mylohyoid** and the **anterior belly of the digastric muscle**.

Course of the Trigeminal Nerve

The trigeminal nerve leaves the anterior aspect of the pons as a small motor root and a large sensory root. The nerve

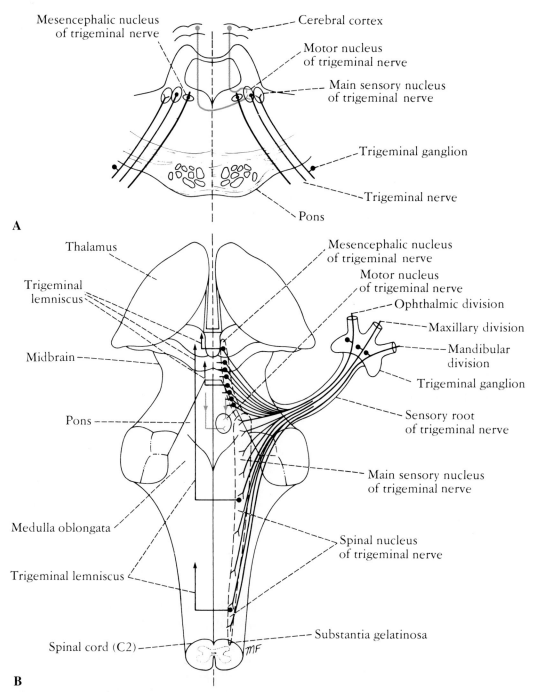

Figure 11–7   A. Trigeminal nerve nuclei seen in a coronal section of the pons. **B.** Trigeminal nerve nuclei in the brainstem and their central connections.

passes forward out of the posterior cranial fossa and rests on the upper surface of the apex of the petrous part of the temporal bone in the middle cranial fossa. The large sensory root now expands to form the crescent-shaped **trigeminal ganglion**, which lies within a pouch of dura mater called the **trigeminal** or **Meckel's cave**. The ophthalmic, maxillary, and mandibular nerves arise from the anterior border of the ganglion (Fig.11-8). The ophthalmic nerve (V1) con-

tains only sensory fibers and leaves the skull through the superior orbital fissure to enter the orbital cavity. The maxillary nerve (V2) also contains only sensory fibers and leaves the skull through the foramen rotundum. The mandibular nerve (V3) contains both sensory and motor fibers and leaves the skull through the foramen ovale.

The sensory fibers to the skin of the face from each division supply a distinct zone (Fig. 11-9), there being little or

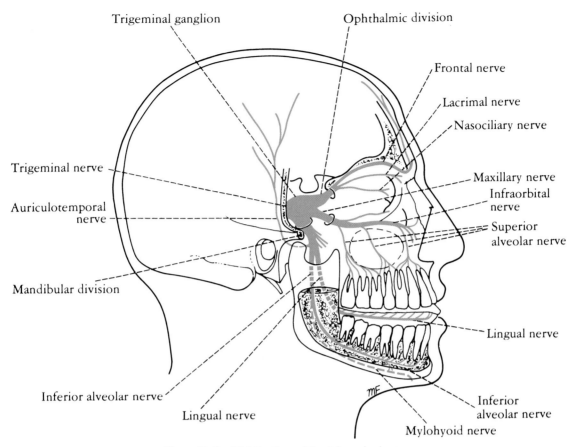

Figure 11–8   Distribution of the trigeminal nerve.

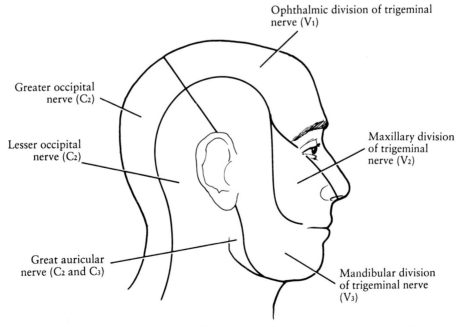

Figure 11–9   Sensory nerve supply to the skin of the head and neck. Note that the skin over the angle of the jaw is supplied by the great auricular nerve (C_2 and C_3) and not by branches of the trigeminal nerve.

no overlap of the dermatomes. (Compare with the overlap of the dermatomes of the spinal nerves.) As noted previously, the motor fibers in the mandibular division are mainly distributed to muscles of mastication.

ABDUCENT NERVE (CRANIAL NERVE VI)

The abducent nerve is a small motor nerve that supplies the **lateral rectus muscle** of the eyeball.

Abducent Nerve Nucleus

The small motor nucleus is situated beneath the floor of the upper part of the fourth ventricle, close to the midline and beneath the **colliculus facialis** (Fig. 11-10A). The nucleus receives afferent corticonuclear fibers from both cerebral hemispheres. It receives the tectobulbar tract from the superior colliculus, by which the visual cortex is connected to the nucleus. It also receives fibers from the medial longitudinal fasciculus, by which it is connected to the nuclei of the third, fourth, and eighth cranial nerves (Fig. 11-9).

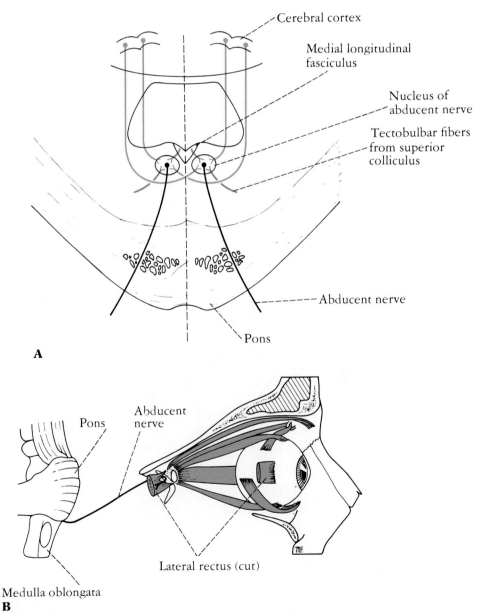

Figure 11–10 **A**. Abducent nerve nucleus and its central connections. **B**. Distribution of the abducent nerve.

Course of the Abducent Nerve

The fibers of the abducent nerve pass anteriorly through the pons and emerge in the groove between the lower border of the pons and the medulla oblongata (Fig. 11-10B). It passes forward through the cavernous sinus, lying below and lateral to the internal carotid artery. The nerve then enters the orbit through the superior orbital fissure. The abducent nerve is entirely a motor nerve and supplies the lateral rectus muscle and is, therefore, responsible for turning the eye laterally.

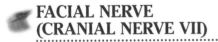

FACIAL NERVE (CRANIAL NERVE VII)

The facial nerve is both a motor and a sensory nerve.

Facial Nerve Nuclei

The facial nerve has three nuclei: (1) the main motor nucleus, (2) the parasympathetic nuclei, and (3) the sensory nucleus.

MAIN MOTOR NUCLEUS

This lies deep in the reticular formation of the lower part of the pons (Fig. 11-11). The part of the nucleus that supplies the muscles of the upper part of the face receives corticonuclear fibers from both cerebral hemispheres. **The part of the nucleus that supplies the muscles of the lower part of the face receives only corticonuclear fibers from the opposite cerebral hemisphere.**

These pathways explain the voluntary control of facial muscles. However, another involuntary pathway exists; it is separate and controls **mimetic or emotional changes in facial expression.** This other pathway forms part of the reticular formation (see p. 305).

PARASYMPATHETIC NUCLEI

These lie posterolateral to the main motor nucleus. They are the **superior salivatory** and **lacrimal nuclei** (Fig. 11-11). The superior salivatory nucleus receives afferent fibers from the hypothalamus through the **descending autonomic pathways.** Information concerning taste also is received from the **nucleus of the solitary tract** from the mouth cavity.

The lacrimal nucleus receives afferent fibers from the hypothalamus for emotional responses and from the sensory nuclei of the trigeminal nerve for reflex lacrimation secondary to irritation of the cornea or conjunctiva.

SENSORY NUCLEUS

This is the upper part of the **nucleus of the tractus solitarius** and lies close to the motor nucleus (Fig. 11-11). Sensations of taste travel through the peripheral axons of nerve cells situated in the **geniculate ganglion** on the seventh cranial nerve. The central processes of these cells synapse on nerve cells in the nucleus. Efferent fibers cross the median plane and ascend to the ventral posterior medial nucleus of the opposite thalamus and also a number of hypothalamic nuclei. From the thalamus, the axons of the thalamic cells pass through the internal capsule and corona radiata to end in the taste area of the cortex in the lower part of the postcentral gyrus (Fig. 11-11).

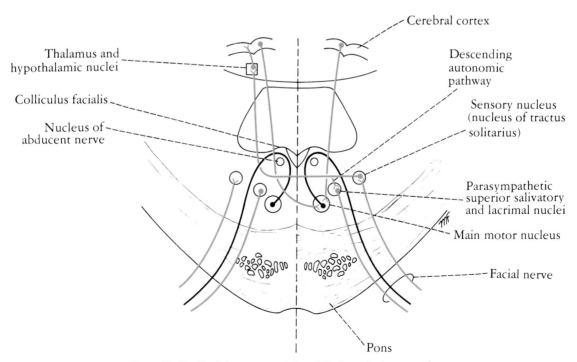

Figure 11–11   Facial nerve nuclei and their central connections.

Course of the Facial Nerve

The facial nerve consists of a motor and a sensory root. The fibers of the motor root first travel posteriorly around the medial side of the abducent nucleus (Fig. 11-11). Then they pass around the nucleus beneath the **colliculus facialis** in the floor of the fourth ventricle and finally pass anteriorly to emerge from the brainstem (Fig. 11-11).

The sensory root (**nervus intermedius**) is formed of the central processes of the unipolar cells of the geniculate ganglion. It also contains the efferent preganglionic parasympathetic fibers from the parasympathetic nuclei.

The two roots of the facial nerve emerge from the anterior surface of the brain between the pons and the medulla oblongata. They pass laterally in the posterior cranial fossa with the vestibulocochlear nerve and enter the internal acoustic meatus in the petrous part of the temporal bone. At the bottom of the meatus, the nerve enters the facial canal and runs laterally through the inner ear. On reaching the medial wall of the tympanic cavity, the nerve expands to form the sensory **geniculate ganglion** (Fig. 11-12) and turns sharply backward above the promontory. At the posterior wall of the tympanic cavity the facial nerve turns

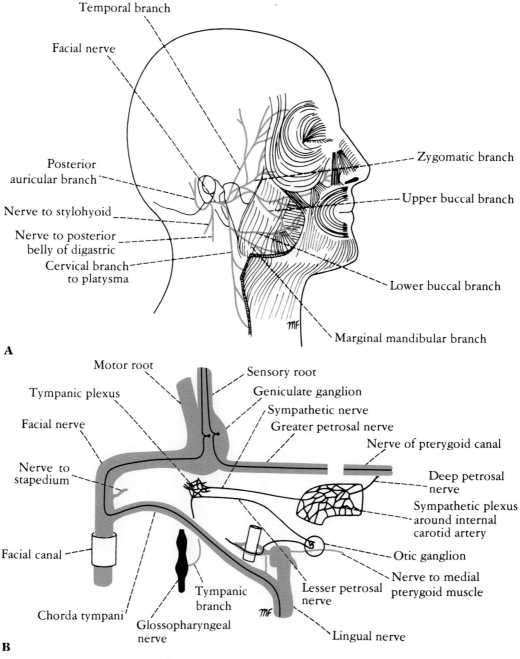

Figure 11–12   A. Distribution of the facial nerve. **B**. Branches of the facial nerve within the petrous part of the temporal bone; the taste fibers are shown in black. The glossopharyngeal nerve is also shown.

downward on the medial side of the aditus of the mastoid antrum, descends behind the pyramid, and emerges from the stylomastoid foramen.

Distribution of the Facial Nerve

The **motor nucleus** supplies the muscles of facial expression, the auricular muscles, the stapedius, the posterior belly of the digastric, and the stylohyoid muscles (Fig. 11-12).

The **superior salivatory nucleus** supplies the submandibular and sublingual salivary glands and the nasal and palatine glands. The **lacrimal nucleus** supplies the lacrimal gland.

The **sensory nucleus** receives taste fibers from the anterior two-thirds of the tongue, the floor of the mouth, and the palate.

VESTIBULOCOCHLEAR NERVE (CRANIAL NERVE VIII)

This nerve consists of two distinct parts, the **vestibular nerve** and the **cochlear nerve**, which are concerned with the transmission of afferent information from the internal ear to the central nervous system (Figs. 11-13 and 11-14).

Vestibular Nerve

The vestibular nerve conducts nerve impulses from the utricle and saccule that provide information concerning the position of the head; the nerve also conducts impulses from the semicircular canals that provide information concerning movements of the head.

The nerve fibers of the vestibular nerve are the central processes of nerve cells located in the **vestibular ganglion**, which is situated in the **internal acoustic meatus**. They enter the anterior surface of the brainstem in a groove between the lower border of the pons and the upper part of the medulla oblongata (Fig. 11-13). When they enter the vestibular nuclear complex, the fibers divide into short ascending and long descending fibers; a small number of fibers pass directly to the cerebellum through the inferior cerebellar peduncle, bypassing the vestibular nuclei.

THE VESTIBULAR NUCLEAR COMPLEX

This complex consists of a group of nuclei situated beneath the floor of the fourth ventricle (Fig. 11-13). Four nuclei may be recognized: (1) the **lateral vestibular nucleus**, (2) the **superior vestibular nucleus**, (3) the **medial vestibular nucleus**, and (4) the **inferior vestibular nucleus** (Fig. 5-7).

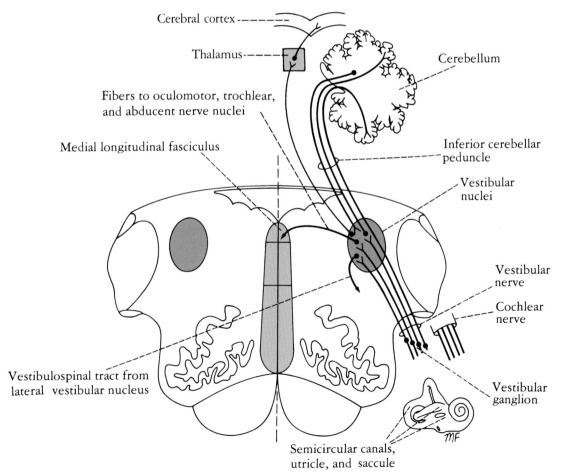

Figure 11–13 Vestibular nerve nuclei and their central connections.

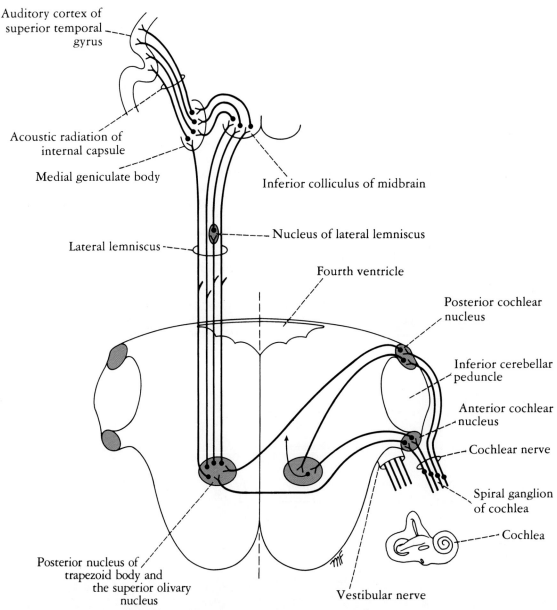

Figure 11–14 Cochlear nerve nuclei and their central connections. The descending pathways have been omitted.

The vestibular nuclei receive afferent fibers from the **utricle** and **saccule** and the **semicircular canals** through the vestibular nerve, and fibers from the cerebellum through the inferior cerebellar peduncle (Fig. 11-13). Efferent fibers from the nuclei pass to the cerebellum through the inferior cerebellar peduncle. Efferent fibers also descend uncrossed to the spinal cord from the lateral vestibular nucleus and form the **vestibulospinal tract** (Fig. 11-13). In addition, efferent fibers pass to the nuclei of the oculomotor, trochlear, and abducent nerves through the medial longitudinal fasciculus.

These connections enable the movements of the head and the eyes to be coordinated so that visual fixation on an object can be maintained. In addition, information received from the internal ear can assist in maintaining balance by influencing the muscle tone of the limbs and trunk.

Ascending fibers also pass upward from the vestibular nuclei to the cerebral cortex, to the vestibular area in the postcentral gyrus, just above the lateral fissure. These fibers are thought to relay in the ventral posterior nuclei of the thalamus. The cerebral cortex probably serves to orient the individual consciously in space.

Cochlear Nerve

The cochlear nerve conducts nerve impulses concerned with sound from the organ of Corti in the cochlea. The

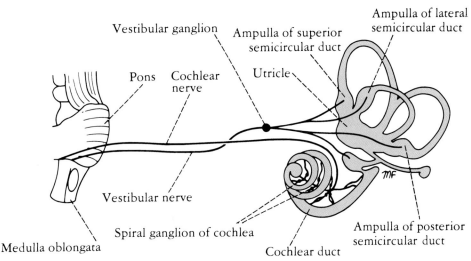

Figure 11–15 Distribution of the vestibulocochlear nerve.

fibers of the cochlear nerve are the central processes of nerve cells located in the **spiral ganglion of the cochlea** (Fig. 11-15). They enter the anterior surface of the brainstem at the lower border of the pons on the lateral side of the emerging facial nerve and are separated from it by the vestibular nerve (Fig. 11-14). On entering the pons the nerve fibers divide, one branch entering the **posterior cochlear nucleus** and the other branch entering the **anterior cochlear nucleus**.

COCHLEAR NUCLEI

The anterior and posterior cochlear nuclei are situated on the surface of the inferior cerebellar peduncle (Fig. 11-14). They receive afferent fibers from the cochlea through the cochlear nerve. The cochlear nuclei send axons (second-order neuron fibers) that run medially through the pons to end in the **trapezoid body** and the olivary nucleus. Here they are relayed in the **posterior nucleus of the trapezoid body** and the superior olivary nucleus on the same or the opposite side. The axons now ascend through the posterior part of the pons and midbrain and form a tract known as the **lateral lemniscus** (Fig. 11-14). Each lateral lemniscus, therefore, consists of third-order neurons from both sides. As these fibers ascend, some of them relay in small groups of nerve cells, collectively known as the **nucleus of the lateral lemniscus** (Fig. 11-14).

On reaching the midbrain, the fibers of the lateral lemniscus either terminate in the **nucleus of the inferior colliculus** or are relayed in the **medial geniculate body** and pass to the **auditory cortex** of the cerebral hemisphere through the **acoustic radiation of the internal capsule** (Fig. 11-14).

The primary auditory cortex (areas 41 and 42) includes the gyrus of Heschl on the upper surface of the superior temporal gyrus. The recognition and interpretation of sounds on the basis of past experience take place in the secondary auditory area.

Nerve impulses from the ear are transmitted along auditory pathways on both sides of the brainstem, with more being projected along the contralateral pathway. Many collateral branches are given off to the reticular activating system of the brainstem (see p. 305). The tonotopic organization present in the organ of Corti is preserved within the cochlear nuclei, the inferior colliculi, and the primary auditory area.

DESCENDING AUDITORY PATHWAYS

Descending fibers originating in the auditory cortex and in other nuclei in the auditory pathway accompany the ascending pathway. These fibers are bilateral and end on nerve cells at different levels of the auditory pathway and on the hair cells of the organ of Corti. It is believed that these fibers serve as a feedback mechanism and inhibit the reception of sound. They may also have a role in the process of auditory sharpening, suppressing some signals and enhancing others.

Course of the Vestibulocochlear Nerve

The vestibular and cochlear parts of the nerve leave the anterior surface of the brain between the lower border of the pons and the medulla oblongata (Fig. 11-15). They run laterally in the posterior cranial fossa and enter the internal acoustic meatus with the facial nerve. The fibers are then distributed to the different parts of the internal ear (Fig. 11-15).

GLOSSOPHARYNGEAL NERVE (CRANIAL NERVE IX)

The glossopharyngeal nerve is a motor and a sensory nerve.

Glossopharyngeal Nerve Nuclei

The glossopharyngeal nerve has three nuclei: (1) the main motor nucleus, (2) the parasympathetic nucleus, and (3) the sensory nucleus.

MAIN MOTOR NUCLEUS

This nucleus lies deep in the reticular formation of the medulla oblongata and is formed by the superior end of the nucleus ambiguus (Fig. 11-16). It receives corticonuclear fibers from both cerebral hemispheres. The efferent fibers supply the **stylopharyngeus muscle**.

PARASYMPATHETIC NUCLEUS

This nucleus is also called the **inferior salivatory nucleus** (see Fig. 11-16). It receives afferent fibers from the hypothalamus through the **descending autonomic pathways**. It also is thought to receive information from the olfactory system through the reticular formation. Information concerning taste also is received from the nucleus of the solitary tract from the mouth cavity.

The efferent preganglionic parasympathetic fibers reach the otic ganglion through the **tympanic branch of the glossopharyngeal nerve**, the **tympanic plexus**, and the **lesser petrosal nerve** (Fig. 11-17). The postganglionic fibers pass to the **parotid salivary gland**.

SENSORY NUCLEUS

This is part of the **nucleus of the tractus solitarius** (Fig. 11-16). Sensations of taste travel through the peripheral

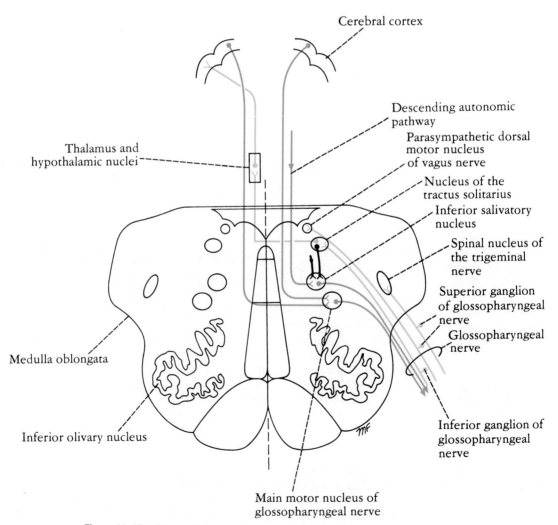

Figure 11–16 Glossopharyngeal nerve nuclei and their central connections.

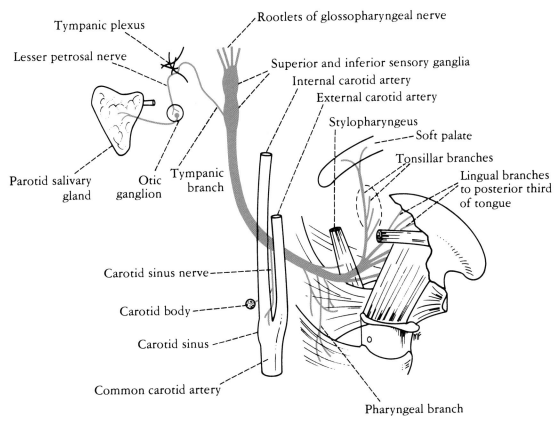

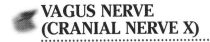

Figure 11–17   Distribution of the glossopharyngeal nerve.

axons of nerve cells situated in the **ganglion** on the glossopharyngeal nerve. The central processes of these cells synapse on nerve cells in the nucleus. Efferent fibers cross the median plane and ascend to the ventral group of nuclei of the opposite thalamus, and also a number of hypothalamic nuclei. From the thalamus, the axons of the thalamic cells pass through the internal capsule and corona radiata to end in the lower part of the postcentral gyrus.

Afferent information that concerns common sensation enters the brainstem through the superior ganglion of the glossopharyngeal nerve, but ends in the **spinal nucleus of the trigeminal nerve**. Afferent impulses from the **carotid sinus**, a baroreceptor situated at the bifurcation of the common carotid artery, also travel with the glossopharyngeal nerve. They terminate in the **nucleus of the tractus solitarius** and are connected to the **dorsal motor nucleus of the vagus nerve**. The carotid sinus reflex that involves the glossopharyngeal and vagus nerves assists in the regulation of arterial blood pressure.

Course of the Glossopharyngeal Nerve

The glossopharyngeal nerve leaves the anterolateral surface of the upper part of the medulla oblongata as a series of rootlets in a groove between the olive and the inferior cerebellar peduncle (Fig. 11-16). It passes laterally in the posterior cranial fossa and leaves the skull through the jugular foramen. The superior and inferior glossopharyngeal sensory ganglia are situated on the nerve here. The nerve then descends through the upper part of the neck in company with the internal jugular vein and the internal carotid artery to reach the posterior border of the stylopharyngeus muscle, which it supplies. The nerve then passes forward between the superior and middle constrictor muscles of the pharynx to give sensory branches to the mucous membrane of the pharynx and the posterior third of the tongue (Fig. 11-17).

VAGUS NERVE (CRANIAL NERVE X)

The vagus nerve is a motor and a sensory nerve.

Vagus Nerve Nuclei

The vagus nerve has three nuclei: (1) the main motor nucleus, (2) the parasympathetic nucleus, and (3) the sensory nucleus.

MAIN MOTOR NUCLEUS

This nucleus lies deep in the reticular formation of the medulla oblongata and is formed by the nucleus ambiguus (Fig. 11-18). It receives corticonuclear fibers from both cerebral hemispheres. The efferent fibers supply the constrictor muscles of the pharynx and the intrinsic muscles of the larynx (Fig. 11-19).

PARASYMPATHETIC NUCLEUS

This nucleus forms the dorsal nucleus of the vagus and lies beneath the floor of the lower part of the fourth ventricle posterolateral to the hypoglossal nucleus (Fig. 11-18). It receives afferent fibers from the hypothalamus through the descending autonomic pathways. It also receives other afferents, including those from the glossopharyngeal nerve (carotid sinus reflex). The efferent fibers are distributed to the involuntary muscle of the bronchi, heart, esophagus, stomach, small intestine, and large intestine as far as the distal one-third of the transverse colon (Fig. 11-19).

SENSORY NUCLEUS

This nucleus is the lower part of the **nucleus of the tractus solitarius**. Sensations of taste travel through the peripheral axons of nerve cells situated in the **inferior ganglion on the vagus nerve.** The central processes of those cells synapse on nerve cells in the nucleus (Fig. 11-18). Efferent fibers cross the

median plane and ascend to the ventral group of nuclei of the opposite thalamus as well as to a number of hypothalamic nuclei. From the thalamus, the axons of the thalamic cells pass through the internal capsule and corona radiata to end in the postcentral gyrus.

Afferent information concerning common sensation enters the brainstem through the superior ganglion of the vagus nerve but ends in the **spinal nucleus of the trigeminal nerve**.

Course of the Vagus Nerve

The vagus nerve leaves the anterolateral surface of the upper part of the medulla oblongata as a series of rootlets in a groove between the olive and the inferior cerebellar peduncle (Fig. 11-18). The nerve passes laterally through the posterior cranial fossa and leaves the skull through the jugular foramen. The vagus nerve possesses two sensory ganglia, a rounded superior ganglion, situated on the nerve within the jugular foramen, and a cylindrical **inferior ganglion**, which lies on the nerve just below the foramen. Below the inferior ganglion the cranial root of the accessory nerve joins the vagus nerve and is distributed mainly in its pharyngeal and recurrent laryngeal branches.

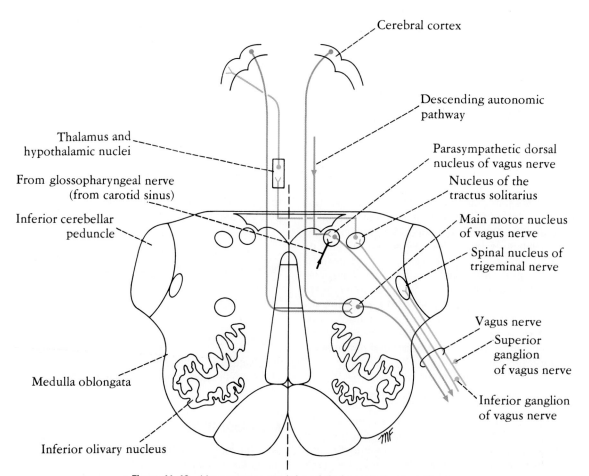

Figure 11–18 Vagus nerve nuclei and their central connections.

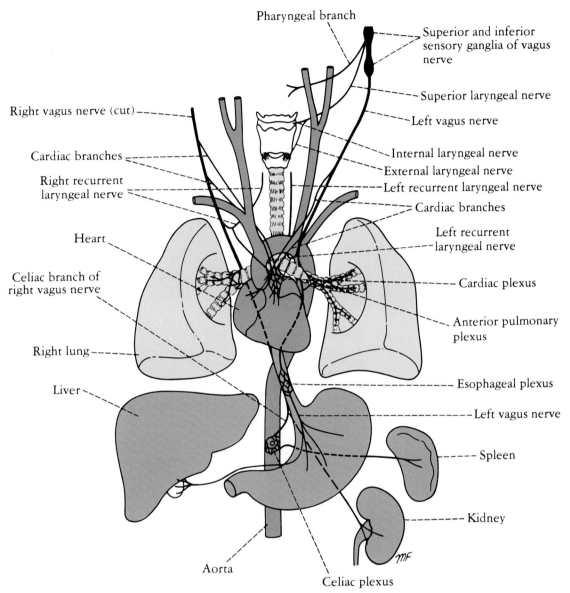

Figure 11–19 Distribution of the vagus nerve.

The vagus nerve descends vertically in the neck within the carotid sheath with the internal jugular vein and the internal and common carotid arteries.

The **right vagus nerve** enters the thorax and passes posterior to the root of the right lung contributing to the pulmonary plexus. It then passes on to the posterior surface of the esophagus and contributes to the **esophageal plexus**. It enters the abdomen through the esophageal opening of the diaphragm. The posterior vagal trunk (which is the name now given to the right vagus) is distributed to the posterior surface of the stomach and by a large celiac branch to the duodenum, liver, kidneys, and small and large intestines as far as the distal third of the

transverse colon. This wide distribution is accomplished through the celiac, superior mesenteric, and renal plexuses.

The **left vagus nerve** enters the thorax and crosses the left side of the aortic arch and descends behind the root of the left lung contributing to the **pulmonary plexus**. The left vagus then descends on the anterior surface of the esophagus contributing to the **esophageal plexus**. It enters the abdomen through the esophageal opening of the diaphragm. The anterior vagal trunk (which is the name now given to the left vagus) divides into several branches, which are distributed to the stomach, liver, upper part of the duodenum, and head of the pancreas.

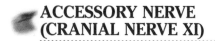
ACCESSORY NERVE (CRANIAL NERVE XI)

The accessory nerve is a motor nerve that is formed by the union of a cranial and a spinal root.

Cranial Root (Part)

The cranial root is formed from the axons of nerve cells of the nucleus ambiguus (Fig. 11-20). The nucleus receives corticonuclear fibers from both cerebral hemispheres. The efferent fibers of the nucleus emerge from the anterior surface of the medulla oblongata between the olive and the inferior cerebellar peduncle.

COURSE OF THE CRANIAL ROOT

The nerve runs laterally in the posterior cranial fossa and joins the spinal root. The two roots unite and leave the skull through the jugular foramen. The roots then separate and the cranial root joins the vagus nerve and is distributed in its pharyngeal and recurrent laryngeal branches to the muscles of the soft palate, pharynx, and larynx.

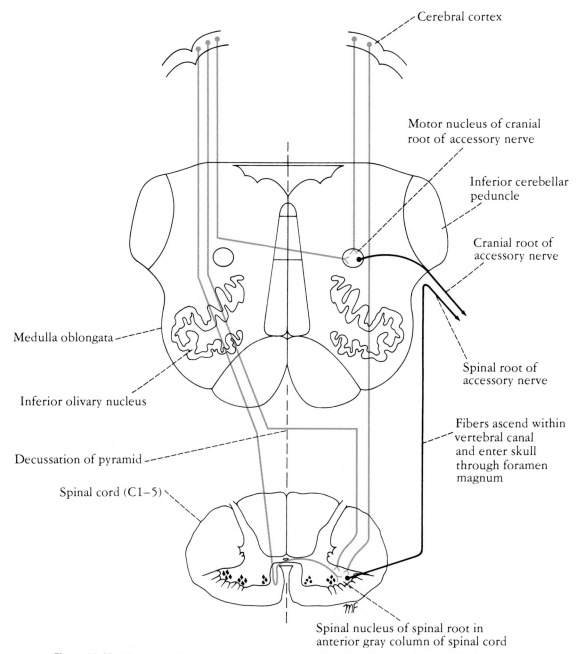

Figure 11–20   Cranial and spinal nuclei of the accessory nerve and their central connections.

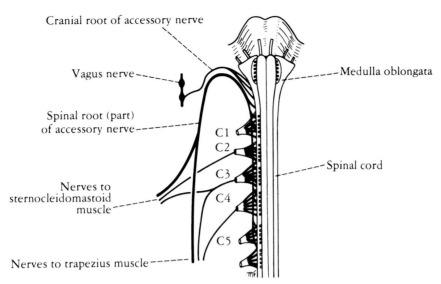

Figure 11–21   Distribution of the accessory nerve.

Spinal Root (Part)

The spinal root is formed from axons of nerve cells in the **spinal nucleus**, which is situated in the anterior gray column of the spinal cord in the upper five cervical segments (Fig. 11-20). The spinal nucleus is thought to receive corticospinal fibers from both cerebral hemispheres.

COURSE OF THE SPINAL ROOT

The nerve fibers emerge from the spinal cord midway between the anterior and posterior nerve roots of the cervical spinal nerves. The fibers form a nerve trunk that ascends into the skull through the foramen magnum. The spinal root passes laterally and joins the cranial root as they pass through the jugular foramen. After a short distance, the spinal root separates from the cranial root and runs downward and laterally and enters the deep surface of the sternocleidomastoid muscle, which it supplies (Fig. 11-21). The nerve then crosses the posterior triangle of the neck and passes beneath the trapezius muscle, which it supplies.

The accessory nerve thus brings about movements of the soft palate, pharynx, and larynx and controls the movement of two large muscles in the neck.

HYPOGLOSSAL NERVE (CRANIAL NERVE XII)

The hypoglossal nerve is a motor nerve and supplies all the intrinsic muscles of the tongue and, in addition, the styloglossus, the hyoglossus, and the genioglossus muscles.

Hypoglossal Nucleus

The hypoglossal nucleus is situated close to the midline immediately beneath the floor of the lower part of the fourth ventricle (Fig. 11-22). It receives corticonuclear fibers from both cerebral hemispheres. **However, the cells responsible for supplying the genioglossus muscle (Fig. 11-23) only receive corticonuclear fibers from the opposite cerebral hemisphere.**

The hypoglossal nerve fibers pass anteriorly through the medulla oblongata and emerge as a series of roots in the groove between the pyramid and the olive (Fig. 11-22).

Course of the Hypoglossal Nerve

The hypoglossal nerve fibers emerge on the anterior surface of the medulla oblongata between the pyramid and the olive (Fig. 11-22). It crosses the posterior cranial fossa and leaves the skull through the hypoglossal canal. The nerve passes downward and forward in the neck between the internal carotid artery and the internal jugular vein until it reaches the lower border of the posterior belly of the digastric muscle. Here, it turns forward and crosses the internal and external carotid arteries and the loop of the lingual artery. It passes deep to the posterior margin of the mylohyoid muscle lying on the lateral surface of the hyoglossus muscle. The nerve then sends branches to the muscles of the tongue (Fig. 11-23).

In the upper part of its course, the hypoglossal nerve is joined by C1 fibers* from the cervical plexus.

The hypoglossal nerve thus controls the movements and shape of the tongue.

---

*The delicate cervical nerve fibers merely run with the hypoglossal nerve for support and later leave it to supply muscles in the neck.

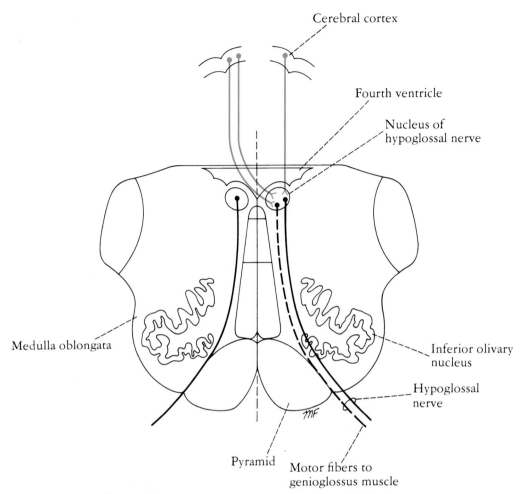

Figure 11–22 Hypoglossal nucleus and its central connections.

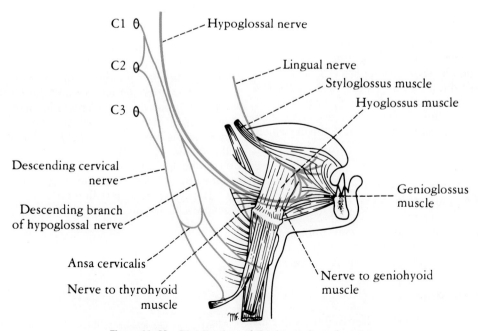

Figure 11–23 Distribution of the hypoglossal nerve.

CLINICAL NOTES

GENERAL CONSIDERATIONS

The 12 pairs of cranial nerves supply information to the brain from outlying receptor organs and bring about changes in peripheral effector organs by means of appropriate motor nerves. Unfortunately for the student, the nerve cells are not arranged simply, as in the spinal cord, but are grouped together to form **nuclei** that are found in different situations at different levels of the brainstem. Moreover, whereas spinal nerves possess afferent somatic fibers, afferent visceral fibers, efferent somatic fibers, and efferent visceral fibers, cranial nerves, in addition, possess special somatic afferent fibers (e.g., visual and auditory) and special visceral afferent fibers (e.g., taste).

When the central connections of the different cranial nerve nuclei were discussed in the previous section, a simplified practical version was given, since many of the precise connections of the cranial nerve nuclei are still not known. Because the delicate movements of the eyes, the larynx, and the face require carefully integrated muscle action and the fine control of muscle tone, it must be assumed that the motor nuclei of the various cranial nerves receive input from the cerebellum, the red nucleus, the reticular formation, and the corpus striatum in the same manner as the lower motor neurons of the spinal cord.

Three points of clinical value should be remembered:

1. Bilateral corticonuclear connections are present for all the cranial motor nuclei **except** that part of the facial nucleus that supplies the muscles of the lower part of the face and that part of the hypoglossal nucleus that supplies the genioglossus muscle.
2. The cranial nerves that possess afferent sensory fibers have cell bodies that are found in ganglia along the course of the nerves; these are equivalent to the posterior root ganglia. In the case of the olfactory nerves, the cells are the olfactory receptors.
3. In situations where the cranial nerve nuclei are close together, it is very rare for a disease process to affect one nucleus only. For example, the cell groups of the nucleus ambiguus serve the glossopharyngeal, the vagus, and the cranial root of the accessory nerve, and functional loss involving all three nerves is a common finding.

CLINICAL EXAMINATION OF CRANIAL NERVES

The systematic examination of the 12 cranial nerves is an important part of the examination of every neurological patient. It may reveal a lesion of a cranial nerve nucleus, or its central connections, or it may show an interruption of the lower motor neurons.

Olfactory Nerve

First, determine that the nasal passages are clear. Then apply some easily recognizable aromatic substance, such as oil of peppermint, oil of cloves, or tobacco, to each nostril in turn. Ask the patient whether he or she can smell anything; then ask the patient to identify the smell. It should be remembered that food flavors depend on the sense of smell and not on the sense of taste.

Bilateral anosmia can be caused by disease of the olfactory mucous membrane, such as the common cold or allergic rhinitis. **Unilateral anosmia** can result from disease affecting the olfactory nerves, bulb, or tract. A lesion of the olfactory cortex on one side is unlikely to produce complete anosmia because fibers from each olfactory tract travel to both cerebral hemispheres. Fractures of the anterior cranial fossa involving the cribriform plate of the ethmoid could tear the olfactory nerves. Cerebral tumors of the frontal lobes or meningiomas of the anterior cranial fossa can produce anosmia by pressing upon the olfactory bulb or tract.

Optic Nerve

First ask the patient whether he or she has noted any change in eyesight. **Visual acuity** should be tested for near and distant vision. Near vision is tested by asking the patient to read a card with a standard size of type. Each eye is tested in turn, with or without spectacles. Distant vision is tested by asking the patient to read Snellen's type at a distance of 20 feet.

The **visual fields** should then be tested. The patient and the examiner sit facing each other at a distance of 2 feet. The patient is asked to cover the right eye and the examiner covers his own left eye. The patient is asked to look into the pupil of the examiner's right eye. A small object is then moved in an arc around the periphery of the field of vision, and the patient is asked whether he or she can see the object. The extent of the patient's field of vision is compared with the normal examiner's field. The other eye then is tested. It is important not to miss loss or impairment of vision in the central area of the field (central scotoma).

LESIONS OF THE VISUAL PATHWAY

Lesions of the optic pathway may have many pathological causes. Expanding tumors of the brain and neighboring structures, such as the pituitary gland and the meninges, and cerebrovascular accidents are commonly responsible. The most widespread effects on vision occur where the nerve fibers of the visual pathway are tightly packed together, such as in the optic nerve or the optic tract.

Circumferential Blindness

This may be caused by hysteria or optic neuritis (Fig. 11-24 [1]). Optic neuritis may occur following spread of infection from the sphenoid and ethmoid sinuses; the nerve is infected as it passes through the optic canal to enter the orbital cavity.

Total Blindness of One Eye

This would follow complete section of one optic nerve (Fig. 11-24 [2]).

Nasal Hemianopia

This would follow a partial lesion of the optic chiasma on its lateral side (Fig.11-24 [3]).

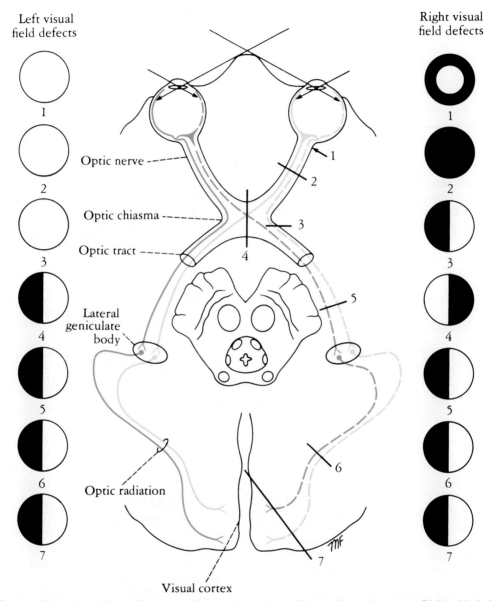

Left visual field defects

Right visual field defects

Optic nerve

Optic chiasma

Optic tract

Lateral geniculate body

Optic radiation

Visual cortex

Figure 11–24 Visual field defects associated with lesions of the optic pathways. 1. Right-sided circumferential blindness due to retrobulbar neuritis. 2. Total blindness of the right eye due to division of the right optic nerve. 3. Right nasal hemianopia due to a partial lesion of the right side of the optic chiasma. 4. Bitemporal hemianopia due to a complete lesion of the optic chiasma. 5. Left temporal hemianopia and right nasal hemianopia due to a lesion of the right optic tract. 6. Left temporal and right nasal hemianopia due to a lesion of the right optic radiation. 7. Left temporal and right nasal hemianopia due to a lesion of the right visual cortex.

Bitemporal Hemianopia

This would follow a sagittal section of the optic chiasma (Fig. 11-24 [4]). This condition is most commonly produced by a tumor of the pituitary gland exerting pressure on the optic chiasma.

Contralateral Homonymous Hemianopia

This would follow division of the optic tract or optic radiation or destruction of the visual cortex on one side; the lesion would produce the same hemianopia for both eyes, that is, homonymous hemianopia (Fig. 11-24 [5, 6, and 7]). If the right optic tract is divided, for example, a left temporal hemianopia and a right nasal hemianopia will occur.

EXAMINATION OF THE FUNDI

The ocular fundus should be examined with an ophthalmoscope. The patient is asked to look at a distant object. When the right eye is examined, the physician should use his or her right eye and hold the ophthalmoscope in his or her right hand. The physician should systematically examine the fundus, looking first at the optic disc, then at the retina, then at the blood vessels, and finally at the macula.

The **optic disc** is creamy pink and the lateral margin is seen clearly. The center of the disc is paler and hollowed out.

The **retina** is pinkish red and there should be no hemorrhages or exudates.

The **blood vessels** should consist of four main arteries with their accompanying veins. Carefully examine the arteriovenous crossings. The veins should not be indented by the arteries.

The **macula** is examined by asking the patient to look directly at the light of the ophthalmoscope. It should look slightly darker than the surrounding retina.

EXAMINATION OF THE EXTRAOCULAR MUSCLES

To examine the extraocular muscles, the patient's head is fixed, and the patient is asked to move the eyes, in turn, to the left, to the right, upward, and downward, as far as possible in each direction. He or she should then be asked to look upward and laterally, upward and medially, downward and medially, and downward and laterally.

The pupillary reactions to convergence associated with accommodation and the direct and consensual pupillary reactions to light are tested. The nervous pathways involved in the pupillary reflexes are described on page 335.

Oculomotor Nerve

The oculomotor nerve supplies all the extraocular muscles except the superior oblique and the lateral rectus. It also supplies the striated muscle of the levator palpebrae superioris and the smooth muscle concerned with accommodation, namely, the sphincter pupillae and the ciliary muscle.

In a complete lesion of the oculomotor nerve, the eye cannot be moved upward, downward, or inward. At rest, the eye looks laterally (external strabismus) owing to the activity of the lateral rectus and downward owing to the activity of the superior oblique. The patient sees double (diplopia).

There is drooping of the upper eyelid (ptosis) due to paralysis of the levator palpebrae superioris. The pupil is widely dilated and nonreactive to light owing to paralysis of the sphincter pupillae and unopposed action of the dilator (supplied by the sympathetic). Accommodation of the eye is paralyzed.

Incomplete lesions of the oculomotor nerve are common and may spare the extraocular muscles or the intraocular muscles. The condition in which the innervation of the extraocular muscles is spared with selective loss of the autonomic innervation of the sphincter pupillae and ciliary muscle is called **internal ophthalmoplegia**. The condition in which the sphincter pupillae and the ciliary muscle are spared with paralysis of the extraocular muscles is called **external ophthalmoplegia**.

The possible explanation for the involvement of the autonomic nerves and the sparing of the remaining fibers is that the parasympathetic autonomic fibers are superficially placed within the oculomotor nerve and are likely to be first affected by compression. The nature of the disease also plays a role. For example, in cases of diabetes with impaired nerve conduction (diabetic neuropathy), the autonomic fibers are unaffected whereas the nerves to the extraocular muscles are paralyzed.

The conditions most commonly affecting the oculomotor nerve are diabetes, aneurysm, tumor, trauma, inflammation, and vascular disease. See lesions of the oculomotor nerve in the midbrain (Benedikt's syndrome) on page 215.

Trochlear Nerve

The trochlear nerve supplies the superior oblique muscle, which rotates the eye downward and laterally.

In lesions of the trochlear nerve the patient complains of double vision on looking straight downward, because the images of the two eyes are tilted relative to each other. This is because the superior oblique is paralyzed, and the eye turns medially as well as downward. In fact the patient has great difficulty in turning the eye downward and laterally.

The conditions most often affecting the trochlear nerve include stretching or bruising as a complication of head injuries (the nerve is long and slender), cavernous sinus thrombosis, aneurysm of the internal carotid artery, and vascular lesions of the dorsal part of the midbrain. See lesions of the trochlear nerve in the midbrain on page 215.

Abducent Nerve

The abducent nerve supplies the lateral rectus muscle, which rotates the eye laterally.

In a lesion of the abducent nerve the patient cannot turn the eye laterally. When the patient is looking straight ahead, the lateral rectus is paralyzed, and the unopposed medial rectus pulls the eyeball medially, causing **internal strabismus**. There is also diplopia.

Lesions of the abducent nerve include damage due to head injuries (the nerve is long and slender), cavernous sinus thrombosis or aneurysm of the internal carotid artery, and vascular lesions of the pons.

Lesions of the medial longitudinal fasciculus will disconnect the oculomotor nucleus that innervates the medial rectus muscle from the abducent nucleus that innervates the lateral rectus muscle. When the patient is asked to look laterally to the right or left, the ipsilateral lateral rectus contracts, turning the eye laterally, but the contralateral medial rectus fails to contract and the eye looks straight forward.

Bilateral internuclear ophthalmoplegia can occur with multiple sclerosis, occlusive vascular disease, trauma, or brainstem tumors. Unilateral internuclear ophthalmoplegia can follow an infarct of a small branch of the basilar artery.

Trigeminal Nerve

The trigeminal nerve has sensory and motor roots. The sensory root passes to the trigeminal ganglion, from which emerge the ophthalmic (V1), maxillary (V2), and mandibular (V3) divisions. The motor root joins the mandibular division.

The sensory function may be tested by using cotton and a pin over each area of the face supplied by the divisions of the trigeminal nerve (Fig. 11-9). Note that there is very little overlap of the dermatomes and that the skin covering the angle of the jaw is innervated by branches from the cervical plexus (C_2 and C_3). In lesions of the ophthalmic division, the cornea and conjunctiva will be insensitive to touch.

The motor function may be tested by asking the patient to clench his or her teeth. The masseter and the temporalis muscles can be palpated and felt to harden as they contract.

TRIGEMINAL NEURALGIA

This severe, stabbing pain over the face is of unknown cause and involves the pain fibers of the trigeminal nerve. Pain is felt most commonly over the skin areas innervated by the mandibular and maxillary divisions of the trigeminal nerve; only rarely is pain felt in the area supplied by the ophthalmic division.

Facial Nerve

The facial nerve supplies the muscles of facial expression, supplies the anterior two-thirds of the tongue with taste fibers, and is secretomotor to the lacrimal, submandibular, and sublingual glands.

To test the facial nerve, the patient is asked to show the teeth by separating the lips with the teeth clenched. Normally, equal areas of the upper and lower teeth are revealed on both sides. If a lesion of the facial nerve is present on one side, the mouth is distorted. A greater area of teeth is revealed on the side of the intact nerve, since the mouth is pulled up on that side. Another useful test is to ask the patient to close both eyes firmly. The examiner then attempts to open the eyes by gently raising the patient's upper lids. On the side of the lesion the orbicularis oculi is paralyzed so that the eyelid on that side is easily raised.

The sensation of taste on each half of the anterior two-thirds of the tongue can be tested by placing small amounts of sugar, salt, vinegar, and quinine on the tongue for the sweet, salt, sour, and bitter sensations.

FACIAL NERVE LESIONS

The facial nerve may be injured or may become dysfunctional anywhere along its long course from the brainstem to the face. Its anatomical relationship to other structures greatly assists in the localization of the lesion. If the abducent nerve (supplies the lateral rectus muscle) and the facial nerve are not functioning, this would suggest a lesion in the pons of the brain. If the vestibulocochlear nerve (for balance and hearing) and the facial nerve are not functioning, this suggests a lesion in the internal acoustic meatus. If the patient is excessively sensitive to sound in one ear, the lesion probably involves the nerve to the stapedius muscle, which arises from the facial nerve in the facial canal.

Loss of taste over the anterior two-thirds of the tongue indicates that the facial nerve is damaged proximal to the point where it gives off the chorda tympani branch in the facial canal.

A firm swelling of the parotid salivary gland associated with impaired function of the facial nerve is strongly indicative of a cancer of the parotid gland with involvement of the nerve within the gland.

Deep lacerations of the face may involve branches of the facial nerve.

The part of the facial nucleus that controls the muscles of the upper part of the face receives corticonuclear fibers from both cerebral hemispheres. Therefore it follows that with a lesion involving the upper motor neurons only the muscles of the lower part of the face will be paralyzed (Fig. 11-25). However, in patients with a lesion of the facial nerve motor nucleus or the facial nerve itself, that is, a lower motor neuron lesion, all the muscles on the affected side of the face will be paralyzed (Fig. 11-25). The lower eyelid will droop, and the angle of the mouth will sag. Tears will flow over the lower eyelid, and saliva will dribble from the corner of the mouth. The patient will be unable to close the eye and will be unable to expose the teeth fully on the affected side.

In patients with hemiplegia, the emotional movements of the face are usually preserved. This indicates that the upper motor neurons controlling these **mimetic movements** have a course separate from that of the main corticobulbar fibers. A lesion involving this separate pathway alone results in a loss of emotional movements, but voluntary movements are preserved. A more extensive lesion will produce both mimetic and voluntary facial paralysis.

Bell's Palsy

Bell's palsy is a dysfunction of the facial nerve, as it lies within the facial canal; it is usually unilateral. The site of the dysfunction will determine the aspects of facial nerve function that do not work.

The swelling of the nerve within the bony canal causes pressure on the nerve fibers; this results in a temporary loss of function of the nerve producing a lower motor neuron type of facial paralysis. The cause of Bell's palsy is not known; it sometimes follows exposure of the face to a cold draft.

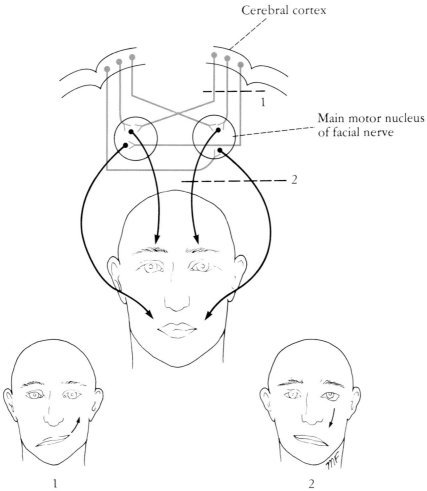

Figure 11–25 Facial expression defects associated with lesions of: 1. The upper motor neurons. 2. Lower motor neurons.

Vestibulocochlear Nerve

The vestibulocochlear nerve innervates the utricle and saccule, which are sensitive to static changes in equilibrium; the semicircular canals, which are sensitive to changes in dynamic equilibrium; and the cochlea, which is sensitive to sound.

DISTURBANCES OF VESTIBULAR NERVE FUNCTION

Disturbances of vestibular nerve function include giddiness (**vertigo**) and **nystagmus** (see p. 240). Vestibular nystagmus is an uncontrollable rhythmic oscillation of the eyes and the fast phase is away from the side of the lesion. This form of nystagmus is essentially a disturbance in the reflex control of the extraocular muscles, which is one of the functions of the semicircular canals. Normally, the nerve impulses pass reflexly from the canals through the vestibular nerve, the vestibular nuclei, and the medial longitudinal fasciculus, to the third, fourth, and sixth cranial nerve nuclei, which control the extraocular muscles; the cerebellum assists in coordinating the muscle movements.

Vestibular function can be investigated with **caloric tests**. These involve the raising and lowering of the temperature in the external auditory meatus, which induces convection currents in the endolymph of the semicircular canals (principally the lateral semicircular canal) and stimulates the vestibular nerve endings.

The causes of vertigo include diseases of the labyrinth of which Menière's disease is an example. Lesions of the vestibular nerve, the vestibular nuclei, and the cerebellum can also be responsible. Multiple sclerosis, tumors, and vascular lesions of the brainstem also cause vertigo.

DISTURBANCES OF COCHLEAR NERVE FUNCTION

Disturbances of cochlear function are manifested as **deafness** and **tinnitus**. The patient's ability to hear a whispered voice or a vibrating tuning fork should be tested; each ear should be tested separately.

Loss of hearing may be due to a defect of the auditory-conducting mechanism in the middle ear, damage to the receptor cells in the spiral organ of Corti in the cochlea, a lesion of the cochlear nerve, a lesion of the central auditory pathways, or the cortex of the temporal lobe.

Lesions of the internal ear include **Menière's disease**, **acute labyrinthitis**, and **trauma** following head injury. Lesions of the cochlear nerve include **tumor (acoustic neuroma)** and **trauma**. Lesions in the central nervous system include **tumors of the midbrain** and **multiple sclerosis**. Only bilateral temporal lobe lesions cause deafness.

Glossopharyngeal Nerve

The glossopharyngeal nerve supplies the stylopharyngeus muscle and sends secretomotor fibers to the parotid gland. Sensory fibers innervate the posterior one-third of the tongue for general sensation and taste.

The integrity of this nerve may be evaluated by testing the patient's general sensation and that of taste on the posterior third of the tongue.

Isolated lesions of the glossopharyngeal nerve are rare and usually also involve the vagus nerve.

Vagus Nerve

The vagus nerve innervates many important organs, but the examination of this nerve depends upon testing the function of the branches to the pharynx, soft palate, and larynx. The **pharyngeal** or **gag reflex** may be tested by touching the lateral wall of the pharynx with a spatula. This should immediately cause the patient to gag; that is, the pharyngeal muscles will contract. The afferent neuron of the pharyngeal reflex runs in the glossopharyngeal nerve, and the efferent neurons run in the glossopharyngeal (to the stylopharyngeus muscle) and vagus nerves (pharyngeal constrictor muscles). Unilateral lesions of the vagus will show little or no gag reflex on that side.

The innervation of the soft palate may be tested by asking the patient to say "ah." Normally, the soft palate rises and the uvula moves backward in the midline.

All the muscles of the larynx are supplied by the recurrent laryngeal branch of the vagus, except the cricothyroid muscle, which is supplied by the external laryngeal branch of the superior laryngeal branch of the vagus. Hoarseness or absence of the voice may occur as a symptom of vagal nerve palsy. The movements of the vocal cords may be tested by means of a laryngoscopic examination. Lesions involving the vagus nerve in the posterior cranial fossa commonly involve the glossopharyngeal, accessory, and hypoglossal nerves also.

Accessory Nerve

The accessory nerve supplies the sternocleidomastoid and the trapezius muscles by means of its spinal root. The patient should be asked to rotate the head to one side against resistance, causing the sternocleidomastoid of the opposite side to come into action. Then the patient should be asked to shrug the shoulders, causing the trapezius muscles to come into action.

Lesions of the spinal part of the accessory nerve will result in paralysis of the sternocleidomastoid and trapezius muscles. The sternocleidomastoid muscle will atrophy and there will be weakness in turning the head to the opposite side. The trapezius muscle will also atrophy and the shoulder will droop on that side; there will also be weakness and difficulty in raising the arm above the horizontal.

Lesions of the spinal part of the accessory nerve may occur anywhere along its course and may result from tumors or trauma from stab or gunshot wounds in the neck.

Hypoglossal Nerve

The hypoglossal nerve supplies the intrinsic muscles of the tongue and the styloglossus, hyoglossus, and genioglossus muscles. To test the integrity of the nerve the patient is asked to put out the tongue; if there is a lower motor neuron lesion, the tongue will be observed to deviate toward the paralyzed side. The tongue will be smaller on the side of the lesion, owing to muscle atrophy, and fasciculation may accompany or precede the atrophy. Remember that the greater part of the hypoglossal nucleus receives corticonuclear fibers from both cerebral hemispheres. However, the part of the nucleus that supplies the genioglossus receives corticonuclear fibers only from the opposite cerebral hemisphere. If a patient has a lesion of the corticonuclear fibers, there will be no atrophy or fibrillation of the tongue and on protrusion the tongue will deviate to the side opposite the lesion. (Note that the genioglossus is the muscle that pulls the tongue forward.)

Lesions of the hypoglossal nerve may occur anywhere along its course and may result from tumor, demyelinating diseases, syringomyelia, and vascular accidents. Injury of the nerve in the neck may also follow stab and gunshot wounds.

Clinical Problem Solving

1. A 60-year-old woman was seen as an outpatient because she had suddenly developed double vision. She was watching her favorite television program the day before when it suddenly occurred. She had no other symptoms. After a complete physical examination, it was found that her right eye, when at rest, was turned medially and she was unable to turn it laterally. A moderate amount of glucose was found in her urine and she had an abnormally elevated blood glucose level. When closely questioned, she admitted that recently she had noticed having to pass water more frequently, especially at night. She also said she often felt thirsty. She had lost 28 pounds during the past 2 years. Using your knowledge of neuroanatomy, explain the problem in

her right eye. Do you think there is any connection between her glucosuria, high blood glucose, polyuria, polydipsia, and weight loss and her eye condition?

2. An 18-year-old man was admitted to the hospital unconscious after a serious motorcycle accident. After a complete physical examination was performed and lateral and anteroposterior radiographs of the skull were taken, it was found that the patient had a fracture involving the anterior cranial fossa. It also was noted that he had a slight but continuous blood-stained watery discharge from his left nostril. Three days later, he recovered consciousness and a further physical examination revealed that he could no longer smell. This was tested by asking him to recognize the smell of coffee, oil of cloves, and oil of peppermint. Using your knowledge of neuroanatomy, diagnose what is wrong with this patient. Is it possible for normal individuals with an acute sense of smell to be unable to recognize common scents? Could a tumor that had destroyed the olfactory cortex of one cerebral hemisphere be responsible for the anosmia in this patient?

3. A 72-year-old man with a known history of cerebrovascular problems visited his physician because 3 days previously he had begun to have trouble reading the paper. He complained that the print started to tilt and that he was beginning to see double. He also said that he found it difficult to see the steps when he descended the staircase to the physician's office. On physical examination, the patient had weakness of movement of the right eye both downward and laterally. Using your knowledge of neuroanatomy, explain this patient's signs and symptoms. If we assume that a cranial nerve nucleus is the site of the lesion, is it the right one or the left one that is involved?

4. A 73-year-old man consulted his physician because he was becoming deaf. His only other complaints were that he didn't think he was as tall as he used to be and he was annoyed to find that each year he had to buy a size larger hat. The physician diagnosed osteitis deformans (Paget's disease) and explained to the medical students that this is a disease of bones involving bone absorption and new bone formation. These bony changes lead to enlargement of the skull, deformities of the vertebral column, and bowing of the long bones of the legs. The physician asked the students whether there was any connection between the bone disease and the patient's deafness and which other cranial nerve they would be particularly interested in testing. How would you have answered these questions?

5. A neurologist was visited by a 25-year-old man who complained of a feeling of heaviness in both legs and giddiness on walking. On examination, it was found that the patient had widely disseminated lesions involving the corticospinal tracts, the posterior white column, and the optic nerves. A diagnosis of multiple sclerosis was made. This disease of unknown origin primarily involves the white matter of the brain and spinal cord. Do you think this patient's symptoms of vertigo could be accounted for by this disease?

6. A 54-year-old woman with left-sided hemiplegia was examined by a fourth-year medical student. He very carefully tested each cranial nerve and noted any defects. During the examination, he stood behind the patient and gently grasped the trapezius muscles between his fingers and thumbs and asked the patient to shrug her shoulders against resistance. He was surprised to find that there was no evidence of weakness in either trapezius muscle and there was no muscle wasting. Would you expect to find evidence of weakness or wasting in the trapezius muscles of a patient with hemiplegia?

7. A 35-year-old man was admitted to the hospital with a complaint of severe pain of the right side of the forehead and the right eye. The pain had started 3 weeks previously and had progressively increased since then. One week ago he started to see double and this morning his wife noticed that his right eye was turning out laterally. The physician in charge made a careful neurological workup on this patient and found a lateral deviation of the right eye, dilatation of the right pupil with loss of direct and consensual light reflexes, paralysis of accommodation on the right, and paralysis of all right-sided ocular movement except laterally. He initially advised the patient to have CT and MRI scans of the skull and later ordered a right-sided carotid arteriogram. The film showed an aneurysm of the internal carotid artery on the right side. Explain the signs and symptoms of this patient. Relate the signs and symptoms to the aneurysm.

8. During ward rounds, the neurologist demonstrated the signs and symptoms of neurosyphilis to a group of students. The patient was a 62-year-old man. The physician asked the students to note that both the patient's pupils were small and fixed and were not altered by shining a light in the eyes or shading the eyes. It was noted, however, that the pupils narrowed when the patient was asked to look from a distant object to the tip of his nose. Moreover, the pupils dilated again when he looked in the distance. "This is a good example of the Argyll Robertson pupil," said the physician. Using your knowledge of neuroanatomy, explain this curious pupillary reaction.

9. Describe the effects of a lesion at the following points along the visual pathway of the right eye:
   (a) Section of the right optic nerve
   (b) Midline section of the optic chiasma
   (c) Section of the right optic tract
   (d) Section of the right optic radiation
   (e) Destruction of the cortex of the right occipital pole

10. A 58-year-old woman was diagnosed as having an advanced carcinoma of the nasopharynx with neoplastic infiltration of the posterior cranial fossa. How would you test for the integrity of the ninth, tenth, and eleventh cranial nerves?

11. A 32-year-old woman with syringomyelia was found on physical examination to have impairment of appreciation of pain and temperature of the face but preservation of light touch. Using your knowledge of neuroanatomy, explain this dissociated sensory loss in the face.

12. A 51-year-old man complaining of an agonizing, stabbing pain over the middle part of the right side of his face was seen in the emergency department. The stabs would last a few seconds and were repeated several times. "The pain is the worst I have ever experienced," he told the physician. A draft of cold air on the right side of his face or the touching of a few hairs in the right temporal region of his scalp could trigger the pain. The patient had no other complaints and said he felt otherwise very fit. A complete physical examination of the cranial nerves revealed nothing abnormal. In particular, there was no evidence of sensory or motor loss of the right trigeminal nerve. The patient indicated the area on the right side of his face in which he experienced the pain; it was seen to be in the distribution of the maxillary division of the trigeminal nerve. Using your knowledge of neuroanatomy, make the diagnosis.

13. A physician turned to a group of students and said, "I think this patient has an advanced neoplasm in the posterior cranial fossa with involvement of the medulla oblongata and in particular the nuclei of the vagus nerve." What are the nuclei of the vagus nerve? Is it possible to have abnormal movements of the vocal cords in a patient with hemiplegia? Is it possible to have a solitary lesion of the vagal nuclei without involvement of other cranial nerve nuclei?

Answers to Clinical Problem Solving

1. The medial strabismus of her right eye, the diplopia, and the inability to turn the right eye laterally were due to paralysis of the right lateral rectus muscle caused by a lesion of the abducent nerve. Yes, there is a connection between the eye condition and the other symptoms. The glucosuria, high blood glucose, polyuria, polydipsia, and weight loss are the classic signs and symptoms of diabetes mellitus. The lesion of the abducent nerve was an example of diabetic neuropathy, a complication of untreated or poorly treated diabetes. Once the patient's diabetes was carefully controlled, the right lateral rectus palsy disappeared after three months.

2. This man suffered from anosmia secondary to a lesion involving both olfactory tracts. The watery discharge from the nose was due to a leak of cerebrospinal fluid through the fractured cribriform plate of the ethmoid bone. It was the fracture and the associated hemorrhage that had damaged both olfactory tracts. Yes, many normal persons with an acute sense of smell cannot name common scents. No, a lesion of one olfactory cortex cannot produce complete anosmia because both olfactory tracts communicate with each other through the anterior commissure.

3. This patient has a paralysis of the right superior oblique muscle resulting from a lesion of the trochlear nerve. Since the trochlear nerves decussate on emergence from the midbrain, the left trochlear nucleus is the site of the lesion. This patient had a thrombosis of a small artery supplying the left trochlear nucleus. The difficulty in reading, the diplopia, and the difficulty in walking down stairs were due to the paralysis of the right superior oblique muscle.

4. As the result of the great increase in the thickness of the bones due to new bone formation in osteitis deformans, mental deterioration may occur owing to compression of the cerebral hemispheres. Those cranial nerves that pass through relatively small foramina in the skull are likely to be compressed by the new bone growth. The nerves commonly involved are the vestibulocochlear and facial nerves, following narrowing of the internal acoustic meatus. The olfactory and optic nerves also may be compressed as they pass through the cribriform plate and the optic canal, respectively.

5. Yes. Multiple sclerosis may affect white matter in widely disseminated areas of the central nervous system. Although remissions may occur, it is inevitably progressive. Thirty years later, when this patient died, numerous areas of sclerosis were found throughout the brainstem and white matter of the spinal cord. It was noted that the region of the vestibular nuclei beneath the floor of the fourth ventricle was involved in the disease process.

6. No. The trapezius muscle is supplied by the spinal part of the accessory nerve. The spinal nucleus of this nerve in the upper five cervical segments of the spinal cord receives cortical fibers from both cerebral hemispheres. This would account for the absence of muscular weakness in this patient with a left-sided hemiplegia. For a muscle to atrophy (except for disuse atrophy), the integrity of the monosynaptic reflex arc must be destroyed. This was not the case in this patient.

7. The severe pain over the forehead and the right eye was due to irritation of the ophthalmic division of the trigeminal nerve by the slowly expanding aneurysm of the internal carotid artery as it was lying in the cavernous sinus. The double vision (diplopia) and the lateral deviation of the right eye were due to the unopposed action of the lateral rectus muscle (supplied by the abducent nerve). The dilatation of the right pupil, with loss of direct and consensual light reflexes, paralysis of accommodation, and paralysis of all right-sided ocular movement except laterally, were due to pressure on the right oculomotor nerve by the aneurysm. The nerve at this point is situated in the lateral wall of the cavernous sinus. Note that the lateral movement of the eyeball was accomplished by contracting the lateral rectus muscle (abducent nerve) and the inferolateral movement was due to the contraction of the superior oblique muscle (trochlear nerve).

8. The Argyll Robertson pupil is a common finding in neurosyphilis, although it may occur in other diseases. The lesion is believed to be located where the pretectal fibers pass to the parasympathetic oculomotor nuclei on both sides of the midbrain. This lesion effectively destroys the direct and consensual light reflexes of both eyes but leaves the pathway for the accommodation reflex intact. (For details of pathway, see p. 335.)

9. (a) Complete blindness of the right eye
   (b) Bitemporal hemianopia
   (c) Left homonymous hemianopia
   (d) Left homonymous hemianopia
   (e) Left homonymous hemianopia, usually with some macular sparing owing to the very large area of the cortex allotted to the macula

10. The glossopharyngeal nerve supplies the posterior one-third of the tongue with fibers that subserve common sensations and taste. This may be tested easily. The vagus nerve, by means of its pharyngeal branch, supplies many muscles of the soft palate and these may be tested by asking the patient to say "ah" and observing that normally the uvula is elevated in the midline. A lesion of the vagus nerve would result in the uvula being elevated to the opposite side. Additional tests may be carried out by observing the movements of the vocal cords through a laryngoscope.

   The spinal part of the accessory nerve may be tested by asking the patient to shrug her shoulders by using the trapezius muscles or to rotate her head so that she looks upward to the opposite side by contracting the sternocleidomastoid muscles. Both muscles are innervated by the spinal part of the accessory nerve.

11. The afferent fibers entering the central nervous system through the trigeminal nerve pass either to the main sensory nucleus in the pons or to the spinal nucleus situated in the medulla oblongata and the first two cervical segments of the spinal cord. The sensations of touch and pressure are served by the main sensory nucleus, while those of pain and temperature are served by the more inferiorly placed spinal nucleus. In this patient, the lesion of syringomyelia was situated in the medulla oblongata and the cervical part of the spinal cord and the main sensory nucleus in the pons was intact.

12. This patient exhibited the classic history of right-sided trigeminal neuralgia involving the maxillary division of that cranial nerve. The temporal region of the scalp, supplied by the auriculotemporal branch of the mandibular division of that nerve, was the trigger area for the initiation of the intense pain. Clearly, knowledge of the distribution of the branches of the trigeminal nerve and the diseases that can affect this nerve is essential for a physician to be able to make the diagnosis.

13. The vagal nuclei are the (a) main motor nucleus, (b) parasympathetic nucleus, and (c) sensory nucleus. The main motor and parasympathetic nuclei are controlled by both cerebral hemispheres, so that hemiplegia will have no effect on the movement of the vocal cords. The vagal nuclei are practically continuous with the nuclei of the glossopharyngeal and accessory nerves and these usually are involved together in lesions of the medulla oblongata.

Review Questions

Directions: Each of the numbered items in this section is followed by answers that are positively phrased. Select the ONE lettered answer that is the EXCEPTION.

1. The cranial nerve nuclei listed below have the following descending tracts terminating on them **except:**
   (a) The inferior salivatory nucleus of the glossopharyngeal nerve receives the descending tracts from the hypothalamus.
   (b) The nucleus of the abducent nerve receives crossed and uncrossed corticobulbar tracts.
   (c) The nucleus of the facial nerve supplying the muscles of the lower part of face receives crossed and uncrossed corticobulbar tracts.
   (d) The trigeminal motor nucleus receives crossed and uncrossed corticobulbar tracts.
   (e) The nucleus of the trochlear nerve receives crossed and uncrossed corticobulbar tracts.

2. The nuclei associated with the facial nerve include the following **except:**
   (a) Nucleus of the tractus solitarius
   (b) Superior salivatory nucleus
   (c) Nucleus ambiguus
   (d) Main motor nucleus
   (e) Lacrimal nucleus

3. A patient with unilateral upper motor neuron paralysis of the facial muscles can smile with both sides of his face in response to a joke, but not voluntarily. This can be explained by the following facts **except:**
   (a) The corticobulbar fibers controlling voluntary movement of the facial muscles have been destroyed.
   (b) Reticular fibers, possibly originating in the hypothalamus and descending to the motor nuclei of the facial nerves, are intact.
   (c) The facial nerves are intact.
   (d) The main motor nuclei of the facial nerves are intact.
   (e) There is a lesion involving the lower motor neurons.

Directions: Each of the numbered items or incomplete statements in this section is followed by answers or by completions of the statement. Select the ONE lettered answer or completion that is BEST in each case.

4. The following structures participate in the reception of sound
   (a) trapezoid body
   (b) medial lemniscus
   (c) nucleus of the trigeminal lemniscus
   (d) inferior temporal gyrus
   (e) lateral geniculate body
5. The cerebral cortex is necessary for the following visual reflexes
   (a) corneal reflex
   (b) accommodation reflex
   (c) consensual light reflex
   (d) pupillary light reflex
   (e) visual body reflex
6. The nasal field of the right eye is projected to the
   (a) left lateral geniculate body
   (b) both banks of the left calcarine fissure
   (c) left optic tract
   (d) temporal retina of the right eye
   (e) left optic radiation
7. Right pupillary constriction associated with light directed at the left eye requires the
   (a) right optic radiation
   (b) left optic nerve
   (c) left Edinger-Westphal nucleus
   (d) left oculomotor nerve
   (e) right optic nerve
8. Select the lettered statement concerning the hypoglossal nerve that is **correct:**
   (a) A lesion involving the hypoglossal nerve will result in deviation of the tongue toward the same side as the lesion, when the tongue is protruded.
   (b) The hypoglossal nerve conducts taste impulses from the posterior third of the tongue.
   (c) The hypoglossal nerve emerges from the brainstem between the olive and the inferior cerebellar peduncle.
   (d) The hypoglossal nerve carries with it fibers from the third and fourth cervical nerves.
   (e) The fibers of the accessory nerve wind round the motor nucleus of the hypoglossal nerve beneath the floor of the fourth ventricle.
9. Select the lettered statement concerning the trigeminal nuclei that is **correct:**
   (a) The main sensory nucleus lies within the medulla oblongata.
   (b) The spinal nucleus extends inferiorly as far as the fifth cervical segment.
   (c) Proprioceptive impulses from the muscles of mastication reach the mesencephalic nucleus along

fibers that are part of the unipolar neurons of the nucleus.
   (d) The sensations of pain and temperature terminate in the main sensory nucleus.
   (e) The trigeminal lemniscus contains only efferent fibers from the ipsilateral sensory nuclei of the trigeminal nerve.

Directions: Each of the numbered items in this section is followed by answers that are positively phrased. Select the ONE lettered answer that is an EXCEPTION.

10. The cranial nerves listed below are associated with the following functions **except:**
    (a) The spinal part of accessory nerve shrugs the shoulder.
    (b) The oculomotor nerve closes the eye.
    (c) The trigeminal nerve is responsible for chewing.
    (d) The facial nerve receives the sensation of taste from the anterior two-thirds of the tongue.
    (e) The glossopharyngeal nerve receives the sensation of touch from the posterior third of the tongue.
11. The following statements concerning the cranial nerves involved in the process of vision are correct **except:**
    (a) The nerve fibers of the optic nerve are surrounded by Schwann cells.
    (b) The optic nerve is surrounded by an extension of the subarachnoid space.
    (c) Internal ophthalmoplegia is a condition in which the oculomotor nerve supply to the sphincter pupillae and the ciliary muscle is lost but the innervation of the extraocular muscles is spared.
    (d) External ophthalmoplegia is a condition in which the oculomotor nerve supply to the extraocular muscles is lost but the innervation of the sphincter pupillae and the ciliary muscle are spared.
    (e) The optic nerve leaves the orbital cavity through the optic canal in the lesser wing of the sphenoid bone.
12. The following statements concerning the cranial nerves listed below are correct **except:**
    (a) The main sensory nucleus of the trigeminal nerve lies in the brainstem lateral to the motor nucleus.
    (b) Proprioceptive impulses from the facial muscles end in the mesencephalic nucleus of the trigeminal nerve.
    (c) The facial nerve leaves the posterior cranial fossa with the vestibulocochlear nerve and enters the internal acoustic meatus.
    (d) The superior salivatory nucleus of the facial nerve innervates the parotid salivary gland.
    (e) The olfactory receptor cells are located in the mucous membrane of the nasal cavity above the level of the superior concha.

Directions: Read the case histories then answer the questions. You will be required to select ONE BEST lettered answer.

A 64-year-old man visited his physician because he had noticed a swelling on the right side of his neck. He mentioned that he had suffered from a chronic cough for six months and was rapidly losing weight.

13. On physical examination the following possible signs emerged **except:**
    (a) The right half of his tongue was wrinkled and wasted.
    (b) When he was asked to protrude his tongue, it turned to the right.
    (c) The swelling on the right side of his neck was high up deep to the right sternocleidomastoid muscle and was hard and fixed.
    (d) A chest radiograph revealed an advanced bronchogenic carcinoma of the right lung.

    (e) The patient had no taste sensation on the anterior two-thirds of the tongue on the right side.

14. The physician made the following correct conclusions **except:**
    (a) The patient had numerous lung metastases in the deep cervical lymph nodes on the right side.
    (b) There was a lesion of the right hypoglossal nerve at some point between the nucleus in the medulla oblongata and the tongue muscles supplied.
    (c) One of the metastases had invaded the right hypoglossal nerve in the neck.
    (d) The loss of weight could be explained by the presence of the advanced carcinoma in the lung.
    (e) The tongue was wrinkled because the mucous membrane was atrophied.

Answers to Review Questions

1. C
2. C
3. E
4. A
5. B
6. D
7. B
8. A
9. C
10. B
11. A
12. D

13. E. The taste sensation from the mucous membrane covering the anterior two-thirds of the tongue is conducted in the facial nerves and the chorda tympani nerves, which are a considerable distance from the metastases in the deep cervical lymph nodes in the neck.

14. E. The wasted right half of the tongue and the pointing of the protruded tongue to the right side indicated a lesion of the right hypoglossal nerve. The tongue muscles on the right side had atrophied and diminished in size resulting in the wrinkling of the overlying normal mucous membrane.

ADDITIONAL READING

Altschuler, R.A., et al. *Neurobiology of Hearing. The Central Auditory System*. New York, Raven Press,1991.

Ashworth, B., and Isherwood, I. *Clinical Neuro-Ophthalmology* (2nd ed.). Oxford: Blackwell, 1981.

Baker, R., Evinger, C., and McCrea, R. A. Some thoughts about the three neurons in the vestibular ocular reflex. *Ann. N.Y. Acad. Sci.* 374:171, 1981.

Bender, M. B., and Bodis-Wollner, I. Visual dysfunction in optic tract lesions. *Ann. Neurol.* 3:187, 1978.

Brandt, T. *Vertigo: Its Multisensory Syndromes*. London: Springer-Verlag, 1991.

Brazis, P. W., Masden, J. C., and Biller, J. *Localization in Clinical Neurology* (2nd ed.). Boston: Little, Brown, 1990.

Büttner, V., and Dichgans, J. The Vestibulo-ocular Reflex and Related Functions. In S. Lessell and J. T. W. Van Dalen (eds.), *Neuro-Ophthalmology*. Vol. 3. Amsterdam: Elsevier, and New York: Oxford University Press, 1984. P. 205.

Doty, R.L. *Handbook of Olfaction and Gustation*. New York, Marcel Dekker, Inc.,1994.

Dubner, R., Sessle, B. J., and Storey, A. T. Jaw, Facial, and Tongue Reflexes. In R. Dubner, B. J. Sessle, and A. T. Storey (eds.), *The Neural Basis of Oral and Facial Function*. Amsterdam: Elsevier, 1978. P. 246.

Farah, M.J., and Ratcliff, G. *The Neuropsychology of High Level Vision*. Hillsdale, NJ, Lawrence Erlbaum Assoc., Inc., 1994.

Fitzgerald, M. J. T., Comerford, P. T., and Tuffery, A. Sources of innervation of the neuromuscular spindles in sternomastoid and trapezius. *J. Anat.* 134:471, 1982.

Frisen, L. The neurology of visual activity. *Brain* 103:639, 1980.

Hussein, M., Wilson, L. A., and Illingworth, R. Patterns of sensory loss following fractional posterior fossa Vth nerve section for trigeminal neuralgia. *J. Neurol. Neurosurg. Psychiatry* 45:786, 1982.

Judge, R. D., and Zuidema, G. D. *Physical Diagnosis: A Physiologic Approach to Clinical Examination* (2nd ed.). Boston: Little, Brown, 1968.

Kroenke, K., et al. Causes of persistent dizziness: A prospective study of 100 patients in ambulatory care. *Ann. Intern. Med.* 117:898, 1992.

Margo, C. E., et al. *Diagnostic Problems in Clinical Ophthalmology.* Philadelphia, W.B. Saunders Co.,1994.

Masterson, R. B. Neural mechanisms for sound localization. *Annu. Rev. Physiol.* 46:275, 1984.

McLaughlin, S., and Margolskee, R. The Sense of Taste. *Am. Sci.* 82:538, 1994.

Merritt, H. H. *A Textbook of Neurology* (5th ed.). Philadelphia: Lea & Febiger, 1973.

Moran, D. T., Rowley, J. C., Jafek, B. W., and Lovell, M. A. The fine structure of the olfactory mucosa in man. *J. Neurocytol.* 11:721, 1982.

Ongeboer de Visser, B. W. The corneal reflex: Electrophysiological and anatomical data in man. *Prog. Neurobiol.* 15:71, 1980.

Parker, D. E. The vestibular apparatus. *Sci. Am.* 243:98, 1980.

Rinn, W. E. The neuropsychology of facial expression: A review of the neurological and psychological mechanisms for producing facial expressions. *Psych. Bull.* 95:52, 1984.

Rudge, P. *Clinical Neurology.* Edinburgh: Churchill Livingstone, 1983.

Sawchenko, P. E. Central connections of the sensory and motor nuclei of the vagus nerve. *J. Auton. Nerv. Syst.* 9:13, 1983.

Sears, E. S., and Franklin, G. M. *Diseases of the Cranial Nerves in Neurology.* New York: Grune & Stratton, 1980. P. 471.

Snell, R. S. *Clinical Anatomy for Medical Students* (6th ed.). Philadelphia: Lippincott Wiliams & Wilkins, 2000.

Snell, R. S., and Lemp, M. A. *Clinical Anatomy of the Eye.* 2nd ed.Boston: Blackwell, 1998.

Spillane, J. D. *An Atlas of Clinical Neurology* (2nd ed.). New York and London: Oxford University Press, 1975.

Sullivan, S.L., Ressler, K.J., and Buck, L.B. Spatial Patterning and Information Coding in the Olfactory System. *Curr. Opin. Genet. Dev.* 5:516-523, 1995.

Walton, J. N. *Brain's Diseases of the Nervous System* (9th ed.). New York and London: Oxford University Press, 1984.

Warr, W. B. Parallel Ascending Pathways from the Cochlear Nucleus. In William D. Neff (ed.), *Contributions to Sensory Physiology.* Vol. 7. New York: Academic, 1982. P. 1.

Williams, P. L., et al.(eds.). *Gray's Anatomy* (38th Brit. ed.). New York, Edinburgh: Churchill Livingstone, 1995.

Wilson, V. J., and Peterson, B. W. Central Pathways for Vestibular Reflexes. In B. V. Brooks (ed.), *Handbook of Physiology,* Section 1: The Nervous System. Vol. 2, Part 1. Bethesda, Maryland: American Physiological Society, 1981. P. 671.

CHAPTER 12

The Thalamus and Its Connections

A 61-year-old man with hypertension was seen in the emergency department, having apparently suffered a stroke. A neurologist was called and made a complete examination of the patient. The patient was conscious and was unable to feel any sensation down the right side of his body. There was no evidence of paralysis on either side of the body and the reflexes were normal. The patient was admitted to the hospital for observation.

Three days later, the patient appeared to be improving and there was evidence of return of sensation to the right side of his body. The patient, however, seemed to be excessively sensitive to testing for sensory loss. On light pinprick on the lateral side of the right leg, the patient suddenly shouted out because of excruciating burning pain, and he asked that the examination be stopped. Although the patient experienced very severe pain with the mildest stimulation, the threshold for pain sensitivity was raised and the interval between applying the pinprick and the start of the pain was longer than normal; also the pain persisted after the stimulus had been removed. Moreover, the patient volunteered the information that the pain appeared to be confined to the skin and did not involve deeper structures. Later, it was found that heat and cold stimulation excited the same degree of discomfort.

The neurologist made the diagnosis of analgesia dolorosa or Roussy-Dejerine syndrome involving the left thalamus. This condition of thalamic overreaction is most commonly caused by infarction of the lateral nuclei of the thalamus due to hypertensive vascular disease or thrombosis. Understanding the functional role of the thalamus in the sensory system, and knowing the central connections of the thalamus, are necessary in making a diagnosis of thalamic disease.

CHAPTER OUTLINE

CHAPTER OBJECTIVES

The thalamus is situated at the rostral end of the brainstem and functions as an important relay and integrative station for information passing to all areas of the cerebral cortex, the basal ganglia, the hypothalamus, and the brainstem. The objective of this chapter is to give a brief account of a very complex area of the nervous system and to emphasize that the thalamus lies at the center of many afferent and efferent neuronal loops to other parts of the nervous system.

GENERAL APPEARANCES OF THE THALAMUS

The thalamus is a large, egg-shaped mass of gray matter that forms the major part of the diencephalon. There are two thalami and one is situated on each side of the third ventricle (Figs. 12-1 and 7-3). The anterior end of the thalamus is narrow and rounded and forms the posterior boundary of the interventricular foramen. The posterior end is expanded to form the **pulvinar**, which overhangs the superior colliculus (Fig. 12-2). The inferior surface is continuous with the tegmentum of the midbrain. The medial surface of the thalamus forms part of the lateral wall of the third ventricle and is usually connected to the opposite thalamus by a band of gray matter (Fig. 12-2), the **interthalamic connection** (interthalamic adhesion).

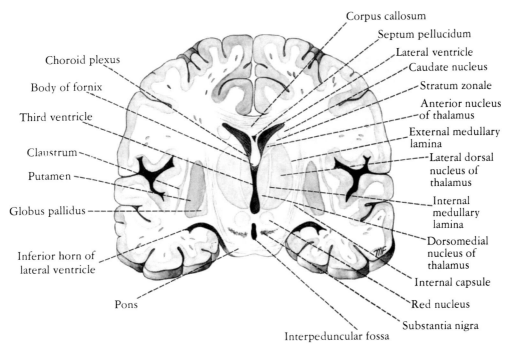

Figure 12–1 Coronal section of the cerebral hemispheres, showing the position and relations of the thalamus.

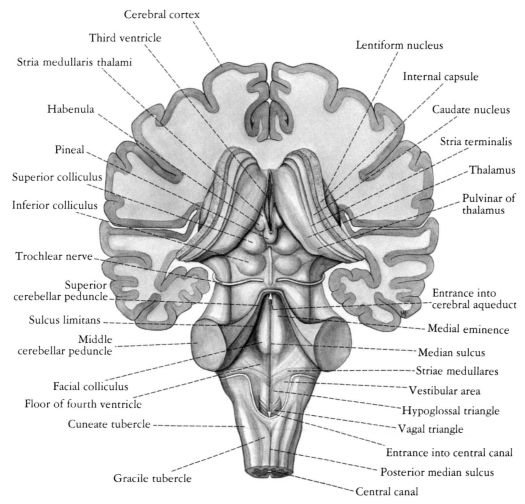

Figure 12–2 Posterior view of the brainstem, showing the thalamus and the tectum of the midbrain.

SUBDIVISIONS OF THE THALAMUS

The thalamus is covered on its superior surface by a thin layer of white matter, called the **stratum zonale** (Fig. 12-1), and on its lateral surface by another layer, the **external medullary lamina** (Fig. 12-1). The gray matter of the thalamus is divided by a vertical sheet of white matter, the **internal medullary lamina**, into medial and lateral halves (Figs. 12-1 and 12-3). The internal medullary lamina consists of nerve fibers that pass from one thalamic nucleus to another. Anterosuperiorly, the internal medullary lamina splits so that it is Y-shaped. The thalamus thus is subdivided into three main parts; the **anterior part** lies between the limbs of the Y, and the **medial** and **lateral parts** lie on the sides of the stem of the Y (Fig. 12-3).

Each of the three parts of the thalamus contains a group of thalamic nuclei (Fig. 12-3). Moreover, smaller nuclear

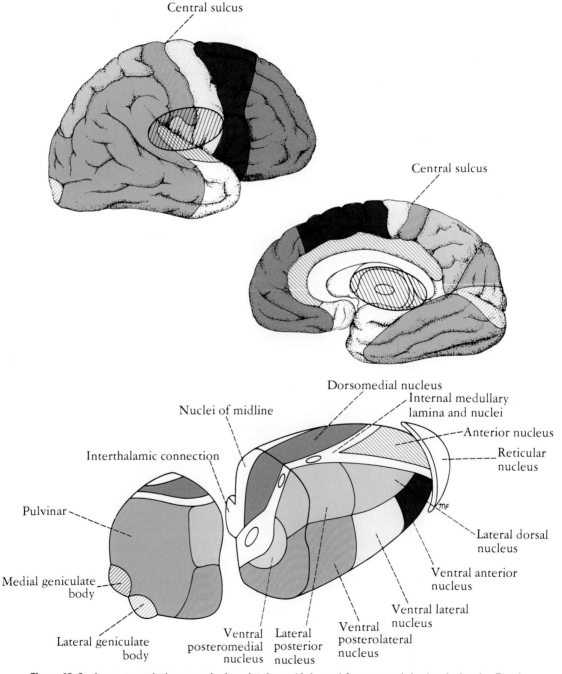

Figure 12–3 Important thalamocortical projections. (Adapted from an original painting by Frank H. Netter, M.D., from *The CIBA Collection of Medical Illustrations,* copyright by CIBA Pharmaceutical Company, Division of CIBA-GEIGY Corporation.)

groups are situated within the internal medullary lamina, and some are located on the medial and lateral surfaces of the thalamus.

Anterior Part

This part of the thalamus contains the **anterior thalamic nuclei** (Fig. 12-3). They receive the mammillothalamic tract from the mammillary nuclei. These anterior thalamic nuclei also receive reciprocal connections with the cingulate gyrus and hypothalamus. The function of the anterior thalamic nuclei is closely associated with that of the limbic system and is concerned with emotional tone and the mechanisms of recent memory.

Medial Part

This part of the thalamus contains the large **dorsomedial nucleus** and several smaller nuclei (Fig. 12-3). The dorsomedial nucleus has two-way connections with the whole prefrontal cortex of the frontal lobe of the cerebral hemisphere. It also has similar connections with the hypothalamic nuclei. It is interconnected with all other groups of thalamic nuclei. The medial part of the thalamus is responsible for the integration of a large variety of sensory information, including somatic, visceral, and olfactory information, and the relation of this information to one's emotional feelings and subjective states.

Lateral Part

The nuclei are subdivided into a dorsal tier and a ventral tier (Fig. 12-3).

DORSAL TIER OF THE NUCLEI

This tier includes the **lateral dorsal nucleus**, the **lateral posterior nucleus**, and the **pulvinar**. The details of the connections of these nuclei are not clear. They are known, however, to have interconnections with other thalamic nuclei, and with the parietal lobe, cingulate gyrus, and occipital and temporal lobes.

VENTRAL TIER OF THE NUCLEI

This tier consists of the following in a craniocaudal sequence:

1. **Ventral anterior nucleus** (Fig. 12-3). This nucleus is connected to the reticular formation, the substantia nigra, the corpus striatum, and the premotor cortex as well as to many of the other thalamic nuclei. Since this nucleus lies on the pathway between the corpus striatum and the motor areas of the frontal cortex, it probably influences the activities of the motor cortex.
2. **Ventral lateral nucleus** (Fig. 12-3). This nucleus has connections similar to those of the ventral anterior nucleus but, in addition, has a major input from the cerebellum and a minor input from the red nucleus. Its main

projections pass to the motor and premotor regions of the cerebral cortex. Here again this thalamic nucleus probably influences motor activity.
3. **Ventral posterior nucleus**. This nucleus is subdivided into the **ventral posteromedial nucleus** and the **ventral posterolateral nucleus** (Fig. 12-3). The ventral posteromedial nucleus receives the ascending trigeminal and gustatory pathways, while the ventral posterolateral nucleus receives the important ascending sensory tracts, the medial and spinal lemnisci. The thalamocortical projections from these important nuclei pass through the posterior limb of the internal capsule and corona radiata to the primary somatic sensory areas of the cerebral cortex in the postcentral gyrus (areas 3, 1, and 2).

Other Nuclei of the Thalamus

These nuclei include the intralaminar nuclei, the midline nuclei, the reticular nucleus, and the medial and lateral geniculate bodies.

The **intralaminar nuclei** are small collections of nerve cells within the internal medullary lamina (Fig. 12-3). They receive afferent fibers from the reticular formation as well as fibers from the spinothalamic and trigeminothalamic tracts; they send efferent fibers to other thalamic nuclei, which in turn project to the cerebral cortex, and fibers to the corpus striatum. The nuclei are believed to influence the levels of consciousness and alertness in an individual.

The **midline nuclei** consist of groups of nerve cells adjacent to the third ventricle and in the interthalamic connection (Fig. 12-3). They receive afferent fibers from the reticular formation. Their precise functions are unknown.

The **reticular nucleus** is a thin layer of nerve cells sandwiched between the external medullary lamina and the posterior limb of the internal capsule (Fig. 12-3). Afferent fibers converge on this nucleus from the cerebral cortex and the reticular formation and its output is mainly to other thalamic nuclei. The function of this nucleus is not fully understood, but it may be concerned with a mechanism by which the cerebral cortex regulates thalamic activity.

The **medial geniculate body** forms part of the auditory pathway and is a swelling on the posterior surface of the thalamus beneath the pulvinar (Fig. 12-3). Afferent fibers to the medial geniculate body form the **inferior brachium** and come from the inferior colliculus. It will be remembered that the inferior colliculus receives the termination of the fibers of the lateral lemniscus. The medial geniculate body receives auditory information from both ears but predominantly from the opposite ear.

The efferent fibers leave the medial geniculate body to form the auditory radiation, which passes to the auditory cortex of the superior temporal gyrus. The **lateral geniculate body** forms part of the visual pathway and is a swelling on the undersurface of the pulvinar of the thalamus (Fig. 12-3). The nucleus consists of six layers of nerve cells and is the terminus of all but a few fibers of the optic tract (except the fibers passing to the pretectal nucleus). The fibers are the axons of the ganglion cell layer of the retina and come from the temporal half of the ipsilateral eye and from the nasal half of the contralateral eye, the latter fibers crossing the midline in the optic chiasma. Each lateral geniculate body, therefore, receives visual information from the opposite field of vision.

The efferent fibers leave the lateral geniculate body to form the visual radiation, which passes to the visual cortex of the occipital lobe.

CONNECTIONS OF THE THALAMUS

The following important neuronal loops exist between the thalamic nuclei and other areas of the central nervous system:

1. Every thalamic nucleus (except the reticular nucleus) sends axons to different parts of the cerebral cortex (Fig. 12-3) and every part of the cerebral cortex sends reciprocal fibers back to the thalamic nuclei. This would indicate that information received by the thalamus is always shared with the cerebral cortex and that the cortex and thalamus can modify each other's activities.

2. The thalamus is an important relay station for two sensory-motor axonal loops involving the cerebellum and the basal nuclei: (a) the cerebellar-rubro-thalamic-cortical-ponto-cerebellar loop and (b) the corticalstriatal-pallidal-thalamic-cortical loop, both of which are necessary for normal voluntary movement.

A summary of the various thalamic nuclei, their nervous connections, and their functions is provided in Table 12-1. The main connections of the various thalamic nuclei are summarized in Figure 12-4.

Table 12–1 The Various Thalamic Nuclei, Their Nervous Connections, and Their Functions

Thalamic Nucleus	Afferent Neuronal Loop	Efferent Neuronal Loop	Function
Anterior	Mammillothalamic tract, cingulate gyrus, hypothalamus	Cingulate gyrus, hypothalamus	Emotional tone, mechanisms of recent memory
Dorsomedial	Prefrontal cortex, hypothalamus, other thalamic nuclei	Prefrontal cortex, hypothalamus, other thalamic nuclei	Integration of somatic, visceral, and olfactory information and relation to emotional feelings and subjective states
Lateral dorsal, lateral posterior, pulvinar	Cerebral cortex, other thalamic nuclei	Cerebral cortex, other thalamic nuclei	Unknown
Ventral anterior	Reticular formation, substantia nigra, corpus striatum, premotor cortex, other thalamic nuclei	Reticular formation, substantia nigra, corpus striatum, premotor cortex, other thalamic nuclei	Influences activity of motor cortex
Ventral lateral	As in ventral anterior nucleus but also major input from cerebellum and minor input from red nucleus		Influences motor activity of motor cortex
Ventral posteromedial (VPM)	Trigeminal lemniscus, gustatory fibers	Primary somatic sensory (areas 3, 1, and 2) cortex	Relays common sensations to consciousness
Ventral posterolateral (VPL)	Medial and spinal lemnisci	Primary somatic sensory (areas 3, 1, and 2) cortex	Relays common sensations to consciousness
Intralaminar	Reticular formation, spinothalamic and trigeminothalamic tracts	To cerebral cortex via other thalamic nuclei, corpus striatum	Influences levels of consciousness and alertness
Midline	Reticular formation	Unknown	Unknown
Reticular	Cerebral cortex, reticular formation	Other thalamic nuclei	? Cerebral cortex regulates thalamus
Medial geniculate body	Inferior colliculus, lateral lemniscus from both ears but predominantly the contralateral ear	Auditory radiation to superior temporal gyrus	Hearing
Lateral geniculate body	Optic tract	Optic radiation to visual cortex of occipital lobe	Visual information from opposite field of vision

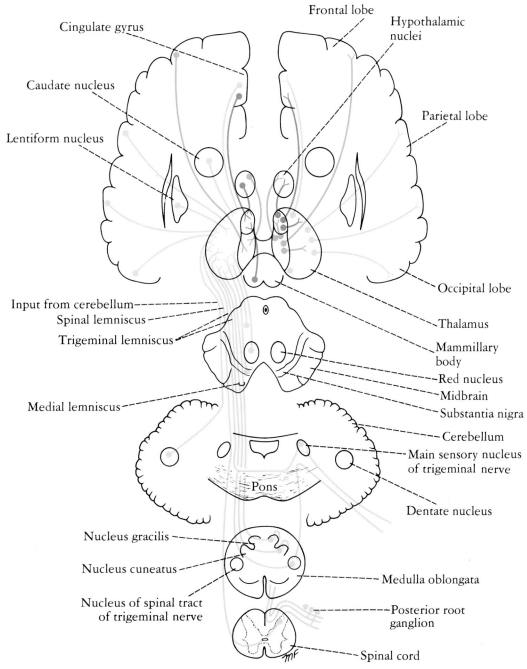

Figure 12–4 Main connections of the thalamus. On the left are shown the afferent fibers and on the right the efferent fibers.

FUNCTION OF THE THALAMUS

It is not considered essential for a practicing physician to have a detailed knowledge of all the thalamic nuclei and their connections. Although an enormous amount of research has been devoted to this area, we still know very little about the functional significance of many of the nuclei.

The following basic principles should be committed to memory:

1. The thalamus is made up of complicated collections of nerve cells that are centrally placed in the brain and are interconnected.
2. A vast amount of sensory information of all types (except smell) converges on the thalamus and presumably is

integrated through the interconnections between the nuclei. The resulting information pattern is distributed to other parts of the central nervous system. It is probable that olfactory information is first integrated at a lower level with taste and other sensations and is relayed to the thalamus from the amygdaloid complex and hippocampus through the mammillothalamic tract.

3. Anatomically and functionally, the thalamus and the cerebral cortex are closely linked. The fiber connections have been established, and it is known that following removal of the cortex the thalamus can appreciate crude sensations. However, the cerebral cortex is required for the interpretation of sensations based on past experiences. For example, if the sensory cortex is destroyed, one can still appreciate the presence of a hot object in the hand; however, appreciation of the shape, weight, and exact temperature of the object would be impaired.

4. The thalamus possesses certain very important nuclei whose connections have been clearly established. These include the ventral posteromedial nucleus, the ventral posterolateral nucleus, the medial geniculate body, and the lateral geniculate body. Their positions and connections should be learned.

5. The ventroanterior and the ventrolateral nuclei of the thalamus form part of the basal nuclei circuit and thus are involved in the performance of voluntary movements. These nuclei receive input from the globus pallidus and send fibers to the prefrontal, supplemental, and premotor areas of the cerebral cortex.

6. The large dorsomedial nucleus has extensive connections with the frontal lobe cortex and hypothalamus. There is considerable evidence that this nucleus lies on the pathway that is concerned with subjective feeling states and the personality of the individual.

7. The intralaminar nuclei are closely connected with the activities of the reticular formation and they receive much of their information from this source. Their strategic position enables them to control the level of overall activity of the cerebral cortex. The intralaminar nuclei are thus able to influence the levels of consciousness and alertness in an individual.

CLINICAL NOTES

Since the thalamus is such an important relay and integrative center, it follows that disease of this area of the central nervous system will have profound effects. The thalamus may be invaded by neoplasm, undergo degeneration following disease of its arterial supply, or be damaged by hemorrhage.

LESIONS OF THE THALAMUS

Sensory Loss

These lesions usually result from thrombosis or hemorrhage of one of the arteries supplying the thalamus. Damage to the ventral posteromedial nucleus and the ventral posterolateral nucleus will result in the loss of all forms of sensation, including light touch, tactile localization and discrimination, and muscle joint sense from the opposite side of the body.

The thalamus is centrally located among other important nervous structures. Usually, a thalamic lesion results in dysfunction of neighboring structures, producing symptoms and signs that overshadow those produced by the thalamic disease. For example, a vascular lesion of the thalamus may also involve the midbrain, with resulting coma, or a lateral extension of thalamic disease may involve the internal capsule and produce extensive motor as well as sensory deficits.

Thalamic Pain

Thalamic pain may occur as the patient is recovering from a thalamic infarct. Spontaneous pain, which is often excessive (thalamic overreaction), occurs on the opposite side of the body. The painful sensation may be aroused by light touch or by cold, and may fail to respond to powerful analgesic drugs.

ABNORMAL INVOLUNTARY MOVEMENTS

Choreoathetosis with ataxia may follow vascular lesions of the thalamus. It is not certain whether these signs in all cases are due to the loss of function of the thalamus or to involvement of the neighboring caudate and lentiform nuclei. The ataxia may arise as the result of the loss of appreciation of muscle and joint movement owing to a thalamic lesion.

THALAMIC HAND

The contralateral hand is held in an abnormal posture in some patients with thalamic lesions. The wrist is pronated and flexed, the metacarpophalangeal joints are flexed, and the interphalangeal joints are extended. The fingers can be moved actively, but the movements are slow. The condition is due to altered muscle tone in the different muscle groups.

Clinical Problem Solving

1. A 45-year-old man who had suddenly developed a weakness of the left leg 12 hours previously was admitted to a medical ward. On examination, he was found to have paralysis of the left leg and weakness of the muscles of the left arm. The muscles of the affected limbs showed increased tone and there was an exaggeration of the tendon reflexes on the left side of the body. There was also considerable sensory loss on the left side of the body, involving both the superficial and deep sensations. During the examination the patient would exhibit spontaneous jerking movements of the left leg. When asked to touch the tip of his nose with the left index finger, he demonstrated considerable intention tremor. The same test with the right arm showed nothing abnormal. Three days later, the patient started to complain of agonizing pain down the left leg. The pain would start spontaneously or be initiated by the light touch of the bed sheet. What is your diagnosis? How can you explain the various signs and symptoms?

Answers to Clinical Problem Solving

1. This man had a thrombosis of the thalamogeniculate branch of the right posterior cerebral artery. This resulted in a degenerative lesion within the right thalamus causing the impairment of superficial and deep sensations on the left side of the body. The contralateral hemiparesis, involving the left leg and left arm with increased muscle tone, was produced by edema in the nearby posterior limb of the right internal capsule causing blocking of the corticospinal fibers. As the edema resolved, the paralysis and spasticity improved, The choreoathetoid movements of the left leg and the intention tremor of the left arm were probably due to damage to the right thalamus or to the right dentatothalamic nerve fibers. The agonizing pain felt down the left leg was due to the lesion in the right thalamus.

Review Questions

Directions: Each of the numbered items in this section is followed by answers that are positively phrased. Select the ONE lettered answer that is an EXCEPTION.

1. The following statements concerning the thalamus are correct **except:**
   (a) All types of sensory information, with the exception of smell, reach the thalamic nuclei via afferent fibers.
   (b) Very few afferent fibers reach the thalamic nuclei from the cerebral cortex.
   (c) The intralaminar nuclei of the thalamus are closely connected with the reticular formation.
   (d) The intralaminar nuclei can influence the levels of consciousness and alertness.
   (e) The thalamus is covered on its superior surface by a thin layer of white matter called the stratum zonale.

2. The following statements concerning the thalamus are correct **except:**
   (a) The external medullary lamina is an area of gray matter lying on the lateral surface of the thalamus.
   (b) The Y-shaped internal medullary lamina subdivides the thalamus into three main parts.
   (c) The ventral posteromedial nucleus receives the ascending trigeminal and gustatory pathways.
   (d) The cerebellar-rubro-thalamic-cortical-pontocerebellar neuron pathway is important in voluntary movement.
   (e) The mammillary body-thalamus-amygdaloid nucleus-dentate gyrus neuron pathway is not important in maintaining posture.

3. The following statements concerning the thalamic nuclei are correct **except:**
   (a) The ventral posterolateral nucleus receives the ascending sensory tracts of the medial and spinal lemnisci.
   (b) The intralaminar nuclei lie within the internal medullary lamina.
   (c) The projections of the posterolateral nucleus ascend to the postcentral gyrus.
   (d) The reticular nucleus is part of the reticular formation.
   (e) The projections of the ventral posterolateral nucleus ascend to the postcentral gyrus through the posterior limb of the internal capsule.

4. The following statements concerning the medial geniculate body are correct **except:**
   (a) The medial geniculate body receives auditory information from the inferior colliculus and from the lateral lemniscus.

(b) Efferent fibers from the medial geniculate body form the inferior brachium.

(c) The medial geniculate body receives auditory information from both ears but predominantly from the opposite ear.

(d) The medial geniculate body projects to the auditory cortex of the superior temporal gyrus.

(e) The medial geniculate body is a swelling on the posterior surface of the thalamus.

5. The following statements concerning the lateral geniculate body are correct **except:**

(a) The lateral geniculate body receives most of the fibers of the optic tract.

(b) Each lateral geniculate body receives visual information from the opposite field of vision.

(c) The lateral geniculate body has a nucleus made up of six layers of nerve cells.

(d) The lateral geniculate body is part of the midbrain at the level of the red nucleus.

(e) The afferent fibers to the lateral geniculate body are the axons of the ganglion cells of the retina.

Answers to Review Questions

1. B
2. A
3. D

4. B
5. D

ADDITIONAL READING

Ajmone Marsan, C. The thalamus: Data on its functional anatomy and on some aspects of thalamocortical integration. *Arch. Ital. Biol.* 103:847, 1965.

Angevine, J. B., Jr., Locke, S., and Yakovlev, P. Limbic nuclei of thalamus and connections of limbic cortex; thalamocortical projections of the magnocellular medial dorsal nucleus in man. *Arch. Neurol.* 10:165, 1964.

Bertrand, G., Jasper, H. H., and Wong, A. Microelectrode study of the human thalamus, functional organization in the ventrobasal complex. *Confin. Neurol.* 29:81, 1967.

Carpenter, M. B. Ventral Tier Thalamic Nuclei. In D. Williams (ed.), *Modern Trends in Neurology.* London and Washington, D.C.: Butterworth, 1967. P. 1.

Craig, A.D., Bushnell, M.C., Zhang, E.T., and Blomqvist, A. A thalamic nucleus specific for pain and temperature sensation. *Nature* 372:770-773,1994.

Dejerine, J., and Roussy, G. Le syndrome thalamique. *Rev. Neurol.* 14: 521-532,1906.

Guyton, A. C., and Hall, J.E. *Textbook of Medical Physiology* (9th ed.). Philadelphia and London: Saunders, 1996.

Houser, C. R., Vaughn, J. E., Barber, R. P., and Roberts, E. GABA neurons are the major cell type of the nucleus reticularis thalami. *Brain Res.* 200:341, 1980.

Jones, E. G. *The Thalamus.* New York: Plenum, 1985.

Jones, E.G. The Anatomy of Sensory Relay Functions in the Thalamus. pp.29-53 in Holstege, E.(ed.), *Role of the Forebrain in Sensation and Behavior.* Elsevier, 1991.

Markowitsch, H. J. Thalamic mediodorsal nucleus and memory: A critical evaluation of studies in animals and man. *Neurosci. Behav. Rev.* 6:351, 1982.

Purpura, D., and Yahr, M. D. *The Thalamus.* New York: Columbia University Press, 1986.

Scheibel, M. A., and Scheibel, A. B. The organization of the nucleus reticularis thalami; a Golgi study. *Brain Res.* 1:43, 1966.

Steriade, M. Mechanisms Underlying Cortical Activation: Neuronal Organization and Properties of the Midbrain Reticular Core and Intralaminar Thalamic Nuclei. In O. Pompeiano and C. A. Marsan (eds.), *Awareness.* New York: Raven, 1981; p. 327.

Van Buren, J. M., and Borke, R. C. *Variations and Connections of the Human Thalamus.* Berlin and Vienna: Springer, 1972.

CHAPTER 13

The Hypothalamus and Its Connections

A 16-year-old girl was taken by her mother to a pediatrician because she was rapidly losing weight. The mother stated that the weight loss started about 1 year ago. The child's eating habits had changed from eating practically anything put before her to being a very choosy eater. Her personality had also changed and she feared meeting strangers. Her relatives had noticed that she was impatient and irritable and would cry a great deal. On being urged to eat more food, the girl countered by saying she was getting fat and must diet to improve her figure. Although she would not admit to having anything wrong with her, she admitted that menstruation had ceased 3 months previously.

On being questioned by the pediatrician, she admitted to calorie counting and sometimes, when she felt she had overeaten, she went to the toilet and forced herself to vomit by sticking her fingers down her throat. On physical examination, the girl showed obvious signs of weight loss with hollow facial features, prominent bones, and wasted buttocks. Apart from having cold extremities and a low blood pressure of 85/60 mm Hg, no further abnormalities were discovered.

The pediatrician made the diagnosis of anorexia nervosa and admitted the patient to the local hospital. Psychological treatment included getting the confidence of the patient by using nursing personnel who understood the condition. The primary treatment is to restore the patient's weight by persuading the individual to eat adequate amounts of food.

Anorexia nervosa is a disorder of feeding and endocrine function that is normally controlled by the hypothalamus. However, there is strong evidence that it is also of psychogenic origin.

CHAPTER OUTLINE

CHAPTER OBJECTIVES

The hypothalamus controls body homeostasis. The purpose of this chapter is to present to the student the location and boundaries of the hypothalamus and to briefly discuss the various nuclei that make up this important area. The main connections of the nuclei are also considered, with special emphasis on the connections between the hypothalamus and the pituitary gland. Some of the common clinical problems involving the hypothalamus are also considered.

The hypothalamus, although small (0.3% of the total brain), is a very important part of the central nervous system. It controls the autonomic nervous system and the endocrine system and thus indirectly controls body homeostasis. The hypothalamus is well placed for this purpose, lying in the center of the limbic system. It is the site of numerous converging and diverging neuronal pathways and through its adequate blood supply it is able to sample the blood chemistry. The hypothalamus makes appropriate controlling responses following the integration of its nervous and chemical inputs.

The hypothalamus is that part of the diencephalon that extends from the region of the optic chiasma to the caudal border of the mammillary bodies. It lies below the thalamus and forms the floor and the inferior part of the lateral walls of the third ventricle (Fig. 13-1). Anterior to the hypothalamus is an area that for functional reasons is often included in the hypothalamus. Because it extends forward from the optic chiasma to the lamina terminalis and the anterior commissure, it is referred to as the preoptic area. Caudally, the hypothalamus merges into the tegmentum of the midbrain. The lateral boundary of the hypothalamus is formed by the internal capsule.

When observed from below (Fig. 13-2), the hypothalamus is seen to be related to the following structures, from anterior to posterior: (1) the optic chiasma, (2) the tuber cinereum and the infundibulum, and (3) the mammillary bodies.

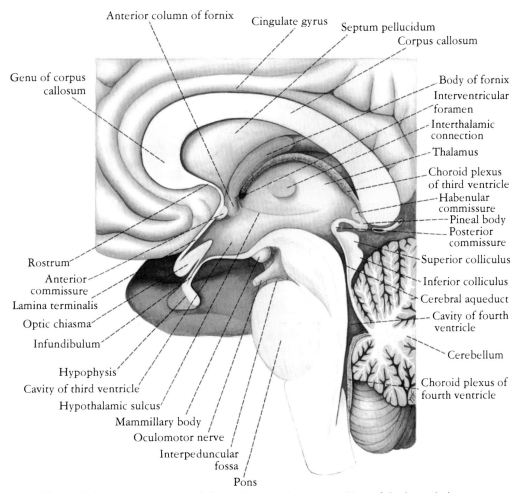

Anterior column of fornix   Cingulate gyrus   Septum pellucidum

Corpus callosum

Genu of corpus callosum

Body of fornix

Interventricular foramen

Interthalamic connection

Thalamus

Choroid plexus of third ventricle

Habenular commissure

Pineal body

Posterior commissure

Superior colliculus

Inferior colliculus

Cerebral aqueduct

Cavity of fourth ventricle

Cerebellum

Choroid plexus of fourth ventricle

Rostrum

Anterior commissure

Lamina terminalis

Optic chiasma

Infundibulum

Hypophysis

Cavity of third ventricle

Hypothalamic sulcus

Mammillary body

Oculomotor nerve

Interpeduncular fossa

Pons

Figure 13–1 Sagittal section of the brain, showing the position of the hypothalamus.

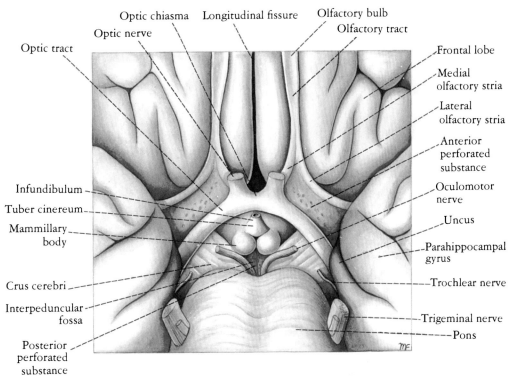

Optic chiasma   Longitudinal fissure   Olfactory bulb

Optic nerve

Olfactory tract

Optic tract

Frontal lobe

Medial olfactory stria

Lateral olfactory stria

Anterior perforated substance

Oculomotor nerve

Uncus

Parahippocampal gyrus

Trochlear nerve

Trigeminal nerve

Pons

Infundibulum

Tuber cinereum

Mammillary body

Crus cerebri

Interpeduncular fossa

Posterior perforated substance

Figure 13–2 Inferior surface of the brain, showing parts of the hypothalamus.

HYPOTHALAMIC NUCLEI

Microscopically, the hypothalamus is composed of small nerve cells that are arranged in groups or nuclei, many of which are not clearly segregated from one another. For functional reasons the **preoptic area** is included as part of the hypothalamus. For purposes of description, the nuclei are divided by an imaginary parasagittal plane into medial and lateral zones (Fig. 13-3). Lying within the plane are the columns of the fornix and the mammillothalamic tract, which serve as markers (Figs. 13-3 and 13-4).

Medial Zone

In the medial zone, the following hypothalamic nuclei can be recognized, from anterior to posterior: (1) part of the

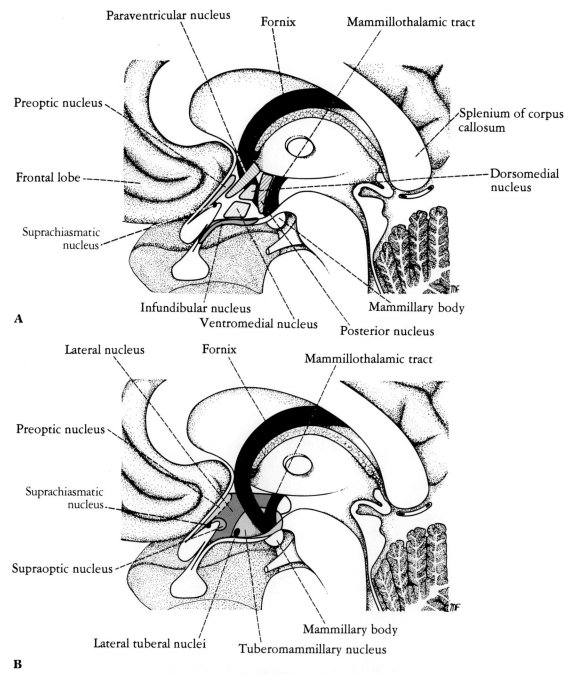

Figure 13–3 Sagittal section of the brain, showing the hypothalamic nuclei. **A.** Medial zone nuclei lying medial to the plane of the fornix and the mammillothalamic tract. **B.** Lateral zone nuclei lying lateral to the plane of the fornix and the mammillothalamic tract.

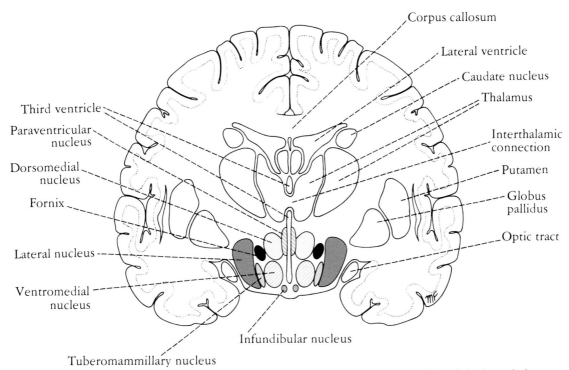

Figure 13–4   Coronal section of the cerebral hemispheres, showing the position of the hypothalamic nuclei.

preoptic nucleus; (2) the **anterior nucleus**, which merges with the preoptic nucleus; (3) part of the **suprachiasmatic nucleus**; (4) the **paraventricular nucleus**; (5) the **dorsomedial nucleus**; (6) the **ventromedial nucleus**; (7) the **infundibular (arcuate) nucleus**; and (8) the **posterior nucleus**.

Lateral Zone

In the lateral zone, the following hypothalamic nuclei can be recognized, from anterior to posterior: (1) part of the **preoptic nucleus**, (2) part of the **suprachiasmatic nucleus**, (3) the **supraoptic nucleus**, (4) the **lateral nucleus**, (5) the **tuberomamillary nucleus**, and (6) the **lateral tuberal nuclei**.

Some of the nuclei, for example, the preoptic nucleus, the suprachiasmatic nucleus, and the mammillary nuclei, overlap both zones. It should be emphasized that most of the hypothalamic nuclei have ill-defined boundaries. With the use of modern technology, including histochemical, immunochemical, and anterograde and retrograde tracer studies, groups of neurons and their connections are being more precisely identified. Unfortunately, as new nuclear groups are discovered and given names the reader has difficulty coming to terms with the old and new nomenclature. Only the major nuclear groups with well established names and their connections are described in this account.

Hypothalamic Lines of Communication

The hypothalamus receives information from the rest of the body through (1) Nervous connections, (2) Bloodstream, and (3) Cerebrospinal fluid. The neurons of the hypothalamic nuclei respond and exert their control via the same routes. The cerebrospinal fluid may serve as a conduit between the neurosecretory cells of the hypothalamus and distant sites of the brain.

AFFERENT NERVOUS CONNECTIONS OF THE HYPOTHALAMUS

The hypothalamus, which lies in the center of the limbic system, receives many afferent fibers from the viscera, the olfactory mucous membrane, the cerebral cortex, and the limbic system.

The afferent connections are numerous and complex; the main pathways (Fig. 13-5) are as follows:

1. **Somatic and Visceral afferents**. General somatic sensation, gustatory and visceral sensations, reach the hypothalamus through collateral branches of the lemniscal afferent fibers and the tractus solitarius, and through the reticular formation.
2. **Visual afferents** leave the optic chiasma and pass to the suprachiasmatic nucleus.

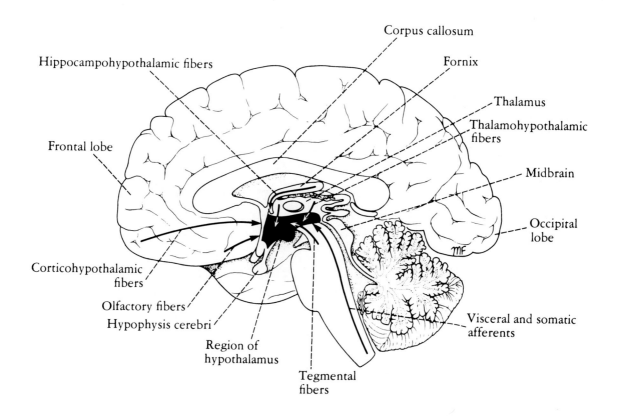

Figure 13–5 Sagittal section of the brain, showing the main afferent pathways entering the hypothalmus.

3. **Olfaction** travels through the medial forebrain bundle.
4. **Auditory afferents** have not been identified but since auditory stimuli can influence the activities of the hypothalamus they must exist.
5. **Corticohypothalamic fibers** arise from the frontal lobe of the cerebral cortex and pass directly to the hypothalamus.
6. **Hippocampohypothalamic fibers** pass from the hippocampus through the fornix to the mammillary body. Many neurophysiologists regard the hypothalamus as the main output pathway of the limbic system.

7. **Amygdalohypothalamic fibers** pass from the amygdaloid complex to the hypothalamus through the stria terminalis and by a route that passes inferior to the lentiform nucleus.
8. **Thalamohypothalamic fibers** arise from the dorsomedial and midline thalamic nuclei.
9. **Tegmental fibers** arise from the midbrain.

The main afferent nervous connections of the hypothalamus are summarized in Table 13-1.

Table 13–1   The Main Afferent and Efferent Nervous Connections of the Hypothalamus

Pathway	Origin	Destination
Afferent		
Medial and spinal lemnisci, tractus solitarius, reticular formation	Viscera and somatic structures	Hypothalamic nuclei
Visual fibers	Retina	Suprachiasmatic nucleus
Medial forebrain bundle	Olfactory mucous membrane	Hypothalamic nuclei
Auditory fibers	Inner ear	Hypothalamic nuclei
Corticohypothalamic fibers	Frontal lobe of cerebral cortex	Hypothalamic nuclei
Hippocampohypothalamic fibers; possibly main output pathway of limbic system	Hippocampus	Nuclei of mammillary body
Amygdalohypothalamic fibers	Amygdaloid complex	Hypothalamic nuclei
Thalamohypothalamic fibers	Dorsomedial and midline nuclei of thalamus	Hypothalamic nuclei
Tegmental fibers	Tegmentum of midbrain	Hypothalamic nuclei
Efferent		
Descending fibers in reticular formation to brainstem and spinal cord	Preoptic, anterior, posterior, and lateral nuclei of hypothalamus	Craniosacral parasympathetic and thoracolumbar sympathetic outflows
Mammillothalamic tract	Nuclei of mammillary body	Anterior nucleus of thalamus; relayed to cingulate gyrus
Mammillotegmental tract	Nuclei of mammillary body	Reticular formation in tegmentum of midbrain
Multiple pathways	Hypothalamic nuclei	Limbic system

EFFERENT NERVOUS CONNECTIONS OF THE HYPOTHALAMUS
··

The efferent connections of the hypothalamus are also numerous and complex, and only the main pathways (Fig. 13-6) are described here:

1. **Descending fibers to the brainstem and spinal cord** influence the peripheral neurons of the autonomic nervous system. They descend through a series of neurons in the reticular formation. The hypothalamus is connected to the parasympathetic nuclei of the oculomotor, facial, glossopharyngeal, and vagus nerves in the brainstem. In a similar manner, the reticulospinal fibers connect the hypothalamus with sympathetic cells of origin in the lateral gray horns of the first thoracic segment to the second lumbar segment of the spinal cord and the sacral parasympathetic outflow at the level of the second, third, and fourth sacral segments of the spinal cord.

2. The **mammillothalamic tract** arises in the mammillary body and terminates in the anterior nucleus of the thalamus. Here the pathway is relayed to the cingulate gyrus.

3. The **mammillotegmental tract** arises from the mammillary body and terminates in the cells of the reticular formation in the tegmentum of the midbrain.

4. Multiple pathways to the **limbic system**.

The main efferent nervous connections of the hypothalamus are summarized in Table 13-1.

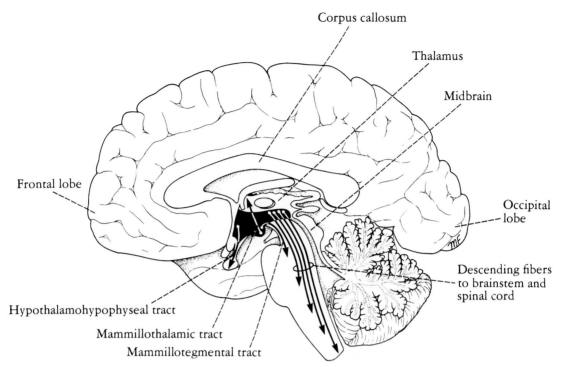

Figure 13–6 Sagittal section of the brain, showing the main efferent pathways leaving the hypo-thalamus.

CONNECTIONS OF THE HYPOTHALAMUS WITH THE HYPOPHYSIS CEREBRI

The hypothalamus is connected to the hypophysis cerebri (pituitary gland) by two pathways: (1) nerve fibers that travel from the supraoptic and paraventricular nuclei to the posterior lobe of the hypophysis, and (2) long and short portal blood vessels that connect sinusoids in the median eminence and infundibulum with capillary plexuses in the anterior lobe of the hypophysis (Fig. 13-7). These pathways enable the hypothalamus to influence the activities of the endocrine glands.

Hypothalamohypophyseal Tract

The hormones **vasopressin** and **oxytocin** are synthesized in the nerve cells of the supraoptic and paraventricular nuclei. The hormones are passed along the axons together with carrier proteins called **neurophysins** and are released at the axon terminals (Fig. 13-7). Here the hormones are absorbed into the bloodstream in fenestrated capillaries of the posterior lobe of the hypophysis. The hormone vasopressin (antidiuretic hormone) is produced mainly in the nerve cells of the supraoptic nucleus. Its function is to cause **vasoconstriction**. It also has an important **antidiuretic function**, causing an increased absorption of water in the distal convoluted tubules and collecting tubules of the kidney. The other hormone is oxytocin, which is produced mainly in the paraventricular nucleus. Oxytocin stimulates the contraction of the smooth muscle of the uterus and causes contraction of the myoepithelial cells that surround the alveoli and ducts of the breast. Toward the end of pregnancy oxytocin is produced in large amounts and stimulates labor contractions of the uterus. Later, when the baby suckles at the breast, a nervous reflex from the nipple stimulates the hypothalamus to produce more of the hormone. This promotes contraction of the myoepithelial cells and assists in the expression of the milk from the breasts.

The supraoptic nucleus, which produces vasopressin, acts as an **osmoreceptor**. Should the osmotic pressure of the blood circulating through the nucleus be too high, the nerve cells increase their production of vasopressin and the antidiuretic effect of this hormone will increase the reab-sorption of water from the kidney. By this means, the osmotic pressure of the blood will return to normal limits.

Hypophyseal Portal System

Neurosecretory cells situated mainly in the medial zone of the hypothalamus are responsible for the production of the **releasing hormones** and **release-inhibitory hormones**. The hormones are packaged into granules and transported along the axons of these cells into the median eminence and infundibulum. Here, the granules are released by exo-cytosis onto fenestrated capillaries at the upper end of the hypophyseal portal system.

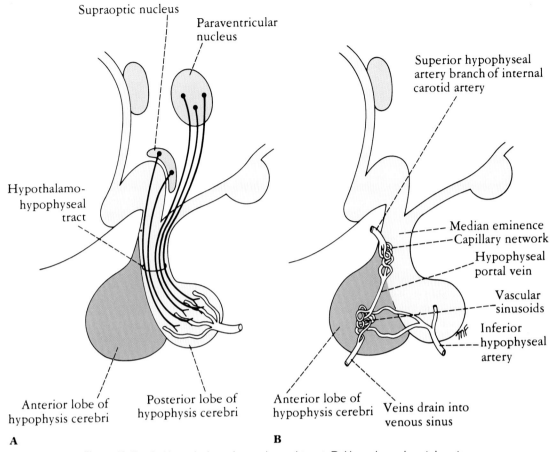

Figure 13–7   A. Hypothalamohypophyseal tract. **B.** Hypophyseal portal system.

The hypophyseal portal system is formed on each side from the superior hypophyseal artery, which is a branch of the internal carotid artery (Fig. 13-7). The artery enters the median eminence and divides into tufts of capillaries. These capillaries drain into long and short descending vessels that end in the anterior lobe of the hypophysis by dividing into vascular sinusoids that pass between the secretory cells of the anterior lobe.

The portal system carries the releasing hormones and the release-inhibiting hormones to the secretory cells of the anterior lobe of the hypophysis. The releasing hormones stimulate the production and release of **adrenocorticotropic hormone** (ACTH), **follicle-stimulating hormone** (FSH), **luteinizing hormone** (LH), **thyrotropic hormone** or **thyroid-stimulating hormone** (TSH), and **growth hormone** (GH). The release of inhibiting hormones inhibits the release of the **melanocyte-stimulating hormone** (MSH) and **luteotropic hormone** (LTH). Luteotropic hormone (also known as the **lactogenic hormone** or **prolactin**) stimulates the corpus luteum to secrete progesterone and the mammary gland to produce milk. The growth hormone inhibitory hormone (somatostatin) inhibits the release of growth hormone. A summary of the hypothalamic releasing and inhibitory hormones and their effects on the anterior lobe of the hypophysis are shown in Table 13-2.

The neurons of the hypothalamus that are responsible for the production of the releasing hormones and the release-inhibiting hormones are influenced by the afferent fibers passing to the hypothalamus. They also are influenced by the level of the hormone produced by the target organ controlled by the hypophysis. Should the level of thyroxine in the blood, for example, fall, then the releasing factor for the thyrotropic hormone would be produced in increased quantities. Table 13-3 summarizes the presumed nuclear origin of the pituitary releasing and inhibitory hormones in the hypothalamus.

FUNCTIONS OF THE HYPOTHALAMUS

Table 13-4 summarizes the functions of the main hypothalamic nuclei.

Autonomic Control

The hypothalamus has a controlling influence on the autonomic nervous system and appears to integrate the autonomic and neuroendocrine systems, thus preserving body

Table 13–2 The Hypothalamic Releasing and Inhibitory Hormones and Their Effects on the Anterior Lobe of the Hypophysis (Pituitary)

Hypothalamic Regulatory Hormone	Anterior Pituitary Hormone	Functional Result
Growth hormone–releasing hormone (GHRH)	Growth hormone (GH)	Stimulates linear growth in epiphyseal cartilages
Growth hormone–inhibiting hormone (GHIH) or somatostatin	Growth hormone (reduced production)	Reduces linear growth in epiphyseal cartilages
Prolactin-releasing hormone (PRH)	Prolactin (luteotropic hormone, LTH)	Stimulates lactogenesis
Prolactin-inhibiting hormone (PIH), dopamine	Prolactin (luteotropic hormone, LTH) (reduced production)	Reduces lactogenesis
Corticotropin-releasing hormone (CRH)	Adrenocorticotropic hormone (ACTH)	Stimulates adrenal gland to produce corticosteroids and sex hormones
Thyrotropin-releasing hormone (TRH)	Thyroid-stimulating hormone (TSH)	Stimulates thyroid gland to produce thyroxine
Luteinizing hormone–releasing hormone (LHRH), ? follicle-stimulating releasing hormone (FRH)	Luteinizing hormone (LH) and follicle-stimulating hormone (FSH)	Stimulates ovarian follicles and production of estrogen and progesterone

Table 13–3 The Presumed Nuclear Origin of the Hypophysis (Pituitary) Releasing and Inhibitory Hormones in the Hypothalamus

Hypothalamic Regulatory Hormone	Presumed Nuclear Origin
Growth hormone–releasing hormone (GHRH)	Infundibular or arcuate nucleus
Growth hormone–inhibiting hormone (GHIH) or somatostatin	Suprachiasmatic nucleus
Prolactin-releasing hormone (PRH)	?
Prolactin-inhibiting hormone (PIH)	?
Corticotropin-releasing hormone (CRH)	Paraventricular nuclei
Thyrotropin-releasing hormone (TRH)	Paraventricular and dorsomedial nuclei and adjacent areas
Luteinizing hormone–releasing hormone (LHRH)	Preoptic and anterior nuclei

Table 13–4 Functions of the Main Hypothalamic Nuclei

Hypothalamic Nucleus	Presumed Function
Supraoptic nucleus	Synthesizes vasopressin (antidiuretic hormone)
Paraventricular nucleus	Synthesizes oxytocin
Preoptic and anterior nuclei	Control parasympathetic system
Posterior and lateral nuclei	Control sympathetic system
Anterior hypothalamic nuclei	Regulate temperature (response to heat)
Posterior hypothalamic nuclei	Regulate temperature (response to cold)
Lateral hypothalamic nuclei	Initiate eating and increases food intake (hunger center)
Medial hypothalamic nuclei	Inhibit eating and reduces food intake (satiety center)
Lateral hypothalamic nuclei	Increase water intake (thirst center)
Suprachiasmatic nucleus	Controls circadian rhythms

homeostasis. Essentially, the hypothalamus should be regarded as a higher nervous center for the control of lower autonomic centers in the brainstem and spinal cord (Fig. 13-8).

Electrical stimulation of the hypothalamus in animal experiments shows that the anterior hypothalamic area and the preoptic area influence parasympathetic responses; these include lowering of the blood pressure, slowing of the heart rate, contraction of the bladder, increased motility of the gastrointestinal tract, increased acidity of the gastric juice, salivation, and pupillary constriction.

Stimulation of the posterior and lateral nuclei causes sympathetic responses, which include elevation of blood pressure, acceleration of the heart rate, cessation of peristalsis in the gastrointestinal tract, pupillary dilation, and hyperglycemia. These responses would lead one to believe that there exist in the hypothalamus areas that might be termed "parasympathetic and sympathetic centers." However, it has been shown that considerable overlap of function occurs in these areas.

Endocrine Control

The nerve cells of the hypothalamic nuclei, by producing the releasing factors or release-inhibiting factors (Table 13-2), control the hormone production of the anterior lobe of the

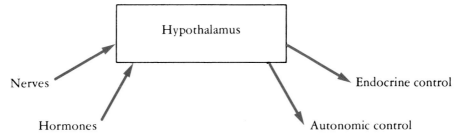

Figure 13–8 Diagram depicting the hypothalamus as the chief center of the brain for controlling the internal milieu of the body.

hypophysis (pituitary gland). The anterior lobe hormones include **growth hormone, prolactin** (luteotropic hormone), **adrenocorticotropic hormone, thyroid-stimulating hormone, luteinizing hormone**, and **follicle-stimulating hormone**. Some of these hormones act directly on body tissues, while others, such as adrenocorticotropic hormone, act through an endocrine organ, which in turn produces additional hormones that influence the activities of general body tissues. It should be pointed out that each stage is controlled by negative and positive feedback mechanisms.

Neurosecretion

The secretion of vasopressin and oxytocin by the supraoptic and paraventricular nuclei is discussed on page 386 and 387.

Temperature Regulation

The anterior portion of the hypothalamus controls those mechanisms that dissipate heat loss. Experimental stimulation of this area causes dilatation of skin blood vessels and sweating, which lower the body temperature. Stimulation of the posterior portion of the hypothalamus results in vasoconstriction of the skin blood vessels and inhibition of sweating; there also may be shivering, in which the skeletal muscles produce heat.

Normally the hypothalamus sets the body temperature at 98.0–98.6° F when measured orally and one degree higher when measured rectally. The temperature set can be altered in response to extremes in environmental temperatures or in infection, for example.

Regulation of Food and Water Intake

Stimulation of the lateral region of the hypothalamus initiates the feeling of hunger and results in an increase in food intake. This lateral region sometimes is referred to as the **hunger center**. Bilateral destruction of this center results in anorexia with the consequent loss in body weight. Stimulation of the medial region of the hypothalamus inhibits eating and reduces food intake. This area is referred to as the **satiety center**. Bilateral destruction of the satiety center produces an uncontrolled voracious appetite causing extreme obesity.

Experimental stimulation of other areas in the lateral region of the hypothalamus causes an immediate increase in the desire to drink water; this area is referred to as the **thirst center**. In addition, the hypothalamus exerts a careful control on the osmolarity of the blood through the secretion of vasopressin (antidiuretic hormone) by the posterior lobe of the hypophysis. This hormone causes a great increase in the reabsorption of water in the distal convoluted tubules and collecting tubules of the kidneys.

Emotion and Behavior

Emotion and behavior are a function of the hypothalamus, the limbic system, and the prefrontal cortex. Some authorities believe that the hypothalamus is the integrator of afferent information received from other areas of the nervous system, and brings about the physical expression of emotion; it can produce an increase in the heart rate, elevate the blood pressure, cause dryness of the mouth, flushing or pallor of the skin, and sweating, and can often produce a massive peristaltic activity of the gastrointestinal tract.

Control of Circadian Rhythms

The hypothalamus controls many circadian rhythms, including body temperature, adrenocortical activity, eosinophil count, and renal secretion. Sleeping and wakefulness, although dependent on the activities of the thalamus, the limbic system, and the reticular activating system, are also controlled by the hypothalamus. Lesions of the anterior part of the hypothalamus seriously interfere with the rhythm of sleeping and waking. The suprachiasmatic nucleus, which receives afferent fibers from the retina, appears to play an important role in controlling the biological rhythms. Nerve impulses generated in response to variations in the intensity of light are transmitted via this nucleus to influence the activities of many of the hypothalamic nuclei.

CLINICAL NOTES

GENERAL CONSIDERATIONS

In summary, the activities of the hypothalamus are modified by information received along numerous afferent pathways from different parts of the central nervous system (especially from the limbic system and the prefrontal cortex) and by the plasma levels of circulating hormones. It exerts its influence on bodily functions through the autonomic nervous system and the endocrine system.

Although small, the hypothalamus should not be interpreted as a structure of little importance. It is the chief center of the brain for maintaining the internal milieu of the body (Fig. 13-8). There is hardly a tissue in the body that escapes its influence.

The connections of the hypothalamus are extremely complicated and only the major pathways should be committed to memory for use in clinical work.

CLINICAL DISORDERS ASSOCIATED WITH HYPOTHALAMIC LESIONS

The hypothalamus may be the site of inflammation, neoplasm, or vascular disorder. Because of its deep-seated central position, it can be pressed upon by tumors of the surrounding brain tissue or may be compressed as the result of the development of internal hydrocephalus. Its widespread influence on many homeostatic and behavioral functions means that a lesion of the hypothalamus will produce a large number of different syndromes. Thus, it is important to remember that an acute lesion is more likely to produce signs and symptoms than is a slowly growing tumor.

Obesity and Wasting

Severe obesity can occur as the result of hypothalamic lesions. It is generally associated with genital hypoplasia or atrophy.

Wasting is less common than obesity in hypothalamic disease. Severe cachexia is suggestive of damage to the hypophysis (pituitary gland).

Sexual Disorders

In children there may be sexual retardation and, rarely, sexual precocity with hypothalamic lesions. After puberty, the patient with hypothalamic disease may have impotence or amenorrhea.

Hyperthermia and Hypothermia

Hyperthermia can follow lesions of the hypothalamus caused by head injury or following surgical operations in the region of the hypothalamus. The patient with hyperthermia is otherwise normal and has no signs of malaise, which occurs with pyrexia secondary to infections.

Hypothermia also can follow a lesion of the hypothalamus.

Diabetes Insipidus

This disease results from a lesion of the supraoptic nucleus or from the interruption of the nervous pathway to the posterior lobe of the hypophysis. Characteristically, the patient passes large volumes of urine of low specific gravity. As a result, the patient is extremely thirsty and drinks large quantities of fluids. The condition must be distinguished from diabetes mellitus, in which there is glucosuria.

Disturbances of Sleep

The occurrence of either frequent short periods of sleep during the waking hours or insomnia has been observed in patients with hypothalamic lesions.

Emotional Disorders

Attacks of unexplained weeping or laughter, uncontrollable rage, depressive reactions, or even maniacal outbursts all have been observed in patients with hypothalamic lesions.

Clinical Problem Solving

1. A 17-year-old boy was admitted into the medical ward for observation. The tentative diagnosis was *Fröhlich's syndrome.* He had a 3-month history of severe headaches. More recently, he had had attacks of vomiting, and 1 week ago he had noticed problems with his eyesight. The patient said that he had difficulty seeing objects on the lateral side of both eyes. His parents were concerned that he was putting on weight because he was especially fat over the lower part of the trunk. On physical examination, the boy was found to be 6 feet 3 inches tall; he had

   excessive trunk obesity. The testes and penis were small, and pubic and axillary hair was absent. A lateral radiograph of the skull showed enlargement of the sella turcica with erosion of the dorsum sellae. An examination of the eye fields confirmed that the patient had partial bitemporal hemianopia. Using your knowledge of neuroanatomy, explain the symptoms and signs of this patient.

2. A 40-year-old woman was involved in an automobile accident in which she sustained severe head injuries.

Following a slow but uneventful recovery, she was released from the hospital without any residual signs or symptoms. Six months later, the patient started to complain of frequency of micturition and was passing very large quantities of pale urine. She also said that she always seemed thirsty and would often drink 10 glasses of water in one morning. Using your knowledge of neuroanatomy and neurophysiology, do you think there is any connection between the urinary symptoms and her automobile accident?

3. Do you think it is possible that a patient with hydrocephalus could have a malfunctioning hypothalamus? If so, explain the connection.
4. Sherrington once stated in a scientific publication in 1947 that the hypothalamus should be regarded as the "head ganglion" of the autonomic nervous system. What is the relationship that exists between the hypothalamus and the autonomic nervous system?
5. Explain what is meant by the terms the *hypothalamohypophyseal tract* and the *hypophyseal portal system*.

Answers to Clinical Problem Solving

1. This boy was suffering from Fröhlich's syndrome secondary to a chromophobe adenoma of the anterior lobe of the hypophysis. This space-occupying lesion had gradually eroded the sella turcica of the skull and had compressed the optic chiasma, producing bitemporal hemianopia. The size of the tumor was causing a raised intracranial pressure that was responsible for the headaches and attacks of vomiting. Pressure on the hypothalamus interfered with its function and resulted in the characteristic accumulation of fat in the trunk, especially the lower part of the abdomen. The hypogonadism and absence of secondary sex characteristics could have been due to pressure of the tumor on the hypothalamic nuclei and the consequent loss of control on the anterior lobe of the hypophysis, or it may have been due to the direct effect of the tumor pressing on the neighboring cells of the anterior lobe of the hypophysis.
2. Yes, there is a connection between the accident and the urinary symptoms. This patient is suffering from diabetes insipidus caused by traumatic damage either to the posterior lobe of the hypophysis or to the supraoptic nucleus of the hypothalamus. In any event, production of vasopressin was inhibited. It should be pointed out that a

lesion of the posterior lobe of the hypophysis is usually not followed by diabetes insipidus, since the vasopressin produced by the neurons of the supraoptic nucleus escapes directly into the bloodstream. The action of vasopressin on the distal convoluted tubules and collecting tubules of the kidney is fully explained on page 386.
3. Yes, it is possible. Hydrocephalus, caused by blockage of the three foramina in the roof of the fourth ventricle or by blockage of the cerebral aqueduct, will result in a rise in pressure in the third ventricle, with pressure on the hypothalamus. This pressure on the hypothalamus, which is situated in the floor and lower part of the lateral walls of the third ventricle, if great enough, could easily cause malfunctioning of the hypothalamus.
4. The hypothalamus is the main subcortical center regulating the parasympathetic and sympathetic parts of the autonomic system. It exerts its influence through descending pathways in the reticular formation.
5. The hypothalamohypophyseal tract is described on page 386, and the hypophyseal portal system is described on page 386. Remember that the hypothalamus exerts its control over metabolic and visceral functions through the hypophysis cerebri and the autonomic system.

Review Questions

Directions: Each of the numbered items in this section is followed by answers that are positively phrased. Select the ONE lettered answer that is an EXCEPTION.

1. The following statements concerning the hypothalamus are correct **except:**
   (a) The hypothalamus lies below the thalamus in the tectum of the midbrain.
   (b) The hypothalamus lies in the center of the limbic system.
   (c) The nuclei of the hypothalamus are divided by an imaginary plane formed by the columns of the fornix and the mammillothalamic tract into medial and lateral groups.
   (d) The suprachiasmatic nucleus overlaps both medial and lateral groups of nuclei and receives nerve fibers from the retina.
   (e) The lateral boundary of the hypothalamus is formed by the internal capsule.
2. The following statements concerning the hypothalamus are correct **except:**
   (a) When seen from the inferior aspect, the hypothalamus is related to the following structures, from anterior to posterior: (a) the optic chiasma, (b) the tuber cinereum, and (c) the mammillary bodies.
   (b) The margins of the different nuclei can be clearly seen with the naked eye.

(c) The mammillary body overlaps both the medial and lateral groups of nuclei.

(d) The preoptic area of the hypothalamus is located between the lamina terminalis and the optic chiasma.

(e) The blood-brain barrier is absent in the median eminence of the hypothalamus, thus permitting the neurons to sample the chemical content of the plasma directly.

3. The following statements concerning the afferent fibers passing to the hypothalamus are correct **except:**

(a) Fibers pass from the hippocampus to the mammillary bodies, bringing information from the limbic system.

(b) Olfactory impulses reach the hypothalamus through the medial forebrain bundle.

(c) The dorsomedial nucleus does not receive axons from the posterior lobe of the pituitary.

(d) The pineal gland sends fibers via the habenular commissure to the hypothalamus.

(e) The hypothalamus receives many afferent fibers from the viscera via the reticular formation.

4. The following statements concerning the hypothalamus are correct **except:**

(a) Somatic afferent fibers reach the hypothalamic nuclei via the medial and spinal lemnisci.

(b) The hypothalamus integrates the autonomic and neuroendocrine systems, thus preserving homeostasis.

(c) The nerve cells of the hypothalamus produce releasing and release-inhibiting hormones that control the production of various hormones in the anterior lobe of the hypophysis.

(d) The anterior portion of the hypothalamus controls those mechanisms that dissipate heat loss.

(e) The hunger center is probably located in the posterior hypothalamic nuclei.

5. The following statements concerning the functional activities of the hypothalamus are correct **except:**

(a) The lateral hypothalamic nuclei are concerned with fluid intake.

(b) The hypothalamus probably brings about the physical changes associated with emotion, such as increased heart rate and flushing or pallor of the skin.

(c) The corticotropin-releasing hormone (CRH) is produced in the anterior nucleus of the hypothalamus.

(d) The suprachiasmatic nucleus plays an important role in controlling circadian rhythms.

(e) The hypothalamus controls the lower autonomic centers by means of pathways through the reticular formation.

6. The following statements concerning the hypothalamo-hypophyseal tract are correct **except:**

(a) Oxytocin inhibits the contraction of the smooth muscle of the uterus.

(b) The nerve cells of the supraoptic and paraventricular nuclei produce the hormones vasopressin and oxytocin.

(c) The hormones travel in the axons of the tract with protein carriers called neurophysins.

(d) Vasopressin stimulates the distal convoluted tubules and collecting tubules of the kidney, causing increased absorption of water from the urine.

(e) The hormones leave the axons and are absorbed into the bloodstream in the capillaries of the posterior lobe of the hypophysis.

7. The following statements concerning the hypophyseal portal system are correct **except:**

(a) The portal system carries releasing hormones and release-inhibiting hormones to the secretory cells of the anterior lobe of the hypophysis.

(b) The production of the releasing hormones and the release-inhibiting hormones can be influenced by the level of the hormone produced by the target organ controlled by the hypophysis.

(c) The blood vessels commence superiorly in the median eminence and end inferiorly in the vascular sinusoids of the anterior lobe of the hypophysis cerebri.

(d) Afferent nerve fibers entering the hypothalamus influence the production of the releasing hormones by the nerve cells.

(e) The neuroglial cells of the hypothalamus are responsible for the production of the release-inhibiting hormones.

Answers to Review Questions

1. A
2. B
3. D
4. E

5. C
6. A
7. E

ADDITIONAL READING ....

Adams, J. H., Daniel, P. M., and Prichard, M. Observations on the portal circulation of the pituitary gland. *Neuroendocrinology* 1:193, 1966.

Bisset, G. W., Hilton, S. M., and Poisner, A. M. Hypothalamic pathways for the independent release of vasopressin and oxytocin. *Proc. R. Soc. Lond. [Biol.]* 166:422, 1966.

Boulant, J. A. Hypothalamic Neurons Regulating Body Temperature. pp 105-126 In: *Handbook of Physiology. Section 4: Environmental Physiology.* Oxford Univ. Press, 1997.

Buijs, R. M. Vasopressin and oxytocin—their role in neurotransmission. *Pharmacol. Ther.* 22:127, 1983.

Buijs, R.M., Kalsbeek, A., Romijn, H.J., Pennertz, C.M., and Mirmiran, M. (eds). *Hypothalamic Integration of Circadian Rhythm*s. Elsevier, 1997.

Burgus, R., and Guillemin, R. Hypothalamic releasing factors. *Annu. Rev. Biochem.* 39:499, 1970.

Craig, C. R., and Stitzel, R. E. *Modern Pharmacology* (4th ed.). Boston: Little, Brown, 1994.

Ganten, D., and Pfaff, D. *Morphology of Hypothalamus and Its Connections.* Berlin: Springer-Verlag, 1986.

Grossman, S. P. A reassessment of the brain mechanisms that control thirst. *Neurosci. Behav. Rev.* 8:95, 1984.

Guyton, A. C., and Hall, J.E. *Textbook of Medical Physiology* (9th ed.). Philadelphia: Saunders, 1996.

Haymaker, W., Anderson, E., and Nauta, W. J. H. *The Hypothalamus.* Springfield, Illinois: Thomas, 1969.

Swaab, D.F., Hofman, M.A., Mirmiran, M., Ravid, R., and Van Leewen, F. (eds). *The Human Hypothalamus in Health and Disease.* Elsevier, 1993.

Swanson, L. W., and Sawchenko, P. E. Hypothalamic integration: Organization of the paraventricular and supraoptic nuclei. *Annu. Rev. Neurosci.* 6:269, 1983.

Williams, P.L., et al. *Gray's Anatomy* (38th Br. Ed.). New York and Edinburgh: Churchill Livingstone, 1995.

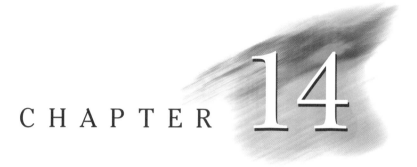

The Autonomic Nervous System

A 46-year-old man who had recently undergone right-sided pneumonectomy for carcinoma of the bronchus was seen by his thoracic surgeon for follow-up after the operation. The patient said that he felt surprisingly fit and was gaining some of the weight that he had lost prior to the operation. His wife commented that about 1 week ago the upper lid of his right eye tended to droop slightly when he was tired at the end of the day.

After a careful physical examination, the surgeon noticed that in addition to the ptosis of the right eye, the patient's right pupil was constricted and that his face was slightly flushed on the right side. Further examination revealed that the skin on the right side of the face appeared to be warmer and drier than normal. Palpation of the deep cervical group of lymph nodes revealed a large hard fixed node just above the right clavicle.

Based on his clinical findings, the surgeon made the diagnosis of a right-sided Horner's syndrome. These findings were not present before the operation. The presence of the enlarged right-sided deep cervical lymph node indicated that the bronchial carcinoma had metastasized to the lymph node in the neck and was spreading to involve the cervical part of the sympathetic trunk on the right side. This observation would explain the abnormal eye and facial skin findings.

Knowledge of the sympathetic innervation of the structures of the head and neck enabled the surgeon to make an accurate diagnosis in this patient.

C H A P T E R   O B J E C T I V E S

The autonomic nervous system and the endocrine system control the internal environment of the body. The object of this chapter is to give the reader a practical basic account of the structure, physiology, and pharmacology of the autonomic nervous system. The information reported is extensively used in clinical practice. The examples of autonomic innervation given in this chapter are important and are commonly used by examiners to construct good questions.

The autonomic nervous system exerts control over the functions of many organs and tissues in the body, including heart muscle, smooth muscle, and the exocrine glands. Along with the endocrine system, it brings about fine internal adjustments necessary for the optimal internal environment of the body.

The autonomic nervous system, like the somatic nervous system, has afferent, connector, and efferent neurons. The afferent impulses originate in visceral receptors and travel via afferent pathways to the central nervous system, where they are integrated through connector neurons at different levels and then leave via efferent pathways to visceral effector organs. The majority of the activities of the autonomic system do not impinge on consciousness.

The efferent pathways of the autonomic system are made up of preganglionic and postganglionic neurons. The cell bodies of the preganglionic neurons are situated in the lateral gray column of the spinal cord and in the motor nuclei of the third, seventh, ninth, and tenth cranial nerves. The axons of these cell bodies synapse on the cell bodies of the postganglionic neurons that are collected together to form **ganglia** outside the central nervous system.

The control exerted by the autonomic system is extremely rapid; it is also widespread, since one preganglionic axon may synapse with several postganglionic neurons. Large collections of afferent and efferent fibers and their associated ganglia form **autonomic plexuses** in the thorax, abdomen, and pelvis.

The visceral receptors include chemoreceptors, baroreceptors, and osmoreceptors. Pain receptors are present in viscera and certain types of stimuli, such as lack of oxygen or stretch, can cause extreme pain.

ORGANIZATION OF THE AUTONOMIC NERVOUS SYSTEM

The autonomic nervous system is distributed throughout the central and peripheral nervous systems. It is divided into two parts, the **sympathetic** and the **parasympathetic;** and, as emphasized above, consists of both afferent and efferent fibers. This division between sympathetic and parasympathetic is made on the basis of anatomical differences, differences in the neurotransmitters, and differences in the physiological effects. Both divisions operate in conjunction with one another and it is the balance in the activities that maintains a stable internal environment.

Sympathetic Part of the Autonomic System

The sympathetic system is the larger of the two parts of the autonomic system and is widely distributed throughout the body, innervating the heart and lungs, the muscle in the walls of many blood vessels, the hair follicles and the sweat glands, and many abdominopelvic viscera.

The function of the sympathetic system is to prepare the body for an emergency. The heart rate is increased, arterioles of the skin and intestine are constricted, those of skeletal muscle are dilated, and the blood pressure is raised. There is a redistribution of blood so that it leaves the skin and gastrointestinal tract and passes to the brain, heart, and skeletal muscle. In addition the sympathetic nerves dilate the pupils; inhibit smooth muscle of the bronchi, intestine, and bladder wall; and close the sphincters. The hair is made to stand on end and sweating occurs.

The sympathetic system consists of the efferent outflow from the spinal cord, two ganglionated sympathetic trunks, important branches, plexuses, and regional ganglia.

EFFERENT NERVE FIBERS (SYMPATHETIC OUTFLOW)

The lateral gray columns (horns) of the spinal cord from the first thoracic segment to the second lumbar segment (sometimes third lumbar segment) possess the cell bodies of the sympathetic connector neurons (Fig. 14-1). The myelinated axons of these cells leave the cord in the anterior nerve roots and pass via the **white rami communicantes** (the white rami are white because the nerve fibers are covered with white myelin) to the **paravertebral ganglia** of the **sympathetic trunk.** Once these fibers (preganglionic) reach the ganglia in the sympathetic trunk, they are distributed as follows:

1. They synapse with an excitor neuron in the ganglion (Fig. 14-1 and 14-2). The gap between the two neurons is bridged by the neurotransmitter **acetylcholine (Ach).** The postganglionic nonmyelinated axons leave the ganglion and pass to the thoracic spinal nerves as **gray rami communicantes** (the gray rami are gray because the nerve fibers are devoid of myelin). They are distributed in branches of the spinal nerves to smooth muscle in the blood vessel walls, sweat glands, and arrector muscles of the hairs of the skin.
2. They travel cephalad in the sympathetic trunk to synapse in ganglia in the cervical region (Fig. 14-2). The postganglionic nerve fibers pass via gray rami communicantes to join the cervical spinal nerves. Many of the preganglionic fibers entering the lower part of the sympathetic trunk from the lower thoracic and upper two lumbar segments of the spinal cord travel caudad to synapse in ganglia in the lower lumbar and sacral regions. Here again, the postganglionic nerve fibers pass via gray rami communicantes to join the lumbar, sacral, and coccygeal spinal nerves (Fig. 14-2).
3. They may pass through the ganglia of the sympathetic trunk without synapsing. These myelinated fibers leave the sympathetic trunk as the **greater splanchnic, lesser splanchnic,** and **lowest** or **least splanchnic nerves.** The greater splanchnic nerve is formed from branches from the fifth to the ninth thoracic ganglia. It descends obliquely on the sides of the bodies of the thoracic vertebrae and pierces the crus of the diaphragm to synapse

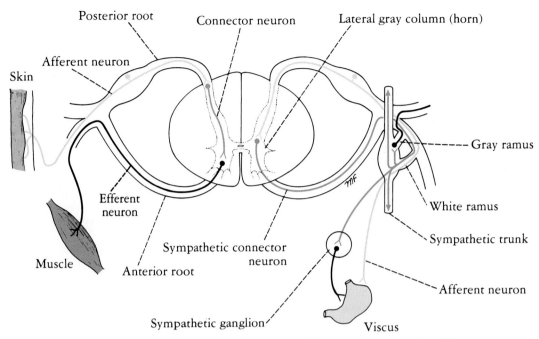

Figure 14-1 General arrangement of the somatic part of the nervous system (on left) compared with the autonomic part of the nervous system (on right).

with excitor cells in the ganglia of the **celiac plexus,** the **renal plexus,** and the suprarenal medulla. The lesser splanchnic nerve is formed from branches of the tenth and eleventh thoracic ganglia. It descends with the greater splanchnic nerve and pierces the diaphragm to join excitor cells in ganglia in the lower part of the **celiac plexus.** The lowest splanchnic nerve (when present) arises from the twelfth thoracic ganglion, pierces the diaphragm, and synapses with excitor neurons in the ganglia of the **renal plexus.** The splanchnic nerves, therefore, are formed of preganglionic fibers. The postganglionic fibers arise from the excitor cells in the peripheral plexuses and are distributed to the smooth muscle and glands of the viscera. A few preganglionic fibers, traveling in the greater splanchnic nerve, end directly on the cells of the **suprarenal medulla.** These medullary cells, which may be regarded as modified sympathetic excitor neurons, are responsible for the secretion of epinephrine and norepinephrine.

The ratio of preganglionic to postganglionic sympathetic fibers is about 1:10 permitting a wide control of involuntary structures.

AFFERENT NERVE FIBERS

The afferent myelinated nerve fibers travel from the viscera through the sympathetic ganglia without synapsing. They pass to the spinal nerve via white rami communicantes and reach their cell bodies in the posterior root ganglion of the corresponding spinal nerve (Fig. 14-1). The central axons then enter the spinal cord and may form the afferent component of a local reflex arc or ascend to higher centers, such as the hypothalamus.

SYMPATHETIC TRUNKS

The sympathetic trunks are two ganglionated nerve trunks that extend the whole length of the vertebral column (Fig. 14-2). In the neck, each trunk has 3 ganglia; in the thorax, 11 or 12; in the lumbar region, 4 or 5; and in the pelvis, 4 or 5. In the neck, the trunks lie anterior to the transverse processes of the cervical vertebrae; in the thorax, they are anterior to the heads of the ribs or lie on the sides of the vertebral bodies; in the abdomen, they are anterolateral to the sides of the bodies of the lumbar vertebrae; and in the pelvis, they are anterior to the sacrum. Below, the two trunks end by joining together to form a single ganglion, the **ganglion impar.**

Parasympathetic Part of the Autonomic System

The activities of the parasympathetic part of the autonomic system are directed toward conserving and restoring energy. The heart rate is slowed, pupils are constricted, peri-

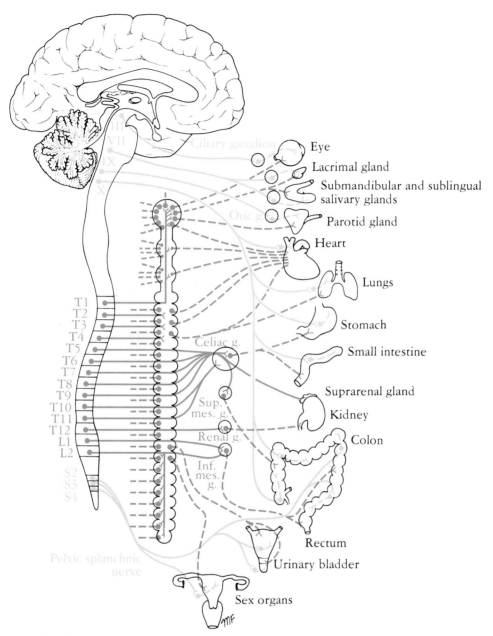

Figure 14–2 Efferent part of the autonomic nervous system. Preganglionic parasympathetic fibers are shown in solid blue, postganglionic parasympathetic fibers in interrupted blue. Preganglionic sympathetic fibers are shown in solid red, postganglionic sympathetic fibers in interrupted red.

stalsis and glandular activity is increased, sphincters are opened, and the bladder wall is contracted.

EFFERENT NERVE FIBERS (CRANIOSACRAL OUTFLOW)

The connector nerve cells of the parasympathetic part of the autonomic nervous system are located in the brainstem and the sacral segments of the spinal cord (Fig. 14-2).

Those nerve cells located in the brainstem form nuclei in the following cranial nerves: the **oculomotor** (parasympathetic or Edinger-Westphal nucleus), the **facial** (superior salivatory nucleus and lacrimatory nucleus), the **glossopharyngeal** (inferior salivatory nucleus), and the **vagus** nerves (dorsal nucleus of the vagus). The axons of these connector nerve cells are myelinated and emerge from the brain within the cranial nerves.

The sacral connector nerve cells are found in the gray matter of the **second, third,** and **fourth sacral segments of the spinal cord.** These cells are not sufficiently numerous to form a lateral gray horn, as do the sympathetic connector neurons in the thoracolumbar region. The myelinated axons leave the spinal cord in the anterior nerve roots of the corresponding spinal nerves. They then leave the sacral nerves and form the **pelvic splanchnic nerves** (Fig. 14-2).

The myelinated efferent fibers of the craniosacral outflow are preganglionic and synapse in peripheral ganglia located close to the viscera they innervate. Here, again, acetylcholine is the neurotransmitter. The cranial parasympathetic ganglia are the **ciliary, pterygopalatine, submandibular,** and **otic** (Fig. 14-2). In certain locations the ganglion cells are placed in nerve plexuses, such as the **cardiac plexus, pulmonary plexus, myenteric plexus (Auerbach's plexus),** and **mucosal plexus (Meissner's plexus)**; the last two plexuses are associated with the gastrointestinal tract. The pelvic splanchnic nerves synapse in ganglia in the **hypogastric plexuses.** Characteristically, the postganglionic parasympathetic fibers are nonmyelinated and of relatively short length as compared with sympathetic postganglionic fibers.

The ratio of preganglionic to postganglionic fibers is about 1:3 or less, which is much more restricted than in the sympathetic part of the system.

AFFERENT NERVE FIBERS

The afferent myelinated fibers travel from the viscera to their cell bodies, located either in the sensory ganglia of the cranial nerves or in the posterior root ganglia of the sacrospinal nerves. The central axons then enter the central nervous system and take part in the formation of local reflex arcs, or pass to higher centers of the autonomic nervous system, such as the hypothalamus.

The afferent component of the autonomic system is identical to the afferent component of somatic nerves, and it forms part of the general afferent segment of the entire nervous system. The nerve endings in the autonomic afferent component may not be activated by such sensations as heat or touch but rather by stretch or lack of oxygen. Once the afferent fibers gain entrance to the spinal cord or brain, they are thought to travel alongside, or mixed with, the somatic afferent fibers.

 ## THE LARGE AUTONOMIC PLEXUSES*

Large collections of sympathetic and parasympathetic efferent nerve fibers and their associated ganglia, together with visceral afferent fibers, form autonomic nerve plexuses in the thorax, abdomen, and pelvis. Branches from these plexuses innervate the viscera. In the thorax there are the cardiac, pulmonary, and esophageal plexuses. In the abdomen the plexuses are associated with the aorta and its branches, and subdivisions of these autonomic plexuses are named according to the branch of the aorta along which they are lying: celiac, superior mesenteric, inferior mesenteric, and aortic plexuses. In the pelvis there are the superior and inferior hypogastric plexuses.

 ## AUTONOMIC GANGLIA

The autonomic ganglion is the site where preganglionic nerve fibers synapse on postganglionic neurons (Fig. 14-3). Ganglia are situated along the course of efferent nerve fibers of the autonomic nervous system. Sympathetic ganglia form part of the sympathetic trunk or are prevertebral in position (e.g., celiac and superior mesenteric ganglia). Parasympathetic ganglia, on the other hand, are situated close to or within the walls of the viscera.

An autonomic ganglion consists of a collection of multipolar neurons together with capsular or satellite cells and a connective tissue capsule. Nerve bundles are attached to each ganglion and consist of preganglionic nerve fibers that enter the ganglion, postganglionic nerve fibers that have arisen from neurons within the ganglion and are leaving the ganglion, and afferent and efferent nerve fibers that pass through the ganglion without synapsing. The preganglionic fibers are myelinated, small, and relatively slow-conducting B fibers. The postganglionic fibers are unmyelinated, smaller, and slower-conducting C fibers.

The structure of synapses in autonomic ganglia shows the characteristic membrane thickening and small clear vesicles. In addition, there are some larger granular vesicles. The smaller vesicles contain acetylcholine; the content of the granular vesicles is unknown.

Although an autonomic ganglion is the site where preganglionic fibers synapse on postganglionic neurons, the

---

*An **autonomic nerve plexus** is a collection of nerve fibers that form a network; nerve cells may be present within such a network. A **ganglion** is a knotlike mass of nerve cells found outside the central nervous system. The term must be distinguished from the ganglion within the central nervous system consisting of nuclear groups (e.g., basal ganglia).

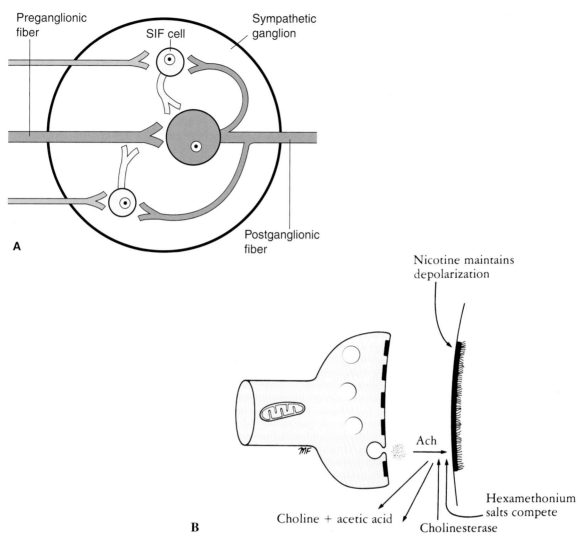

Figure 14–3 A. An autonomic ganglion as an integrator. Shows small intensely fluorescent (SIF) cells. **B.** The liberation of acetylcholine (ACh) at an autonomic synapse.

presence of small interneurons has been recognized. These cells exhibit catecholamine fluorescence and are referred to as **small intensely fluorescent (SIF)** cells. In some ganglia these interneurons receive preganglionic cholinergic fibers so that they may modulate ganglionic transmission. In other ganglia they receive collateral branches and may serve some integrative function (Fig. 14-3). Many SIF cells contain **dopamine** which is thought to be their transmitter.

PREGANGLIONIC TRANSMITTERS

As the preganglionic nerve fibers approach their termination, they wind around and between the dendritic processes of the postganglionic neuron, making multiple synaptic contacts. When the wave of excitation reaches the synaptic contacts, the synaptic transmitter is liberated,

crosses the synaptic cleft, and excites the postganglionic neuron (Fig. 14-3B and 14-4).

The synaptic transmitter that excites the postganglionic neurons in both sympathetic and parasympathetic ganglia is **acetylcholine (Ach).** The action of acetylcholine in autonomic ganglia is quickly terminated by hydrolysis by **acetylcholinesterase.**

FAST, SLOW, AND INHIBITORY SYNAPTIC POTENTIALS

Nicotinic and **muscarinic** receptors are present on the dendrites and cell bodies of the postganglionic neurons. Acetylcholine activation of the postsynaptic nicotinic receptors, results in a depolarization of the membrane, an influx of Na+ and Ca2+ ions, and the generation of the fast excitatory postsynaptic potential (fast **EPSP**). Usually, sev-

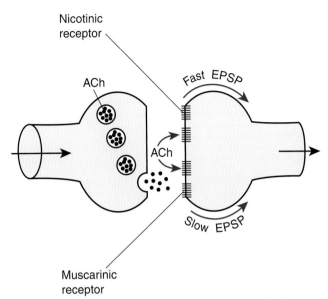

Figure 14–4 Example of the release of acetylcholine from a presynapic terminal. A single presynapic stimulus evokes a fast excitatory postsynaptic potential (fast **EPSP**) at a nicotinic receptor. Further stimulation may lead to a slow excitatory postsynaptic potential (slow **EPSP**) or a slow inhibitory postsynaptic potential (slow **IPSP**)at a muscarinic receptor.

eral presynaptic axon terminals must fire simultaneously and summation has to occur for transmission along the postsynaptic axon to take place. The fast EPSP reaches a maximum within about 15 ms.

Acetylcholine activation of the postsynaptic muscarinic receptors results in the development of the slow excitatory postsynaptic potential (slow **EPSP**), which lasts for 2-5 sec. The underlying mechanism is complicated and the slow potential occurs when the Na+ and Ca2+ channels are open and M-type K+ channels close; this leads to membrane depolarization. Late slow **EPSP** lasting as long as 1-2 min. can also be produced by neuropeptide transmitters.

The activation of postsynaptic muscarinic receptors may also result in the development of the slow inhibitory postsynaptic potential (slow **IPSP**), which lasts about 10 sec. The IPSP results from the opening of K+ channels, permitting K+ ions to flow out into the synaptic space producing hyperpolarization.

The existence of these complex postsynaptic potentials in both sympathetic and parasympathetic ganglia (Fig. 14-4) illustrates how the post synaptic membrane potential can be altered and ganglionic transmission modulated.

GANGLION STIMULATING AGENTS

Stimulating drugs such as nicotine, lobeline, and dimethylphenol piperazinium stimulate sympathetic and parasympathetic ganglia by activating the nicotinic receptors on the postsynaptic membrane and producing a fast EPSP.

GANGLION BLOCKING AGENTS

There are two types of ganglion blocking agents—depolarizing and nonpolarizing. **Nicotine** acts as a blocking agent in high concentrations, by first stimulating the postganglionic neuron and causing depolarization, and then by maintaining depolarization of the excitable membrane. During this latter phase the postganglionic neuron will fail to respond to the administration of any stimulant, regardless of the type of receptor it activates.

Hexamethonium and **tetraethylammonium** block ganglia by competing with acetylcholine at the nicotinic receptor sites.

POSTGANGLIONIC NERVE ENDINGS

The postganglionic fibers terminate on the effector cells without special discrete endings. The axons run between the gland cells and the smooth and cardiac muscle fibers and lose their covering of Schwann cells. At sites where transmission occurs, clusters of vesicles are present within the axoplasm (Fig. 3-40). The site on the axon may lie at some distance from the effector cell so that the transmission time may be slow at these endings. The diffusion of the transmitter through the large extracellular distance also permits a given nerve to have an action on a large number of effector cells.

POSTGANGLIONIC TRANSMITTERS

Parasympathetic postganglionic nerve endings liberate **acetylcholine** as their transmitter substance (Fig. 14-5). All neurons that release acetylcholine at their endings are called **cholinergic** (work like acetylcholine). The acetylcholine traverses the synaptic cleft and binds reversibly with the cholinergic receptor on the postsynaptic membrane. Within 2 to 3 msec it is hydrolyzed into acetic acid and choline by the enzyme **acetylcholinesterase,** which is located on the surface of the nerve and receptor membranes. The choline is reabsorbed into the nerve ending and used again for synthesis of acetylcholine.

Most sympathetic postganglionic nerve endings liberate **norepinephrine*** as their transmitter substance. In addition, some sympathetic postganglionic nerve endings, particularly those that end on cells of sweat glands and the blood vessels in skeletal muscle, release **acetylcholine.**

Sympathetic endings that use norepinephrine are called **adrenergic endings.** There are two major kinds of receptors in the effector organs, called **alpha** and **beta receptors.**

---

*In the United States **norepinephrine** is the name given to the transmitter in the sympathetic nervous system and **epinephrine** is the name given to the suprarenal medullary hormone. In many other parts of the world these two substances are called **noradrenaline** and **adrenaline**, respectively.

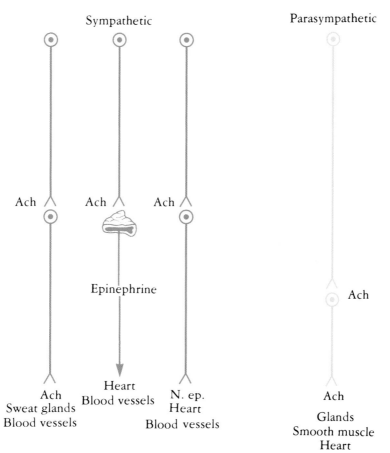

Sympathetic   Parasympathetic

Ach   Ach   Ach

Epinephrine   Ach

Ach   N. ep.   Ach
Sweat glands   Heart   Heart
Blood vessels   Blood vessels   Blood vessels   Glands
                                                 Smooth muscle
Heart
Blood vessels   Heart

Figure 14–5   Efferent parts of the autonomic nervous system and the chemical transmitter substances released at the nerve endings. ACh = acetylcholine; N. ep. = norepinephrine.

Two subgroups of alpha receptors (alpha-1 and alpha-2 receptors) and two subgroups of beta receptors (beta-1 and beta-2 receptors) have been described. Norepinephrine has a greater effect on alpha receptors than on beta receptors. **Phenylephrine** is a pure alpha stimulator. The bronchodilating drugs such as **metaproterenol** and **albuterol** mainly act on beta-2 receptors. As a general rule, alpha receptor sites are associated with most of the excitatory functions of the sympathetic system (e.g., smooth muscle contraction, vasoconstriction, diaphoresis), whereas the beta receptor sites are associated with most of the inhibitory functions (e.g., smooth muscle relaxation). Beta-2 receptors are mainly in the lung, and stimulation results in bronchodilatation. Beta-1 receptors are in the myocardium, where they are associated with excitation.

The action of norepinephrine on the receptor site of the effector cell is terminated by reuptake into the nerve terminal, where it is stored in presynaptic vesicles for reuse. Some of the norepinephrine escapes from the synaptic cleft into the general circulation and is subsequently metabolised in the liver.

OTHER POSTGANGLIONIC TRANSMITTERS

Sympathetic and parasympathetic postganglionic neurons have been shown to liberate substances other than acetyl choline or norepinephrine at their endings; these include adenosine triphosphate (ATP), neuropeptide **Y,** and substance **P.** These substances may be released alone or from neurons that release acetylcholine or norepinephrine; they have their own specific receptors. The function of these transmitters is probably to modulate the effects of the primary transmitter.

BLOCKING OF CHOLINERGIC RECEPTORS

In the case of the parasympathetic and the sympathetic postganglionic nerve endings that liberate acetylcholine as the transmitter substance, the receptors on the effector cells are **muscarinic.** This means that the action can be blocked

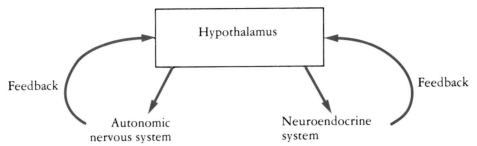

Figure 14–6 Hypothalamus as the control center for the autonomic nervous system and the neuroendocrine system.

by **atropine.** Atropine competitively antagonizes the muscarinic action by occupying the cholinergic receptor sites on the effector cells.

BLOCKING OF ADRENERGIC RECEPTORS

The alpha-adrenergic receptors can be blocked by agents such as **phenoxybenzamine** and the beta-adrenergic receptors can be blocked by agents such as **propranolol.** The synthesis and storage of norepinephrine at sympathetic endings can be inhibited by **reserpine.**

HIGHER CONTROL OF THE AUTONOMIC NERVOUS SYSTEM

The hypothalamus has a controlling influence on the autonomic nervous system and appears to integrate the autonomic and neuroendocrine systems, thus preserving body homeostasis (Fig. 14-6). Essentially, the hypothalamus should be regarded as a higher nervous center for the control of lower autonomic centers in the brainstem and spinal cord.

Stimulation of the anterior region of the hypothalamus can influence parasympathetic responses, whereas stimulation of the posterior part of the hypothalamus gives rise to sympathetic responses. In addition, lower brainstem centers such as **vasopressor, vasodilator, cardioaccelerator, cardiodecelerator,** and **respiratory centers** have been found in the reticular formation as the result of experimental stimulation in lower animals. It is believed that the various levels of control are exerted as the result of interconnections of the different regions by ascending and descending pathways. The neurons of the thoracolumbar outflow of the sympathetic part of the system and the neurons of the craniosacral outflow of the parasympathetic part of the system receive their control through the descending tracts of the reticular formation.

Stimulation of different parts of the cerebral cortex and the limbic system produces autonomic effects, and it is assumed that this is brought about through the hypothalamus. The autonomic nervous system can be brought under voluntary control to some extent. This is seen, for example, in young individuals who may blush easily when embarrassed. As they mature they are usually able to consciously train themselves to control this response. It should also be noted that the higher centers of the brain can abnormally influence the activities of the autonomic nervous system and induce disease such as cardiac palpitations (arrhythmias) and even myocardial infarction.

THE "ENTERIC NERVOUS SYSTEM"

Two important plexuses of nerve cells and fibers extend continuously along the length of the gastrointestinal tract from the esophagus to the anal canal. The submucous or Meissner's plexus lies between the mucous membrane and the circular muscle layer and the myenteric or Auerbach's plexus lies between the circular and longitudinal muscle layers. The submucous plexus is mainly concerned with the control of the glands of the mucous membrane whereas the myenteric plexus controls the muscle and movements of the gut wall.

No longer can these plexuses be regarded as simply parasympathetic plexuses containing preganglionic and postganglionic nerve fibers and nerve cells. It has been shown that contractions of the smooth muscle in the gut wall can occur in the absence of the myenteric plexus, but the coordinated purposeful contractions, as seen with peristalsis and segmental movements, require the presence of a nerve plexus, even though this may be isolated from the central nervous system.

Different types of neurons have been recognized in the plexuses. Some neurons are bipolar or unipolar and are thought to be sensory and involved in local reflex activity; other neurons send axons to the celiac and mesenteric plexuses. Preganglionic parasympathetic fibers synapse on nerve cells that give rise to postganglionic fibers that innervate the smooth muscle and glands. Postganglionic sympathetic fibers have been seen to terminate on parasympathetic nerve cells and probably exert an inhibitory role in parasympathetic activity. Internuncial neurons are also present. It is interesting to note that the nerve cells and their processes are surrounded by neuroglia-like cells that closely resemble astrocytes in the central nervous system. It has been suggested that while the enteric plexuses can coordinate the activities of the gut wall, the parasympathetic and sympathetic inputs modulate these activities.

FUNCTIONS OF THE AUTONOMIC NERVOUS SYSTEM

The autonomic nervous system, along with the endocrine system, maintains body homeostasis. The endocrine control is slower and exerts its influence by means of blood-borne hormones.

The autonomic nervous system functions for the most part at the subconscious level. We are not aware, for example, that our pupils are dilating or that our arteries are constricting. The system should not be regarded as an isolated portion of the nervous system, for we know that it can play a role with somatic activity in expressing emotion and that certain autonomic activities, such as micturition, can be brought under voluntary control. The various activities of the autonomic and endocrine systems are integrated within the hypothalamus.

The sympathetic and parasympathetic components of the autonomic system cooperate in maintaining the stability of the internal environment. The sympathetic part prepares and mobilizes the body in an emergency (Fig. 14-7), when there is sudden severe exercise, fear, or rage. The parasympathetic part aims at conserving and storing energy, for example, in the promotion of digestion and the absorption of food by increasing the secretions of the glands of the gastrointestinal tract and stimulating peristalsis (Fig. 14-8).

The sympathetic and parasympathetic parts of the autonomic system usually have antagonistic control over a viscus. For example, the sympathetic activity will increase the heart rate, whereas the parasympathetic will slow the heart rate. The sympathetic activity will make the bronchial smooth muscle relax but the muscle is contracted by parasympathetic activity.

It should be pointed out, however, that many viscera do not possess this fine dual control from the autonomic system. For example, the smooth muscle of the hair follicles (the arrector pili muscle) is made to contract by the sympathetic activity, and there is no parasympathetic control.

The activities of some viscera are kept under a constant state of inhibition by one or the other components of the autonomic nervous system. The heart in a trained athlete is maintained at a slow rate by the activities of the parasympathetic system. This is of considerable importance, because the heart is a more efficient pump when contracting slowly than when contracting very quickly, thus permitting adequate diastolic filling of the ventricles.

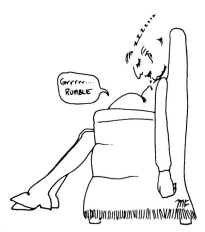

Figure 14–8 There is nothing like a good, large meal and a comfortable armchair to facilitate the activities of the parasympathetic part of the autonomic nervous system.

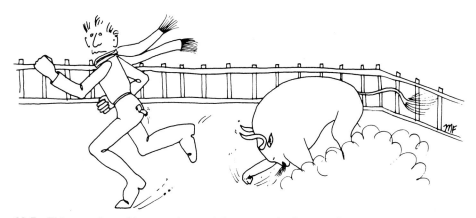

Figure 14–7 This man is making good use of the sympathetic part of his autonomic nervous system.

IMPORTANT ANATOMICAL, PHYSIOLOGICAL, AND PHARMACOLOGICAL DIFFERENCES BETWEEN THE SYMPATHETIC AND PARASYMPATHETIC PARTS OF THE AUTONOMIC NERVOUS SYSTEM (TABLE 14-1)

1. The sympathetic efferent nerve fibers originate (Fig. 14-2) from nerve cells in the lateral gray column of the spinal cord between the first thoracic and second lumbar segments (the **thoracic outflow**). The parasympathetic efferent nerve fibers originate from nerve cells in the third, seventh, ninth, and tenth cranial nerves and in the gray matter of the second, third, and fourth sacral segments of the cord (the **craniosacral outflow**).

2. The sympathetic ganglia are located either in the paravertebral sympathetic trunks or in the prevertebral ganglia, such as the celiac ganglion (Fig. 14-2). The parasympathetic ganglion cells are located as small ganglia close to the viscera or within plexuses within the viscera.

3. The sympathetic part of the autonomic system has long postganglionic fibers, whereas the parasympathetic system has short fibers (Fig. 14-5).

4. The sympathetic part of the system has a widespread action on the body as the result of the preganglionic fibers synapsing on many postganglionic neurons and the suprarenal medulla releasing the sympathetic transmitters epinephrine and norepinephrine, which are distributed throughout the body through the bloodstream (Fig. 14-5). The parasympathetic part of the autonomic system has a more discrete control, since the preganglionic fibers synapse on only a few postganglionic neurons and there is no comparable organ to the suprarenal medulla.

5. The sympathetic postganglionic endings liberate norepinephrine at most endings and acetylcholine at a few endings (e.g., sweat glands). The parasympathetic postganglionic endings liberate acetylcholine (Fig. 14-5).

6. The sympathetic part of the autonomic system prepares the body for emergencies and severe muscular activity, whereas the parasympathetic part conserves and stores energy.

To assist with the learning of the different actions of these two components of the autonomic system, it might be helpful to imagine the sympathetic activity to be maxi-

Table 14–1   Comparison of Anatomical, Physiological, and Pharmacological Characteristics of the Sympathetic and Parasympathetic Parts of the Autonomic Nervous System

	Sympathetic	Parasympathetic
Action	Prepares body for emergency	Conserves and restores energy
Outflow	T1–L2 (3)	Cranial nerves III, VII, IX, and X; S2, S3 and 4
Preganglionic fibers	Myelinated	Myelinated
Ganglia	Paravertebral (sympathetic trunks), prevertebral (e.g., celiac, superior mesenteric, inferior mesenteric)	Small ganglia close to viscera (e.g., otic, ciliary) or ganglion cells in plexuses (e.g., cardiac, pulmonary)
Neurotransmitter within ganglia	Acetylcholine	Acetylcholine
Ganglion blocking agents	Hexamethonium and tetraethylammonium by competing with acetylcholine	Hexamethonium and tetraethylammonium by competing with acetylcholine
Postganglionic fibers	Long, nonmyelinated	Short, nonmyelinated
Characteristic activity	Widespread due to many postganglionic fibers and liberation of epinephrine and norepinephrine from suprarenal medulla	Discrete action with few postganglionic fibers
Neurotransmitter at postganglionic endings	Norepinephrine at most endings and acetylcholine at few endings (sweat glands)	Acetylcholine at all endings
Blocking agents on receptors of effector cells	Alpha-adrenergic receptors—phenoxybenzamine, beta-adrenergic receptors—propranolol	Atropine, scopolamine
Agents inhibiting synthesis and storage of neurotransmitter at postganglionic endings	Reserpine	
Agents inhibiting hydrolysis of neurotransmitter at site of effector cells		Acetylcholinesterase blockers (e.g., neostigmine)
Drugs mimicking autonomic activity	Sympathomimetic drugs Phenylephrine: alpha receptors Isoproterenol: beta receptors	Parasympathomimetic drugs Pilocarpine Methacholine
Higher control	Hypothalamus	Hypothalamus

Table 14–2	Effects of Autonomic Nervous System on Organs of the Body		
Organ		**Sympathetic Action**	**Parasympathetic Action**
Eye	Pupil	Dilates	Constricts
	Ciliary muscle	Relaxes	Contracts
Glands	Lacrimal, parotid, sub-mandibular, sublingual, nasal	Reduces secretion by causing vaso-constriction of blood vessels	Increases secretion
	Sweat	Increases secretion	
Heart	Cardiac muscle	Increases force of contraction	Decreases force of contraction
	Coronary arteries (mainly con-trolled by local metabolic factors)	Dilates (beta receptors), constricts (alpha receptors)	
Lung	Bronchial muscle	Relaxes (dilates bronchi)	Contracts (constricts bronchi), increases secretion
	Bronchial secretion		
	Bronchial arteries	Constricts	Dilates
Gastrointestinal tract	Muscle in walls	Decreases peristalsis	Increases peristalsis
	Muscle in sphincters	Contracts	Relaxes
	Glands	Reduces secretion by vasoconstric-tion of blood vessels	Increases secretion
Liver		Break down glycogen into glucose	
Gallbladder		Relaxes	Contracts
Kidney		Decreases output due to constric-tion of arteries	
Urinary bladder	Bladder wall (detrusor)	Relaxes	Contracts
	Sphincter vesicae	Contracts	Relaxes
Erectile tissue of penis and clitoris			Relaxes, causes erection
Ejaculation		Contracts smooth muscle of vas deferens, seminal vesicles, and prostate	
Systemic arteries			
Skin		Constricts	
Abdominal		Constricts	
Muscle		Constricts (alpha receptors), di-lates (beta receptors), dilates (cholinergic)	
Erector pili muscles		Contracts	
Suprarenal			
Cortex		Stimulates	
Medulla		Liberates epinephrine and norepi-nephrine	

mal in a man who finds himself suddenly alone in a field with a bull that is about to charge (Fig. 14-7). His hair will stand on end with fear; his skin will be pale as the result of vasoconstriction, which causes a redistribution of blood away from the skin and viscera to the heart muscle and skeletal muscle. His upper eyelids will be raised and his pupils widely dilated so that he can see where to run. His heart rate will rise and the peripheral resistance of the ar-terioles will be increased, causing a rise in blood pressure. His bronchi will dilate to permit maximum respiratory flow of air. His peristaltic activity will be inhibited and his gut sphincters will be contracted. His vesical sphincter will also be contracted (this is certainly not the time to be thinking of defecation or micturition). Glycogen will be converted into glucose for energy and he will sweat to lose body heat.

On the other hand, the parasympathetic activity will be great in a man who has fallen asleep in an armchair after a satisfying meal (Fig. 14-8). His heart rate will be slow and his

blood pressure will not be high. His upper eyelids will droop or be closed and his pupils will be constricted. His breathing will be noisy owing to bronchial constriction. His abdomen may rumble owing to excessive peristaltic activity. He may feel the inclination to defecate or micturate.

SOME IMPORTANT AUTONOMIC INNERVATIONS (TABLE 14-2)

Eye
UPPER LID

The upper lid is raised by the levator palpebrae superioris muscle. The major part of this muscle is formed by skeletal muscle innervated by the oculomotor nerve. A small part is composed of smooth muscle fibers innervated by sympa-thetic postganglionic fibers from the superior cervical sym-pathetic ganglion (Fig. 14-9).

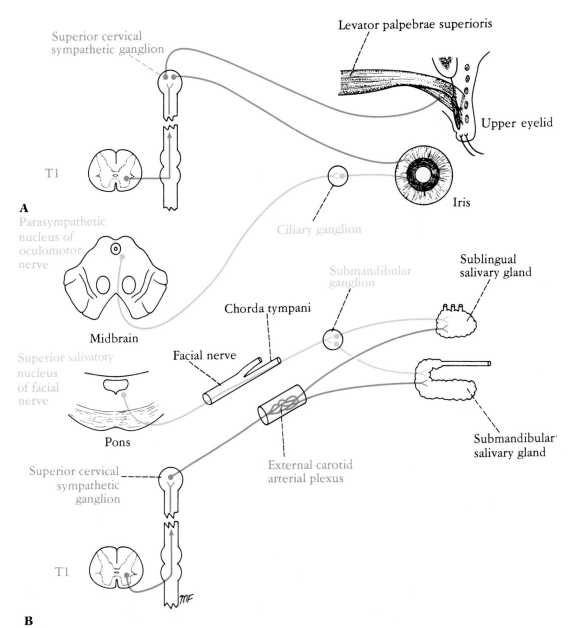

Figure 14–9 Autonomic innervation of: **A.** The upper eyelid and iris. **B.** The sublingual and submandibular salivary glands.

IRIS

The smooth muscle fibers of the iris consist of circular and radiating fibers. The circular fibers form the sphincter pupillae and the radial fibers form the dilator pupillae.

The sphincter pupillae is supplied by parasympathetic fibers from the parasympathetic nucleus (Edinger-Westphal nucleus) of the oculomotor nerve (Fig. 14-9). After synapsing in the **ciliary ganglion,** the postganglionic fibers pass forward to the eyeball in the **short ciliary nerves.** (The ciliary muscle of the eye is also supplied by the short ciliary nerves; see p. 337.)

The dilator pupillae is supplied by postganglionic fibers from the superior cervical sympathetic ganglion (Fig. 14-9).

The postganglionic fibers reach the orbit along the internal carotid and ophthalmic arteries. They pass uninterrupted through the ciliary ganglion and reach the eyeball in the **short ciliary nerves.** Other sympathetic fibers reach the eyeball in the **long ciliary nerves.**

Lacrimal Gland

The parasympathetic secretomotor nerve supply to the lacrimal gland originates in the **lacrimatory nucleus** of the facial nerve (Fig. 14-10). The preganglionic fibers reach the **pterygopalatine ganglion** through the **nervus intermedius** and its **great petrosal branch** and through the **nerve of the**

pterygoid canal. The postganglionic fibers leave the ganglion and join the maxillary nerve. They then pass into its **zygomatic branch** and the **zygomaticotemporal nerve.** They reach the lacrimal gland within the **lacrimal nerve.**

The sympathetic postganglionic fibers arise from the superior cervical sympathetic ganglion and travel in the plexus of nerves around the internal carotid artery. They join the **deep petrosal nerve, the nerve of the pterygoid canal, the maxillary nerve, the zygomatic nerve,** and **zygomaticotemporal nerve,** and, finally, the lacrimal nerve. They function as vasoconstrictor fibers.

Salivary Glands
SUBMANDIBULAR AND SUBLINGUAL GLANDS

The parasympathetic secretomotor supply originates in the **superior salivatory nucleus** of the facial nerve (Fig. 14-9). The preganglionic fibers pass to the **submandibular ganglion** and other small ganglia close to the duct through the **chorda tympani nerve** and the **lingual nerve.**

Postganglionic fibers reach the submandibular gland either directly or along the duct. Postganglionic fibers to the sublingual gland travel through the lingual nerve.

Sympathetic postganglionic fibers arise from the superior cervical sympathetic ganglion and reach the glands as a plexus of nerves around the external carotid, facial, and lingual arteries. They function as vasoconstrictor fibers.

PAROTID GLAND

Parasympathetic secretomotor fibers from the **inferior salivatory nucleus** of the glossopharyngeal nerve supply the gland (Fig. 14-10). The preganglionic nerve fibers pass to the otic ganglion through the **tympanic branch of the glossopharyngeal nerve** and the **lesser petrosal nerve.** Postganglionic fibers reach the gland through the auriculotemporal nerve.

Sympathetic postganglionic fibers arise from the superior cervical sympathetic ganglion and reach the gland as a plexus of nerves around the external carotid artery. They function as vasoconstrictor fibers.

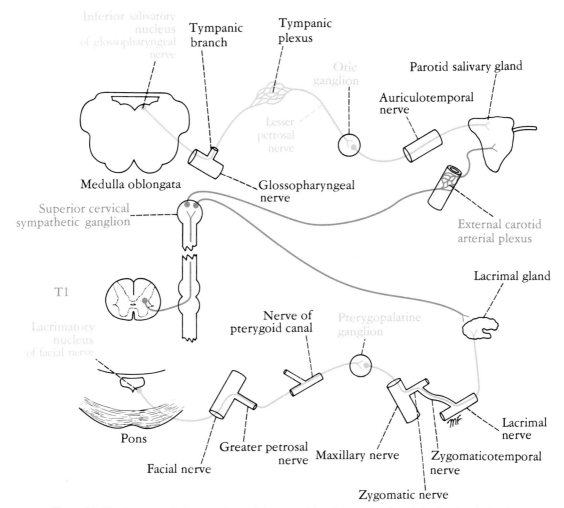

Figure 14–10 Autonomic innervation of the parotid salivary gland and the lacrimal gland.

Heart

The sympathetic postganglionic fibers arise from the cervical and upper thoracic portions of the sympathetic trunks (Fig. 14-11). Postganglionic fibers reach the heart by way of the **superior, middle,** and **inferior cardiac branches** of the cervical portion of the sympathetic trunk and a number of **cardiac branches** from the thoracic portion of the sympathetic trunk. The fibers pass through the **cardiac plexuses** and terminate on the **sinoatrial** and **atrioventricular nodes,** on cardiac muscle fibers, and on coronary arteries. Activation of these nerves results in cardiac acceleration, increased force of contraction of the cardiac muscle, and dilatation of the coronary arteries. The coronary dilatation is mainly produced in response to local metabolic needs rather than by direct nerve stimulation of the coronary arteries.

The parasympathetic preganglionic fibers originate in the **dorsal nucleus of the vagus nerve** and descend into the thorax in the vagus nerves. The fibers terminate by synapsing with postganglionic neurons in the **cardiac plexuses.** Postganglionic fibers terminate on the **sinoatrial** and **atrioventricular nodes** and on the coronary arteries. Activation of these nerves results in a reduction in the rate and force of contraction of the myocardium and a constriction of the coronary arteries. Here again, the coronary constriction is mainly produced by the reduction in local metabolic needs rather than by neural effects.

Lungs

The sympathetic postganglionic fibers arise from the second to the fifth thoracic ganglia of the sympathetic trunk (Fig. 14-11). The fibers pass through the pulmonary plexuses and enter the lung, where they form networks around the bronchi and blood vessels. The sympathetic fibers produce bronchodilatation and slight vasoconstriction.

The parasympathetic preganglionic fibers arise from the **dorsal nucleus of the vagus** and descend to the thorax within the vagus nerves. The fibers terminate by synapsing with postganglionic neurons in the pulmonary plexuses. The postganglionic fibers enter the lung, where they form networks around the bronchi and blood vessels. The parasympathetic fibers produce bronchoconstriction and slight vasodilatation, and increase glandular secretion.

Gastrointestinal Tract

STOMACH AND INTESTINE AS FAR AS THE SPLENIC FLEXURE

Preganglionic parasympathetic fibers enter the abdomen in the **anterior (left)** and **posterior (right) vagal trunks** (Fig. 14-12). The fibers are distributed to many abdominal viscera and to the gastrointestinal tract from the stomach to the splenic flexure of the colon. The fibers that pass to the gastrointestinal tract terminate on postganglionic neu-

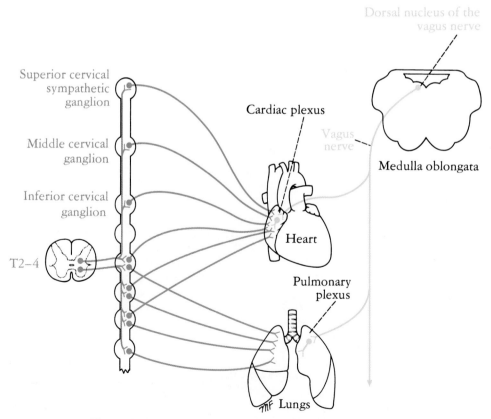

Figure 14–11   Autonomic innervation of the heart and lungs.

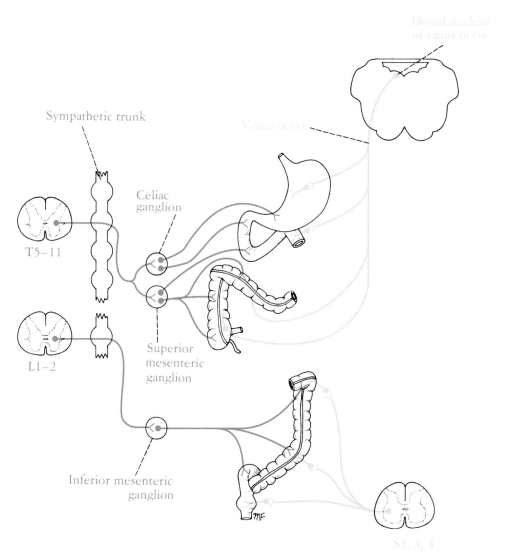

Figure 14–12   Autonomic innervation of the gastrointestinal tract.

rons in the **myenteric (Auerbach's)** and **submucosal (Meissner's) plexuses.** The postganglionic fibers supply the smooth muscle and glands. The parasympathetic nerves stimulate peristalsis and relax the sphincters; they also stimulate secretion.

Sympathetic preganglionic nerve fibers pass through the thoracic part of the sympathetic trunk and enter the **greater** and **lesser splanchnic nerves.** These descend into the abdomen and synapse with postganglionic neurons in the **celiac** and **superior mesenteric ganglia.** The postganglionic nerve fibers are distributed to the stomach and intestine as nerve plexuses around the branches of the celiac and superior mesenteric arteries. The sympathetic nerves inhibit peristalsis and cause contraction of the sphincters; they also inhibit secretion (see the enteric nervous system, p. 404).

DESCENDING COLON, PELVIC COLON, AND RECTUM

The preganglionic parasympathetic fibers originate in the gray matter of the spinal cord from the second to the fourth sacral segments (Fig. 14-12). The fibers pass through the **pelvic splanchnic nerves** and the nerve plexuses around the branches of the inferior mesenteric artery. They terminate on postganglionic neurons in the myenteric (Auerbach's) and submucosal (Meissner's) plexuses. The postganglionic fibers supply the smooth muscle and glands. The parasympathetic nerves stimulate peristalsis and secretion.

The sympathetic preganglionic nerve fibers pass through the lumbar part of the sympathetic trunk and synapse with postganglionic neurons in the **inferior mesenteric plexus.** Postganglionic fibers are distributed to the bowel as nerve plexuses around the branches of the inferior mesenteric arteries. The sympathetic nerves inhibit peristalsis and secretion.

Gallbladder and Biliary Ducts

The gallbladder and biliary ducts receive postganglionic parasympathetic and sympathetic fibers from the hepatic plexus. Parasympathetic fibers derived from the vagus are thought to be motor fibers to the smooth muscle of the gallbladder and bile ducts and inhibitory to the sphincter of Oddi.

Autonomic afferent fibers are also present. Some of the fibers are believed to leave the hepatic plexus and join the right phrenic nerve, thus partially explaining the phenomenon of referred shoulder pain in the presence of gallbladder disease (see p. 420).

Kidney

Preganglionic sympathetic fibers pass through the lower thoracic part of the sympathetic trunk and the lowest thoracic splanchnic nerve to join the **renal plexus** around the renal artery (Fig. 14-13). The preganglionic fibers synapse with postganglionic neurons in the renal plexus. The postganglionic fibers are distributed to the branches of the renal artery. The sympathetic nerves are vasoconstrictor in action to the renal arteries within the kidney.

Preganglionic parasympathetic fibers enter the renal plexus from the vagus. Here they synapse with postganglionic neurons whose fibers are distributed to the kidney along the branches of the renal artery. The parasympathetic nerves are thought to be vasodilator in action.

Medulla of Suprarenal Gland

Preganglionic sympathetic fibers descend to the gland in the **greater splanchnic nerve,** a branch of the thoracic part of the sympathetic trunk (Fig. 14-13). The nerve fibers terminate on the secretory cells of the medulla, which are comparable to postganglionic neurons. Acetylcholine is the transmitter substance between the nerve endings and the secretory cells, as at any other preganglionic endings. The sympathetic nerves stimulate the secretory cells of the medulla to increase the output of epinephrine and norepinephrine. There is no parasympathetic innervation of the medulla of the suprarenal gland.

Involuntary Internal Sphincter of the Anal Canal

The circular smooth muscle coat is thickened at the upper end of the anal canal to form the involuntary internal sphincter. The sphincter is innervated by postganglionic sympathetic fibers from the **hypogastric plexuses** (Fig. 14-14). Each hypogastric plexus receives sympathetic fibers from the **aortic plexus** and from the lumbar and pelvic parts of the sympathetic trunks. The sympathetic nerves cause the internal anal sphincter to contract.

Urinary Bladder

The muscular coat of the bladder is composed of smooth muscle, which at the bladder neck is thickened to form the

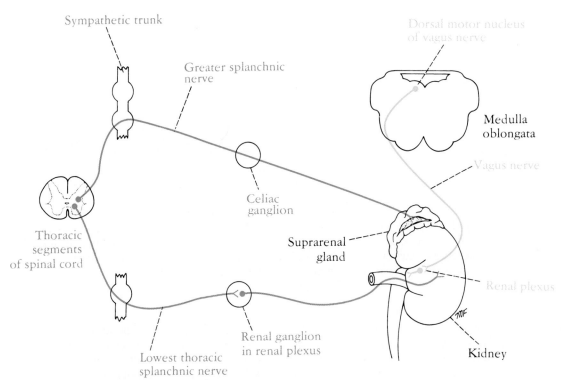

Figure 14–13 Autonomic innervation of the kidney and suprarenal gland.

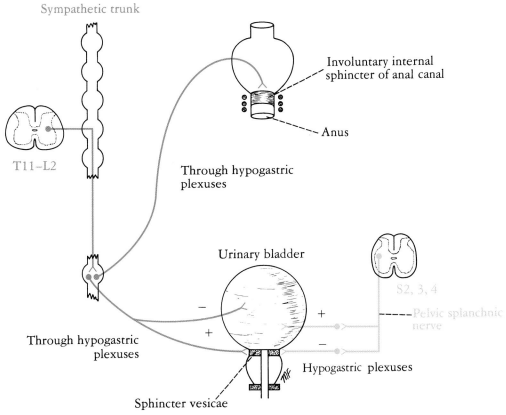

Figure 14–14   Autonomic innervation of the sphincters of the anal canal and urinary bladder.

sphincter vesicae. The nerve supply of the smooth muscle is from the hypogastric plexuses (Fig. 14-14). The sympathetic postganglionic fibers originate in the first and second lumbar ganglia of the sympathetic trunk and travel to the hypogastric plexuses. The parasympathetic preganglionic fibers arise as the pelvic splanchnic nerves from the second, third, and fourth sacral nerves; they pass through the hypogastric plexuses to reach the bladder wall, where they synapse with postganglionic neurons.

The sympathetic nerves to the detrusor muscle have little or no action on the smooth muscle of the bladder wall and are distributed mainly to the blood vessels. The sympathetic nerves to the sphincter vesicae play only a minor role in causing contraction of the sphincter in maintaining urinary continence. However, in the male, the sympathetic innervation of the sphincter causes active contraction of the bladder neck during ejaculation (brought about by sympathetic action), thus preventing seminal fluid from entering the bladder. The parasympathetic nerves stimulate the contraction of the smooth muscle of the bladder wall and in some way inhibit the contraction of the sphincter vesicae.

Erection of the Penis and Clitoris

In erection, the genital **erectile tissue** becomes engorged with blood. The initial vascular engorgement is controlled by the parasympathetic part of the autonomic nervous system. The parasympathetic preganglionic fibers originate in the gray matter of the second, third, and fourth sacral seg-

ments of the spinal cord (Fig. 14-15). The fibers enter the hypogastric plexuses and synapse on the postganglionic neurons. The postganglionic fibers join the internal pudendal arteries and are distributed along their branches, which enter the erectile tissue. The parasympathetic nerves cause vasodilatation of the arteries and greatly increase the blood flow to the erectile tissue.

Ejaculation

Preganglionic sympathetic fibers leave the spinal cord at the first and second lumbar segments (Fig. 14-15). Many of these fibers synapse with postganglionic neurons in the first and second lumbar ganglia. Other fibers may synapse in ganglia in the lower lumbar or pelvic parts of the sympathetic trunks. The postganglionic fibers are then distributed to the **vas deferens,** the **seminal vesicles,** and the **prostate** through the **hypogastric plexuses.** The sympathetic nerves stimulate the contractions of the smooth muscle in the walls of these structures and cause the spermatozoa, together with the secretions of the seminal vesicles and prostate, to be discharged into the urethra.

Uterus

Preganglionic sympathetic nerve fibers leave the spinal cord at segmental levels T12 and L1 and are believed to synapse with ganglion cells in the sympathetic trunk or possibly in the inferior hypogastric plexuses (Fig. 14-16). The

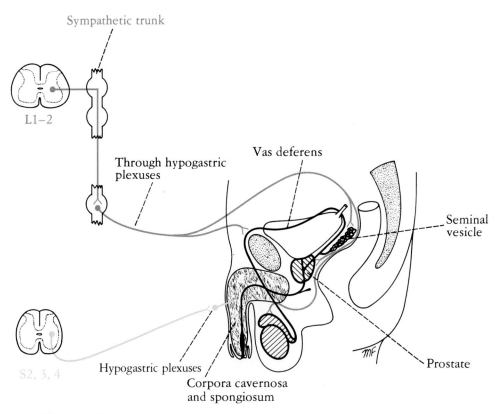

Figure 14–15   Autonomic innervation of the male reproductive tract.

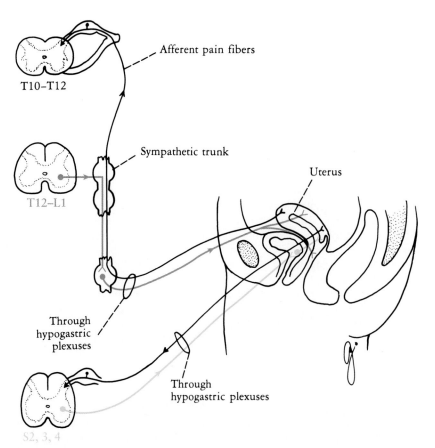

Figure 14–16   Autonomic innervation of the uterus; the pathway taken by the afferent sensory fibers is also shown.

postganglionic fibers supply the smooth muscle of the uterus. Parasympathetic preganglionic fibers leave the spinal cord at levels S2, 3, and 4 and synapse with ganglion cells in the inferior hypogastric plexuses (Fig. 14-16). Although it is recognized that the uterine muscle is largely under hormonal control, sympathetic innervation may cause uterine contraction and vasoconstriction, whereas parasympathetic fibers have the opposite effect.

Afferent pain fibers from the fundus and the body of the uterus ascend to the spinal cord through the hypogastric plexuses, entering it through the posterior roots of the tenth, eleventh, and twelfth thoracic spinal nerves (Fig. 14-16). Fibers from the cervix run in the pelvic splanchnic nerves, and enter the spinal cord through the posterior roots of the second, third, and fourth sacral nerves.

Arteries of the Upper Limb

The arteries of the upper limb are innervated by sympathetic nerves. The preganglionic fibers originate from cell bodies in the second to the eighth thoracic segments of the spinal cord (Fig. 14-17). They pass to the sympathetic trunk through white rami and ascend in the trunk to synapse in the middle cervical, inferior cervical, first thoracic, or stellate ganglia. The postganglionic fibers join the nerves that form the brachial plexus and are distributed to the arteries within the branches of the plexus. The sympathetic nerves cause vasoconstriction of cutaneous arteries and vasodilatation of arteries that supply skeletal muscle.

Arteries of the Lower Limb

The arteries of the lower limb are also innervated by sympathetic nerves (Fig. 14-17). The preganglionic fibers originate from cell bodies in the lower three thoracic and upper two or three lumbar segments of the spinal cord. The preganglionic fibers pass to the lower thoracic and upper lumbar ganglia of the sympathetic trunk through white rami. The fibers synapse in the lumbar and sacral ganglia, and the

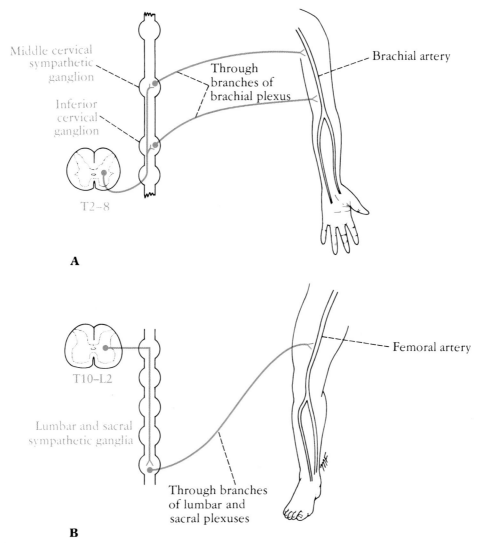

Figure 14–17 Sympathetic innervation of the arteries of: **A.** The upper limb. **B.** The lower limb.

postganglionic fibers reach the arteries through branches of the lumbar and sacral plexuses.

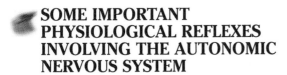

SOME IMPORTANT PHYSIOLOGICAL REFLEXES INVOLVING THE AUTONOMIC NERVOUS SYSTEM

Visual Reflexes

DIRECT AND CONSENSUAL LIGHT REFLEXES

Afferent nervous impulses travel from the retina through the optic nerve, optic chiasma, and optic tract (Fig. 11-3). A small number of fibers leave the optic tract and synapse on nerve cells in the **pretectal nucleus,** which lies close to the superior colliculus. The impulses are passed by axons of the pretectal nerve cells to the parasympathetic nuclei (Edinger-Westphal nuclei) of the oculomotor nerve on both sides. Here the fibers synapse and the parasympathetic nerves travel through the oculomotor nerve to the **ciliary ganglion** in the orbit. Finally, postganglionic parasympathetic fibers pass through the **short ciliary nerves** to the eyeball and to the constrictor pupillae muscle of the iris. Both pupils constrict in the consensual light reflex because the pretectal nucleus sends fibers to the parasympathetic nuclei on both sides of the midbrain.

ACCOMMODATION REFLEX

When the eyes are directed from a distant to a near object, contraction of the medial recti brings about convergence of the ocular axes, the lens thicken to increase its refractive power by contraction of the ciliary muscle, and the pupils constrict to restrict the light waves to the thickest central part of the lens. The afferent impulses travel through the optic nerve, the optic chiasma, the optic tract, the lateral geniculate body, and the optic radiation to the visual cortex (Fig. 11-3). The visual cortex is connected to the eyefield of the frontal cortex. From here, cortical fibers descend through the internal capsule to the oculomotor nuclei in the midbrain. The oculomotor nerve travels to the medial recti muscles. Some of the descending cortical fibers synapse with the parasympathetic nuclei (Edinger-Westphal nuclei) of the oculomotor nerve on both sides. The parasympathetic preganglionic fibers then travel through the oculo-

motor nerve to the **ciliary ganglion** in the orbit where they synapse. Finally, postganglionic parasympathetic fibers pass through the **short ciliary nerves** to the ciliary muscle and the constrictor pupillae muscle of the iris.

Cardiovascular Reflexes

These include the carotid sinus and aortic arch reflexes and the Bainbridge right atrial reflex.

CAROTID SINUS AND AORTIC ARCH REFLEXES

The carotid sinus, located in the bifurcation of the common carotid artery, and the aortic arch serve as baroreceptors. As the blood pressure rises, nerve endings situated in the walls of these vessels are stimulated. The afferent fibers from the carotid sinus ascend in the glossopharyngeal nerve and terminate in the **nucleus solitarius** (Figs. 11-16 and 11-17). The afferent fibers from the aortic arch ascend in the vagus nerve. Connector neurons in the medulla oblongata activate the parasympathetic nucleus (dorsal nucleus) of the vagus, which slows the heart rate. At the same time, reticulospinal fibers descend to the spinal cord and inhibit the preganglionic sympathetic outflow to the heart and cutaneous arterioles. The combined effect of stimulation of the parasympathetic action on the heart and inhibition of the sympathetic action on the heart and peripheral blood vessels reduces the rate and force of contraction of the heart and reduces the peripheral resistance of the blood vessels. Consequently, the blood pressure falls. The blood pressure of the individual is thus modified by the afferent information received from the baroreceptors. The modulator of the autonomic nervous system, namely, the hypothalamus, in turn, can be influenced by other, higher centers in the central nervous system.

BAINBRIDGE RIGHT ATRIAL REFLEX

This reflex is initiated when the nerve endings in the wall of the right atrium and in the walls of the venae cavae are stimulated by a rise of venous pressure. The afferent fibers ascend in the vagus to the medulla oblongata and terminate on the **nucleus of the tractus solitarius** (Fig. 11-18). Connector neurons inhibit the parasympathetic nucleus (dorsal) of the vagus, and reticulospinal fibers stimulate the thoracic sympathetic outflow to the heart, resulting in cardiac acceleration.

CLINICAL NOTES

GENERAL CONSIDERATIONS

From the foregoing description, it must now be clear to the reader that the autonomic nervous system is not an isolated part of the nervous system. It should be regarded as the part of the nervous system that, with the endocrine sys-

tem, is particularly involved in maintaining the stability of the internal environment of the body. Its activities are modified by the hypothalamus, whose function is to integrate vast amounts of afferent information received from other areas of the nervous system, and to translate changing hormonal levels of the bloodstream into appropriate nervous and hormonal activities.

INJURIES TO THE AUTONOMIC NERVOUS SYSTEM

Sympathetic Injuries

The sympathetic trunk in the neck can be injured by stab and bullet wounds. Traction injuries to the first thoracic root of the brachial plexus can damage sympathetic nerves destined for the stellate ganglion. All these conditions can produce a preganglionic type of Horner's syndrome (see below). Injuries to the spinal cord or cauda equina can disrupt the sympathetic control of the bladder (see p. 418).

Parasympathetic Injuries

The oculomotor nerve is vulnerable in head injuries (herniated uncus) and can be damaged by compression by aneurysms in the junction between the posterior cerebral artery and posterior communicating artery. The preganglionic parasympathetic fibers traveling in this nerve are situated in the periphery of the nerve and can be damaged. Surface aneurysmal compression characteristically causes dilatation of the pupil and loss of the visual light reflexes.

The autonomic fibers in the facial nerve can be damaged by fractures of the skull involving the temporal bone. The vestibulocochlear nerve is closely related to the facial nerve in the internal acoustic meatus so that clinical findings involving both nerves are common. Involvement of the parasympathetic fibers in the facial nerve may produce impaired lacrimation in addition to paralysis of the facial muscles.

The glossopharyngeal and vagus nerves are at risk in stab and bullet wounds of the neck. The parasympathetic secretomotor fibers to the parotid salivary gland leave the glossopharyngeal nerve just below the skull so that they are rarely damaged.

The parasympathetic outflow in the sacral region of the spinal cord (S2, 3, and 4) may be damaged by spinal cord and cauda equina injuries, leading to disruption of bladder, rectal, and sexual functions (see p. 418).

Degeneration and Regeneration of Autonomic Nerves

The structural changes are identical to those found in other areas of the peripheral and central parts of the nervous system. Functional recoveries following sympathectomy operations can be explained only by the assumption either that the operative procedure was inadequate and nerve fibers were left intact or regenerated or that alternative nervous pathways existed and were left undisturbed.

The denervation of viscera supplied by autonomic nerves is followed by their increased sensitivity to the agent that was previously the transmitter substance. One explanation is that following nerve section there may be an increase in the number of receptor sites on the postsynaptic membrane. Another possibility, which applies to endings where norepinephrine is the transmitter, is that the reuptake of the transmitter by the nerve terminal is interfered with in some way.

DISEASES INVOLVING THE AUTONOMIC NERVOUS SYSTEM

Horner's Syndrome

This syndrome consists of (1) constriction of the pupil (miosis), (2) slight drooping of the eyelid (ptosis), (3) enophthalmos,* (4) vasodilation of skin arterioles, and (5) loss of sweating (anhydrosis)—all resulting from an interruption of the sympathetic nerve supply to the head and neck. Pathological causes include lesions in the brainstem or cervical part of the spinal cord that interrupt the reticulospinal tracts descending from the hypothalamus to the sympathetic outflow in the lateral gray column of the first thoracic segment of the spinal cord. Such lesions include **multiple sclerosis** and **syringomyelia.** Traction on the stellate ganglion due to a **cervical rib,** or involvement of the ganglion in a metastatic lesion, may interrupt the peripheral part of the sympathetic pathway.

All patients with Horner's syndrome have miosis and ptosis. However, a distinction should be made between lesions occurring at the first neuron (the descending reticulospinal fibers within the central nervous system), the second neuron (the preganglionic fibers), and the third neuron (postganglionic fibers). For example, the clinical signs suggestive of a first-neuron defect (central Horner's syndrome) could include contralateral hyperesthesia of the body and loss of sweating of the entire half of the body. Signs suggesting a second-neuron involvement (preganglionic Horner's syndrome) include loss of sweating limited to the face and neck, and the presence of flushing or blanching of the face and neck. Signs suggesting third-neuron involvement (postganglionic Horner's syndrome) include facial pain or ear, nose, or throat disease.

The presence or absence of other localizing signs and symptoms may assist in differentiating the three types of Horner's syndrome.

Argyll Robertson Pupil

This condition is characterized by a small pupil, which is of fixed size and does not react to light, but does contract with accommodation. It is usually caused by a neurosyphilitic lesion interrupting the fibers that run from the pretectal nucleus to the parasympathetic nuclei (Edinger-Westphal nuclei) of the oculomotor nerve on both sides. The fact that the pupil constricts with accommodation implies that the connections between the parasympathetic nuclei and the constrictor pupillae muscle of the iris are intact.

Adie's Tonic Pupil Syndrome

In this condition the pupil has a decreased or absent light reflex, a slow or delayed contraction to near vision, and a slow or delayed dilatation in the dark. This benign syndrome, which probably results from a disorder of the

---

*The enophthalmos of Horner's syndrome is often apparent but not real and is caused by the ptosis. However, the smooth muscle, the orbitalis, situated at the back of the orbit, is paralyzed and involvement may be responsible.

parasympathetic innervation of the constrictor pupillae muscle, must be distinguished from the Argyll Robertson pupil (above), which is caused by neurosyphilis. Adie's syndrome can be confirmed by looking for hypersensitivity to cholinergic agents. Drops commonly used for this test are 2.5% methacholine (Mecholyl) or 0.1% pilocarpine. The Adie's tonic pupil should constrict when these drops are put in the eye. These cholinergic agents do not cause pupillary constriction in mydriasis caused by oculomotor lesion or in drug-related mydriasis.

Frey's Syndrome

Frey's syndrome is an interesting complication that sometimes follows penetrating wounds of the parotid gland. During the process of healing, the postganglionic parasympathetic secretomotor fibers traveling in the auriculotemporal nerve grow out and join the distal end of the great auricular nerve, which supplies the sweat glands of the overlying facial skin. By this means, a stimulus intended for saliva production instead produces sweat secretion.

A similar syndrome may follow injury to the facial nerve. During the process of regeneration, parasympathetic fibers normally destined for the submandibular and sublingual salivary glands are diverted to the lacrimal gland. This produces watering of the eyes associated with salivation, the so-called **crocodile tears.**

HIRSCHSPRUNG'S DISEASE (MEGACOLON)

Hirschsprung's disease is a congenital condition in which there is a failure of development of the myenteric plexus (Auerbach's plexus) in the distal part of the colon. The involved part of the colon possesses no parasympathetic ganglion cells and peristalsis is absent. This effectively blocks the passage of feces and the proximal part of the colon becomes enormously distended.

URINARY BLADDER DYSFUNCTION FOLLOWING SPINAL CORD INJURIES

Injuries to the spinal cord are followed by disruption of the nervous control of micturition. The normal bladder is innervated as follows:

Sympathetic innervation is from the first and second lumbar segments of the spinal cord.

Parasympathetic innervation is from the second, third, and fourth sacral segments of the spinal cord.

Sensory nerve fibers enter the spinal cord at the above segments.

The **atonic bladder** occurs during the phase of spinal shock immediately following the injury and may last from a few days to several weeks. The bladder wall muscle is relaxed, the sphincter vesicae is tightly contracted (loss of inhibition from higher levels), and the sphincter urethrae is relaxed. The bladder becomes greatly distended and finally overflows. Depending on the level of the cord injury, the patient may or may not be aware that the bladder is full; there is no voluntary control.

The **automatic reflex bladder** occurs after the patient has recovered from spinal shock, provided that the cord lesion lies above the level of the parasympathetic outflow (S2, 3, and 4). This is the type of bladder normally found in infancy. Since the descending fibers in the spinal cord are sectioned, there is no voluntary control. The bladder fills and empties reflexly. Stretch receptors in the bladder wall are stimulated as the bladder fills, and the afferent impulses pass to the spinal cord (S2, 3, and 4). Efferent impulses pass down to the bladder muscle, which contracts; the sphincter vesicae and the urethral sphincter both relax. This simple reflex occurs every 1 to 4 hours.

The **autonomous bladder** is the condition that occurs if the sacral segment of the spinal cord is destroyed or if the cauda equina is severed. The bladder has no reflex control or voluntary control. The bladder wall is flaccid, and the capacity of the bladder is greatly increased. It fills to capacity and overflows, which results in continual dribbling. The bladder may be partially emptied by manual compression of the lower part of the anterior abdominal wall, but infection of the urine and back pressure effects on the ureters and kidneys are inevitable.

Defecation Following Spinal Cord Injuries

The act of defecation involves a coordinated reflex that results in the emptying of the descending colon, pelvic colon, rectum, and anal canal. It is assisted by a rise in the intraabdominal pressure brought about by contraction of the muscles of the anterior abdominal wall. The involuntary internal sphincter of the anal canal normally is innervated by postganglionic sympathetic fibers from the hypogastric plexuses and the voluntary external sphincter of the anal canal is innervated by the inferior rectal nerve. The desire to defecate is initiated by stimulation of the stretch receptors in the wall of the rectum.

Following severe spinal cord injuries (or cauda equina injuries), the patient is not aware of rectal distention. Moreover, the parasympathetic influence on the peristaltic activity of the descending colon, sigmoid colon, and rectum is lost. In addition, control over the abdominal musculature and sphincters of the anal canal may be severely impaired. The rectum, now an isolated structure, responds by contracting when the pressure within its lumen rises. This local reflex response is much more efficient if the sacral segments of the spinal cord and the cauda equina are intact. At best, however, the force of the contractions of the rectal wall is small and constipation and impaction are the usual outcome. The treatment of patients with spinal cord injuries is to empty the rectum with biweekly enemas; the use of suppositories also may be helpful.

Erection and Ejaculation Following Spinal Cord Injuries

As described previously, erection of the penis or clitoris is controlled by the parasympathetic nerves that originate from the second, third, and fourth sacral segments of the spinal cord. Bilateral damage to the reticulospinal tracts in the spinal cord above the second sacral segment of the spinal cord will result in loss of erection. Later, when the effects of spinal shock have disappeared, spontaneous or reflex erection may occur if the sacral segments of the spinal cord are intact.

Ejaculation is controlled by sympathetic nerves that originate in the first and second lumbar segments of the spinal cord. Ejaculation brings about a flow of seminal fluid into the prostatic urethra. The final ejection of the fluid from the penis is the result of the rhythmic contractions of the bulbospongiosus muscles, which compress the urethra. The bulbospongiosus muscles are innervated by the pudendal nerve (S2, 3, and 4). Discharge of the seminal fluid into the bladder is prevented by the contraction of the sphincter vesicae, which is innervated by the sympathetic nerves (L1 and 2). As in the case of erection, severe bilateral damage to the spinal cord results in loss of ejaculation. Later, reflex ejaculation may be possible in patients with spinal cord transections in the thoracic or cervical regions. Some individuals have a normal ejaculation without external emission and the seminal fluid passes into the bladder, owing to paralysis of the sphincter vesicae.

Disease Caused by Botulinum Toxin

A very small amount of this toxin binds irreversibly to the nerve plasma membranes and prevents the release of acetylcholine at cholinergic synapses and neuromuscular junctions, producing an atropine-like syndrome with skeletal muscle weakness.

Disease Caused by Black Widow Spider Venom

The venom causes a brief release of acetylcholine at the nerve endings followed by a permanent blockade.

Disease Caused by Anticholinesterase Agents

Acetylcholinesterase, which is responsible for hydrolyzing and limiting the action of acetylcholine at nerve endings, can be blocked by certain drugs. Physostigmine, neostigmine, pyridostigmine, and carbamate and organophosphate insecticides are effective acetylcholinesterase inhibitors. Their use results in an excessive stimulation of the cholinergic receptors, producing the "SLUD syndrome"—salivation, lacrimation, urination, and defecation.

SYMPATHECTOMY AS A METHOD OF TREATING ARTERIAL DISEASE

Raynaud's Disease

This is a vasospastic disorder involving the digital arteries of the upper limb. The disorder is usually bilateral and an attack is provoked by exposure to cold. There is pallor or cyanosis of the fingers as well as severe pain. Gangrene of the tips of the fingers may occur.

In mild cases of Raynaud's disease, the treatment is the avoidance of cold and no smoking (smoking causes vasoconstriction). In more severe cases, drugs that inhibit sympathetic activity, such as reserpine, bring about arterial vasodilatation with consequent increase in blood flow to the fingers. Cervicothoracic preganglionic sympathectomy has been used but the long-term results are disappointing.

Intermittent Claudication

This condition, which is common in men, is due to arterial occlusive disease of the leg. Ischemia of the muscles produces a cramplike pain on exercise. Lumbar preganglionic sympathectomy may be advocated as a form of treatment, in order to bring about vasodilatation and an increase in blood flow through the collateral circulation. Preganglionic sympathectomy is performed by removing the upper three lumbar ganglia and the intervening parts of the sympathetic trunk.

Hypertension

In the past severe essential hypertension was treated by bilateral thoracolumbar sympathectomy to reduce the vasomotor control over the peripheral resistance and thus lower the blood pressure. Today, chemical blocking agents of the sympathetic system are widely used with great success and the resulting reduction in the force of myocardial contraction reduces the arterial blood pressure.

REFERRED VISCERAL PAIN

Most viscera are innervated only by autonomic nerves. It therefore follows that visceral pain is conducted along afferent autonomic nerves. Visceral pain is diffuse and poorly localized, whereas somatic pain is intense and discretely localized. Visceral pain frequently is referred to skin areas that are innervated by the same segments of the spinal cord as the painful viscus (Fig. 14-18). The explanation for referred pain is not known. One theory is that the nerve fibers from the viscus and the dermatome ascend in the central nervous system along a common pathway and the cerebral cortex is incapable of distinguishing between the sites of origin. Another theory is that under normal conditions the viscus does not give rise to painful stimuli, whereas the skin area repeatedly receives noxious stimuli. Because both afferent fibers enter the spinal cord at the same segment, the brain interprets the information as coming from the skin rather than from the viscus. Pain arising from the gastrointestinal tract is referred to the midline. This can probably be explained since the tract arises embryologically as a midline structure and receives a bilateral nerve supply.

Cardiac Pain

Pain originating in the heart as the result of acute myocardial ischemia is assumed to be caused by oxygen deficiency and the accumulation of metabolites, which stimulate the sensory nerve endings in the myocardium. The afferent nerve fibers ascend to the central nervous system through the cardiac branches of the sympathetic trunk and enter the spinal cord through the posterior roots of the

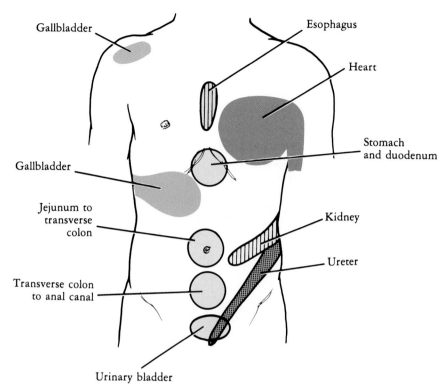

Figure 14–18 Some areas of referred pain from the viscera. In the case of the heart the pain is usually referred to the left side of the thorax; occasionally it is referred to both sides.

upper four thoracic nerves. The nature of the pain varies considerably, from a severe crushing pain to nothing more than a mild discomfort.

The pain is **not felt in the heart**, but is referred to the skin areas supplied by the corresponding spinal nerves. The skin areas supplied by the upper four intercostal nerves and by the intercostobrachial nerve (T2) are therefore affected. The intercostobrachial nerve communicates with the medial cutaneous nerve of the arm and is distributed to skin on the medial side of the upper part of the arm. A certain amount of spread of nervous information must occur within the central nervous system, for the pain is sometimes felt in the neck and the jaw.

Myocardial infarction involving the inferior wall or diaphragmatic surface of the heart often gives rise to discomfort in the epigastrium just below the sternum. One must assume that the afferent pain fibers from the heart ascend in the sympathetic nerves and enter the spinal cord in the posterior roots of the seventh, eighth, and ninth thoracic spinal nerves and give rise to referred pain in the T7, T8 and T9 thoracic dermatomes in the epigastrium.

Since the heart and the thoracic part of the esophagus probably have similar afferent pain pathways, it is not surprising that pain from **acute esophagitis** can mimic the pain of myocardial infarction.

Stomach Pain

Referred pain from the stomach is commonly felt in the epigastrium. The afferent pain fibers from the stomach ascend in company with the sympathetic nerves and pass through the celiac plexus and the greater splanchnic nerves. The sensory fibers enter the spinal cord at segments T5 through T9 and give rise to referred pain in the dermatomes T5 through T9 on the lower chest and abdominal walls.

Appendicular Pain

Visceral pain from the appendix is produced by distension of its lumen or spasm of its muscle. It travels in nerve fibers that accompany sympathetic nerves through the superior mesenteric plexus and the lesser splanchnic nerve to the spinal cord (T10 segment). The vague referred pain is felt in the region of the umbilicus, which is innervated by the tenth intercostal nerve (T10 dermatome). Later, when the inflammatory process involves the parietal peritoneum in the right iliac fossa, which is innervated by the twelfth thoracic and first lumbar spinal nerves, the now somatic pain becomes severe and dominates the clinical picture. The somatic pain is localized precisely to the right lower quadrant of the anterior abdominal wall (T12 and L1 dermatomes).

Gallbladder Pain

Visceral pain impulses from the gallbladder (acute cholecystitis, gallstone colic) travel in nerve fibers that accompany sympathetic fibers through the celiac plexus and the greater splanchnic nerves to the spinal cord (segments T5 through T9). The vague referred pain is felt in the dermatomes (T5 through T9) on the lower chest and upper abdominal walls. Should the inflammatory process spread to involve the parietal peritoneum of the anterior abdominal wall or peripheral diaphragm, the now severe somatic pain will be felt in the right upper quadrant of the anterior abdominal wall and through to the back below the inferior angle of the scapula. Involvement of the central diaphragmatic parietal peritoneum, which is innervated by the phrenic nerve (C3 through C5), may give rise to referred pain to the tip of the shoulder, since the skin in this area is innervated by the supraclavicular nerves (C3 and C4).

Some areas of referred pain from viscera are shown in Figure 14-18.

CAUSALGIA

Causalgia is a painful condition of the arm or leg accompanied by trophic changes in the affected skin and nails. It commonly follows crushing or partial division of the median nerve in the arm or the tibial nerve in the leg. It is thought that the descending impulses in the sympathetic postganglionic fibers in some way evoke ascending impulses in the afferent pain fibers at the site of injury. In many instances sympathectomy has relieved the pain of causalgia.

Clinical Problem Solving

1. A 35-year-old man was getting off the back of a truck when it started to move. Having placed his feet on the ground, he grabbed a rail on the truck with his right hand and held on. The truck continued along the road for one block before it stopped. In the meantime, the man had been dragged along the road as he held onto the truck. He was seen in the emergency department in a state of shock, with cuts and abrasions to his legs. On careful examination of his right arm, the following muscles were found to be paralyzed: the flexor carpi ulnaris, the flexor digitorum profundus, the palmar and dorsal interossei, and the thenar and hypothenar muscles. There was also loss of sensation on the medial side of the arm, forearm, and hand. The deep tendon reflex for the biceps brachii was present but the triceps reflex was absent. It also was noted that the pupil of the right eye was constricted and there was drooping of the right upper eyelid. The right eyeball seemed to be less prominent than the left. The skin of the right cheek felt warmer and drier and was redder in color than the left cheek. Using your knowledge of neuroanatomy, explain the clinical findings.

2. A 3-year-old boy with a history since infancy of chronic constipation and abdominal distention was taken to a pediatrician. The child's mother said that the constipation was getting progressively worse. It was not responding to laxatives, and she was finding it necessary to give her son an enema once a week to relieve his abdominal distention. On physical examination, the child's abdomen was obviously distended and a doughlike mass could be palpated along the course of the descending colon in the left iliac fossa. Examination of the rectum showed it to be empty and not dilated. Following an enema and repeated colonic irrigation with saline solution, the patient was given a barium enema followed by a radiographic examination. The radiograph showed a grossly distended descending colon and an abrupt change in lumen diameter where the descending colon joined the sigmoid colon. It was interesting to note that the child failed to empty the colon of the barium. Using your knowledge of the autonomic nerve supply to the colon, what is the diagnosis? How would you treat this patient?

3. A nervous 25-year-old woman attended her physician because she was experiencing attacks of painful discoloration of the fourth and fifth fingers of both hands. She said that her symptoms had started 2 years previously, during the winter, and affected first her right hand and in subsequent attacks, her left hand as well. Initially, her fingers turned white on exposure to cold and then became deep blue. The color change was confined to the distal half of each finger and was accompanied by an aching pain. Holding her hands over a hot stove or going into a hot room was the only treatment that relieved the pain. As the pain disappeared, she said, her fingers became red and swollen. She told her physician that she had noticed that her fingers were moist with sweat during some of the attacks. Using your knowledge of neuroanatomy, make the diagnosis. What is the autonomic nerve supply to the blood vessels of the upper limb? How would you treat this patient?

4. An obese 45-year-old mother of six children was examined by her physician because her symptoms were suggestive of gallbladder disease. She complained of having severe attacks of colicky pain beneath the right costal margin, which often radiated through to the back beneath the right scapula. The physician turned to a medical student and said, "Note that the patient complains of referred pain to the back." What did he mean by that statement? Explain the phenomenon of referred pain to the back and sometimes the right shoulder in gallbladder disease.

5. Examination of a patient with neurosyphilis indicated that the pupil of her left eye was small and fixed and did not react to light, but contracted when the patient was asked to look at a near object. What is the innervation of the iris? Using your knowledge of neuroanatomy, state where you believe the neurological lesion to be situated to account for these defects.

6. A 36-year-old man was admitted to the emergency department following a gunshot wound to the lower back. Radiographic examination revealed that the bullet was lodged in the vertebral canal at the level of the third lumbar vertebra. A complete neurological examination revealed the symptoms and signs that indicate a complete

lesion of the cauda equina. What is the autonomic nerve supply to the bladder? Is this patient going to have any interference with bladder function?

7. A 40-year-old black man was found, on routine medical examination, to have essential hypertension. His blood pressure readings were 180 systolic and 100 diastolic (mm Hg). How would you treat this patient medically? What is the action of the various types of drugs that are commonly used in the treatment of hypertension?

8. What transmitter substances are liberated at the following nerve endings: (a) preganglionic sympathetic, (b) preganglionic parasympathetic, (c) postganglionic parasympathetic, (d) postganglionic sympathetic fibers to the heart muscle, and (e) postganglionic sympathetic fibers to the sweat glands of the hand?

Answers to Clinical Problem Solving

1. As a result of holding onto the moving truck with the right hand, this man had sustained a severe traction injury of the eighth cervical and first thoracic roots of the brachial plexus. The various paralyzed forearm and hand muscles together with the sensory loss were characteristic of Klumpke's paralysis. In this case, the pull on the first thoracic nerve was so severe that the white ramus communicantes to the inferior cervical sympathetic ganglion was torn. This effectively cut off the preganglionic sympathetic fibers to the right side of the head and neck, causing a right-sided Horner's syndrome (preganglionic type). This was exemplified by (a) constriction of the pupil, (b) drooping of the upper lid, and (c) enophthalmos. The arteriolar vasodilatation, due to loss of sympathetic vasoconstrictor fibers, was responsible for the red, hot cheek on the right side. The dryness of the skin of the right cheek also was due to the loss of the sympathetic secretomotor supply to the sweat glands.

2. This 3-year-old boy has Hirschsprung's disease, a congenital condition in which there is a failure of development of the myenteric plexus (Auerbach's plexus) in the distal part of the colon. The proximal part of the colon is normal but becomes greatly distended due to the accumulation of feces. In this patient, the lower sigmoid colon, later at operation, was shown to have no parasympathetic ganglion cells. Thus, this segment of the bowel had no peristalsis and effectively blocked the passage of feces. Once the diagnosis had been confirmed by performing a biopsy of the distal segment of the bowel, the treatment was to remove the aganglionic segment of the bowel by surgical resection.

3. This patient has given a classic history of Raynaud's disease. The disease is much more common in women than in men, especially those who have a nervous disposition. The initial pallor of the fingers is due to spasm of the digital arterioles. The cyanosis that follows is due to local capillary dilatation due to accumulation of metabolites. Since there is no blood flow through the capillaries, deoxygenated hemoglobin accumulates within them. It is during this period of prolonged cyanosis that the patient experiences severe aching pain. On exposing the fingers to warmth, the vasospasm disappears and oxygenated blood flows back into the very dilated capillaries. There

is now a reactive hyperemia and an increase in the formation of tissue fluid that is responsible for the swelling of the affected fingers. The sweating of the fingers during the attack probably is due to the excessive sympathetic activity, which may be responsible in part for the arteriolar vasospasm.

The arteries of the upper limb are innervated by sympathetic nerves. The preganglionic fibers originate from the cell bodies in the second to the eighth thoracic segments of the spinal cord. They ascend in the sympathetic trunk to synapse in the middle cervical, inferior cervical, and first thoracic or stellate ganglia. The postganglionic fibers join the nerves that form the brachial plexus and are distributed to the digital arteries within the branches of the brachial plexus.

In this patient the attacks were relatively mild. The patient should be reassured and told to keep her hands warm as much as possible. However, should the condition worsen the patient should be treated with drugs, such as reserpine, that inhibit sympathetic activity. This would result in arterial vasodilatation with consequent increase in blood flow to the fingers.

4. The patient was suffering from gallstone colic. The visceral pain originated from the cystic duct or bile duct and was due to stretching or spasm of the smooth muscle in its wall. The pain afferent fibers pass through the celiac ganglia and ascend in the greater splanchnic nerve to enter the fifth to the ninth thoracic segments of the spinal cord. The pain was referred to the fifth through the ninth thoracic dermatomes on the right side, that is, to the skin over and inferior to the right scapula.

Referred pain to the right shoulder in gallbladder disease is discussed on page 421.

5. This patient has an Argyll Robertson pupil, which is a small fixed pupil that does not react to light, but contracts with accommodation. The condition usually is due to a syphilitic lesion. The innervation of the iris is described on page 408. The neurological lesion in this patient interrupted the fibers running from the pretectal nucleus to the parasympathetic nuclei of the oculomotor nerve on both sides.

6. The urinary bladder is innervated by sympathetic fibers from the first and second lumbar segments of the spinal

cord and by parasympathetic fibers from the second, third, and fourth sacral segments of the spinal cord. In this patient, the cauda equina was sectioned at the level of the third lumbar vertebra. This meant that the preganglionic sympathetic fibers that descend in the anterior roots of the first and second lumbar nerves were left intact, since they leave the vertebral canal to form the appropriate spinal nerves above the level of the bullet. The preganglionic parasympathetic fibers were, however, sectioned as they descended in the vertebral canal within the anterior roots of the second, third, and fourth sacral nerves. The patient would, therefore, have an autonomous bladder and would be without any external reflex control. The bladder would fill to capacity and then overflow. Micturition could be activated by powerful con-

traction of the abdominal muscles by the patient, assisted by manual pressure on his anterior abdominal wall in the suprapubic region.

7. The precise cause of essential hypertension is unknown. Nevertheless, the objective of the treatment is to lower the blood pressure and keep it, if possible, within normal limits before the complications of cerebral hemorrhage, renal failure, or heart failure develop. The best way to accomplish this in patients with mild hypertension is to reduce the plasma fluid volume by the use of diuretics. Beta-receptor blocking agents are now extensively used. These reduce the rate and force of contraction of the cardiac muscle and lower the cardiac output.

8. (a) Acetylcholine, (b) acetylcholine, (c) acetylcholine, (d) norepinephrine, and (e) acetylcholine.

Review Questions

Directions: Each of the numbered items in this section is followed by answers that are positively phrased. Select the ONE lettered answer that is an EXCEPTION.

1. The following statements concerning the autonomic nervous system are correct **except:**
   (a) The enteric nervous system is made up of the submucous plexus of Meissner and the myenteric plexus of Auerbach.
   (b) The nerve fibers of the enteric nervous system are naked axons.
   (c) The activities of the parasympathetic part of the autonomic nervous system aim at conserving and restoring energy.
   (d) The parasympathetic part of the autonomic system contains both afferent and efferent nerve fibers.
   (e) The pretectal nucleus is concerned with the light reflex.

2. The following statements concerning the autonomic nervous system are correct **except:**
   (a) An Argyll Robertson pupil indicates that the accommodation reflex for near vision is normal but that the light reflex is lost.
   (b) White rami communicantes are limited to the thoracic part of the sympathetic trunk.
   (c) Gray rami communicantes contain postganglionic sympathetic fibers.
   (d) The greater splanchnic nerves are formed of myelinated axons.
   (e) The lesser splanchnic nerves arise from the tenth and eleventh ganglia of the thoracic part of the sympathetic trunks.

3. The following general statements concerning the autonomic nervous system are correct **except:**
   (a) The hypothalamus has great control over the autonomic nervous system.
   (b) The cerebral cortex has no control over the autonomic nervous system.
   (c) A patient with Adie's Tonic Pupil syndrome has a decreased or absent light reflex and a slow or delayed pupillary contraction to near vision, and a slow or delayed dilatation in the dark.
   (d) Pain arising in the gastrointestinal tract is referred to the midline.
   (e) Visceral pain frequently is referred to skin areas that are innervated by the same segment of the spinal cord as the painful viscus.

4. The following statements concerning the Horner's syndrome are correct **except:**
   (a) The pupil is constricted.
   (b) There is ptosis of the upper eyelid.
   (c) The patient has vasoconstriction of the facial skin arterioles.
   (d) There is an absence of facial sweating.
   (e) There is enophthalmos.

Directions: Each of the numbered items or incomplete statements in this section is followed by answers or completions of the statement. Select the ONE lettered answer or completion that is BEST in each case.

5. The sympathetic outflow
   (a) arises from nerve cells that are situated in the posterior gray column (horn) of the spinal cord
   (b) has preganglionic nerve fibers that leave the spinal cord in the posterior roots of the spinal nerves
   (c) is restricted to T1-L2 segments of the spinal cord
   (d) receives descending fibers from supraspinal levels that pass down the spinal cord in the posterior white column
   (e) has many preganglionic nerve fibers that synapse in the posterior root ganglia of the spinal nerves.

6. Norepinephrine is secreted at the endings of the
   (a) preganglionic sympathetic fibers
   (b) preganglionic parasympathetic fibers
   (c) postganglionic parasympathetic fibers
   (d) postganglionic sympathetic fibers
   (e) preganglionic fibers to the suprarenal medulla
7. The parasympathetic innervation controlling the parotid salivary gland arises from the
   (a) facial nerve
   (b) oculomotor nerve
   (c) vagus nerve
   (d) carotid plexus
   (e) glossopharyngeal nerve
8. Which of the following statements best describes the parasympathetic part of the autonomic nervous system?
   (a) It is associated with the thoracolumbar part of the spinal cord.
   (b) Effects are local and discrete due to preganglionic neurons synapsing with few postganglionic neurons.
   (c) It has short preganglionic axons.
   (d) It is active during an emotional crisis.
   (e) Its activity mobilizes glucose from glycogen.
9. Anticholinesterase drugs act at synapses by
   (a) mimicking the action of acetylcholine at its receptor sites
   (b) preventing the release of acetylcholine
   (c) increasing the secretion of acetylcholine
   (d) blocking the breakdown of acetylcholine
   (e) preventing the uptake of acetylcholine by the nerve ending
10. Atropine has the following effect on the autonomic nervous system:
   (a) It is an anticholinesterase drug.
   (b) It increases the activity of norepinephrine.
   (c) It blocks the action of acetylcholine on effector sites in the parasympathetic system.
   (d) It blocks norepinephrine reuptake by presynaptic terminals in the sympathetic system.
   (e) It blocks norepinephrine receptor sites.
11. The parasympathetic outflow in the spinal cord occurs at levels
   (a) S1 and 2
   (b) S3, 4, and 5
   (c) S1, 2, and 3
   (d) S2, 3, and 4
   (e) L1 and 2

Directions: Each of the numbered items in this section is followed by answers that are positively phrased. Select the ONE lettered answer that is an EXCEPTION.

12. The following statements concerning autonomic innervation of the urinary bladder are correct **except:**
   (a) The parasympathetic part brings about contraction of the bladder wall muscle and relaxation of the sphincter vesicae.
   (b) The sympathetic part in the male causes contraction of the sphincter vesicae and prevents reflux of semen into the bladder during ejaculation.
   (c) The afferent fibers from the bladder reach the spinal cord at the first and second lumbar segments and the second, third, and fourth sacral segments.
   (d) The sympathetic part causes contraction of the sphincter urethrae.
   (e) The sympathetic part innervates the blood vessels supplying the bladder wall.
13. The following statements concerning autonomic innervation of the heart are correct **except:**
   (a) The parasympathetic part causes constriction of the coronary arteries.
   (b) The postganglionic fibers terminate on the sinoatrial and atrioventricular nodes.
   (c) The sympathetic postganglionic fibers liberate acetylcholine at their nerve endings.
   (d) The sympathetic nerves cause cardiac acceleration and increased force of contraction of the heart.
   (e) The local metabolic needs of the cardiac muscle control the degree of dilatation of the coronary arteries rather than the neural control.

Directions: Matching Questions
Match the numbered glands with the most appropriate lettered autonomic ganglion listed below. Each lettered option may be selected once, more than once, or not at all.

14. Submandibular gland   (a) Otic ganglion
15. Lacrimal gland   (b) Submandibular ganglion
16. Nasal glands   (c) Pterygopalatine ganglion
17. Parotid gland   (d) Ciliary ganglion
18. Sublingual gland   (e) None of the above

Match the numbered autonomic ganglia with the most appropriate lettered viscus or muscle listed below. Each lettered option may be selected once, more than once, or not at all.

19. Superior cervical ganglion
20. Ciliary ganglion
21. Celiac ganglion
22. Inferior mesenteric ganglion
23. Superior mesenteric ganglion
   (a) Levator palpebrae superioris (smooth muscle only)
   (b) Vermiform appendix
   (c) Constrictor pupillae
   (d) Descending colon
   (e) None of the above

Match the numbered cranial nerves with the appropriate lettered nuclei listed below. Each lettered option may be selected once, more than once, or not at all.

24. Facial nerve
25. Oculomotor nerve
26. Glossopharyngeal nerve
27. Hypoglossal nerve
    (a) Inferior salivatory nucleus
    (b) Edinger-Westphal nucleus
    (c) Lacrimatory nucleus
    (d) None of the above

In Figure 14-19, match the numbered areas of referred pain with the appropriate lettered viscus originating the pain listed below. Each lettered option may be selected once, more than once, or not at all.

28. Number 1
29. Number 2
30. Number 3
31. Number 4
    (a) Heart
    (b) Appendix
    (c) Gallbladder
    (d) Stomach
    (e) None of the above

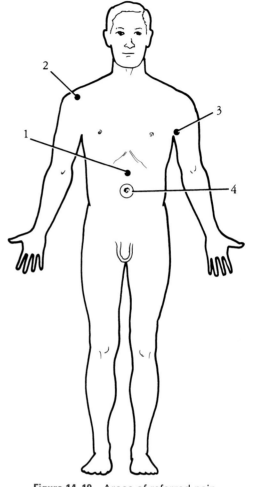

Figure 14–19   Areas of referred pain.

Answers to Review Questions

1. B
2. B
3. B
4. C
5. C
6. D
7. E
8. B
9. D
10. C
11. D
12. D
13. C
14. B
15. C
16. C

17. A.
18. B
19. A
20. C
21. E
22. D
23. B
24. C
25. B
26. A
27. D
28. D
29. C
30. A
31. B

ADDITIONAL READING

Appenzeller, D. *The Autonomic Nervous System.*(4th ed.). Amsterdam: Elsevier Biomedical Press, 1990.

Bors, E., Porter, R. W. Neurosurgical considerations in bladder dysfunction. Urol. Int. 25:114, 1970.

Buckley, N., Caufield, M. In G. Brunstock and C.H.V. Hoyle (eds.), *Transmission: Acetylcholine in Autonomic Neuroeffector Mechanisms.* Chur, Switzerland: Harwood Academic Publishers, pp.257-322,1992.

Bulygin, I. A. A consideration of the general principles of organization of sympathetic ganglia. *J.Auton. Nerv. Syst.* 8:303, 1983.

Craig, C. R., Stitzel, R. E. *Modern Pharmacology* (4th ed.). Boston: Little, Brown, 1994.

Eccles, J. C. *The Physiology of Synapses.* Berlin and Vienna: Springer, 1964.

Elfvin, L.G., Lindh, B., Hokfelt, T. The Chemical Neuroanatomy of Sypathetic Ganglia. *Annu. Rev. Neurosci.* 16:471-507,1993.

Fitzgerald, G. A. Peripheral presynaptic adrenoreceptor regulation of norepinephrine release in humans. *Fed. Proc.* 43:1379, 1984.

Furness, J.B., Costa, M. The Types of Nerves in the Enteric Nervous System. *Neuroscience* 5:1-20,1980.

Gershon, M. D. The enteric nervous system. *Annu. Rev. Neurosci.* 4:227, 1981.

Gershon, M.D. *The Second Brain.* New York: Harper Collins.1998.

Goodman, L. S., Gilman, A. *The Pharmacological Basis of Therapeutics* (3rd ed.). New York and London: Macmillan, 1965.

Grundy, D. *Gastrointestinal Motility.* Lancaster and Boston: MTP Press, 1985.

Kandel,E.R., Schwartz, J.H., Jessell,T.M. *Principles of Neural Science*, 4th Ed. McGraw-Hill, New York,2000.

Karczmar, A. G., Koketsu, K., Nishi, S. (eds.) *Autonomic and Enteric Ganglia.* New York: Plenum, 1986.

Kuntz, A. *The Autonomic Nervous System.* Philadelphia: Lea & Febiger, 1953.

Kuru, M. Nervous control of micturition. *Physiol. Rev.* 45:425, 1965.

Lepor, H., Gregerman, M., Crosby, R., Mostofi, F. K., Walsh, P. C. Precise localization of the autonomic nerves from the pelvic plexus to the corpora cavernosa: A detailed anatomical study of the adult male pelvis. *J. Urol.* 133:207, 1985.

Limbird, L.E. (ed.). *The Alpha-2 Adrenergic Receptors.* Clifton, N.J. Humana,1988.

Merritt, H., Moore, M. The Argyll Robertson pupil. *Arch. Neurol. Psychiatry* 30:357, 1933.

Mitchell, G. A. G. *Anatomy of the Autonomic Nervous System.* Edinburgh: Livingstone, 1953.

Mitchell, G. A. G. *Cardiovascular Innervation.* Edinburgh: Livingstone, 1956.

Nathan, P. W., Smith, M. C. The location of descending fibers to sympathetic neurons supplying the eye and sudomotor neurons supplying the head and neck. *J. Neurol. Neurosurg. Psychiatry* 49:187, 1986.

Perkins, J.D. (ed.). *The Beta-Adrenergic Receptors.* Clifton, N.J. Humana, 1991

Pick, J. *The Autonomic Nervous System: Morphological, Comparative, Clinical and Surgical Aspects.* Philadelphia: Lippincott, 1970.

Procacci, P., Zoppi, M. Pathophysiology and Clinical Aspects of Visceral and Referred Pain. In J. J. Bonica, D. Lindblom, A. Iggo, L. E. Jones, and C. Benedetti (eds.), *Advances in Pain Research and Therapy.* Vol. 5. New York: Raven, 1983. P. 643.

Snell, R. S. *Clinical Anatomy for Medical Students* (6th ed.). Philadelphia. Lippincott, Williams, & Wilkins, 2000.

Snell, R. S. The histochemical appearances of cholinesterase in the parasympathetic nerves supplying the submandibular and sublingual salivary glands of the rat. *J. Anat. (Lond.)* 92:534, 1958.

Snell, R. S. The histochemical appearances of cholinesterase in the superior cervical sympathetic ganglion and the changes which occur after preganglionic nerve section. *J. Anat. (Lond.)* 92:408, 1958.

Snell, R. S., Lemp, M. A. *Clinical Anatomy of the Eye* (2nd ed.). Boston: Blackwell Scientific, 1998.

Snell, R. S., Smith, M. S. *Clinical Anatomy for Emergency Medicine.* St. Louis: Mosby, 1993.

Snider, S. R., Kuchel, O. Dopamine: An important hormone of the sympathoadrenal system. *Endocrinol. Rev.* 4:291, 1983.

Westfall, T. C. Evidence that noradrenergic transmitter release is regulated by presynaptic receptors. *Fed. Proc.* 43:1352, 1984.

CHAPTER 15

The Meninges of the Brain and Spinal Cord

A 44-year-old woman was seen by a neurologist because she was experiencing intense pain in the right eye. On physical examination, she was found to have a slight medial strabismus of the right eye and the right pupil was smaller than normal. Further examination revealed numbness over the right cheek. A CT scan showed the presence of an aneurysm of the right internal carotid artery within the cavernous sinus. The aneurysm was about the size of a pea.

The location of the carotid aneurysm within the cavernous sinus explained the ocular pain; pressure on the right abducent nerve was responsible for the paralysis of the lateral rectus muscle, producing the medial strabismus. The small pupil of the right eye was caused by the aneurysm pressing on the sympathetic plexus surrounding the carotid artery and producing paralysis of the dilator pupillae muscle. The numbness experienced over the right cheek was due to pressure of the aneurysm on the right maxillary division of the trigeminal nerve, as it passed forward through the lateral wall of the sinus.

This patient illustrates the necessity of knowing the relationships between the structures within the skull, especially in regions like the cavernous sinus, where so many important neural structures lie close to one another.

CHAPTER OBJECTIVES

The objective of this chapter is to describe the structure and function of the three meninges that surround the brain and spinal cord. Particular attention is paid to the venous sinuses within the skull and how the meninges contribute to their walls. The relationship of the meninges to the different forms of cerebral hemorrhage is fully discussed.

MENINGES OF THE BRAIN

The brain and spinal cord are surrounded by three membranes, or meninges: the dura mater, the arachnoid mater, and the pia mater.

Dura Mater

The dura mater of the brain is conventionally described as two layers, the endosteal layer and the meningeal layer (Fig. 15-1). These are closely united except along certain lines, where they separate to form **venous sinuses.**

The **endosteal layer** is nothing more than the periosteum covering the inner surface of the skull bones. At the foramen magnum it does **not** become continuous with the dura mater of the spinal cord. Around the margins of all the foramina in the skull it becomes continuous with the **periosteum** on the outside of the skull bones. At the sutures, it is continuous with the **sutural ligaments** (Fig. 15-1). It is most strongly adherent to the bones over the base of the skull.

The **meningeal layer** is the dura mater proper. It is a dense, strong fibrous membrane covering the brain (Figs. 15-2 and 15-3) and is continuous through the foramen magnum with the dura mater of the spinal cord. It provides tubular sheaths for the cranial nerves as the latter pass through the foramina in the skull. Outside the skull, the sheaths fuse with the epineurium of the nerves (Fig. 15-2).

The meningeal layer sends inward four septa, which divide the cranial cavity into freely communicating spaces that lodge the subdivisions of the brain (Figs. 15-1 and 15-3). The function of these septa is to restrict the displacement of the brain associated with acceleration and deceleration, when the head is moved.

The **falx cerebri** is a sickle-shaped fold of dura mater that lies in the midline between the two cerebral hemispheres (Figs. 15-1 and 15-3). Its narrow anterior end is attached to the internal frontal crest and the crista galli. Its broad posterior part blends in the midline with the upper surface of the **tentorium cerebelli.** The **superior sagittal sinus** runs in its upper fixed margin; the **inferior sagittal sinus** runs in its lower concave free margin; and the **straight sinus** runs along its attachment to the tentorium cerebelli.

The **tentorium cerebelli** is a crescent-shaped fold of dura mater that roofs over the posterior cranial fossa (Fig. 15-4; see also Fig. 15-1). It covers the upper surface of the cerebellum and supports the occipital lobes of the cerebral hemispheres. In the anterior edge there is a gap, the **tentorial notch,** for the passage of the midbrain (Fig. 15-4), which produces an inner free border and an outer attached or fixed border. The fixed border is attached to the posterior clinoid processes, the superior borders of the petrous bones, and the margins of the grooves for the transverse sinuses on the occipital bone. The free border runs forward at its two ends, crosses the attached border, and is affixed to the anterior clinoid process on each side. At the point

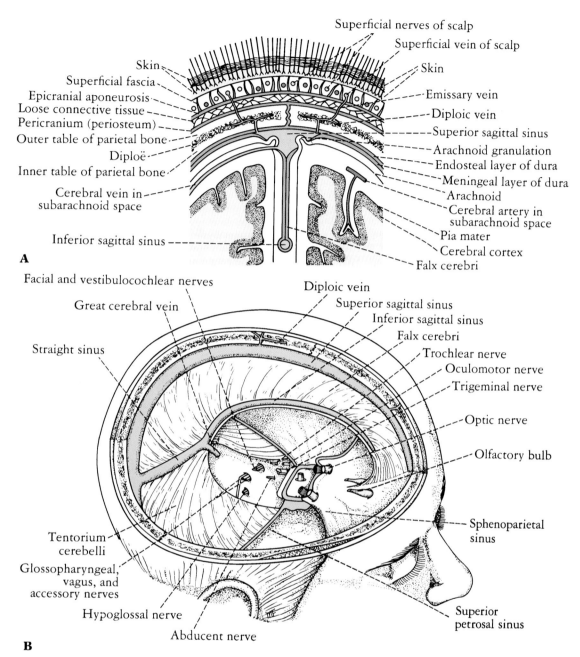

Figure 15–1 **A.** Coronal section of the upper part of the head showing the layers of the scalp, sagittal suture of the skull, falx cerebri, venous sinuses, arachnoid granulations, emissary veins, and relation of the cerebral blood vessels to the subarachnoid space. **B.** Interior of the skull, showing the dura mater and its contained venous sinuses.

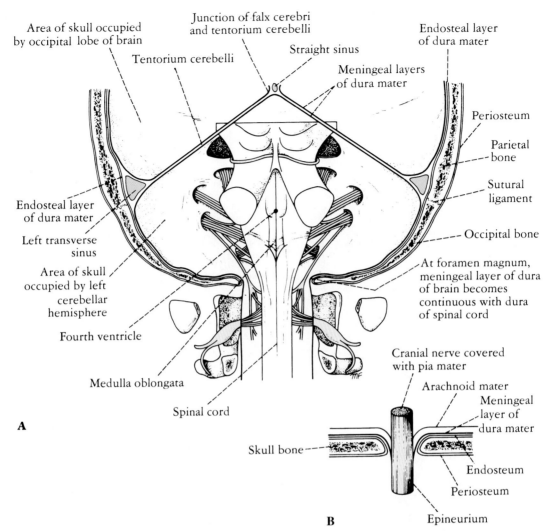

Figure 15–2 **A.** Posterior view of the interior of the skull after removal of the occipital and parietal bones shows the arrangement of the endosteal and meningeal layers of the dura mater. The brainstem has been left in situ. **B.** The arrangement of the meninges as a cranial nerve passes through a foramen in the skull.

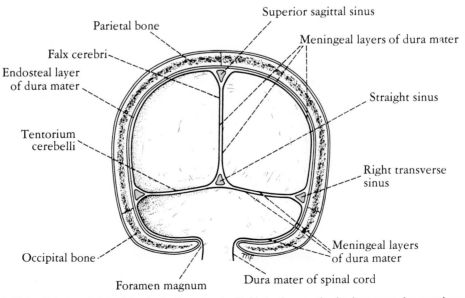

Figure 15–3 Falx cerebri and the tentorium cerebelli. Note the continuity between the meningeal layer of dura mater within the skull and the dura mater of the spinal cord at the foramen magnum.

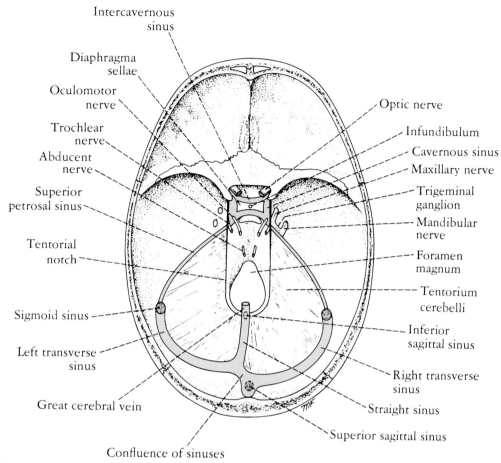

Figure 15–4 Superior view of the diaphragma sellae and tentorium cerebelli. Note the position of the cranial nerves and venous sinuses.

where the two borders cross, the third and fourth cranial nerves pass forward to enter the lateral wall of the cavernous sinus (Fig. 15-4).

Close to the apex of the petrous part of the temporal bone, the lower layer of the tentorium is pouched forward beneath the superior petrosal sinus, to form a recess for the trigeminal nerve and the trigeminal ganglion.

The falx cerebri and the falx cerebelli are attached to the upper and lower surfaces of the tentorium, respectively. The straight sinus runs along its attachment to the falx cerebri; the superior petrosal sinus, along its attachment to the petrous bone; and the **transverse sinus,** along its attachment to the occipital bone (Figs. 15-1 and 15-4).

The **falx cerebelli,** a small, sickle-shaped fold of dura mater attached to the internal occipital crest, projects forward between the two cerebellar hemispheres. Its posterior fixed margin contains the **occipital sinus.**

The **diaphragma sellae** is a small, circular fold of dura mater that forms the roof for the sella turcica (Figs. 15-4 and 15-6). A small opening in its center allows passage of the stalk of the **hypophysis cerebri** (Fig. 15-6).

Dural Nerve Supply

Branches of the trigeminal, vagus, and the first three cervical spinal nerves and branches from the sympathetic trunk pass to the dura.

The dura possesses numerous sensory endings that are sensitive to stretching, which produces the sensation of headache. Stimulation of the sensory endings of the trigeminal nerve above the level of the tentorium cerebelli produces referred pain to an area of skin on the same side of the head. Stimulation of the dural endings below the level of the tentorium produces pain referred to the back of the neck and the back of the scalp along the distribution of the greater occipital nerve.

Dural Arterial Supply

Numerous arteries supply the dura mater from the **internal carotid, maxillary, ascending pharyngeal, occipital,** and **vertebral arteries.** From the clinical standpoint, the most important is the **middle meningeal artery,** which can be damaged in head injuries (Fig. 15-5).

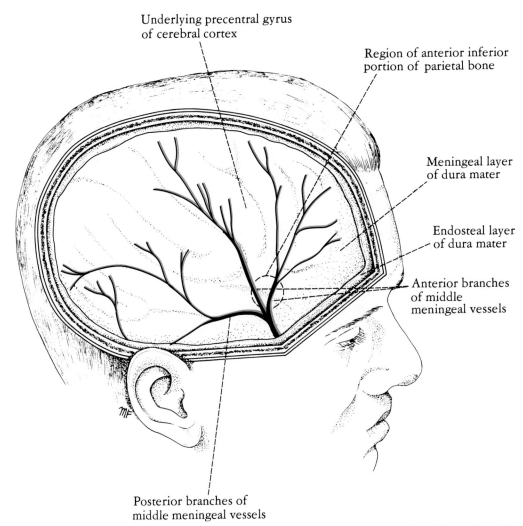

Underlying precentral gyrus
of cerebral cortex

Region of anterior inferior
portion of parietal bone

Meningeal layer
of dura mater

Endosteal layer
of dura mater

Anterior branches
of middle
meningeal vessels

Posterior branches of
middle meningeal vessels

Figure 15–5 Right side of the head, showing the relations of the middle meningeal vessels to the layers of the dura mater and the skull.

The **middle meningeal artery** arises from the maxillary artery in the infratemporal fossa. It enters the cranial cavity through the **foramen spinosum** and then lies between the meningeal and endosteal layers of dura. The artery then runs forward and laterally in a groove on the upper surface of the squamous part of the temporal bone. The anterior branch deeply grooves or tunnels the anterior-inferior angle of the parietal bone (Fig. 15-5), and its course corresponds roughly to the line of the underlying precentral gyrus of the brain. The posterior branch curves backward and supplies the posterior part of the dura mater (Fig. 15-7).

The **meningeal veins** lie in the endosteal layer of dura (Fig. 15-5). The middle meningeal vein follows the branches of the middle meningeal artery and drains into the pterygoid venous plexus or the sphenoparietal sinus. The veins lie lateral to the arteries.

Dural Venous Sinuses

The venous sinuses of the cranial cavity are situated between the layers of the dura mater (Figs. 15-6 and 15-7; see also Figs. 15-3 and 15-4). Their main function is to receive blood from the brain through the cerebral veins and the cerebrospinal fluid from the subarachnoid space through the **arachnoid villi** (Fig.16-18). The blood in the dural sinuses ultimately drains into the internal jugular veins in the neck. The dural sinuses are lined by endothelium, and their walls are thick but devoid of muscular tissue. They have no valves. **Emissary veins,** which are also valveless, connect the dural venous sinuses with the **diploic veins** of the skull and with the veins of the scalp (Fig. 15-1).

The **superior sagittal sinus** occupies the upper fixed border of the falx cerebri (Figs. 15-1 and 15-4). It begins anteriorly at the foramen cecum, where it occasionally re-

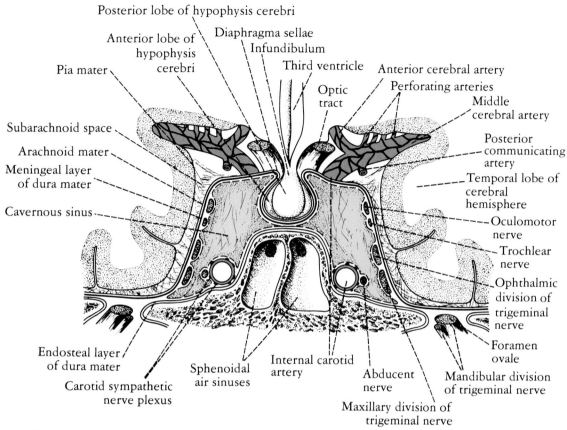

Figure 15–6 Coronal section through the body of the sphenoid bone, showing the hypophysis cerebri and cavernous sinuses. Note the position of the internal carotid artery and the cranial nerves.

ceives a vein from the nasal cavity. It runs posteriorly, grooving the vault of the skull, and at the internal occipital protuberance it deviates to one or the other side (usually the right) and becomes continuous with the corresponding **transverse sinus.** The sinus communicates through small openings with two or three irregularly shaped **venous lacunae** on each side (Fig. 15-7). Numerous arachnoid villi and granulations project into the lacunae, which also receive the diploic and meningeal veins (Fig. 15-1).

The superior sagittal sinus receives in its course the **superior cerebral veins** (Figs. 15-1 and 17-5). At the internal occipital protuberance it is dilated to form the **confluence of the sinuses** (Fig. 15-4). Here, the superior sagittal sinus usually becomes continuous with the right transverse sinus; it is connected to the opposite transverse sinus and receives the **occipital sinus.**

The **inferior sagittal sinus** occupies the free lower margin of the falx cerebri (Fig. 15-1). It runs backward and joins the **great cerebral vein** at the free margin of the tentorium cerebelli, to form the straight sinus (Figs. 15-1 and 15-4). It receives a few cerebral veins from the medial surface of the cerebral hemispheres.

The **straight sinus** occupies the line of junction of the falx cerebri with the tentorium cerebelli (Figs. 15-1 and

15-4). It is formed by the union of the **inferior sagittal sinus** with the **great cerebral vein.** It ends by turning to the left (sometimes to the right) to form the **transverse sinus.**

The **transverse sinuses** are paired structures and they begin at the internal occipital protuberance (Figs. 15-3 and 15-4). The right sinus is usually continuous with the superior sagittal sinus, and the left is continuous with the straight sinus. Each sinus occupies the attached margin of the tentorium cerebelli, grooving the occipital bone and the posteroinferior angle of the parietal bone. They receive the **superior petrosal sinuses, the inferior cerebral and cerebellar veins,** and the **diploic veins.** They end by turning downward as the **sigmoid sinuses** (Fig. 15-4).

The **sigmoid sinuses** are a direct continuation of the transverse sinuses. Each sinus turns downward and medially and grooves the mastoid part of the temporal bone (Fig. 15-4). It is here that the sinus lies posterior to the mastoid antrum. The sinus then turns forward and then inferiorly through the posterior part of the jugular foramen, to become continuous with the **superior bulb** of the **internal jugular vein.**

The **occipital sinus** is a small sinus occupying the attached margin of the falx cerebelli. It commences near

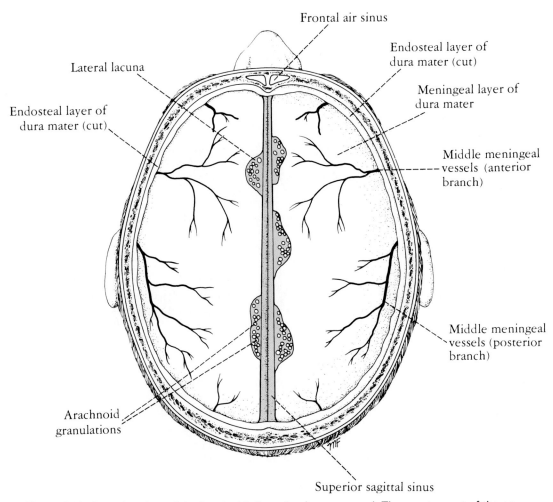

Figure 15–7 Superior view of the head with the calvarium removed. The greater part of the endosteal layer of dura mater has been removed, exposing the underlying meningeal layer of dura and the interior of the superior sagittal venous sinus.

the foramen magnum, where it communicates with the **vertebral veins** and drains into the **confluence of sinuses.**

The **cavernous sinuses** are situated in the middle cranial fossa on each side of the body of the sphenoid bone (Fig. 15-6). Numerous trabeculae cross their interior, giving them a spongy appearance, hence the name. Each sinus extends from the superior orbital fissure in front to the apex of the petrous part of the temporal bone behind.

The **internal carotid artery,** surrounded by its **sympathetic nerve plexus,** runs forward through the sinus (Fig. 15-6). The **abducent nerve** also passes through the sinus. The internal carotid artery and the nerves are separated from the blood by an endothelial covering.

The **third** and **fourth cranial nerves,** and the **ophthalmic** and **maxillary divisions of the trigeminal nerve,** run forward in the lateral wall of the sinus (Fig. 15-6). They lie between the endothelial lining and the dura mater.

The tributaries are the **superior** and **inferior ophthalmic veins,** the **inferior cerebral veins,** the **sphenoparietal sinus,** and the **central vein of the retina.**

The sinus drains posteriorly into the **superior** and **inferior petrosal sinuses,** and inferiorly into the **pterygoid venous plexus.**

The two sinuses communicate with each other by means of the **anterior** and **posterior intercavernous sinuses,** which run in the diaphragma sellae anterior and posterior to the stalk of the hypophysis cerebri (Fig. 15-4). Each sinus has an important communication with the facial vein through the superior ophthalmic vein. (This is a route by which infection can travel from the facial skin to the cavernous sinus.)

The **superior** and **inferior petrosal sinuses** are small sinuses situated on the superior and inferior borders of the petrous part of the temporal bone on each side of the skull (Fig. 15-4). Each superior sinus drains the cavernous sinus into the transverse sinus, and each inferior sinus drains the cavernous sinus into the internal jugular vein.

ARACHNOID MATER

The arachnoid mater is a delicate, impermeable membrane covering the brain and lying between the pia mater internally and the dura mater externally (Fig. 15-1). It is separated from the dura by a potential space, the **subdural space,** filled by a film of fluid; it is separated from the pia by the **subarachnoid space,** which is filled with **cerebrospinal fluid.** The outer and inner surfaces of the arachnoid are covered with flattened mesothelial cells.

The arachnoid bridges over the sulci on the surface of the brain, and in certain situations the arachnoid and pia are widely separated to form the **subarachnoid cisternae.** The **cisterna cerebellomedullaris** lies between the inferior surface of the cerebellum and the roof of the fourth ventricle. The **cisterna interpeduncularis** lies between the two cerebral peduncles. All the cisternae are in free communication with one another and with the remainder of the subarachnoid space.

In certain areas, the arachnoid projects into the venous sinuses to form **arachnoid villi.** The arachnoid villi are most numerous along the superior sagittal sinus. Aggregations of arachnoid villi are referred to as **arachnoid granulations** (Fig. 15-7). Arachnoid villi serve as sites where the cerebrospinal fluid diffuses into the bloodstream.

The arachnoid is connected to the pia mater across the fluid-filled subarachnoid space by delicate strands of fibrous tissue.

Structures passing to and from the brain to the skull or its foramina must pass through the subarachnoid space. All the cerebral arteries and veins lie in the space, as do the cranial nerves (Figs. 15-1 and 15-6). The arachnoid fuses with the epineurium of the nerves at their point of exit from the skull (Fig. 15-2B). In the case of the **optic nerve,** the arachnoid forms a sheath for the nerve, which extends into the orbital cavity through the optic canal and fuses with the sclera of the eyeball (Fig. 15-8). Thus, the subarachnoid space extends around the optic nerve as far as the eyeball.

The **cerebrospinal fluid** is produced by the **choroid plexuses** within the lateral, third, and fourth ventricles of the brain. It escapes from the ventricular system of the brain through the three foramina in the roof of the fourth ventricle and so enters the subarachnoid space. It now circulates both upward over the surfaces of the cerebral hemispheres and downward around the spinal cord. The spinal subarachnoid space extends down as far as the **second sacral vertebra** (see p. 437). Eventually, the fluid enters the bloodstream by passing into the arachnoid villi and diffusing through their walls.

In addition to removing waste products associated with neuronal activity, the cerebrospinal fluid provides a fluid medium in which the brain floats. This mechanism effectively protects the brain from trauma. In addition, the fluid is now believed to play a role in hormonal transport.

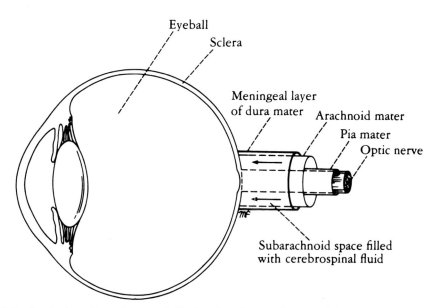

Figure 15–8 Sagittal section of the eyeball, showing the attachment of the meninges to the sclera. Note the extension of the subarachnoid space around the optic nerve to the eyeball.

PIA MATER

The pia mater is a vascular membrane covered by flattened mesothelial cells. It closely invests the brain, covering the gyri and descending into the deepest sulci (Fig. 15-1). It extends out over the cranial nerves and fuses with their epineurium. The cerebral arteries entering the substance of the brain carry a sheath of pia with them.

The pia mater forms the **tela choroidea** of the roof of the third and fourth ventricles of the brain, and it fuses with the ependyma to form the choroid plexuses in the lateral, third, and fourth ventricles of the brain.

MENINGES OF THE SPINAL CORD

Dura Mater

The dura mater is a dense, strong, fibrous membrane that encloses the spinal cord and the cauda equina (Figs. 15-9 and 1-6). It is continuous above through the foramen magnum with the meningeal layer of dura covering the brain. Inferiorly, it ends on the filum terminale at the level of the lower border of the second sacral vertebra. The dural sheath lies loosely in the vertebral canal and is separated

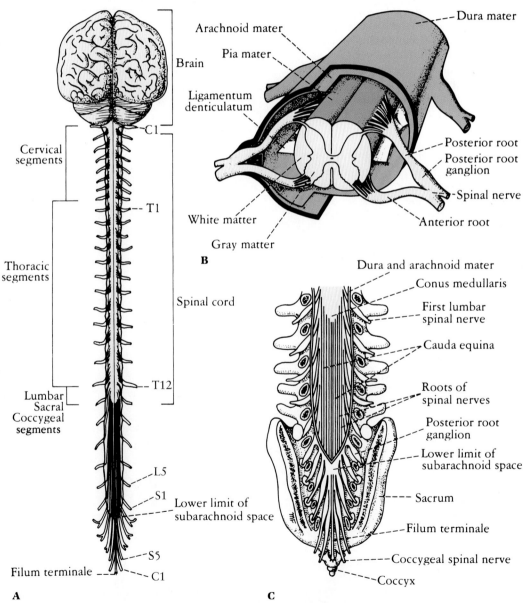

Figure 15–9 **A**. Brain, spinal cord, spinal nerve roots, and spinal nerves as seen on their posterior aspect. **B**. Transverse section through the thoracic region of the spinal cord, showing the anterior and posterior roots of a spinal nerve and the meninges. **C**. Posterior view of the lower end of the spinal cord and cauda equina, showing their relationship with the lumbar vertebrae, sacrum, and coccyx.

from the wall of the canal by the **extradural space.** This contains loose areolar tissue and the **internal vertebral venous plexus.** The dura mater extends along each nerve root and becomes continuous with the connective tissue surrounding each spinal nerve (epineurium). The inner surface of the dura mater is in contact with the arachnoid mater (See Fig. 4-1).

Arachnoid Mater

The arachnoid mater is a delicate impermeable membrane that covers the spinal cord and lies between the pia mater internally and dura mater externally (Fig. 15-9). It is separated from the pia mater by a wide space, the **subarachnoid space**, which is filled with **cerebrospinal fluid**. The subarachnoid space is crossed by a number of fine strands of connective tissue. The arachnoid mater is continuous

above through the foramen magnum with the arachnoid covering the brain. Inferiorly, it ends on the filum terminale at the level of the lower border of the second sacral vertebra (Fig.15-9). The arachnoid mater continues along the spinal nerve roots, forming small lateral extensions of the subarachnoid space.

Pia Mater

The pia mater, a vascular membrane that closely covers the spinal cord (Fig. 15-9), is thickened on either side between the nerve roots to form the **ligamentum denticulatum**, which passes laterally to adhere to the arachnoid and dura. It is by this means that the spinal cord is suspended in the middle of the dural sheath. The pia mater extends along each nerve root and becomes continuous with the connective tissue surrounding each spinal nerve (Fig.15-9).

CLINICAL NOTES

FUNCTIONAL SIGNIFICANCE OF THE MENINGES

The meninges of the brain and spinal cord form three concentric membranous coverings. The outermost, the dura mater, by virtue of its toughness serves to protect the underlying nervous tissue. The dura protects the cranial nerves by forming a sheath that covers each cranial nerve for a short distance as it passes through foramina in the skull. The dura mater also provides each spinal nerve root with a protective sheath.

In the skull, the falx cerebri, which is a vertical sheet of dura between the cerebral hemispheres, and the tentorium cerebelli, which is a horizontal sheet that projects forward between the cerebrum and cerebellum, serve to limit excessive movements of the brain within the skull.

The arachnoid mater is a much thinner impermeable membrane and loosely covers the brain. The interval between the arachnoid and pia mater, the subarachnoid space, is filled with cerebrospinal fluid. The cerebrospinal fluid gives buoyancy to the brain and protects the nervous tissue from mechanical forces applied to the skull.

The pia mater is a vascular membrane that closely invests and supports the brain and spinal cord.

EXCESSIVE MOVEMENTS OF THE BRAIN RELATIVE TO THE SKULL AND MENINGES IN HEAD INJURIES

When a moving patient's head is suddenly halted, the momentum of the brain causes it to travel onward until its movement is resisted by the skull or the strong septa of the dura mater. In lateral movements, the lateral surface of one hemisphere hits the side of the skull and the medial surface of the opposite hemisphere hits the side of the falx cerebri. In superior movements, the superior surfaces of the cerebral hemispheres hit the vault of the skull and the superior surface of the corpus callosum hits the sharp free edge of the

falx cerebri; the superior surface of the cerebellum presses against the inferior surface of the tentorium cerebelli.

Movements of the brain relative to the skull and dural septa may seriously injure the cranial nerves that are tethered as they pass through the various foramina. Furthermore, the fragile cortical veins that drain into the dural sinuses may be torn, resulting in severe **subdural** or **subarachnoid hemorrhage.** The tortuous arteries, with their strong walls, are rarely damaged.

INTRACRANIAL HEMORRHAGE AND THE MENINGES
Epidural Hemorrhage

Epidural hemorrhage results from injuries to the meningeal arteries or veins. The most common artery to be damaged is the **anterior division of the middle meningeal artery.** A comparatively minor blow to the side of the head, resulting in fracture of the skull in the region of the anterior-inferior portion of the parietal bone, may sever the artery. Arterial or venous injury is especially liable to occur if the vessels enter a bony canal in this region. Bleeding occurs and strips up the meningeal layer of dura from the internal surface of the skull. The intracranial pressure rises, and the enlarging blood clot exerts local pressure on the underlying motor area in the precentral gyrus. Blood also passes laterally through the fracture line, to form a soft swelling under the temporalis muscle.

In order to stop the hemorrhage, the torn artery or vein must be ligated or plugged. The burr hole through the skull wall should be placed about 1 1/2 inches (4 cm) above the midpoint of the zygomatic arch.

SUBDURAL HEMORRHAGE

Subdural hemorrhage results from tearing of the **superior cerebral veins** at their point of entrance into the superior sagittal sinus. The cause is usually a blow on the front or the back of the head, causing excessive anteroposterior displacement of the brain within the skull. Acute and chronic forms of the condition occur.

CT Scans of Epidural and Subdural Hematomas

The different appearances of the blood clots in these two conditions as seen on CT scans is related to the anatomy of the area (Fig.15-10). In an epidural hemorrhage the blood strips up the meningeal layer of the dura from the endosteal layer of dura (periosteum of the skull), producing a **lens-shaped** hyper dense collection of blood that compresses the brain and displaces the midline structures to the opposite side. The shape of the blood clot is determined by the adherence of the meningeal layer of dura to the periosteal layer of dura.

In patients with subdural hematoma the blood accumulates in the extensive potential space between the meningeal layer of dura and the arachnoid, producing a long **crescent-shaped,** hyperdense rim of blood that extends from anterior to posterior along the inner surface of the skull. With a large

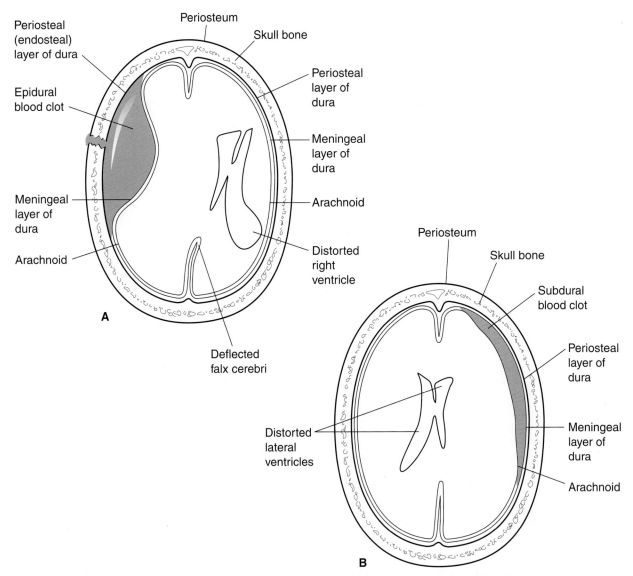

Figure 15–10 Diagrammatic representation of an epidural hemorrhage and a subdural hemorrhage. **A.** Epidural hemorrhage from the middle meningeal artery or vein on the left side. The hematoma is lens-shaped and occupies the space between the endosteal layer of dura (periosteum of the skull) and the meningeal layer of dura (true dura-hence the name epidural). **B.** Subdural hemorrhage from the cerebral veins at the site of entrance into the venous sinus on right side. The hematoma is crescent shaped and occupies the space between the meningeal layer of dura and the arachnoid, i.e., beneath the dura.

hematoma, the brain sulci are obliterated, and the midline structures are displaced to the opposite side.

Subarachnoid and Cerebral Hemorrhages

Subarachnoid and cerebral hemorrhages are described on page 437.

INTRACRANIAL HEMORRHAGE IN THE INFANT

Intracranial hemorrhage may occur during birth and may result from excessive molding of the head. Bleeding may occur from the cerebral veins or the venous sinuses. Excessive anteroposterior compression of the head often tears the anterior attachment of the falx cerebri from the tentorium cerebelli. Bleeding then takes place from the great cerebral veins, the straight sinus, or the inferior sagittal sinus.

The Shaken-Baby Syndrome is described on page 22.

HEADACHE

The brain itself is insensitive to pain. It follows that headaches are due to the stimulation of receptors outside the brain.

Meningeal Headaches

The dura mater receives its sensory nerve supply from the trigeminal and the first three cervical nerves. The dura above the tentorium is innervated by the trigeminal nerve, and the headache is referred to the forehead and face. The dura below the tentorium is innervated by the cervical nerves, and the headache is referred to the back of the head and neck. **Meningitis,** or inflammation of the meninges, causes severe headache over the entire head and back of the neck.

Headaches Caused by Cerebral Tumors

An expanding tumor with its associated raised intracranial pressure produces severe, continuous, and progressive headache, caused by the irritation and stretching of the dura. A tumor above the tentorium tends to produce a headache referred to the front of the head, while a tumor below the tentorium produces a headache referred to the back of the head.

Migraine Headache

This is a common form of headache, which may be unilateral or bilateral, recurring at intervals, and associated with prodromal visual disturbances. The prodromal visual disturbances are thought to be due to sympathetic vasoconstriction of the cerebral arteries supplying the visual cortex. The headache is due chiefly to the dilatation and stretching of other cerebral arteries and branches of the external carotid artery. The disease therefore appears to affect arteries both inside and outside the skull and its cause is unknown, although genetic, hormonal, and biochemical factors may initiate an attack. It is has been found that B-blockers bring about relief in some patients due to the reduction in cerebral vasodilation.

Alcoholic Headache

This type of headache is due to the direct toxic affect of alcohol on the meninges.

Headaches Due to Diseases of the Teeth, Paranasal Sinuses, and Eyes

Dental infection and sinusitis are common causes of headache. The pain is referred to the skin of the face and the forehead along the branches of the trigeminal nerve. Tonic spasm of the ciliary muscle of the eye, when attempting to focus on an object for prolonged periods (e.g., reading small print), may cause severe orbital headache. This commonly occurs in individuals who need lenses for the correction of presbyopia.

Clinical Problem Solving

1. In an automobile accident, which structures present within the skull limit damage to the cerebral hemispheres and other parts of the brain? Which blood vessels are damaged more commonly, the cerebral arteries or the cerebral veins? Are cranial nerves likely to be damaged in head injuries? If so, which ones are damaged most commonly and what is the reason for their increased susceptibility?
2. While performing an autopsy on a patient who had died of a meningioma, the pathologist explained to a group of students that these tumors arise from the arachnoid mater. She explained that they occur in those areas in which the arachnoid pierces the dura to form the arachnoid villi that project into the dural venous sinuses. She then asked the students where they would expect to find meningiomas. How would you answer that question?
3. A 10-year-old girl was admitted to hospital for surgical correction of medial strabismus of the right eye. Twenty-four hours after successful completion of the operation it was noted that her right eyeball was projecting forward excessively (proptosis) and the conjunctiva of the right eye was inflamed. A watery, purulent discharge could be expressed from beneath the eyelids. The ophthalmologist was greatly concerned because he did not want the complication of cavernous sinus thrombosis to occur. What is the connection between infection of the eye and

cavernous sinus thrombosis? Is cavernous sinus thrombosis a serious condition?

4. A 41-year-old man was found, on examination, to have paralysis of the lateral rectus muscle of his left eye; the left pupil was dilated but reacted slowly to light, and there was some anesthesia of the skin over the left side of the forehead. A carotid arteriogram revealed the presence of an aneurysm of the right internal carotid artery situated in the cavernous sinus. Using your knowledge of anatomy, explain the clinical findings on physical examination.

5. A 45-year-old woman was found on ophthalmoscopic examination to have edema of both optic discs (*bilateral papilledema*) and congestion of the retinal veins. The cause of the condition was found to be a rapidly growing intracranial tumor. Using your knowledge of anatomy, explain the papilledema. Why does the patient exhibit bilateral papilledema?

6. A pediatrician was observing a 6-year-old boy playing with his toys. He noted that the child had perfectly normal use of his arms but that his legs were stiff and, when he walked, he tended to cross his legs and had a scissor-like gait. A diagnosis of cerebral diplegia* secondary to birth injuries was made. Apparently the child was born prematurely and he was a breech presentation. Using your knowledge of anatomy, explain what happens to the fetal skull bones during delivery. Why are the dural venous sinuses likely to be damaged at birth? Why is cere-

bral hemorrhage more likely to occur in a premature baby with a malpresentation?

7. A 25-year-old woman was admitted to the emergency department unconscious. She had apparently been hit on the side of the head by a car while crossing the road. Within an hour, her state of unconsciousness deepened. On examination, she was found to have a large, dough-like swelling over the right temporalis muscle. She also had the signs of right-sided hemiplegia. Later, a right-sided, fixed, dilated pupil developed. A lateral radiograph of the skull showed a fracture line across the groove for the anterior division of the right middle meningeal artery. Her coma deepened, and she died 4 hours after the accident. Using your knowledge of neuroanatomy, make a diagnosis in this case. Explain the clinical findings. How could you account for the homolateral hemiplegia?

8. A 50-year-old woman complaining of a severe headache of 3 days' duration visited her physician. She said that the headache had started getting very severe about 1 hour after she had hit her head on the mantelpiece after bending down to poke the fire. She was admitted to the hospital for observation. Three hours later it was noticed that she was becoming mentally confused and also that she was developing a right-sided hemiplegia on the side of the body opposite the head injury. She had exaggeration of the deep reflexes and a positive Babinski response on the right side. Examination of the cerebrospinal fluid with a spinal tap showed a raised pressure and the presence of blood in the fluid. Radiographic examination showed no fracture of the skull. A CT scan revealed the presence of a subdural hematoma. What exactly is a subdural hematoma?

---

*Congenital cerebral diplegia is believed by some authorities to occur early in fetal life and to be caused by a viral infection that arrests cerebral development.

Answers to Clinical Problem Solving

1. The meninges and the cerebrospinal fluid afford a remarkable degree of protection to the delicate brain. The dural partitions, especially the falx cerebri and the tentorium cerebelli, limit the extent of brain movement within the skull.

    The thin-walled cerebral veins are liable to be damaged during excessive movements of the brain relative to the skull, especially at the point where the veins join the dural venous sinuses. The thick-walled cerebral arteries are rarely damaged.

    The small-diameter cranial nerves of long length are particularly prone to damage during head injuries. The trochlear, abducent, and oculomotor nerves are commonly injured.

2. Meningiomas arise from the arachnoid villi found along the dural venous sinuses. They are therefore most commonly found along the superior sagittal sinus and the sphenoparietal sinuses. They are rare below the tentorium cerebelli.

3. The anterior facial vein, the ophthalmic veins, and the cavernous sinus are in direct communication with one another. Infection of the skin of the face alongside the nose, ethmoidal sinusitis, and infection of the orbital contents can lead to thrombosis of the veins and ultimately cavernous sinus thrombosis. If untreated with antibiotics, this condition can be fatal, since the cavernous sinus drains many cerebral veins from the inferior surface of the brain.

4. The internal carotid artery passes forward on the lateral surface of the body of the sphenoid within the cavernous sinus. An aneurysm of the artery may press on the abducent nerve and cause paralysis of the lateral rectus muscle. Further expansion of the aneurysm may cause compression of the oculomotor nerve and the ophthalmic division of the trigeminal nerve as they lie in the lateral wall of the cavernous sinus. This patient had left lateral rectus paralysis and paralysis of the left pupillary constrictor muscle owing to involvement of the abducent and oculomotor

nerves, respectively. The slight anesthesia of the skin over the left side of the forehead was due to pressure on the ophthalmic division of the left trigeminal nerve.

5. The optic nerves are surrounded by sheaths derived from the pia mater, arachnoid mater, and dura mater. There is an extension of the intracranial subarachnoid space forward around the optic nerve to the back of the eyeball. A rise in cerebrospinal fluid pressure due to an intracranial tumor will compress the thin walls of the retinal vein as it crosses the extension of the subarachnoid space in the orbital cavity. This will result in congestion of the retinal vein and bulging of the optic disc, involving both eyes.

6. During the descent of the fetal head through the birth canal during labor, the bones of the calvarium overlap, a process known as molding. If this process is excessive or takes place too rapidly, as in malpresentations or in premature deliveries (when there is rapid birth of a small fetus), an abnormal strain is put on the falx cerebri. This stress involves the superior sagittal sinus, especially if the anteroposterior compression is excessive, and the sinus may tear where it joins the transverse sinus. The great cerebral vein may tear as well. The result is either a subarachnoid or subdural hemorrhage with accompanying brain damage.

7. The initial loss of consciousness was due to concussion or cerebral trauma. The swelling over the right temporalis and the radiographic finding of a fracture over the right middle meningeal artery were due to hemorrhage from the artery into the overlying muscle and soft tissue. This patient had an extradural hemorrhage. The right homolateral hemiplegia was due to the compression of the left cerebral peduncle against the edge of the tentorium cerebelli. This is unusual. A left hemiplegia due to pressure on the right precentral gyrus is more common. The right-sided, fixed, dilated pupil was due to the pressure on the right oculomotor nerve by the hippocampal gyrus, which had herniated through the tentorial notch.

8. A subdural hematoma is an accumulation of blood clot in the interval between the meningeal layer of dura and the arachnoid mater. It results from tearing of the superior cerebral veins at their point of entrance into the superior sagittal sinus. The cause is usually a blow on the front or the back of the head, causing excessive anteroposterior displacement of the brain within the skull. A subdural hematoma can be easily identified by CT as a dense rim of blood extending along the inner table of the skull obliterating the cerebral fissures and displacing the cerebral structures to the opposite side.

Review Questions

Directions: Each of the numbered items in this section is followed by answers that are positively phrased. Select the ONE lettered answer that is an EXCEPTION.

1. The following statements concerning the meninges of the brain are correct **except:**
   (a) Both layers of the dura mater covering the brain are continuous through the foramen magnum with the dura covering the spinal cord.
   (b) The periosteal layer of dura mater is continuous with the sutural ligaments of the skull.
   (c) As each cranial nerve passes through a foramen in the skull, it is surrounded by a tubular sheath of pia, arachnoid, and dura mater.
   (d) The cranial venous sinuses run between the meningeal and endosteal layers of dura mater.
   (e) The meninges extend anteriorly through the optic canal and fuse with the sclera of the eyeball.

2. The following general statements concerning the meninges are correct **except:**
   (a) The cisterna cerebellomedullaris is filled with cerebrospinal fluid and lies between the inferior surface of the cerebellum and the roof of the fourth ventricle.
   (b) The arachnoid mater is permeable to cerebrospinal fluid.
   (c) The cerebrospinal fluid in the arachnoid villi is able to drain into the venous sinuses through small tubules lined with endothelial cells.

   (d) The arachnoid mater surrounding the spinal cord ends inferiorly on the filum terminale at the level of the lower border of the second sacral vertebra.
   (e) The extradural space that separates the dural sheath of the spinal cord and the walls of the vertebral canal is filled with loose areolar tissue and contains the internal vertebral venous plexus.

3. The following statements concerning the tentorium cerebelli are correct **except:**
   (a) The free border is attached anteriorly to the anterior clinoid processes.
   (b) It is formed from the meningeal layer of the dura mater.
   (c) It separates the cerebellum from the occipital lobes of the brain.
   (d) The sigmoid sinus lies within its attached border to the occipital bone.
   (e) In the anterior edge there is the tentorial notch.

4. The following statements concerning headache are correct **except:**
   (a) Brain tissue is insensitive to pain.
   (b) Intracranial pain arises from receptors situated in the dura mater.
   (c) An expanding cerebral tumor located in the posterior cranial fossa would produce pain referred to the face.
   (d) Migraine headache is believed to be due to dilatation of cerebral arteries and branches of the external carotid artery.

(e) Headaches associated with presbyopia are due to tonic spasm of the ciliary muscles of the eyes.

5. The following statements concerning the subarachnoid space are true **except:**
   (a) It is filled with cerebrospinal fluid.
   (b) It extends inferiorly as far as the second sacral vertebra.
   (c) It contains the cerebral arteries and veins.
   (d) The cranial nerves lie outside the subarachnoid space in sheaths derived from the dura mater.
   (e) The arachnoid villi project into the venous sinuses as minute outpouchings of the subarachnoid space.

6. The following statements concerning the cavernous sinus are correct **except:**
   (a) It has passing through it the internal carotid artery and the abducent nerve.
   (b) It has the oculomotor, trochlear, and ophthalmic divisions of the trigeminal nerve in its lateral wall.

(c) It drains directly posteriorly into the straight sinus.
(d) It communicates anteriorly via the superior ophthalmic vein with the facial vein.
(e) It is related medially to the pituitary gland and the sphenoid air sinus.

7. The following structures limit rotatory movements of the brain within the skull **except** the:
   (a) Falx cerebri
   (b) Diaphragma sellae
   (c) Falx cerebelli
   (d) Body of the sphenoid bone
   (e) Petrous part of the temporal bone

8. The following nerves are sensory to the dura mater **except** the:
   (a) Hypoglossal nerve
   (b) Trigeminal nerve
   (c) Third cervical spinal nerve
   (d) Vagus nerve
   (e) First and second cervical spinal nerves

Answers to Review Questions

1.	A		5.	D
2.	B		6.	C
3.	D		7.	B
4.	C		8.	A

ADDITIONAL READING

Bannister, R. *Brain's Clinical Neurology* (6th ed.). London and New York: Oxford University Press, 1985.

Bruyn, G. W. Biochemistry of Migraine. *Headache* 20:235, 1980.

Dalessio, D. J., and Silberstein, S. D. *Wolff's Headache and Other Head Pain* (6th ed.). New York: Oxford University Press, 1993.

Doogan, D. P. Prophylaxis of migraine with beta-blockers. *Practitioner* 227:441, 1983.

Durand, M. L., et al. Acute bacterial meningitis in adults. *N. Engl. J. Med.* 328:21, 1993.

Lance, J. W. *The Mechanism and Management of Headache* (5th ed.). London: Butterworth, 1993.

Snell, R. S. *Clinical Anatomy for Medical Students* (6th ed.). Philadelphia, Lippincott, Williams, & Wilkins, 2000.

Snell, R. S., and Smith, M. S. *Clinical Anatomy for Emergency Medicine.* St. Louis: Mosby, 1993.

Welch, K. M. A. The therapeutics of migraine. *Curr. Opin. Neurol. Neurosurg.* 6:264, 1993.

Williams, P. L., et al., (eds.). *Gray's Anatomy* (38th Brit. ed.). New York Edinburgh, Churchill Livingstone, 1995.

CHAPTER 16

The Ventricular System, the Cerebrospinal Fluid, and the Blood-Brain and Blood-Cerebrospinal Fluid Barriers

A 26-year-old woman involved in an automobile accident was admitted to the emergency department. Her mother, who was also in the car, told the physician that at the time of impact, her daughter's head was thrown forward against the windshield.

On examination, the patient was unconscious and showed evidence of a severe head injury on the left side. After a thorough physical examination, the physician decided to perform a spinal tap. The cerebrospinal fluid pressure was 160 mm of water and two samples of the fluid were collected. The specimens showed red blood cells at the bottom of the tubes and the supernatant fluid was blood-stained. After standing for an hour, the supernatant fluid in both tubes became colorless.

The physician made the diagnosis of subarachnoid hemorrhage secondary to the head injury. The blood could have originated from a severe fracture of the skull, damage to one of the cerebral blood vessels, or a tear involving the brain or covering meninges. The physician was confident that the blood in the cerebrospinal fluid specimens did not originate from an accidental puncture of a vertebral vein during the spinal tap procedure. He eliminated this possibility by removing the two specimens of the fluid. If a local vein had been punctured by the needle, the first specimen would have been blood-stained and the second specimen most probably would have been clear. With this patient, both specimens were uniformly blood-stained, so the blood was in the subarachnoid space.

The management of this patient in the emergency department and the evaluation of the spinal tap specimen depended on knowledge of the cerebrospinal fluid system and the anatomy involved in the spinal tap procedure.

C H A P T E R   O B J E C T I V E S

The central nervous system contains and is surrounded by a clear fluid, the cerebrospinal fluid. The objective of this chapter is to discuss the locations, the functions, the origins, and the fate of this important fluid. Special emphasis is placed on the clinical significance of the fluid.

The structure and significance of the blood-brain and blood-cerebrospinal fluid barriers are also described. The importance of knowing how certain parts of the brain are protected from potentially toxic drugs or other exogenous materials is explained.

VENTRICULAR SYSTEM

The ventricles of the brain are the lateral ventricles, the third ventricle, and the fourth ventricle (Fig. 16-1). The two **lateral ventricles** communicate through the **interventricular foramina** (of Monro) with the **third ventricle**. The third ventricle is connected to the **fourth ventricle** by the **cerebral aqueduct** (**aqueduct of Sylvius**). The fourth ventricle in turn is continuous with the narrow **central canal** of the spinal cord and, through the three foramina in its roof, with the subarachnoid space. The central canal has a small dilatation at its inferior end, referred to as the **terminal ventricle** (see Fig. 16-1).

The ventricles are developmentally derived from the cavity of the neural tube. They are lined throughout with **ependyma** and are filled with **cerebrospinal fluid**.

Lateral Ventricles

There are two lateral ventricles and one is present in each cerebral hemisphere (Fig. 16-2). The ventricle is a roughly C-shaped cavity and may be divided into a **body**, which occupies the parietal lobe and from which **anterior, posterior**, and **inferior horns** extend into the frontal, occipital, and temporal lobes, respectively. The lateral ventricle communicates with the cavity of the third ventricle through the **interventricular foramen** (Figs. 16-2, 16-3, and 16-4). This opening, which lies in the anterior part of the medial wall of the ventricle, is bounded anteriorly by the anterior column of the fornix and posteriorly by the anterior end of the thalamus.

The **body of the lateral ventricle** extends from the interventricular foramen posteriorly as far as the posterior end of the thalamus. Here it becomes continuous with the posterior and the inferior horns. The body of the lateral ventricle has a roof, a floor, and a medial wall (Fig. 16-5).

The **roof** is formed by the undersurface of the **corpus callosum** (Fig. 16-5). The **floor** is formed by the body of the **caudate nucleus** and the lateral margin of the thalamus. The superior surface of the thalamus is obscured in its medial part by the **body of the fornix**. The **choroid plexus**

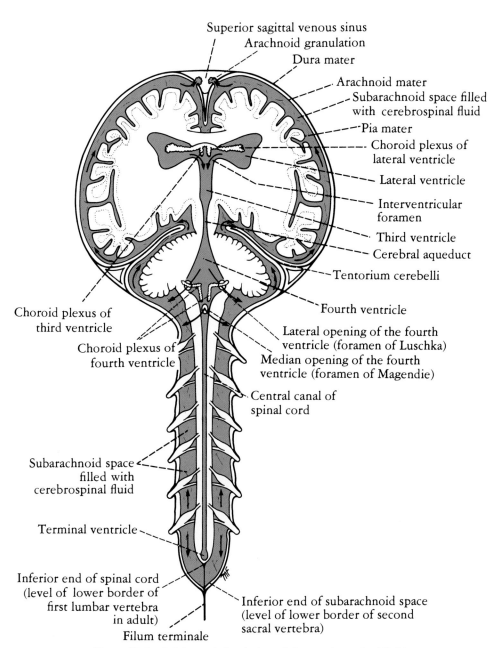

Figure 16–1 Origin and circulation of the cerebrospinal fluid.

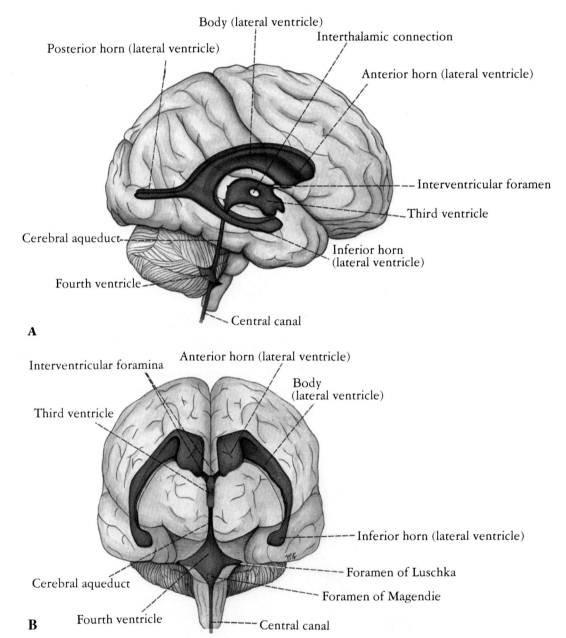

Figure 16–2 Cast of the ventricular cavities of the brain as seen from: **A**. The lateral view. **B**. The anterior view.

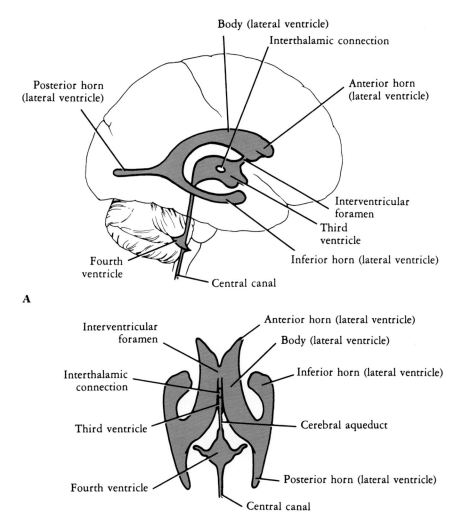

Figure 16–3   Ventricular cavities of the brain. **A.** Lateral view. **B**. Superior view.

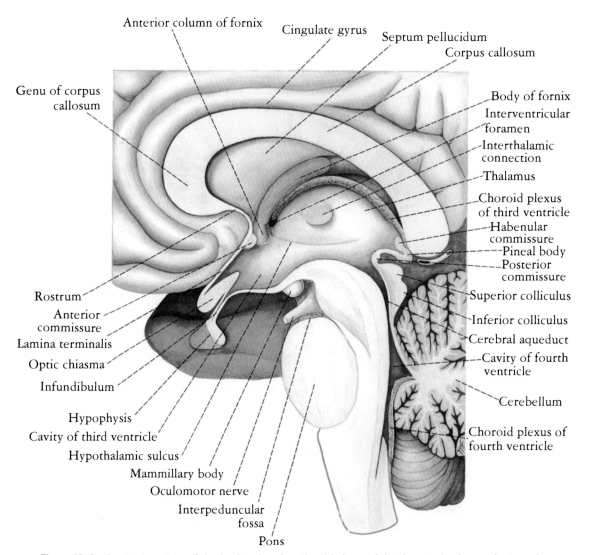

Figure 16–4   Sagittal section of the brain, showing the third ventricle, the cerebral aqueduct, and the fourth ventricle.

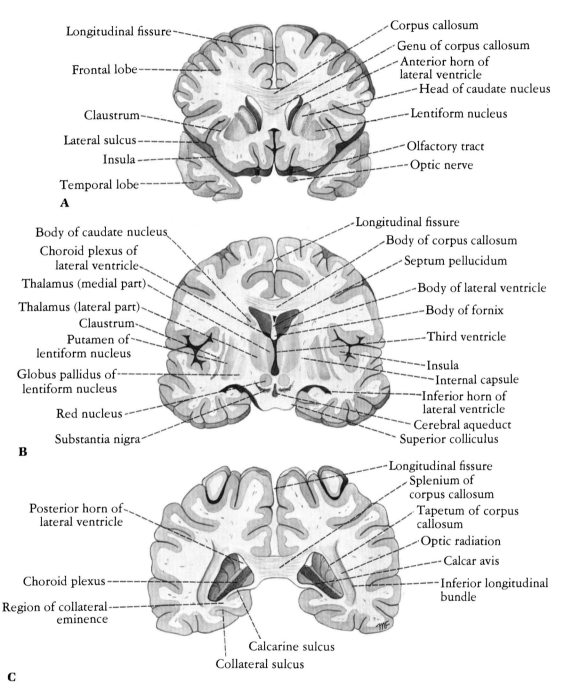

Figure 16–5 Coronal sections of the brain passing through: **A.** The anterior horn of the lateral ventricle. **B.** The body of the lateral ventricle. **C.** The posterior horn of the lateral ventricle.

of the ventricle projects into the body of the ventricle through the slitlike gap between the body of the fornix and the superior surface of the thalamus. This slitlike gap is known as the **choroidal fissure**; through it the blood vessels of the plexus invaginate the pia mater of the tela choroidea and the ependyma of the lateral ventricle. The **medial wall** is formed by the **septum pellucidum** anteriorly; posteriorly the roof and the floor come together on the medial wall (Fig. 16-5).

The **anterior horn of the lateral ventricle** extends forward into the frontal lobe (Figs. 16-2 and 16-3). It is continuous posteriorly with the body of the ventricle at the interventricular foramen. The anterior horn has a roof, a floor, and a medial wall. The **roof** is formed by the undersurface of the anterior part of the **corpus callosum**; the **genu of the corpus callosum** limits the anterior horn anteriorly (Fig. 16-5). The **floor** is formed by the rounded **head of the caudate nucleus**, and medially a small portion is formed by the superior surface of the **rostrum of the corpus callosum**. The **medial wall** is formed by the **septum pellucidum** and the **anterior column of the fornix** (Fig. 16-5).

The **posterior horn of the lateral ventricle** extends posteriorly into the occipital lobe (Figs. 16-2 and 16-3). The **roof** and **lateral wall** are formed by the fibers of the **tapetum of the corpus callosum**. Lateral to the tapetum are the fibers of the **optic radiation** (Fig. 16-5). The **medial wall** of the posterior horn has two elevations. The superior swelling is caused by the splenial fibers of the corpus callosum, called the **forceps major**, passing posteriorly into the occipital lobe; this superior swelling is referred to as the **bulb of the posterior horn**. The inferior swelling is produced by the **calcarine sulcus** and is called the **calcar avis** (Fig. 16-5).

The **inferior horn of the lateral ventricle** extends anteriorly into the temporal lobe (Figs. 16-2 and 16-3). The inferior horn has a roof and a floor (Fig. 16-5).

The **roof** is formed by the inferior surface of the **tapetum of the corpus callosum** and by the **tail of the caudate nucleus** (see Fig. 9-5). The latter passes anteriorly to end in the **amygdaloid nucleus**. Medial to the tail of the caudate nucleus is the **stria terminalis**, which also ends anteriorly in the amygdaloid nucleus.

The **floor** is formed laterally by the **collateral eminence**, produced by the **collateral** fissure, and medially by the hippocampus (see Figs. 9-3 and 9-4). The anterior end of the hippocampus is expanded and slightly furrowed to form the pes **hippocampus**. The hippocampus is composed of gray matter; however, the ventricular surface of the hippocampus is covered by a thin layer of white matter called the **alveus**, which is formed from the axons of the cells of the hippocampus. These axons converge on the medial border of the hippocampus to form a bundle known as the **fimbria**. The fimbria of the hippocampus becomes continuous posteriorly with the **posterior column of the fornix**.

In the interval between the stria terminalis and the fimbria is the temporal part of the choroidal fissure. It is here that the lower part of the **choroid plexus** of the lateral ventricle invaginates the ependyma from the medial side and closes the fissure (see Fig. 16-8B).

CHOROID PLEXUS OF THE LATERAL VENTRICLE

The **choroid plexus** projects into the ventricle on its medial aspect and is a vascular fringe composed of pia mater covered with the ependymal lining of the ventricular cavity (Fig.16-6). The choroid plexus is, in fact, the irregular lateral

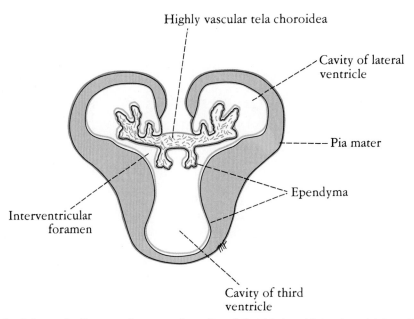

Figure 16–6   Schematic diagram of a coronal section of the third and lateral ventricles at the site of the interventricular foramina, showing the structure of the tela choroidea and its relationship with the ependyma and pia mater.

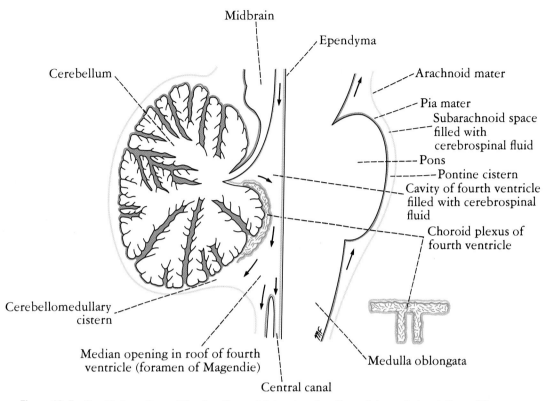

Figure 16–7   Sagittal section of the fourth ventricle, showing the origin and circulation of the cerebrospinal fluid. Note the position of the foramen of Magendie.

edge of the tela choroidea, which is a two-layered fold of pia mater situated between the fornix superiorly and the upper surface of the thalamus (Fig.16-8). At the junction of the body of the lateral ventricle and the inferior horn, the choroid plexus is continued into the inferior horn and projects through the choroidal fissure. The function of the choroid plexus is to produce cerebrospinal fluid.

Third Ventricle

The third ventricle is a slitlike cleft between the two thalami. It communicates anteriorly with the lateral ventricles through the interventricular foramina (of Monro) and posteriorly with the fourth ventricle through the cerebral aqueduct (of Sylvius) (Fig. 16-4). The walls of the third ventricle are described on page 254.

CHOROID PLEXUSES OF THE THIRD VENTRICLE

The choroid plexuses are formed from the tela choroidea situated above the roof of the ventricle (Fig. 16-6). The vascular tela choroidea projects downward on each side of the midline, invaginating the ependymal roof of the ventricle. The two vascular ridges or fringes that hang from the roof of the third ventricle form the choroid plexuses. The function of the choroid plexuses is to produce cerebrospiinal fluid.

The blood supply of the tela choroidea and therefore also of the choroid plexuses of the third and lateral ventri-

cles is derived from the **choroidal branches of the internal carotid and basilar arteries**. The venous blood drains into the internal cerebral veins, which unite to form the great cerebral vein. The great cerebral vein joins the inferior sagittal sinus to form the straight sinus.

Cerebral Aqueduct (Aqueduct of Sylvius)

The cerebral aqueduct, a narrow channel about 3/4-inch (1.8-cm) long, connects the third with the fourth ventricle (Figs. 16-2 and 16-3). It is lined with ependyma and is surrounded by a layer of gray matter called the **central gray**. The direction of flow of cerebrospinal fluid is from the third to the fourth ventricle. There is no choroid plexus in the cerebral aqueduct.

Fourth Ventricle

The fourth ventricle is a tent-shaped cavity filled with cerebrospinal fluid. It is situated anterior to the cerebellum and posterior to the pons and the superior half of the medulla oblongata (Figs. 16-4, 16-7, and 16-9). It is lined with ependyma and is continuous above with the cerebral aqueduct of the midbrain and below with the central canal of the medulla oblongata and the spinal cord (Fig. 16-3). The fourth ventricle possesses lateral boundaries, a roof, and a rhomboid-shaped floor.

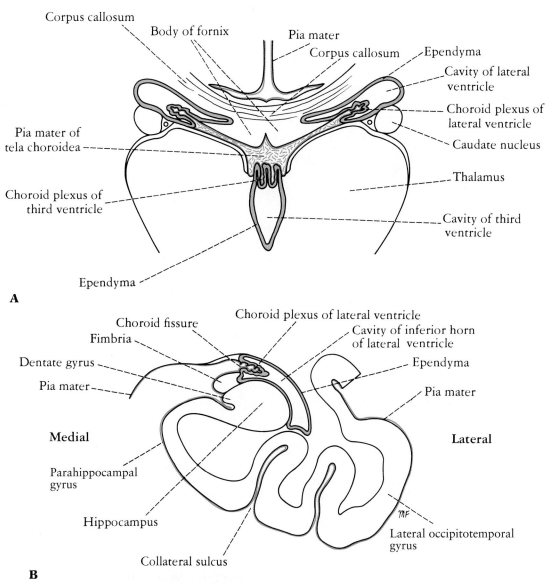

Figure 16–8   Coronal section of: **A**. The cavities of the third and lateral ventricles. **B**. The cavity of the inferior horn of the lateral ventricle.

Lateral Boundaries

The caudal part of each lateral boundary is formed by the inferior cerebellar peduncle (Fig. 16-10). The cranial part of each lateral boundary is formed by the superior cerebellar peduncle.

Roof or Posterior Wall

The tent-shaped roof projects into the cerebellum (Figs. 16-7 and 16-9). The superior part is formed by the medial borders of the two superior cerebellar peduncles and a connecting sheet of white matter called the **superior medullary**

velum (Fig. 16-11). The inferior part of the roof is formed by the **inferior medullary velum**, which consists of a thin sheet devoid of nervous tissue and formed by the ventricular ependyma and its posterior covering of pia mater (Fig. 16-12). This part of the roof is pierced in the midline by a large aperture, the **median aperture** or **foramen of Magendie** (Figs. 16-11 and 16-12). Lateral recesses extend laterally around the sides of the medulla and open anteriorly as the **lateral openings of the fourth ventricle**, or the **foramina of Luschka** (Fig. 16-13). Thus, the cavity of the fourth ventricle communicates with the subarachnoid space through a single median opening and two lateral

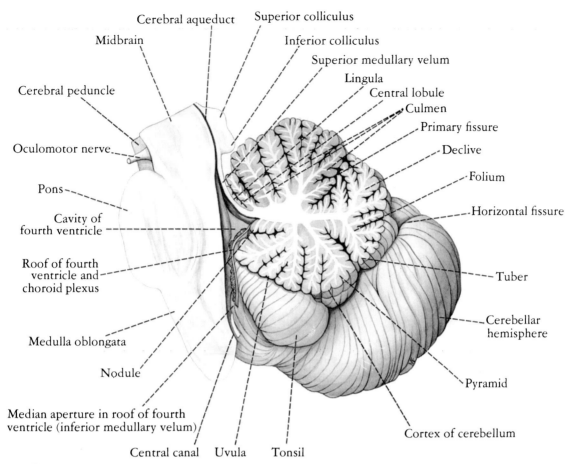

Figure 16–9 Sagittal section through the brainstem and the cerebellum showing the fourth ventricle

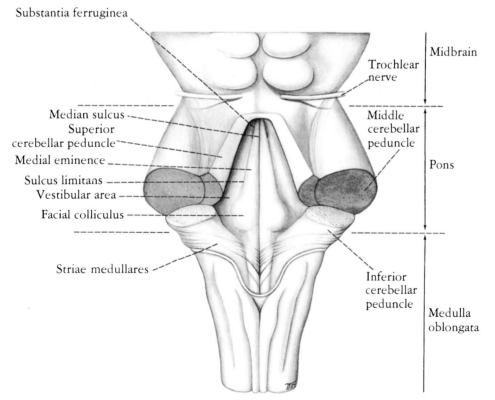

Figure 16–10 Posterior surface of the brainstem showing the floor of the fourth ventricle. The cerebellum has been removed.

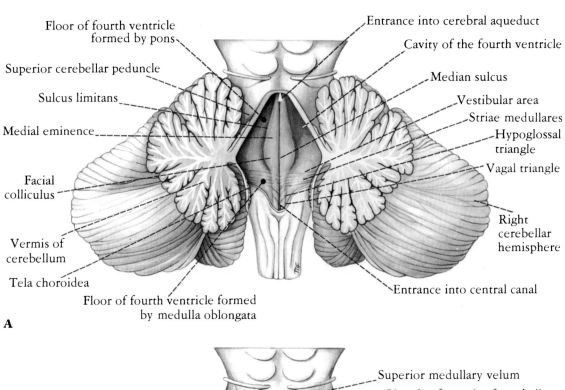

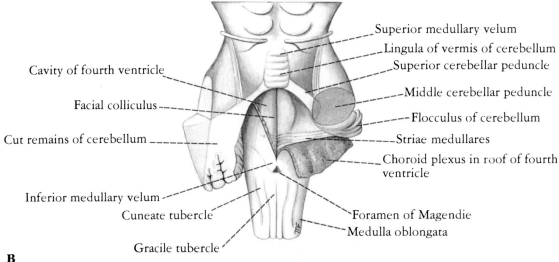

Figure 16–11 Posterior view of the cavity of the fourth ventricle. **A.** The vermis of the cerebellum has been divided in the midline and the cerebellar hemispheres have been displaced laterally. **B.** The greater part of the cerebellum has been removed, leaving the superior and inferior medullary vela. Note that the right half of the inferior medullary velum has been reflected inferiorly to reveal the choroid plexus.

apertures. These important openings permit the cerebrospinal fluid to flow from the ventricular system into the subarachnoid space.

Floor or Rhomboid Fossa

The diamond-shaped floor is formed by the posterior surface of the pons and the cranial half of the medulla oblongata (Fig. 16-10). The floor is divided into symmetrical halves by the **median sulcus**. On each side of this sulcus there is an elevation, the **medial eminence**, which is

bounded laterally by another sulcus, the **sulcus limitans**. Lateral to the sulcus limitans there is an area known as the **vestibular area** (Figs. 16-10 and 16-11). The vestibular nuclei lie beneath the vestibular area.

The **facial colliculus** is a slight swelling at the inferior end of the medial eminence that is produced by the fibers from the motor nucleus of the facial nerve looping over the abducens nucleus (Fig. 16-14). At the superior end of the sulcus limitans there is a bluish-gray area produced by a cluster of nerve cells containing melanin pigment; the cluster of cells is called the **substantia ferruginea**. Strands of nerve fibers,

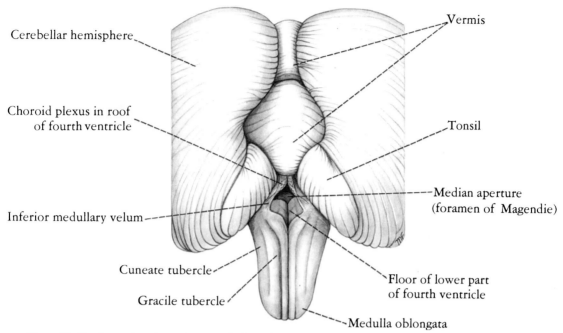

Figure 16–12 Posterior view of the roof of the fourth ventricle. The cerebellum has been displaced superiorly to show the large median aperture (foramen of Magendie).

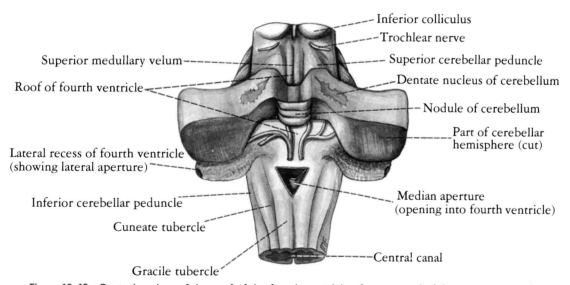

Figure 16–13 Posterior view of the roof of the fourth ventricle after removal of the greater part of the cerebellum. Shows the lateral recess and aperture (foramen of Luschka).

the **stria medullaris**, derived from the arcuate nuclei, emerge from the median sulcus and pass laterally over the medial eminence and the vestibular area and enter the inferior cerebellar peduncle to reach the cerebellum (Fig. 16-10).

Inferior to the stria medullaris the following features should be recognized in the floor of the ventricle. The most medial is the **hypoglossal triangle**, which indicates the po-

sition of the underlying **hypoglossal nucleus** (Fig. 16-11). Lateral to this is the **vagal triangle**, beneath which lies the dorsal motor nucleus of the vagus. The **area postrema** is a narrow area between the vagal triangle and the lateral margin of the ventricle, just rostral to the opening into the central canal. The inferior part of the vestibular area also lies lateral to the vagal triangle.

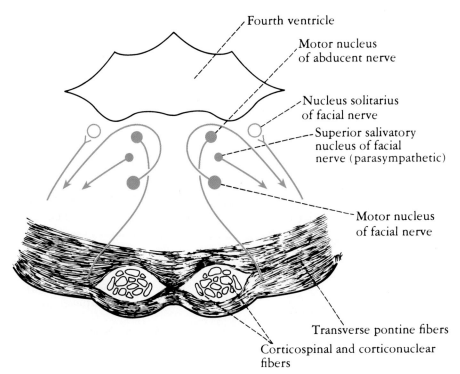

Figure 16–14 Transverse section through the developing pons showing the nuclei of the facial nerve and their relationship to the nucleus of the abducent nerve.

CHOROID PLEXUS OF THE FOURTH VENTRICLE

The choroid plexus has a T shape; the vertical part of the T is double (Fig. 16-7). It is suspended from the inferior half of the roof of the ventricle and is formed from the highly vascular tela choroidea. The tela choroidea is a two-layered fold of pia mater that projects through the roof of the ventricle and is covered by ependyma. The blood supply to the plexus is from the **posterior inferior cerebellar arteries**. The function of the choroid plexus is to produce cerebrospinal fluid.

Central Canal of the Spinal Cord and Medulla Oblongata

The central canal opens superiorly into the fourth ventricle. Inferiorly, it extends through the inferior half of the medulla oblongata and through the entire length of the spinal cord. In the conus medullaris of the spinal cord, it expands to form the **terminal ventricle** (Fig. 16-1). The central canal is closed at its lower end, is filled with cerebrospinal fluid, and is lined with ependyma. The central canal is surrounded by gray matter, the **gray commissure**. There is no choroid plexus in the central canal.

SUBARACHNOID SPACE

The subarachnoid space is the interval between the arachnoid mater and pia mater and therefore is present where these meninges envelop the brain and spinal cord (Fig. 16-1). The space is filled with cerebrospinal fluid and contains the large blood vessels of the brain (Fig. 16-15). It is traversed by a network of fine trabeculae formed of delicate connective tissue. The subarachnoid space completely surrounds the brain and extends along the olfactory nerves to the mucoperiosteum of the nose. The subarachnoid space also extends along the cerebral blood vessels as they enter and leave the substance of the brain and stops where the vessels become an arteriole or a venule.

In certain situations around the base of the brain, the arachnoid does not closely follow the surface of the brain so that the subarachnoid space expands to form **subarachnoid cisterns**. The descriptions of the **cerebellomedullary cistern**, the **pontine cistern**, and the **interpeduncular cistern**, which are the largest cisterns, are on page 435.

Inferiorly, the subarachnoid space extends beyond the lower end of the spinal cord and invests the **cauda equina** (see Fig. 1-16). The subarachnoid space ends below at the

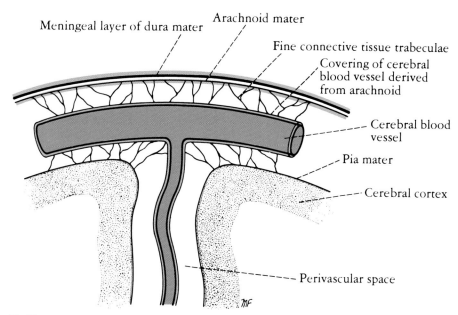

Figure 16–15 Diagram of the subarachnoid space around the cerebral hemisphere showing the relationship of the cerebral blood vessel to the meninges and cerebral cortex.

level of the interval between the second and third sacral vertebrae.

The subarachnoid space surrounds the cranial and spinal nerves and follows them to the point where they leave the skull and vertebral canal. Here the arachnoid mater and pia mater fuse with the perineurium of each nerve.

 CEREBROSPINAL FLUID

The cerebrospinal fluid is found in the ventricles of the brain and in the subarachnoid space around the brain and spinal cord. It is a clear, colorless fluid. It possesses, in solution, inorganic salts similar to those in the blood plasma. The glucose content is about half that of blood and there is only a trace of protein. Only a few cells are present and these are lymphocytes. The normal lymphocyte count is 0 to 3 cells per cubic millimeter. The pressure of the cerebrospinal fluid is kept remarkably constant. In the lateral recumbent position the pressure, as measured by spinal tap, is about 60 to 150 mm of water. This pressure may be raised by straining, coughing, or compressing the internal jugular veins in the neck (see p. 466). The total volume of cerebrospinal fluid in the subarachnoid space and within the ventricles is about 130 ml. Table 16-1 summarizes the physical characteristics and composition of the cerebrospinal fluid.

Functions

The cerebrospinal fluid, which bathes the external and internal surfaces of the brain and spinal cord, serves as a cushion between the central nervous system and the surrounding bones, thus protecting it against mechanical trauma. Because the density of the brain is only slightly greater than that of the cerebrospinal fluid, it provides mechanical buoyancy and support for the brain. The close relationship of the fluid to the nervous tissue and the blood enables it to serve as a reservoir and assist in the regulation of the contents of the skull. For example, if the brain volume

Table 16–1	The Physical Characteristics and Composition of the Cerebrospinal Fluid
Appearance	Clear and colorless
Volume	130 ml
Rate of production	0.5 ml/min
Pressure (spinal tap with patient in lateral recumbent position)	60–150 mm of water
Composition	
Protein	15–45 mg/100 ml
Glucose	50–85 mg/100 ml
Chloride	720–750 mg/100 ml
No. of cells	0–3 lymphocytes/cu mm

or the blood volume increases, the cerebrospinal fluid volume decreases. Since the cerebrospinal fluid is an ideal physiological substrate, it probably plays an active part in the nourishment of the nervous tissue; it almost certainly assists in the removal of products of neuronal metabolism. It is possible that the secretions of the pineal gland influence the activities of the pituitary gland by circulating through the cerebrospinal fluid in the third ventricle (see p. 252).

Box 16-1 summarizes the functions of the cerebrospinal fluid.

Formation

The cerebrospinal fluid is formed mainly in the choroid plexuses of the lateral, third, and fourth ventricles; some originates from the ependymal cells lining the ventricles

---

Box 16–1   The Functions of the Cerebrospinal Fluid

1. Cushions and protects the central nervous system from trauma
2. Provides mechanical buoyancy and support for the brain
3. Serves as a reservoir and assists in the regulation of the contents of the skull
4. Nourishes the central nervous system
5. Removes metabolites from the central nervous system
6. Serves as a pathway for pineal secretions to reach the pituitary gland

---

and from the brain substance through the perivascular spaces.

The choroid plexuses have a much folded surface and each fold consists of a core of vascular connective tissue covered with cuboidal epithelium of the ependyma (Fig. 16-16). Electron-microscopic examination of the epithelial cells shows that their free surfaces are covered with microvilli. The blood of the capillaries is separated from the ventricular lumen by endothelium, a basement membrane, and the surface epithelium. The epithelial cells are fenestrated and permeable to large molecules.

The choroid plexuses actively secrete cerebrospinal fluid and at the same time they actively transport nervous system metabolites from the cerebrospinal fluid into the blood. Active transport also explains the fact that the concentrations of potassium, calcium, magnesium, bicarbonate, and glucose are lower in the cerebrospinal fluid than in the blood plasma.

The cerebrospinal fluid is produced continuously at a rate of about 0.5 ml per minute and with a total volume of about 130 ml; this corresponds to a turnover time of about 5 hours.

Circulation

The circulation begins with its secretion from the choroid plexuses in the ventricles and its production from the brain surface. The fluid passes from the lateral ventricles into the third ventricle through the interventricular foramina (Figs. 16-1 and 16-17). It then passes into the fourth ventricle through the cere-

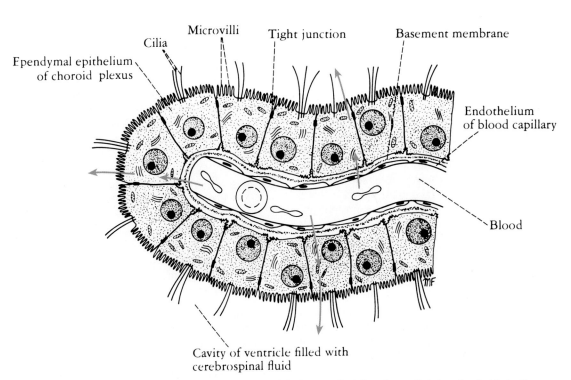

Figure 16–16 Microscopic structure of the choroid plexus, showing the path taken by fluids in the formation of cerebrospinal fluid.

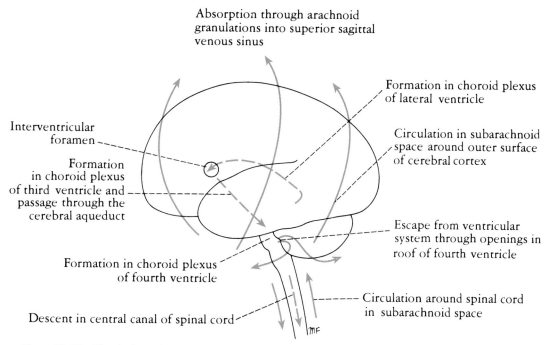

Figure 16–17 Circulation of the cerebrospinal fluid. The dashed line indicates the course taken by fluid within the cavities of the central nervous system.

bral aqueduct. The circulation is aided by the arterial pulsations of the choroid plexuses and by the cilia on the ependymal cells lining the ventricles.

From the fourth ventricle, the fluid passes through the median aperture and the lateral foramina of the lateral recesses of the fourth ventricle and enters the subarachnoid space. The fluid slowly moves through the cerebellomedullary cistern and pontine cisterns and flows superiorly through the tentorial notch of the tentorium cerebelli to reach the inferior surface of the cerebrum (Figs. 16-1 and 16-17). It now moves superiorly over the lateral aspect of each cerebral hemisphere. Some of the cerebrospinal fluid moves inferiorly in the subarachnoid space around the spinal cord and cauda equina. The pulsations of the cerebral and spinal arteries and the movements of the vertebral column, respiration, coughing, and the changing of the positions of the body facilitate this gradual flow of fluid.

The cerebrospinal fluid not only bathes the ependymal and pial surfaces of the brain and spinal cord but also penetrates the nervous tissue along the blood vessels.

Absorption

The main sites for the absorption of the cerebrospinal fluid are the **arachnoid villi** that project into the dural venous sinuses, especially the **superior sagittal sinus** (Fig. 16-18). The arachnoid villi tend to be grouped together to form elevations known as **arachnoid granulations**. Structurally, each arachnoid villus is a diverticulum of the subarachnoid space that pierces the dura mater. The arachnoid diverticulum is capped by a thin cellular layer, which in turn is cov-

ered by the endothelium of the venous sinus. The arachnoid granulations increase in number and size with age and tend to become calcified with advanced age.

The absorption of cerebrospinal fluid into the venous sinuses occurs when the cerebrospinal fluid pressure exceeds the pressure in the sinus. Electron-microscopic studies of the arachnoid villi indicate that fine tubules lined with endothelium permit a direct flow of fluid from the subarachnoid space into the lumen of the venous sinuses. Should the venous pressure rise and exceed the cerebrospinal fluid pressure, compression of the tips of the villi closes the tubules and prevents the reflux of blood into the subarachnoid space. The arachnoid villi thus serve as valves.

Some of the cerebrospinal fluid probably is absorbed directly into the veins in the subarachnoid space and some possibly escapes through the perineural lymph vessels of the cranial and spinal nerves.

Because the production of cerebrospinal fluid from the choroid plexuses is constant, the rate of absorption of cerebrospinal fluid through the arachnoid villi controls the cerebrospinal fluid pressure.

Extensions of the Subarachnoid Space

A sleeve of the subarachnoid space extends around the optic nerve to the back of the eyeball (Fig. 16-19). Here the arachnoid mater and pia mater fuse with the sclera. The central artery and vein of the retina cross this extension of the subarachnoid space to enter the optic nerve, and they may be compressed in patients with raised cerebrospinal fluid pressure.

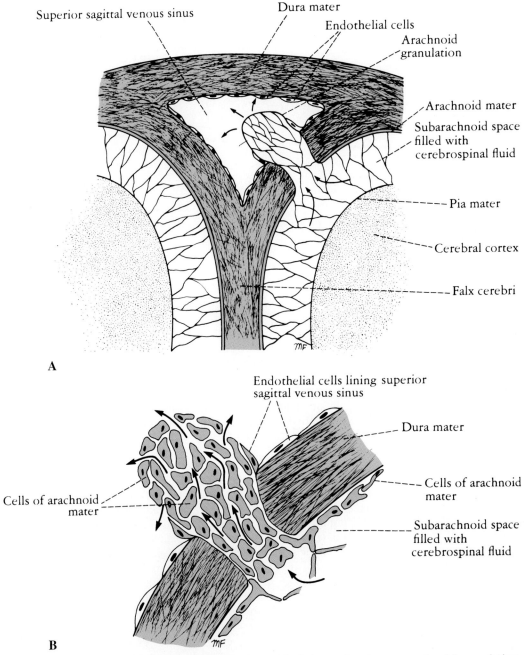

Figure 16–18 **A.** Coronal section of the superior sagittal sinus, showing an arachnoid granulation. **B.** Magnified view of an arachnoid granulation, showing the path taken by the cerebrospinal fluid into the venous system.

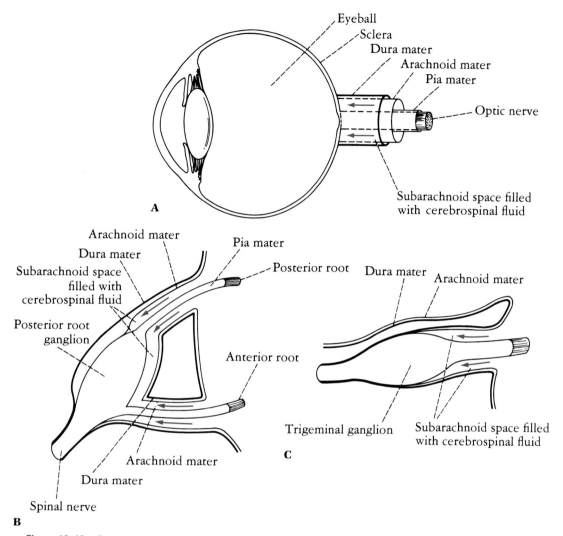

Figure 16–19 Course taken by cerebrospinal fluid around: **A.** The optic nerve. **B.** The roots of a spinal nerve. **C.** The trigeminal nerve.

Small extensions of the subarachnoid space also occur around the other cranial and spinal nerves (Fig. 16-19). It is here that some communication may occur between the subarachnoid space and the perineural lymph vessels.

The subarachnoid space also extends around the arteries and veins of the brain and spinal cord at points where they penetrate the nervous tissue (Fig. 16-15). The pia mater, however, quickly fuses with the outer coat of the blood vessel below the surface of the brain and spinal cord, thus closing off the subarachnoid space.

 BLOOD-BRAIN AND BLOOD-CEREBROSPINAL FLUID BARRIERS

The central nervous system requires a very stable environment in order to function normally. This stability is provided by isolating the nervous system from the blood by the exis-

tence of the so-called blood-brain barrier and the blood-cerebrospinal fluid barrier.

BLOOD-BRAIN BARRIER

The experiments of Paul Ehrlich in 1882 showed that living animals injected intravascularly with vital dyes, such as trypan blue, demonstrated staining of all the tissues of the body except the brain and spinal cord. Later, it was demonstrated that although most of the brain is not stained after the intravenous injection of trypan blue, the following areas do in fact become stained: the pineal gland, the posterior lobe of the pituitary, the tuber cinereum, the wall of the optic recess, and the vascular area postrema* at the lower

---

*Area of the medulla on the floor of the fourth ventricle just rostral to the opening into the central canal.

end of the fourth ventricle. These observations led to the concept of a blood-brain barrier (for which blood-brain-spinal cord barrier would be a more accurate name).

The permeability of the blood-brain barrier is inversely related to the size of the molecules and directly related to their lipid solubility. Gases and water pass readily through the barrier, whereas glucose and electrolytes pass more slowly. The barrier is almost impermeable to plasma proteins and other large organic molecules. Compounds with molecular weights of about 60,000 and higher remain within the blood circulatory system. This would explain why in the early experiments with trypan blue, which quickly binds to the plasma protein albumin, the dye did not pass into the neural tissue in the greater part of the brain.

Structure

Examination of an electron micrograph of the central nervous system shows that the lumen of a blood capillary is separated from the extracellular spaces around the neurons and neuroglia by the following structures: (1) the endothelial cells in the wall of the capillary, (2) a continuous basement membrane surrounding the capillary outside the endothelial cells, and (3) the foot processes of the astrocytes that adhere to the outer surface of the capillary wall (Fig. 16-20).

The use of electron-dense markers such as lanthanum and horseradish peroxidase (Brightman and Reese, 1969) has shown that these substances do not penetrate between the endothelial cells of the capillaries because of the presence of tight junctions that form belts around the cells.

When the dense markers are introduced into the extracellular spaces of the neuropil, they pass between the perivascular foot processes of the astrocytes as far as the endothelial lining of the capillary. On the basis of this evidence, it is now known that the tight junctions between the endothelial cells of the blood capillaries are responsible for the blood-brain barrier* (Fig. 16-20).

Although the blood-brain barrier exists in the newborn, there is evidence that it is more permeable to certain substances than it is in the adult.

The structure of the blood-brain barrier is not identical in all regions of the central nervous system. In fact, in those areas where the blood-brain barrier appears to be absent, the capillary endothelium contains fenestrations across which proteins and small organic molecules may pass from the blood to the nervous tissue (Fig. 16-21). It has been suggested that areas such as the area postrema of the floor of the fourth ventricle and the hypothalamus may serve as sites at which neuronal receptors may sample the chemical content of the plasma directly. The hypothalamus, which is involved in the regulation of the metabolic activity of the body, might bring about appropriate modifications of activity, thereby protecting the nervous tissue.

---

*Peripheral nerves are isolated from the blood in the same manner as the central nervous system. The endothelial cells of the blood capillaries in the endoneurium have tight junctions, so that there is a blood-nerve barrier.

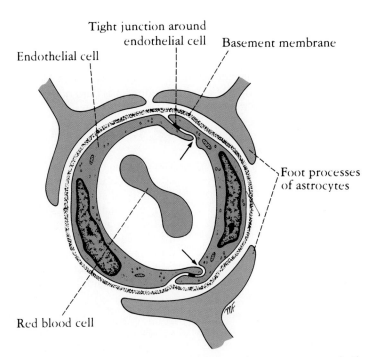

Figure 16–20　Cross section of a blood capillary of the central nervous system in the area where the blood-brain barrier exists.

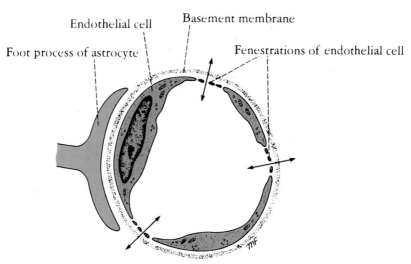

Figure 16–21 Cross section of a blood capillary of the central nervous system where the blood-brain barrier appears to be absent. Note the presence of fenestrations in the endothelial cells.

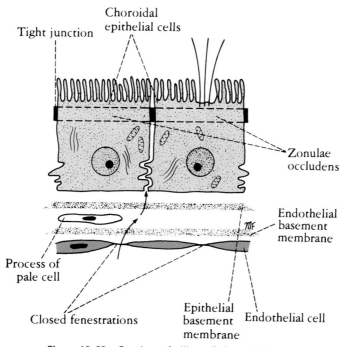

Figure 16–22 Section of villus of choroid plexus.

BLOOD-CEREBROSPINAL FLUID BARRIER

There is free passage of water, gases, and lipid-soluble substances from the blood to the cerebrospinal fluid. Macromolecules such as proteins and most hexoses other than glucose are unable to enter the cerebrospinal fluid. It has been suggested that a barrier similar to the blood-brain barrier exists in the choroid plexuses.

Structure

Electron-microscopic examination of a villus of a choroid plexus shows that the lumen of a blood capillary is separated from the lumen of the ventricle by the following structures: (1) the endothelial cells, which are fenestrated and have very thin walls (the fenestrations are not true perforations but are filled by a thin diaphragm); (2) a continuous basement membrane surrounding the capillary outside the endothelial cells; (3) scattered pale cells with flattened processes; and (4) a continuous basement membrane, upon which rest (5) the choroidal epithelial cells (Fig. 16-22). The use of electron-dense markers has not been entirely successful in localizing the barrier precisely. Horseradish peroxidase injected intravenously appears as a coating on the luminal surface of the endothelial cells and in many areas examined it did pass between the endothelial cells. It is probable that the tight junctions between the choroidal epithelial cells serve as the barrier (Fig. 16-22).

CEREBROSPINAL FLUID-BRAIN INTERFACE

Although vital dyes given by intravenous injection do not gain access to most brain tissues, if the dyes are injected into the subarachnoid space or into the ventricles, they soon enter the extracellular spaces around the neurons and glial cells. Thus there is no comparable physiological barrier between the cerebrospinal fluid and the extracellular compartment of the central nervous system. It is interesting, however, to consider the structures that separate the cerebrospinal fluid from the nervous tissue. Three sites must be examined: (1) the pia-covered surface of the brain and spinal cord, (2) the perivascular extensions of the sub-

arachnoid space into the nervous tissue, and (3) the ependymal surface of the ventricles (Fig. 16-23).

The pia-covered surface of the brain consists of a loosely arranged layer of pial cells resting on a basement membrane (Fig. 16-23). Beneath the basement membrane are the astrocytic foot processes. No intercellular junctions exist between adjacent pial cells or between adjacent astrocytes, so that the extracellular spaces of the nervous tissue are in almost direct continuity with the subarachnoid space.

The prolongation of the subarachnoid space into the central nervous tissue quickly ends below the surface of the brain, where the fusion of the outer covering of the blood vessel with the pial covering of the nervous tissue occurs.

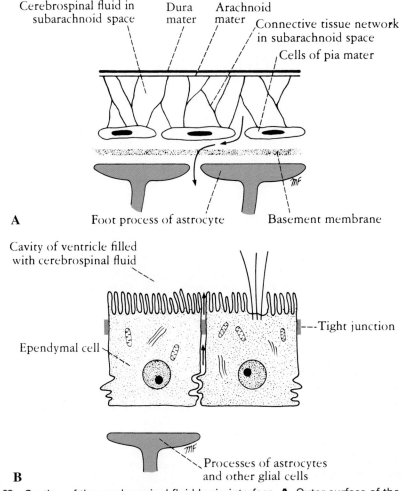

Figure 16–23   Section of the cerebrospinal fluid-brain interface. **A.** Outer surface of the brain. **B**. Ventricular surface of the brain.

The ventricular surface of the brain is covered with columnar ependymal cells with localized tight junctions (Fig. 16-23).

Intercellular channels exist that permit free communication between the ventricular cavity and the extracellular neuronal space. The ependyma does not have a basement membrane and there are no specialized astrocytic foot processes because the neuroglial cells are loosely arranged.

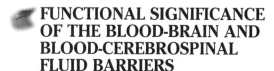

FUNCTIONAL SIGNIFICANCE OF THE BLOOD-BRAIN AND BLOOD-CEREBROSPINAL FLUID BARRIERS

In normal conditions, these two important semipermeable barriers protect the brain and spinal cord from potentially harmful substances while permitting gases and nutriments to enter the nervous tissue.

CLINICAL NOTES

THE OPTIC NERVE, RAISED CEREBROSPINAL FLUID PRESSURE, AND PAPILLEDEMA

The optic nerves are surrounded by sheaths derived from the pia mater, arachnoid mater, and dura mater. There is an extension of the intracranial subarachnoid space forward around the optic nerve to the back of the eyeball (Fig. 16-19). A rise of cerebrospinal fluid pressure caused by an intracranial tumor will compress the thin walls of the retinal vein as it crosses the extension of the subarachnoid space to enter the optic nerve. This will result in congestion of the retinal vein, bulging forward of the optic disc, and edema of the disc; the last condition is referred to as **papilledema**. Since both subarachnoid extensions are continuous with the intracranial subarachnoid space, both eyes will exhibit papilledema. Persistent papilledema leads to optic atrophy and blindness.

HYDROCEPHALUS

Hydrocephalus is an abnormal increase in the volume of the cerebrospinal fluid within the skull. If the hydrocephalus is accompanied by a raised cerebrospinal fluid pressure, then it is due to either (1) an abnormal increase in the formation of the fluid, (2) a blockage of the circulation of the fluid, or (3) a diminished absorption of the fluid. Rarely, hydrocephalus occurs with a normal cerebrospinal fluid pressure and in these patients there is a compensatory hypoplasia or atrophy of the brain substance.

Varieties

Two varieties of hydrocephalus are described: noncommunicating and communicating. In **noncommunicating hydrocephalus**, the raised pressure of the cerebrospinal fluid is due to blockage at some point between its formation at the choroid plexuses and its exit through the foramina in the roof of the fourth ventricle. In **communicating hydrocephalus,** there is no obstruction within or to the outflow from the ventricular system; the cerebrospinal fluid freely reaches the subarachnoid space and is found to be under increased pressure.

Causes

EXCESSIVE FORMATION OF CEREBROSPINAL FLUID
This condition is rare and may occur when there is a tumor of the choroid plexuses.

BLOCKAGE OF THE CIRCULATION OF CEREBROSPINAL FLUID
An obstruction of the interventricular foramen by a tumor will block the drainage of the lateral ventricle on that side. The continued production of cerebrospinal fluid by the choroid plexus of that ventricle will cause distention of that ventricle and atrophy of the surrounding neural tissue.

An obstruction in the cerebral aqueduct may be congenital or result from inflammation or pressure from a tumor. This causes a symmetrical distention of both lateral ventricles and distention of the third ventricle.

Obstruction of the median aperture (foramen of Magendie) in the roof of the fourth ventricle and the two lateral apertures (foramina of Luschka) in the lateral recesses of the fourth ventricle by inflammatory exudate, or by tumor growth, will produce symmetrical dilatation of both lateral ventricles and the third and fourth ventricles.

Sometimes inflammatory exudate secondary to meningitis will block the subarachnoid space and obstruct the flow of cerebrospinal fluid over the outer surface of the cerebral hemispheres. Here, again, the entire ventricular system of the brain will become distended.

DIMINISHED ABSORPTION OF CEREBROSPINAL FLUID
Interference with the absorption of cerebrospinal fluid at the arachnoid granulations may be caused by inflammatory exudate, venous thrombosis or pressure on the venous sinuses, or obstruction of the internal jugular vein.

CLINICAL INVESTIGATION OF THE CEREBRAL VENTRICLES

The size of the cerebral ventricles may be investigated clinically by the use of (1) CT and MRI and, if necessary, (2) intracranial pneumography.

CT and **MRI** are safe and easy to perform. The outline of the ventricles may be demonstrated by using these methods (see Figs. 1-23 and 1-24). Apart from ventricular distention or distortion, the cerebral tumor causing the condition also may be demonstrated.

Intracranial pneumography is essentially the replacement of cerebrospinal fluid within the ventricles and subarachnoid space with air or oxygen. Because the air or gas is less dense than the fluid or neural tissue, the ventricles and cerebral gyri can be visualized. In an **encephalogram**, the air or oxygen is introduced through a spinal tap. Radiographs of the skull are then made. In a **ventriculogram**, the air or oxygen is introduced into the lateral ventricle through a needle inserted through a hole in the skull (in a young child the needle may be inserted through a suture). Radiographs of the skull then are made. In ventriculography, only the ventricles are visualized.

CEREBROSPINAL FLUID PRESSURE AND COMPOSITION IN DISEASE

The examination of cerebrospinal fluid can be of great assistance in making a neurological diagnosis.

The clinical measurement of cerebrospinal fluid pressure by means of a spinal tap is described on page 18. An increase in pressure is usually due to meningitis or an increase in volume of the brain produced by edema, tumor formation, a cerebral abscess, or the presence of a hematoma.

The gross appearance of a specimen of cerebrospinal fluid is of great value. Normally, it is clear and colorless. A cloudy fluid usually indicates the presence of polymorphonuclear leukocytes or an excessive quantity of protein. An increase in the white cells would suggest inflammation of the meninges or encephalitis. An increase in protein content implies a change in the vascular permeability and protein escapes into the cerebrospinal fluid. A raised protein content is seen in tuberculous meningitis, and poliomyelitis. In multiple sclerosis the gamma globulin is elevated due to production of immunoglobulins in the brain and spinal cord.

Normal cerebrospinal fluid does not contain red blood cells. Gross blood in the cerebrospinal fluid is usually caused by contamination brought about by puncture of a vertebral vein by the spinal tap needle. Uniform blood staining is found in subarachnoid hemorrhage. Yellow coloration or **xanthochromia** is caused by the presence of oxyhemoglobin in the fluid some hours after subarachnoid hemorrhage.

Normal cerebrospinal fluid contains fewer than four white cells. In bacterial infections many thousands of cells may be present per cubic millimeter. In viral infections of the nervous system a moderate lymphocyte reaction may occur. A slight rise in lymphocyte count may also occur in cerebral tumors, cerebral infarction, and multiple sclerosis.

The glucose level in the cerebrospinal fluid may disappear completely in acute bacterial meningitis but remains normal in viral infections.

The normal physical characteristics and composition of cerebrospinal fluid are summarized in Table 16-1.

Blockage of the Subarachnoid Space in the Vertebral Canal

A block of the subarachnoid space in the vertebral canal may be caused by a tumor of the spinal cord or the meninges. Performing a spinal tap is of great value in making a diagnosis. The normal pressure of cerebrospinal fluid with the patient lying quietly on his or her side and breathing through the mouth is between 60 mm and 150 mm of water. If the flow of cerebrospinal fluid in the subarachnoid space is blocked, the normal variations in pressure corresponding to the pulse and respiration are reduced or absent. Compression of the internal jugular veins in the neck raises the cerebral venous pressure and inhibits the absorption of cerebrospinal fluid in the arachnoid villi and granulations, thus producing a rise in the manometric reading of the cerebrospinal fluid pressure. If this fails to occur, the subarachnoid space is blocked and the patient is exhibiting a positive **Queckenstedt's sign**. Should the tumor completely occupy the vertebral canal in the region of the cauda equina, no cerebrospinal fluid may flow out of the spinal tap needle.

Normally the cerebrospinal fluid is clear. In the presence of a tumor the cerebrospinal fluid may become yellow and clot spontaneously owing to the rise in protein content.

Tumors of the Fourth Ventricle

Tumors may arise in the vermis of the cerebellum or in the pons and invade the fourth ventricle. **Ependymomas** arising from the ependymal cells lining the ventricle also occur. Tumors in this region may invade the cerebellum and produce the symptoms and signs of cerebellar deficiency, or they may press upon the vital nuclear centers situated beneath the floor of the ventricle; the hypoglossal and vagal nuclei, for example, control movements of the tongue, swallowing, respiration, heart rate, and blood pressure.

Blood-Brain Barrier in the Fetus and Newborn

In the fetus, the newborn child, or premature infant, where these barriers are not fully developed, toxic substances such as bilirubin can readily enter the central nervous system and produce yellowing of the brain and kernicterus. This is not possible in the adult.

Brain Trauma and the Blood-Brain Barrier

Any injury to the brain, whether it be due to direct trauma or to inflammatory or chemical toxins, causes a breakdown of the blood-brain barrier, allowing the free diffusion of large molecules into the nervous tissue. It is believed that this is brought about by actual destruction of the vascular endothelial cells or disruption of their tight junctions.

Drugs and the Blood-Brain Barrier

The systemic administration of **penicillin** results in only a small amount entering the central nervous system. This is fortunate, because penicillin in high concentrations is toxic to nervous tissue. In the presence of meningitis, however, the meninges become more permeable locally, at the site of inflammation, thus permitting sufficient antibiotic to reach the infection. **Chloramphenicol** and the **tetracyclines** readily cross the blood-brain barrier and enter the nervous tissue. The **sulfonamide** drugs also easily pass through the blood-brain barrier.

Lipid-soluble substances such as the anesthetic agent **thiopental** rapidly enter the brain after intravenous injection. On the other hand, water-soluble substances such as exogenous **norepinephrine** cannot cross the blood-brain barrier. **Phenylbutazone** is a drug that becomes bound to plasma protein and the large drug protein molecule is un-able to cross the barrier. Most tertiary amines such as **atropine** are lipid-soluble and quickly enter the brain, whereas the quaternary compounds such as **atropine methylnitrate** do not.

In Parkinson's disease there is a deficiency of the neurotransmitter dopamine in the corpus striatum. Unfortunately, dopamine cannot be used in the treatment, as it will not cross the blood-brain barrier. L-Dopa readily crosses the barrier and has been used with great success.

TUMORS AND THE BLOOD-BRAIN BARRIER

Brain tumors frequently possess blood vessels that have no blood-brain barriers. Anaplastic malignant astrocytomas, glioblastomas, and secondary metastatic tumors lack the normal barriers. However, slow growing tumors often have normal vascular barriers.

Clinical Problem Solving

1. A 55-year-old man was being investigated for signs and symptoms that suggested the presence of a cerebral tumor. Examination of the CT scan showed gross enlargement and distortion of the left lateral ventricle. What other investigation might be carried out in this patient to display the ventricles of the brain? Using your knowledge of neuroanatomy, determine the location of the tumor in this patient.

2. A 3-year-old child had been referred to the children's hospital because the circumference of his head greatly exceeded the normal limit for his age. After a careful history had been taken and a detailed physical examination had been performed, a diagnosis of hydrocephalus was made. What is your definition of hydrocephalus? Name three common causes of hydrocephalus in young children.

3. A 50-year-old man was found on ophthalmoscopic examination to have edema of both optic discs (bilateral papilledema) and congestion of the retinal veins. The cause of the condition was found to be a rapidly growing intracranial tumor. Using your knowledge of neuroanatomy, explain the papilledema. Why does the patient exhibit bilateral papilledema?

4. A 38-year-old man was admitted to the neurosurgery ward with symptoms of persistent headache and vomiting and some unsteadiness in walking. The headache started 6 weeks previously and became progressively worse. On examination it was found that he could not sit up in bed unsupported. The limbs on the right side of the body showed some loss of tone. Examination of the patient when he stood up showed a marked loss of equilibrium. Examination of the cranial nerves showed central deafness of the right ear. Ophthalmoscopic examination showed severe bilateral papilledema. Using your knowl-edge of neuroanatomy, explain the symptoms and signs experienced by this patient and try to make a diagnosis.

5. A 4-year-old girl was found to have tuberculous meningitis. She was immediately admitted to the hospital and administration of streptomycin and isoniazid was commenced. As soon as this therapy was started, she was also administered steroid hormones to reduce the incidence of adhesions. She recovered fully, with no complications. Using your knowledge of neuroanatomy, explain why it is important to prevent the formation of adhesions in the subarachnoid space.

6. A 5-year-old girl with symptoms of headache, general malaise, and vomiting was admitted to the children's hospital. On examination, the body temperature was found to be 104°F and the pulse rate was rapid. Attempts to flex the neck produced pain and resulted in the patient's flexing her hip and knee joints. A spinal tap was performed and the cerebrospinal fluid was seen to be cloudy, and the pressure was raised to 190 mm of water. Microscopic examination of the fluid showed a large number of polymorphonuclear leukocytes. A diagnosis of meningitis was made. Subsequent culture revealed the infection to be a meningococcal meningitis. The resident vaguely remembered reading in a textbook the importance of the blood-brain barrier in the use of antibiotics for the treatment of meningitis. What is the blood-brain barrier? Does the presence of the blood-brain barrier influence your choice and dose of antibiotics to be used in this patient?

7. During a ward round in the children's hospital, the pediatrician informed the students that the 4-day-old baby with jaundice had a serum indirect bilirubin level of 45 mg per 100 ml and that by now the bile pigment was staining the brain a yellow color (kernicterus). The neuronal damage was revealed clinically by lethargy and

poor feeding habits and by occasional muscle spasms. She said the prognosis was very poor. One of the students observed that he could not understand why the bile pigment was having such a dramatic effect on the baby. Recently he had examined a patient who was dying of inoperable carcinoma of the head of the pancreas with total obstruction of the common bile duct. In that patient the skin was a deep yellow but, apart from complaints of the intense skin irritation owing to the high concentra-

tion of bile salts in the blood, and loss of weight, the patient had no symptoms and no neurological abnormalities. Explain why the baby had neuronal damage and the adult did not.

8. Name five areas of the brain where the blood-brain barrier appears to be absent. What do you think is the significance of the fact that in a few areas of the brain the barrier is absent?

Answers to Clinical Problem Solving

1. An MRI shows the outline of the ventricles very well. Occasionally, when these methods show insufficient detail, a ventriculogram can be obtained. This procedure consists of the introduction of air or oxygen into the lateral ventricle through a needle inserted through a burr hole in the skull.

   Since the left lateral ventricle was the only part of the ventricular system that showed distention and distortion, one can assume that the tumor had closed off the left interventricular foramen and therefore was in the vicinity of that foramen. This was confirmed on the CT scan.

2. Hydrocephalus is a condition in which there is an abnormal increase in the volume of cerebrospinal fluid within the skull. Congenital atresia of the cerebral aqueduct, meningitis, tumors, and blockage of the arachnoid granulations by subarachnoid bleeding or inflammatory exudate are common causes of this condition in young children.

3. There is an extension of the intracranial subarachnoid space forward around the optic nerve to the back of the eyeball. A rise in cerebrospinal fluid pressure caused by an intracranial tumor will compress the thin walls of the retinal vein as it crosses the extension of the subarachnoid space to enter the optic nerve. This will result in congestion of the retinal vein, bulging of the optic disc, and edema of the disc. Since both subarachnoid extensions are continuous with the intracranial subarachnoid space, both eyes will exhibit papilledema.

4. This man was operated on and found to have a large astrocytoma of the vermis of the cerebellum. The tumor had severely encroached upon the cavity of the fourth ventricle, producing internal hydrocephalus and pressure on the floor of the ventricle.

   The symptoms of headache and persistent vomiting were produced by a raised intracranial pressure caused by the enlarging tumor. The tumor also blocked off the median and lateral apertures in the roof of the fourth ventricle, causing an internal hydrocephalus, which further raised the intracranial pressure. The bilateral papilledema was secondary to the raised intracranial pressure. The inability to sit up in bed (truncal ataxia) and the loss of equilibrium on standing were due to the tumor involvement of the vermis of the cerebellum. The

loss of tone of the muscles of the right limbs indicated spread of the tumor to involve the right cerebellar hemisphere. Central deafness on the right side was due to involvement of the right eighth cranial nerve nuclei by the tumor mass. The patient died 6 months after neurosurgical exploration.

5. Steroid hormones (e.g., prednisone) inhibit the normal inflammatory reaction and thereby reduce the incidence of fibrous adhesions. It is important to prevent the formation of such adhesions because they can block the openings in the roof of the fourth ventricle, thus preventing the escape of cerebrospinal fluid into the subarachnoid space from within the ventricular system. Adhesions also can prevent the flow of cerebrospinal fluid over the cerebral hemispheres or reduce the absorption of the fluid into the arachnoid granulations. Thus adhesions of the meninges may result in hydrocephalus.

6. The blood-brain barrier is a semipermeable barrier that exists between the blood and the extracellular spaces of the nervous tissue of the brain. It permits the passage of water, gases, glucose, electrolytes, and amino acids, but it is impermeable to substances with a large molecular weight.

   Yes, the presence of the blood-brain barrier does affect the choice and dose of antibiotics. The antibiotic penicillin, when injected intramuscularly into a normal individual, is found in much lower concentrations in the cerebrospinal fluid than in the blood; this is due to the existence of the blood-brain barrier and the blood-cerebrospinal fluid barrier. Inflammation of the meninges results in an increased permeability of the meningeal blood vessels, and consequently the concentration of penicillin rises in the cerebrospinal fluid. It is important, however, for the treatment to be effective in patients with meningitis, to give very large doses of penicillin intravenously.

   By contrast, chloramphenicol and the sulfonamides rapidly cross the blood-brain and blood-cerebrospinal fluid barriers, so that an adequate concentration in the cerebrospinal fluid can easily be maintained.

7. The blood-brain barrier in the newborn child is not fully developed and is more permeable than that in the adult. Indirect bilirubin readily crosses the barrier in the newborn but does not do so in the adult. Once the bile pigment reaches the extracellular spaces of the brain tissue

in the newborn, it passes into the neurons and neuroglial cells. This results in abnormal cell function and eventually neuronal death.

8. The pineal gland, the posterior lobe of the pituitary, the tuber cinereum, the wall of the optic recess, and the vascular area postrema at the inferior end of the fourth ventricle are parts of the brain where the capillary endothelium contains open fenestrations across which proteins and small organic molecules may pass. It is in these areas that the blood-brain barrier appears to be absent.

The significance of the absence of the barrier in the pineal gland is not understood. It is possible that the pinealocytes, in order to function normally, require a close relationship with the blood plasma in order to sample the concentrations of hormones.

The absence of the blood-brain barrier in the region of the hypothalamus may allow this area of the brain to sample the chemical content of the plasma, so that appropriate modifications of metabolic activity may take place, thus protecting the nervous tissue as a whole.

Review Questions

Directions: Each of the numbered items in this section is followed by answers that are positively phrased. Select the ONE lettered answer that is an EXCEPTION.

1. The following statements concerning the ventricular system are correct **except:**
   (a) The aqueduct of Sylvius connects the third ventricle with the fourth ventricle.
   (b) The two lateral ventricles communicate directly with one another through the foramen of Monro.
   (c) The ventricles are developed from the neural tube in the embryo.
   (d) The ventricular system is lined throughout with ependyma.
   (e) The choroid plexuses are found in the lateral ventricles and the third and the fourth ventricles.

2. The following statements concerning the ventricular system are correct **except:**
   (a) The choroid plexus of the lateral ventricle projects into the cavity on its medial side through the choroidal fissure.
   (b) The fourth ventricle has a diamond-shaped floor called the rhomboid fossa.
   (c) The pineal body is suspended from the roof of the fourth ventricle.
   (d) The nerve centers controlling the heart rate and blood pressure lie beneath the floor of the fourth ventricle.
   (e) The foramen of Magendie is an aperture in the inferior medullary velum of the fourth ventricle.

3. The following statements concerning the blood-brain barrier are correct **except:**
   (a) The blood-brain barrier protects the brain from toxic compounds of high molecular weight.
   (b) The blood-brain barrier is absent from the pineal gland.
   (c) The endothelial cells of the blood capillaries are nonfenestrated.
   (d) The endothelial cells of the blood capillaries are held together by localized tight junctions.
   (e) L-Dopa readily passes through the barrier in the treatment of Parkinson's disease.

4. The following statements concerning the blood-brain barrier are correct **except:**
   (a) Chloramphenicol and the tetracyclines cannot cross the barrier.
   (b) In the newborn child the blood-brain barrier is not fully developed.
   (c) Cerebral trauma or inflammation may have a great effect on the integrity of the blood-brain barrier.
   (d) Gases and water pass readily through the barrier.
   (e) Glucose and electrolytes pass slowly through the barrier.

5. The following statements concerning the blood-cerebrospinal fluid barrier are correct **except:**
   (a) The beltlike tight junctions between the choroidal ependymal cells form the barrier.
   (b) The proteins and most hexoses, other than glucose, are unable to cross the barrier.
   (c) Gases and water pass readily through the barrier.
   (d) Lipid soluble substances have difficulty in passing through the barrier.
   (e) The basement membrane of the endothelial cells plays no part in the formation of the barrier.

6. The following structures are associated with the roof of the fourth ventricle **except:**
   (a) The inferior medullary velum
   (b) The choroid plexus
   (c) The superior medullary velum
   (d) The vermis of the cerebellum
   (e) The temporal lobes of the cerebral hemispheres

7. The following statements concerning the cerebrospinal fluid in the fourth ventricle are correct **except:**
   (a) It is produced mainly by the choroid plexuses of the lateral, third, and fourth ventricles.
   (b) It leaves the midbrain through the cerebral aqueduct.
   (c) It enters the spinal cord through the central canal.
   (d) It is dark yellow in color.
   (e) It escapes into the subarachnoid space through the apertures in the roof of the fourth ventricle.

Directions: In the next item, select the ONE BEST lettered answer.

8. The lateral boundaries of the fourth ventricle are formed by
   (a) the tentorium cerebelli
   (b) the sulcus limitans
   (c) the cerebellar peduncles
   (d) the cerebral peduncles
   (e) the striae medullares

Directions: Each of the numbered items in this section is followed by answers that are positive or positively phrased. Select the ONE lettered answer that is an EXCEPTION.

9. The following important nuclei lie beneath the floor of the fourth ventricle **except:**
   (a) The vestibular nuclei
   (b) The trochlear nucleus
   (c) The vagal nucleus
   (d) The hypoglossal nucleus
   (e) The abducent nucleus

10. The following statements concerning the third ventricle are correct **except:**
    (a) It is situated between the thalami.
    (b) It communicates with the lateral ventricles through the interventricular foramina.
    (c) It is continuous with the fourth ventricle through the cerebral aqueduct.
    (d) The choroid plexus is located in the floor.
    (e) The choroid plexus receives its arterial supply through the internal carotid and basilar arteries.

11. The following statements concerning the subarachnoid space are correct **except:**
    (a) The space is the interval between the arachnoid mater and the pia mater.
    (b) The space contains cerebrospinal fluid and the cerebral arteries, but not the cerebral veins.
    (c) In certain situations the space is expanded to form cisterns.
    (d) The fourth ventricle drains into it through three foramina.
    (e) The space surrounds the cranial and spinal nerves to the point where they leave the skull and the vertebral canal.

12. The following statements concerning the formation of the cerebrospinal fluid are correct **except:**
    (a) It is largely formed by the choroid plexuses.
    (b) Some of the fluid may originate from the brain substance.
    (c) It is actively secreted by the ependymal cells covering the choroid plexuses.
    (d) The fluid is produced continuously at a rate of about 0.5 ml per minute.
    (e) The fluid is drained into the subarachnoid space from the lymphatic vessels of the brain and spinal cord.

13. The following statements concerning the cerebrospinal fluid are correct **except:**
    (a) Its circulation through the ventricles is aided by the arterial pulsations of the choroid plexuses.
    (b) It extends inferiorly in the subarachnoid space to the level of the fifth sacral vertebra.
    (c) It exits from the ventricular system through the foramen of Magendie and the foramina of Luschka.
    (d) Its circulation in the subarachnoid space is aided by the pulsations of the cerebral and spinal arteries and the movements of the vertebral column.
    (e) The cerebrospinal fluid pressure in the subarachnoid space rises if the internal jugular veins in the neck are compressed.

14. The following statements concerning absorption of the cerebrospinal fluid are correct **except:**
    (a) The cerebrospinal fluid is passed into the blood by active transport through the cells forming the arachnoid villi.
    (b) The minor sites for the absorption of the cerebrospinal fluid are into the veins in the subarachnoid space and the perineural lymph vessels.
    (c) The arachnoid villi play an important role in the absorption of cerebrospinal fluid.
    (d) The fine tubules found within the arachnoid villi permit direct flow of cerebrospinal fluid into the venous sinuses.
    (e) In communicating hydrocephalus there is no obstruction to the flow of the cerebrospinal fluid within the ventricular system or to the outflow from the ventricular system to the subarachnoid space.

Directions: Matching Questions
In Figure 16-24, match the numbers listed on the left with the appropriate lettered structures listed on the right. Each lettered option may be selected once, more than once, or not at all.

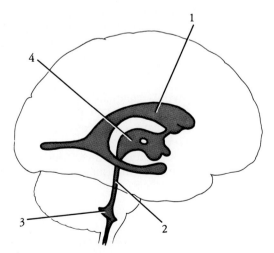

Figure 16–24 Lateral view of the brain showing an outline of ventricular cavities.

15. Number 1
16. Number 2
17. Number 3
18. Number 4
  (a) Cerebral aqueduct
  (b) Body of lateral ventricle
  (c) Third ventricle
  (d) Fourth ventricle
  (e) None of the above

Directions: Read the case histories then answer the questions. You will be required to select ONE BEST lettered answer.

A 24-year-old woman complaining of recent onset of severe headaches and several attacks of morning vomiting was seen by a neurologist. A thorough physical examination revealed findings suggesting that she might have an intracranial tumor involving the cerebellum. The physician ordered an MRI of the patient's brain with particular reference to the contents of the posterior cranial fossa.

19. Figure 16-25 is a coronal MRI (contrast-enhanced) through the fourth ventricle. The radiologist made the following correct observations in his report **except:**
  (a) The bones of the skull show nothing abnormal. The cerebral cortex appeared to be normal.
  (b) The midline structures were not deflected to one or other side.

  (c) The cavity of the fourth ventricle was distorted and larger than normal.
  (d) The body of the lateral ventricle had a normal appearance.

A 21-year-old pregnant woman was invited to a reunion party and during the course of the evening she drank several gin and tonics. The party was followed by several others extending over a 3-week period during which she drank heavily. Six months later, she gave birth to a boy who was diagnosed as having congenital hydrocephalus.

20. The pediatric neurologist carefully questioned the mother and came to the following correct conclusions **except:**
  (a) The consumption of a large amount of alcohol during pregnancy usually has no adverse effects on the developing fetus.
  (b) The high alcoholic intake coincided with the first trimester.
  (c) The alcohol had crossed the placental barrier and entered the fetal circulation.
  (d) The alcohol had probably also crossed the fetal blood-brain barrier and entered the brain.
  (e) The neurologist was of the opinion that the toxic effect of alcohol was probably responsible for the hydrocephalus.

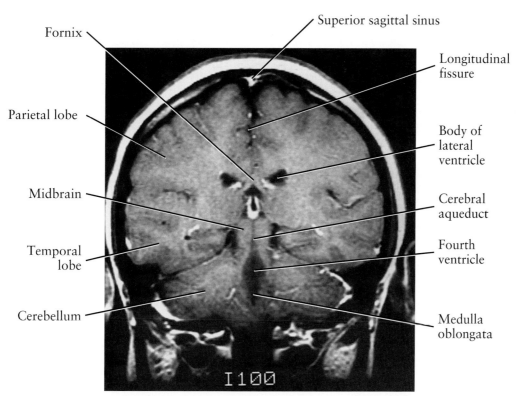

Figure 16–25 A coronal MRI (contrast enhanced) through the hind brain showing the fourth ventricle and the surrounding neural and bony structures.

Answers to Review Questions

1. B
2. C
3. D
4. A
5. D
6. E
7. D
8. C
9. B
10. D
11. B
12. E
13. B
14. A
15. B

16. A
17. D
18. C
19. C. The size and shape of the cavity of the fourth ventricle was within normal limits.
20. A. Many chemical substances when consumed are toxic to the central nervous system, and alcohol in large quantities is one of the worst offenders. During the first trimester, alcohol can readily access the brain at a time when it is particularly vulnerable. Before a physician prescribes a therapeutic drug, he or she must know whether the drug will cross the blood-brain barrier and what effect, if any, that drug will have on the central nervous system.

ADDITIONAL READING

Alksne, J. F., Lovings, E. T. Functional ultrastructure of the arachnoid villus. *Arch. Neurol.* 27:371, 1972.

Bradbury, M. W. B. The structure and function of the blood-brain barrier. *Fed. Proc.* 43:186, 1984.

Bradbury, M.W.B. (ed). *Physiology and Pharmacology of the Blood-Brain Barrier.* New York, Springer, 1992.

Brightman, M. W. The distribution within the brain of ferritin injected into cerebrospinal fluid compartments: II. Parenchymal distribution. *Am. J. Anat.* 117:193, 1965.

Brightman, M. W., Reese, T. W. Junctions between intimately apposed cell membranes in the vertebrate brain. *J. Cell Biol.* 40:648, 1969.

Broadwell, R. D., Brightman, M. W. Entry of peroxidase into neurons of the central and peripheral nervous systems from extracerebral and cerebral blood. *J. Comp. Neurol.* 166:257, 1976.

Cervos-Navarro, J., Artigas, J., Mesulja, B. J. Morphofunctional aspects of the normal and pathological blood-brain barrier. *Acta Neuropathol. (Berl.)* 7(suppl):1, 1983.

Craig, C. R., Stitzel, R. E. *Modern Pharmacology* (4th ed.). Boston: Little, Brown, 1994.

Cserr, H. F. Relationship between cerebrospinal fluid and interstitial fluid of brain. *Fed. Proc.* 33:2075, 1974.

Davson, H. Formation and Drainage of the Cerebrospinal Fluid. In K. Shapiro, A. Marmarov, H. Portnoy (eds.), *Hydrocephalus.* New York: Raven, 1984. P. 3.

Ermisch, A., et al. Peptides and Blood-Brain Barrier Transport. *Physiol. Rev.*, 73,489, 1993.

Fishman, R. A. *Cerebrospinal Fluids in Diseases of the Nervous System.* Philadelphia: Saunders, 1992.

Gaab, M. R., Koos, W. T. Hydrocephalus in infancy and childhood: Diagnosis and indication for operation. *Neuropediatrics* 15:173, 1984.

Klatzo, I. Disturbances of the blood-brain barrier in cerebrovascular disorders. *Acta Neuropathol. (Berl.)* 8(suppl):81, 1983.

Lyons, M.K., Meyer, F.B., Cerebrospinal Fluid Physiology and the Management of Increased Intracranial Pressure. *Mayo Clin. Proc.* 65:684-707,1990.

Neuwelt, E.A. (ed.) *Implications of the Blood-Brain Barrier and its Manipulation.* New York, Plenum Publishing Corp., 1989.

Oldendorf, W. H. Some clinical aspects of the blood-brain barrier. *Hosp. Pract.* 17(2):143, 1982.

Pardridge, W.M. *The Blood-Brain Barrier: Cellular and Molecular Biology.* New York, Raven Press,1993.

Pollay, M. Research into Human Hydrocephalus: A Review. In K. Shapiro, A. Marmarov, H. Portnoy (eds.), *Hydrocephalus.* New York: Raven, 1984. P. 301.

Rhoades, R. A., Tanner, G. A. *Medical Physiology.* Boston: Little, Brown, 1995.

Saunders, N. R., Milgard, K. Development of the blood-brain barrier. *J. Dev. Physiol.* 6:45, 1984.

Westmoreland, B. F., Benarroch, E. E., Daube, J. R., Reagan, T. J., Sandok, B. A. *Medical Neurosciences* (3rd ed.). Boston: Little, Brown, 1994.

Williams, P.L. et al. (eds.) *Gray's Anatomy* (38th Br. Ed.) New York, Edinburgh. Churchill Livingstone, 1995.

Wright, E. M. Transport processes in the formation of cerebrospinal fluid. *Rev. Physiol. Biochem. Pharmacol.* 83:1, 1978.

CHAPTER 17

The Blood Supply of the Brain and Spinal Cord

A 61-year-old woman collapsed in the supermarket and was in a coma when admitted to the emergency department of the local hospital. Twenty-four hours later she recovered consciousness and was found to have paralysis on the left side of her body, mainly involving the lower limb. There was also some sensory loss of the left leg and foot. She was able to swallow normally and did not appear to have difficulty with her speech.

The left-sided hemiplegia and hemianesthesia strongly suggested a cerebrovascular accident involving the right cerebral hemisphere. The limitation of the paralysis and anesthesia to the leg and foot indicated that the right anterior cerebral artery or one of its branches was blocked by a thrombus or embolus. The diagnosis was confirmed by PET, which showed an absence of blood flow through the leg area on the medial surface of the right cerebral hemisphere.

CHAPTER OBJECTIVES

Cerebrovascular accidents (stroke) still remain the third leading cause of morbidity and death in the United States. The purpose of this chapter is to describe the main arteries and veins supplying the brain and spinal cord. Emphasis is placed on knowing the areas of the cerebral cortex and spinal cord supplied by a particular artery and understanding the dysfunction that would result if the artery is blocked.

The circle of Willis is discussed in detail, as well as the blood supply to the internal capsule. This latter important structure contains the major ascending and descending pathways to the cerebral cortex and is commonly disrupted by arterial hemorrhage or thrombosis. Many examination questions concern the areas covered in this chapter.

BLOOD SUPPLY TO THE BRAIN
ARTERIES OF THE BRAIN

The brain is supplied by the two internal carotid and the two vertebral arteries. The four arteries lie within the subarachnoid space, and their branches anastomose on the inferior surface of the brain to form the circle of Willis.

Internal Carotid Artery

The internal carotid artery begins at the bifurcation of the common carotid artery (Fig. 17-1), where it usually possesses a localized dilatation, called the **carotid sinus.** It ascends the neck and perforates the base of the skull by passing through the carotid canal of the temporal bone. The artery then runs horizontally forward through the cavernous

sinus and emerges on the medial side of the anterior clinoid process by perforating the dura mater. It now enters the subarachnoid space by piercing the arachnoid mater and turns posteriorly to the region of the medial end of the lateral cerebral sulcus. Here, it divides into the **anterior** and **middle cerebral arteries** (Figs. 17-1 and 17-2).

BRANCHES OF THE CEREBRAL PORTION

1. The **ophthalmic artery** arises as the internal carotid artery emerges from the cavernous sinus (Fig. 17-1). It enters the orbit through the optic canal below and lateral to the optic nerve. It supplies the eye and other orbital structures and its terminal branches supply the frontal area of the scalp, the ethmoid and frontal sinuses, and the dorsum of the nose.

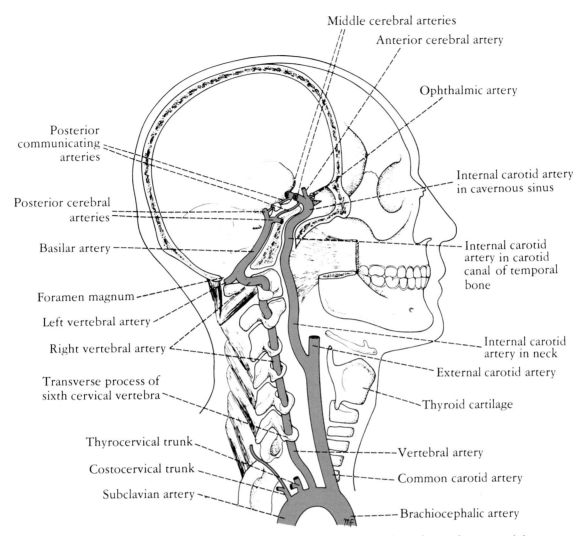

Figure 17–1 Origin and courses of the internal carotid and vertebral arteries as they ascend the neck to enter the skull.

2. The **posterior communicating artery** is a small vessel that originates from the internal carotid artery close to its terminal bifurcation (Figs. 17-1 and 17-2). The posterior communicating artery runs posteriorly above the oculomotor nerve to join the posterior cerebral artery, thus forming part of the **circle of Willis.**

3. The **choroidal artery,** a small branch, also originates from the internal carotid artery close to its terminal bifurcation. The choroidal artery passes posteriorly close to the optic tract, enters the inferior horn of the lateral ventricle, and ends in the choroid plexus. It gives off numerous small branches to surrounding structures, including the crus cerebri, the lateral geniculate body, the optic tract, and the internal capsule.

4. The **anterior cerebral artery** is the smaller terminal branch of the internal carotid artery (Fig. 17-2). It runs forward and medially superior to the optic nerve and enters the longitudinal fissure of the cerebrum. Here, it is joined to the anterior cerebral artery of the opposite side by the **anterior communicating artery.** It curves backward over the corpus callosum, and, finally, anastomoses with the posterior cerebral artery (Figs. 17-3 and 17-8). The **cortical branches** supply all the medial surface of the cerebral cortex as far back as the parieto-occipital sulcus (Fig. 17-3). They also supply a strip of cortex about 1 inch (2.5 cm) wide on the adjoining lateral surface. The anterior cerebral artery thus supplies the "leg area" of the precentral gyrus. A group of **central branches** pierces the anterior perforated substance and helps to supply parts of the lentiform and caudate nuclei and the internal capsule.

5. The **middle cerebral artery,** the largest branch of the internal carotid, runs laterally in the lateral cerebral sulcus (Fig. 17-2). **Cortical branches** supply the entire lateral surface of the hemisphere, except for the narrow strip supplied by the anterior cerebral artery, the occip-

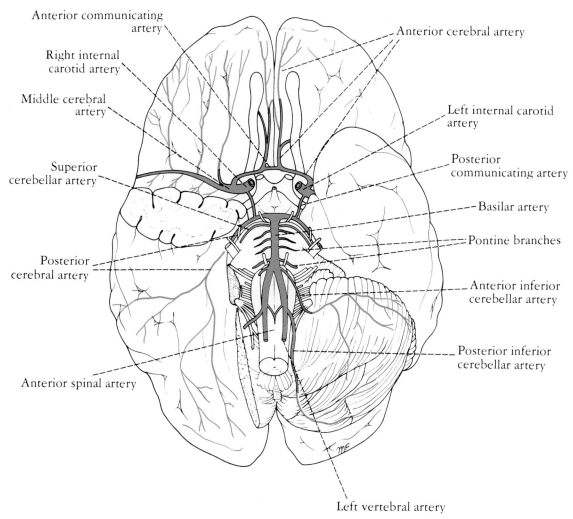

Figure 17–2 Arteries of the inferior surface of the brain. Note the formation of the circle of Willis. Part of the right temporal lobe has been removed to show the course of the middle cerebral artery.

ital pole, and the inferolateral surface of the hemisphere, which are supplied by the posterior cerebral artery (Fig. 17-3). This artery thus supplies all the motor area except the "leg area." **Central branches** enter the anterior perforated substance and supply the lentiform and caudate nuclei and the internal capsule (Fig. 17-4).

Vertebral Artery

The vertebral artery, a branch of the first part of the subclavian artery, ascends the neck by passing through the foramina in the transverse processes of the upper six cervical vertebrae (Fig. 17-1). It enters the skull through the foramen magnum and pierces the dura mater and arachnoid to enter the subarachnoid space. It then passes upward, forward, and medially on the medulla oblongata (Fig. 17-2). At the lower border of the pons, it joins the vessel of the opposite side to form the **basilar artery.**

BRANCHES OF THE CRANIAL PORTION

1. The **meningeal branches** are small and supply the bone and dura in the posterior cranial fossa.
2. The **posterior spinal artery** may arise from the vertebral artery or the posterior inferior cerebellar artery. It descends on the posterior surface of the spinal cord close to the posterior roots of the spinal nerves. The branches are reinforced by radicular arteries that enter the vertebral canal through the intervertebral foramina. For the detailed distribution of this artery, see page 481.
3. The **anterior spinal artery** is formed from a contributory branch from each vertebral artery near its termination (Fig. 17-2). The single artery descends on the anterior surface of the medulla oblongata and spinal cord and is embedded in the pia mater along the anterior median fissure. The artery is reinforced by radicular arteries that enter the vertebral canal through the intervertebral foramina. For the detailed distribution of this artery, see page 481.

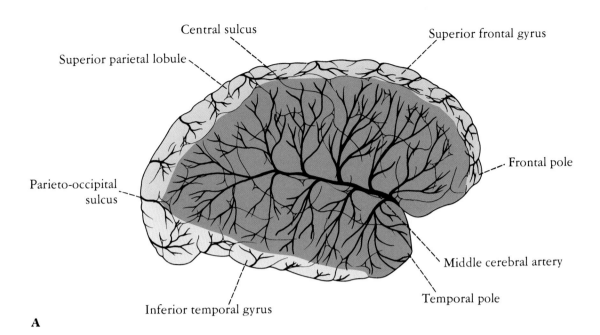

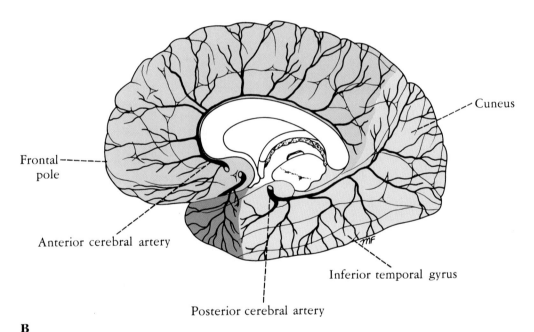

B

Figure 17–3   Areas supplied by the cerebral arteries. **A.** The lateral surface of the right cerebral hemisphere. **B.** The medial surface of the right cerebral hemisphere. The area supplied by the anterior cerebral artery is colored blue, that supplied by the middle cerebral artery is red, and that supplied by the posterior cerebral artery is brown.

4. The **posterior inferior cerebellar artery,** the largest branch of the vertebral artery, passes on an irregular course between the medulla and the cerebellum (Figs. 17-2, 17-12, and 17-14). It supplies the inferior surface of the vermis, the central nuclei of the cerebellum, and the undersurface of the cerebellar hemisphere; it also supplies the medulla oblongata and the choroid plexus of the fourth ventricle.

5. The **medullary arteries** are very small branches that are distributed to the medulla oblongata.

Basilar Artery

The basilar artery, formed by the union of the two vertebral arteries (Fig. 17-1), ascends in a groove on the anterior surface of the pons (Figs. 17-2, 17-13, and 17-14). At the upper

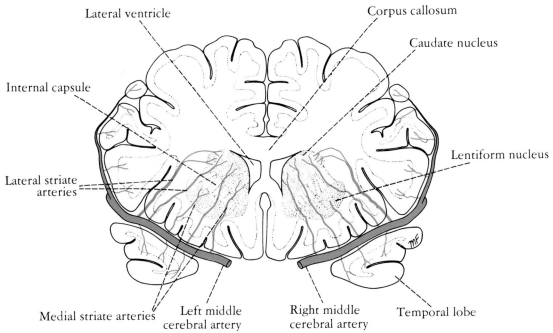

Figure 17–4   Coronal section of the cerebral hemispheres, showing the arterial supply to the deep cerebral structures from the middle cerebral artery.

border of the pons, it divides into the two posterior cerebral arteries.

BRANCHES

1. The **pontine arteries** are numerous small vessels that enter the substance of the pons (Figs. 17-2, 17-13, and 17-14).
2. The **labyrinthine artery** is a long, narrow artery that accompanies the facial and the vestibulocochlear nerves into the internal acoustic meatus and supplies the internal ear. It often arises as a branch of the anterior inferior cerebellar artery.
3. The **anterior inferior cerebellar artery** passes posteriorly and laterally and supplies the anterior and inferior parts of the cerebellum (Figs. 17-2, 17-13, and 17-14). A few branches pass to the pons and the upper part of the medulla oblongata.
4. The **superior cerebellar artery** arises close to the termination of the basilar artery (Figs. 17-2 and 17-11 through 17-14). It winds around the cerebral peduncle and supplies the superior surface of the cerebellum. It also supplies the pons, the pineal gland, and the superior medullary velum.
5. The **posterior cerebral artery** curves laterally and backward around the midbrain and is joined by the posterior communicating branch of the internal carotid artery (Figs. 17-1, 17-2, and 17-11 through 17-14). **Cortical branches** supply the inferolateral and medial surfaces of the temporal lobe and the lateral and medial surfaces of the occipital lobe (Fig. 17-3). Thus the posterior cerebral artery supplies the visual cortex. **Central branches** pierce the brain substance and supply parts of the thalamus and the lentiform nu-

cleus, and the midbrain, the pineal, and the medial geniculate bodies. A **choroidal branch** enters the inferior horn of the lateral ventricle and supplies the choroid plexus; it also supplies the choroid plexus of the third ventricle.

Circle of Willis

The circle of Willis lies in the interpeduncular fossa at the base of the brain. It is formed by the anastomosis between the two internal carotid arteries and the two vertebral arteries (Fig. 17-2). The anterior communicating, anterior cerebral, internal carotid, posterior communicating, posterior cerebral, and basilar arteries all contribute to the circle. The circle of Willis allows blood that enters by either internal carotid or vertebral arteries to be distributed to any part of both cerebral hemispheres. Cortical and central branches arise from the circle and supply the brain substance.

Variations in the sizes of the arteries forming the circle are common and the absence of one or both posterior communicating arteries has been reported.

Arteries to Specific Brain Areas

The **corpus striatum** and the **internal capsule** are supplied mainly by the medial and lateral striate central branches of the middle cerebral artery (Fig. 17-4); the central branches of the anterior cerebral artery supply the remainder of these structures.

The **thalamus** is supplied mainly by branches of the posterior communicating, basilar, and posterior cerebral arteries.

The **midbrain** is supplied by the posterior cerebral, superior cerebellar, and basilar arteries.

The **pons** is supplied by the basilar and the anterior, inferior, and superior cerebellar arteries.

The **medulla oblongata** is supplied by the vertebral, anterior and posterior spinal, posterior inferior cerebellar, and basilar arteries.

The **cerebellum** is supplied by the superior cerebellar, anterior inferior cerebellar, and posterior inferior cerebellar arteries.

Nerve Supply of Cerebral Arteries

The cerebral arteries receive a rich supply of sympathetic postganglionic nerve fibers. These fibers are derived from the superior cervical sympathetic ganglion. Stimulation of these nerves causes vasoconstriction of the cerebral arteries. However, under normal conditions, the local blood flow is mainly controlled by the concentrations of carbon dioxide, hydrogen ions, and oxygen present in the nervous tissue; a rise in the carbon dioxide and hydrogen ion concentrations and a lowering of the oxygen tension bring about a vasodilatation.

VEINS OF THE BRAIN

The veins of the brain have no muscular tissue in their very thin walls, and they possess no valves. They emerge from the brain and lie in the subarachnoid space. They pierce the arachnoid mater and the meningeal layer of the dura and drain into the cranial venous sinuses (Fig. 17-5).

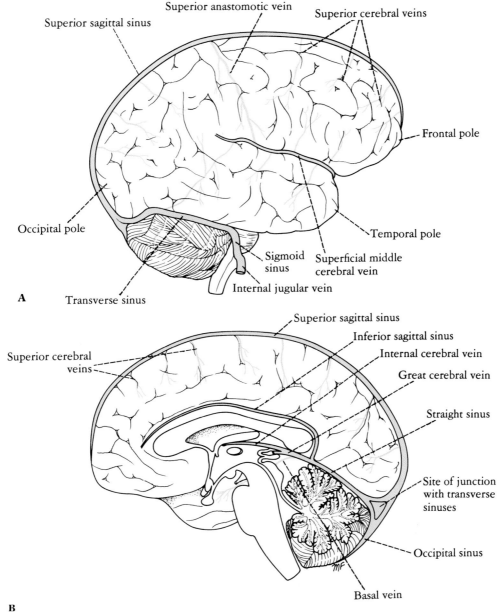

Figure 17–5   Venous drainage of the right cerebral hemisphere. **A.** Lateral surface. **B.** Medial surface.

External Cerebral Veins

The **superior cerebral veins** pass upward over the lateral surface of the cerebral hemisphere and empty into the superior sagittal sinus (Fig. 17-5).

The **superficial middle cerebral vein** drains the lateral surface of the cerebral hemisphere. It runs inferiorly in the lateral sulcus and empties into the cavernous sinus (Fig. 17-5).

The **deep middle cerebral vein** drains the insula and is joined by the **anterior cerebral** and **striate veins** to form the **basal vein.** The basal vein ultimately joins the great cerebral vein, which in turn drains into the straight sinus (Fig. 17-5).

Internal Cerebral Veins

There are two internal cerebral veins and they are formed by the union of the **thalamostriate vein** and the **choroid vein** at the interventricular foramen. The two veins run posteriorly in the tela choroidea of the third ventricle and unite beneath the splenium of the corpus callosum to form the great cerebral vein, which empties into the straight sinus.

Veins of Specific Brain Areas

The **midbrain** is drained by veins that open into the basal or great cerebral veins.

The **pons** is drained by veins that open into the basal vein, cerebellar veins, or neighboring venous sinuses.

The **medulla oblongata** is drained by veins that open into the spinal veins and neighboring venous sinuses.

The **cerebellum** is drained by veins that empty into the great cerebral vein or adjacent venous sinuses.

CEREBRAL CIRCULATION

The blood flow to the brain must deliver oxygen, glucose, and other nutrients to the nervous tissue and remove carbon dioxide, lactic acid, and other metabolic byproducts. The brain has been shown to be supplied with arterial blood from the two internal carotid arteries and the two vertebral arteries. The blood supply to half of the brain is provided by the internal carotid and vertebral arteries on that side, and their respective streams come together in the posterior communicating artery at a point where the pressure of the two is equal and they do not mix (Fig. 17-6). If, however, the internal carotid or vertebral artery is occluded, the blood passes forward or backward across that point to compensate for the reduction in blood flow. The arterial circle also permits the blood to flow across the midline, as shown when the internal carotid or vertebral artery on one side is occluded. It also has been shown that the two streams of blood from the vertebral arteries remain separate and on the same side of the lumen of the basilar artery and do not mix.

Although the cerebral arteries anastomose with one another at the circle of Willis and by means of branches on the

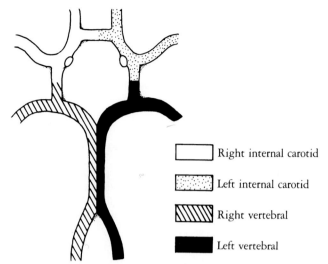

Figure 17–6   Circle of Willis showing the distribution of blood from the four main arteries.

surface of the cerebral hemispheres, once they enter the brain substance, no further anastomoses occur.

The most important factor in forcing the blood through the brain is the arterial blood pressure. This is opposed by such factors as a raised intracranial pressure, increased blood viscosity, and narrowing of the vascular diameter. Cerebral blood flow remains remarkably constant in spite of changes in the general blood pressure. This autoregulation of the circulation is accomplished by a compensatory lowering of the cerebral vascular resistance when the arterial pressure is decreased, and a raising of the vascular resistance when the arterial pressure is increased. Needless to say, this autoregulation does not maintain an adequate blood flow when the arterial blood pressure falls to a very low level.

The diameter of the cerebral blood vessels is the main factor contributing to the cerebrovascular resistance. While it is known that they are innervated by sympathetic postganglionic nerve fibers and that they respond to norepinephrine, they apparently play little or no part in the control of cerebrovascular resistance in normal human beings. The most powerful vasodilator influence on cerebral blood vessels is an increase in carbon dioxide or hydrogen ion concentration; a reduction in oxygen concentration also causes vasodilatation. It has been shown, using PET, that an increase in neuronal activity in different parts of the brain causes a local increase in blood flow. For example, viewing an object will increase the oxygen and glucose consumption in the visual cortex of the occipital lobes. This results in an increase in the local concentrations of carbon dioxide and hydrogen ions and brings about a local increase in blood flow.

The cerebral blood flow in patients can be measured by the intracarotid injection or inhalation of radioactive krypton or xenon. A cerebral blood flow of 50 to 60 ml per 100 g of brain per minute is considered normal.

BLOOD SUPPLY OF THE SPINAL CORD

Arteries of the Spinal Cord

The spinal cord receives its arterial supply from three small arteries, the two posterior spinal arteries and the anterior spinal artery. These longitudinally running arteries are reinforced by small segmentally arranged arteries that arise from arteries outside the vertebral column and enter the vertebral canal through the intervertebral foramina. These vessels anastomose on the surface of the cord and send branches into the substance of the white and gray matter.. Considerable variation exists as to the size and segmental levels at which the reinforcing arteries occur.

POSTERIOR SPINAL ARTERIES

The posterior spinal arteries arise either directly from the vertebral arteries inside the skull or indirectly from the posterior inferior cerebellar arteries. Each artery descends on the anterior surface of the spinal cord close to the posterior nerve roots and gives off branches that enter the substance of the cord (Fig. 17-7). The posterior spinal arteries supply the posterior one-third of the spinal cord.

The posterior spinal arteries are small in the upper thoracic region and the first three thoracic segments of the spinal cord are particularly vulnerable to ischemia should the segmental or radicular arteries in this region be occluded.

ANTERIOR SPINAL ARTERY

The anterior spinal artery is formed by the union of two arteries, each of which arises from the vertebral artery inside the skull. The anterior spinal artery then descends on the anterior surface of the spinal cord within the anterior median fissure (Fig. 17-7). Branches from the anterior spinal artery enter the substance of the cord and supply the anterior two-thirds of the spinal cord.

In the upper and lower thoracic segments of the spinal cord the anterior spinal artery may be extremely small. Should the segmental or radicular arteries be occluded in these regions, the fourth thoracic and the first lumbar segments of the spinal cord would be particularly liable to ischemic necrosis.

SEGMENTAL SPINAL ARTERIES

At each intervertebral foramen the longitudinally running posterior and anterior spinal arteries are reinforced by

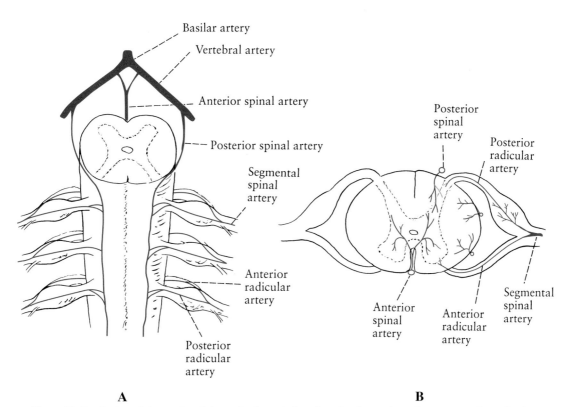

A **B**

Figure 17–7 **A.** Arterial supply of the spinal cord showing the formation of two posterior spinal arteries and one anterior spinal artery. **B.** Transverse section of the spinal cord showing the segmental spinal arteries and the radicular arteries.

small segmental arteries on both sides (Fig. 17-7). The arteries are branches of arteries outside the vertebral column (deep cervical, intercostal, and lumbar arteries). Having entered the vertebral canal, each segmental spinal artery gives rise to **anterior** and **posterior radicular arteries** that accompany the anterior and posterior nerve roots to the spinal cord.

Additional, **feeder arteries** enter the vertebral canal and anastomose with the anterior and posterior spinal arteries; however, the number and size of these arteries vary considerably from one individual to another. One large and important feeder artery, the **great anterior medullary artery of Adamkiewicz,** arises from the aorta in the lower

thoracic or upper lumbar vertebral levels, it is unilateral and in the majority of persons enters the spinal cord from the left side. The importance of this artery lies in the fact that it may be the major source of blood to the lower two-thirds of the spinal cord.

VEINS OF THE SPINAL CORD

The veins of the spinal cord drain into six tortuous longitudinal channels that communicate superiorly within the skull with the veins of the brain and the venous sinuses. They drain mainly into the internal vertebral venous plexus.

CLINICAL NOTES

In spite of the recent decrease in cerebrovascular disease, it has been estimated that it is responsible for about 50 percent of all adult neurological hospital admissions.

CEREBRAL ISCHEMIA

Unconsciousness occurs in 5–10 seconds if the blood flow to the brain is completely cut off. Irreversible brain damage with death of nervous tissue rapidly follows complete arrest of cerebral blood flow. It has been estimated that neuronal function ceases after about 1 minute and that irreversible changes start to occur after about 4 minutes, although this time may be longer if the patient's body has been cooled.* Cardiac arrest due to coronary thrombosis is the most common cause of this condition.

Interruption of Cerebral Circulation

Vascular lesions of the brain are extremely common and the resulting neurological defect will depend on the size of the artery occluded, the state of the collateral circulation, and the area of the brain involved. Clinical studies and the examination of postmortem material have focused attention on the high frequency of lesions in the common carotid, internal carotid, and vertebral arteries in the neck.

CEREBRAL ARTERY SYNDROMES

Anterior Cerebral Artery Occlusion
If the occlusion of the artery is proximal to the anterior communicating artery, the collateral circulation is usually adequate to preserve the circulation. Occlusion distal to the communicating artery may produce the following signs and symptoms:

1. Contralateral hemiparesis and hemisensory loss involving mainly the leg and foot (paracentral lobule of cortex)
2. Inability to identify objects correctly, apathy, and personality changes (frontal and parietal lobes)

Middle Cerebral Artery Occlusion
Occlusion of the artery may produce the following signs and symptoms, but the clinical picture will vary according to the site of occlusion and the degree of collateral anastomoses:

1. Contralateral hemiparesis and hemisensory loss involving mainly the face and arm (precentral and postcentral gyri)
2. Aphasia if the left hemisphere is affected (rarely if the right hemisphere is affected)
3. Contralateral homonymous hemianopia (damage to the optic radiation)
4. Anosognosia if the right hemisphere is affected (rarely if the left hemisphere is affected)

Posterior Cerebral Artery Occlusion
Occlusion of the artery may produce the following signs and symptoms, but the clinical picture will vary according to the site of the occlusion and the availability of collateral anastomoses:

1. Contralateral homonymous hemianopia with some degree of macular sparing (damage to the calcarine cortex, macular sparing due to the occipital pole receiving collateral blood supply from the middle cerebral artery)
2. Visual agnosia (ischemia of the left occipital lobe)
3. Impairment of memory (possible damage to the medial aspect of the temporal lobe)

Internal Carotid Artery Occlusion
The occlusion can occur without causing symptoms or signs or can cause massive cerebral ischemia depending on the degree of collateral anastomoses.

1. The symptoms and signs are those of middle cerebral artery occlusion, including contralateral hemiparesis and hemianesthesia.
2. There is partial or complete loss of sight on the same side but permanent loss is rare (emboli dislodged from the internal carotid artery reach the retina through ophthalmic artery).

*It must be emphasized that brain damage might be reversed if the blood flow can be restored even after 5 minutes.

Vertebrobasilar Artery Occlusion

The vertebral and basilar arteries supply all the parts of the central nervous system in the posterior cranial fossa, and through the posterior cerebral arteries they supply the visual cortex on both sides. The clinical signs and symptoms are extremely varied and may include the following:

1. Ipsilateral pain and temperature sensory loss of the face and contralateral pain and temperature sensory loss of the body
2. Attacks of hemianopia or complete cortical blindness
3. Ipsilateral loss of the gag reflex, dysphagia, and hoarseness as the result of lesions of the nuclei of the glossopharyngeal and vagus nerves
4. Vertigo, nystagmus, nausea, and vomiting
5. Ipsilateral Horner's syndrome
6. Ipsilateral ataxia and other cerebellar signs
7. Unilateral or bilateral hemiparesis
8. Coma

Impairment of Cerebral Blood Flow

Impairment of cerebral blood flow can be caused by a large number of conditions, and the more important can be considered under the following headings: (1) diseases that produce alteration in blood pressure, (2) diseases of arterial walls, and (3) diseases that result in blockage of the arterial lumen.

DISEASES THAT ALTER BLOOD PRESSURE

Postural Hypotension

Patients who get up after being confined to bed for several days, soldiers who stand at attention for long periods on a hot day, and worshipers kneeling in church may experience the accumulation of venous blood in the limbs or impaired venous return to the heart, with a consequent fall in the cardiac output and a lowered arterial blood pressure. The general arterial pressure has to be lowered considerably before the cerebral blood flow is diminished.

Physical and Psychological Shock

The profound and prolonged fall in blood pressure that may follow physical trauma such as an automobile accident or extensive surgery, especially in the elderly, in whom the cerebral arteries are already narrowed by disease, may cause the patient to lose consciousness. Hyperventilation in anxiety states may reduce the cerebral blood flow by lowering the carbon dioxide content of the blood.

Change in Blood Viscosity

In polycythemia vera, the cerebral blood flow is considerably reduced as the result of an increase in the viscosity of the blood.

Carotid Sinus Syndrome

The carotid sinus, situated at the proximal end of the internal carotid artery, is extremely sensitive to changes in arterial blood pressure. Distention of the arterial wall causes a reflex slowing of the heart rate and a fall in blood pressure. This occurs as the result of an increased number of nervous impulses passing up the sinus nerve, a branch of the glossopharyngeal nerve, which connects with the cardioinhibitory and vasomotor centers. Hypersensitivity of the reflex or external pressure may cause the blood pressure to fall suddenly and produce cerebral ischemia and loss of consciousness.

Diseases of the Heart

Any severe cardiac disease, such as coronary thrombosis, auricular fibrillation, or heart block, that results in a marked fall in cardiac output will result in a severe fall in general arterial blood pressure and reduction in cerebral blood flow.

DISEASES OF THE ARTERIAL WALLS

The most common cause of narrowing of the lumen of the arteries that supply the brain is atheroma. This disease may affect the main arteries supplying the brain in their course through the neck as well as their course within the skull. Moreover, the impairment of the cerebral circulation may be worsened by an attack of coronary thrombosis, with its associated hypotension, shock due to surgical procedures, severe anemia, or even rotation of the head with external pressure on the carotid arteries.

Atheromatous degeneration of the cerebral arteries occurs most commonly in middle or old age and often complicates diabetes and hypertension. When actual blockage of an artery occurs, the effect will depend on the size and location of the vessel. The nerve cells and their fibers will degenerate in the avascular area and the surrounding neuroglia will proliferate and invade the area. In patients with generalized narrowing of the cerebral arteries without blockage of a single artery, the brain will undergo a diffuse atrophy. It should be remembered that a very narrow atheromatous artery may be blocked by a thrombus, thus totally closing the lumen.

DISEASES THAT RESULT IN BLOCKAGE OF THE ARTERIAL LUMEN

Embolism of a cerebral artery can occur in two forms: (1) by far the most common, a thrombus, and (2) fat globules. The thrombus may develop anywhere on the endothelial lining from the left side of the heart to the parent vessels of the cerebral arteries. A common site of origin is an atheromatous plaque on the internal carotid, common carotid, or vertebral artery. Another area is the site of endocarditis on the mitral or aortic valve or the endocardial lining of a myocardial infarction following a coronary thrombosis. In women, cerebral thrombosis is more common among those taking oral contraceptives, especially those taking a high-dose estrogen-progesterone combination.

Fat embolism usually follows severe fractures of one of the long bones. Fat globules from the macerated yellow marrow enter the nutrient veins, pass through the pulmonary circulation, and end up blocking multiple small cerebral end arteries.

CEREBRAL ANEURYSMS

Congenital Aneurysms

Congenital aneurysms occur most commonly at the site where two arteries join in the formation of the circle of Willis. At this point, there is a deficiency in the tunica media and this is complicated by the development of atheroma, which so weakens the arterial wall that a local dilatation occurs. The aneurysm may press on neighboring structures, such as the optic nerve or the third, fourth, or sixth cranial nerve, and produce signs or symptoms, or may suddenly rupture into the subarachnoid space. In the latter case, a severe pain in the head suddenly develops, followed by mental confusion. Death may quickly occur, or the patient may survive the first bleeding only to die a few days or weeks later. Clipping or ligating the neck of the aneurysm offers the best chance of recovery.

Other types of aneurysms are rare and include those due to softening of the arterial wall following the lodging of an infected embolus, those due to damage of the internal carotid artery as it lies within the cavernous sinus following a fracture of the skull, and those that are associated with disease of the arterial wall such as atheroma.

Intracranial Hemorrhage

Intracranial hemorrhage can result from trauma or cerebral vascular lesions. Four varieties are considered: (1) epidural, (2) subdural, (3) subarachnoid, and (4) cerebral. Epidural and subdural hemorrhage are described on page 22.

Subarachnoid Hemorrhage

Subarachnoid hemorrhage usually results from leakage or rupture of a congenital aneurysm on the cerebral arterial circle or, less commonly, from an angioma or contusion and laceration of the brain and meninges. The symptoms, which are sudden in onset, will include severe headache, stiffness of the neck, and loss of consciousness. The diagnosis is established by the use of CT. The dense areas of the blood in the subarachnoid space can be identified. The withdrawal of heavily blood-stained cerebrospinal fluid through a lumbar puncture is also diagnostic, but this method has been replaced by the use of CT.

Cerebral Hemorrhage

Cerebral hemorrhage generally is due to rupture of an atheromatous artery and is most common in patients with hypertension. It usually occurs in individuals of middle age and often involves a rupture of the thin-walled lenticulostriate artery, a branch of the middle cerebral artery. The important corticonuclear and corticospinal fibers in the internal capsule are damaged, producing hemiplegia on the opposite side of the body. The patient immediately loses consciousness, and the paralysis is evident when consciousness is regained. In some cases, the hemorrhage bursts into the lateral ventricle, resulting in deeper unconsciousness and corticospinal lesions on both sides of the body. Hemorrhage may also occur into the pons and cerebellum.

CT, MRI, and PET

Computed tomography (CT), magnetic resonance imaging (MRI), and positron emission tomography (PET) are techniques that are indispensable in making the diagnosis of different forms of cerebrovascular disease. The diagnosis can usually be made with speed, accuracy, and safety. An intracranial blood clot can be recognized by its density. These techniques have largely replaced cerebral angiography (see pp. 23 and 26).

Cerebral Angiography

The technique of cerebral angiography is used for the detection of abnormalities of the blood vessels; the detection and localization of space-occupying lesions such as tumors, hematomas, or abscesses; or the determination of the vascular pattern of tumors to aid in the diagnosis of their pathology. With the patient under general anesthesia and in the supine position, the head is centered on a radiographic apparatus that will take repeated radiographs at 2-second intervals. Both anteroposterior and lateral projections are obtained. A radiopaque medium is injected rapidly into the lumen of the common carotid or vertebral artery or is indirectly introduced into one of these arteries through a catheter inserted into the radial or femoral artery. As the radiopaque material is rapidly introduced, a series of films are exposed. By this means, the cerebral arteries, the capillary flush, and the veins may be demonstrated. Examples of normal-appearing carotid and vertebral angiograms are shown in Figures 17-8 through 17-15.

Cerebral angiography is an invasive technique that unfortunately has a morbidity of 0.5 to 2.5 percent. CT and MRI should therefore be used whenever possible. PET is now also used extensively.

Spinal Cord Ischemia

The blood supply to the spinal cord is surprisingly meager considering the importance of this nervous tissue. The posterior and anterior spinal arteries are of small and variable diameter and the reinforcing segmental arteries vary in number and size.

The posterior one-third of the spinal cord receives its arterial supply from the posterior spinal arteries. The anterior two-thirds of the spinal cord is supplied by the small, tenuous anterior spinal artery. This latter artery therefore supplies the anterior white column, the anterior gray horns and the anterior part of the lateral white columns and the root of the posterior horns.

Occlusion of the anterior spinal artery may produce the following signs and symptoms (Fig 17-16).

1. Loss of motor function (paraplegia) below the level of the lesion occurs due to bilateral damage to the corticospinal tracts.
2. Bilateral thermoanesthesia and analgesia below the level of the lesion due to bilateral damage to the spinothalamic tracts.
3. Weakness of the limb muscles may occur due to damage of the anterior gray horns in the cervical or lumbar regions of the cord.
4. Loss of bladder and bowel control due to damage of the descending autonomic tracts.

5. Position sense, vibration, and light touch are normal due to preservation of the posterior white columns that are supplied by the posterior spinal arteries.

Ischemia of the spinal cord can easily follow minor damage to the arterial supply, as the result of nerve block procedures, aortic surgery, or any operation in which severe hypotension occurs. The fourth thoracic and first lumbar segments of the cord are particularly prone to ischemia.

Spinal Cord Ischemia and Thoracic Aortic Dissection

The thoracic region of the spinal cord receives its segmental arteries from the posterior intercostal arteries, which arise directly from the thoracic aorta. In thoracic aortic dissection the expanding blood clot in the aortic wall can block the origins of the posterior intercostal arteries, causing ischemia of the spinal cord.

Spinal Cord Ischemia as a Complication of a Leaking Abdominal Aortic Aneurysm

The lumbar region of the spinal cord receives its segmental arteries from the lumbar arteries, which are branches of the abdominal aorta. The effect of direct pressure on the lumbar arteries by a leaking aneurysm can interfere with the blood supply to the spinal cord.

Clinical Problem Solving

1. A distinguished neurosurgeon, while giving a lecture on cerebrovascular accidents, made the following statement: "It is generally agreed that there are no anastomoses of clinical importance between the terminal end arteries within the brain substance, but there are many important anastomoses between the large arteries, both within and outside the skull, and these may play a major role in determining the extent of brain damage in cerebral vascular disease." Comment on this statement and name the sites at which important arterial anastomoses take place.
2. During examination of a carotid angiogram, the contrast medium had filled the anterior and middle cerebral arteries but had failed to fill the posterior cerebral artery. Careful following of the contrast medium showed it to enter the posterior communicating artery but to extend no farther. Explain this phenomenon in a normal person.
3. A 45-year-old man was admitted to the hospital after collapsing in his home 3 days previously. He was in a partial state of unconsciousness on the floor and was found by a friend. On physical examination, he had right-sided homonymous hemianopia, although careful examination of the fields of vision showed that the macular regions were normal. Right-sided hemianesthesia and hemianalgesia also were present, although the patient complained of severe burning pain in the right leg. During the first 24 hours in the hospital, the patient demonstrated mild right-sided hemiparesis of the flaccid type, which disappeared within 2 days. What is your diagnosis? Be specific in describing the branches of the artery that are involved.
4. During the course of an autopsy on a patient who had recently died of cerebrovascular disease, the pathologist made the comment that in atherosclerosis of the cerebral arteries, the atheromatous plaques tend to occur where the main arteries divide or where the arteries suddenly curve. It is thought that at these sites the pressure flow changes may be a factor in the causation of the disease process. Using your knowledge of anatomy, name as many sites as you can where the main cerebral arteries divide or undergo abrupt change in their course.
5. Having carefully examined a male patient with cerebrovascular disease, the physician met with the family to discuss the nature of the illness, the course of treatment, and the prognosis. The daughter asked the physician what was meant by the term *stroke* and what the common causes are. He was also asked why the clinical findings vary so much from patient to patient. Using your knowledge of the anatomy and physiology of cerebral blood flow, explain why patients with cerebrovascular disease present such a variety of syndromes.
6. The classic sign of cerebrovascular disease is hemiplegia, yet we know that most patients also exhibit sensory deficits of different types. Using your knowledge of the anatomical distribution of the cerebral arteries, discuss the main types of sensory loss that you may find in such patients.
7. During the discussion of the symptoms and signs of a 70-year-old woman who had been admitted to the hospital for treatment of cerebrovascular disease, a fourth-year medical student made the comment that she was surprised to find that many of the signs and symptoms were bilateral in this patient. She said that the three previous patients she had examined had displayed only unilateral signs and symptoms. Using your knowledge of neuroanatomy, explain why some patients exhibit bilateral signs and symptoms while in others the syndrome is clearly unilateral.
8. Neurologists speak frequently of the dominant hemisphere, and if cerebrovascular disease should involve

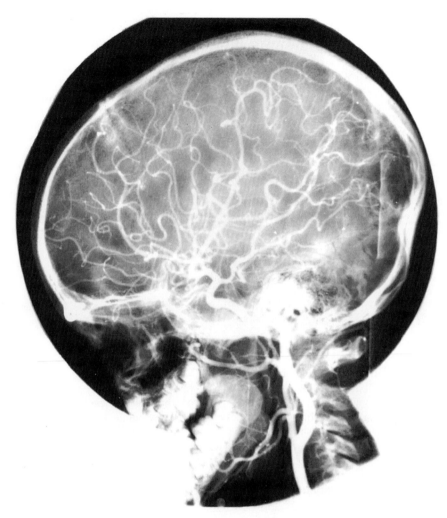

Figure 17–8 Lateral internal carotid arteriogram. Male aged 20 years.

that hemisphere one would expect the patient possibly to have global or total sensorimotor aphasia. Explain this phenomenon.

9. Explain why patients with a thrombosis of the middle cerebral artery often present with homonymous hemianopia as well as hemiplegia and hemianesthesia.

10. During the neurobiology course, the professor of neuroanatomy emphasized the importance of knowing the structure and blood supply of the internal capsule. He explained the arrangement of the ascending and descending tracts within the capsule and showed how they were concentrated into a small area between the thalamus and caudate nucleus medially and the lentiform nucleus laterally. Clearly, an interruption of the blood supply to this vital area would produce widespread neurological defects. What is the blood supply to the internal capsule?

11. A 36-year-old man visited his physician with a complaint that on three occasions during the past 6 months he had fainted at work. During careful questioning, the pa-

tient stated that on each occasion he had fainted while sitting at his desk and while interviewing office personnel; he added that the person being interviewed sat in a chair immediately to the right of the desk. He said that before each fainting attack he felt dizzy; then he lost consciousness, only to recover within a few moments. The previous evening, he had a similar dizzy spell when he turned his head quickly to the right to talk to a friend in the street. The physician noted that the patient wore a stiff collar that was rather close-fitting. When the physician commented on this, the patient stated that he always wore this type of collar to work. No abnormal physical signs were found. Using your knowledge of anatomy and physiology, you would make what diagnosis?

12. A 45-year-old man, a company director, rose to give his annual after-dinner speech to the board when he suddenly experienced an "agonizing, crushing" pain over the sternum. Feeling giddy and weak, he fell back in his chair. A few moments later, he lapsed into uncon-

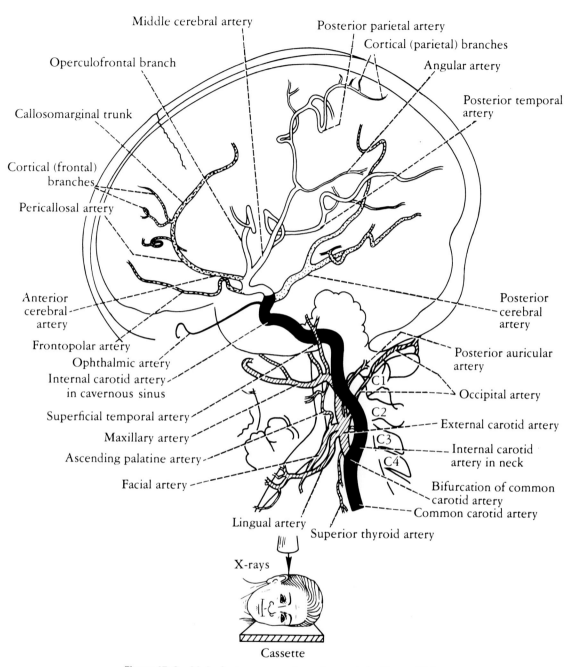

Middle cerebral artery

Operculofrontal branch

Callosomarginal trunk

Cortical (frontal)
branches

Pericallosal artery

Anterior
cerebral
artery

Frontopolar artery

Ophthalmic artery

Internal carotid artery
in cavernous sinus

Superficial temporal artery

Maxillary artery

Ascending palatine artery

Facial artery

Posterior parietal artery

Cortical (parietal) branches

Angular artery

Posterior temporal
artery

Posterior
cerebral
artery

Posterior auricular
artery

C1

C2

C3

C4

Occipital artery

External carotid artery

Internal carotid
artery in neck

Bifurcation of common
carotid artery

Common carotid artery

Lingual artery

Superior thyroid artery

X-rays

Cassette

Figure 17–9   Main features seen in radiograph in Figure 17-8.

sciousness. An attendant at the dinner, who had received some training in cardiopulmonary resuscitation while a member of the armed forces, ran forward and noted that the patient had stopped breathing. He quickly started mouth-to-mouth resuscitation and cardiac compression and kept going until ambulance personnel arrived to take the patient to the hospital. The physician in the intensive care unit at the hospital later told the patient that his life had been saved by the alertness and competence of the attendant at the dinner.

Using your knowledge of neurophysiology, state how long brain tissue can survive when there is complete cardiac arrest and breathing has ceased.

13. A 62-year-old man with a history of hypertension visited his physician because the day before he had temporarily lost the sight in his right eye. He explained that the sight loss was partial and lasted about half an hour. On close questioning, the patient admitted that he had had similar episodes of blindness in the same eye during the previous 6 months, but they had lasted only a few min-

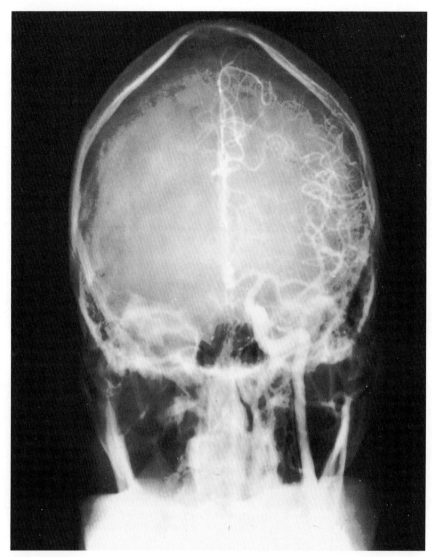

Figure 17–10   Anteroposterior internal carotid arteriogram. Male aged 20 years.

utes. The patient also mentioned that there were days when he could not remember the names of people and things. He also had recently experienced severe right-sided headaches. When asked about his activities, he said that he could not walk as well as he used to and his left leg sometimes felt weak and numb. While performing a careful physical examination, the physician heard with his stethoscope a distinct systolic bruit over the right side of the neck. Given that the patient has vascular disease of the brain, which artery is likely to be involved in the disease process? What special clinical investigations could you perform to confirm the diagnosis?

14. A 39-year-old man was admitted to the hospital with a history of a sudden excruciating, generalized headache while gardening. This was followed, 10 minutes later, by the patient's collapsing to the ground in a state of un-

consciousness. After being carried indoors and placed on a settee, the patient regained consciousness but appeared confused. He complained of a severe headache and a stiff neck. Physical examination revealed some rigidity of the neck but nothing further. A careful neurological examination 3 days later revealed some loss of tone in the muscles of the left leg. Using your knowledge of anatomy, make the diagnosis. What is the reason for the neck rigidity?

15. A 26-year-old man, on leaving a bar after a few drinks, stepped into the road at 1:00 AM and was struck by a passing car. Fortunately, the car was traveling slowly and struck the patient's head a glancing blow. One hour later, a policeman found the patient unconscious on the sidewalk. Physical examination at the local hospital found that the patient had recovered consciousness for a few minutes, but then he had quickly relapsed into an

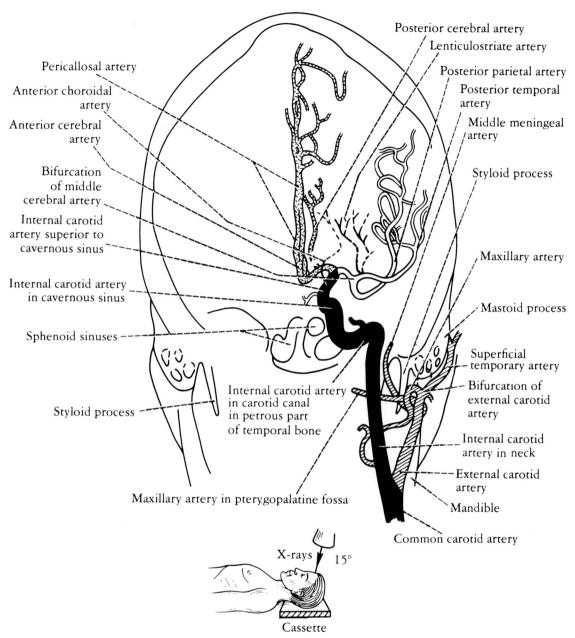

Posterior cerebral artery

Lenticulostriate artery

Posterior parietal artery

Posterior temporal artery

Middle meningeal artery

Styloid process

Maxillary artery

Mastoid process

Superficial temporary artery

Bifurcation of external carotid artery

Internal carotid artery in neck

External carotid artery

Mandible

Common carotid artery

Pericallosal artery

Anterior choroidal artery

Anterior cerebral artery

Bifurcation of middle cerebral artery

Internal carotid artery superior to cavernous sinus

Internal carotid artery in cavernous sinus

Sphenoid sinuses

Styloid process

Internal carotid artery in carotid canal in petrous part of temporal bone

Maxillary artery in pterygopalatine fossa

X-rays 15°

Cassette

Figure 17–11 Main features seen in the radiograph in Figure 17-10.

unconscious state. The right pupil was dilated and the muscle tone of the left leg was found to be less than normal. A positive Babinski sign was obtained on the left side. Examination of the scalp showed a severe bruise over the right temple and a lateral radiograph of the skull showed a fracture of the anterior inferior angle of the parietal bone. A CT scan showed a dense area extending from anterior to posterior along the inner table of the right parietal bone. What is the diagnosis? Let us suppose that the equipment for performing a CT scan was unavailable and that it was decided to perform a

lumbar puncture; this test revealed a raised cerebrospinal fluid pressure and the fluid was very slightly blood-stained. Explain these additional findings.

16. A 50-year-old woman complaining of headaches, drowsiness, and mental confusion visited her physician. On close questioning, the patient distinctly remembered striking her head against a closet door when bending down 3 weeks previously. A CT scan revealed the presence of a large space-occupying lesion over the right frontal lobe of the brain. What is the possible diagnosis?

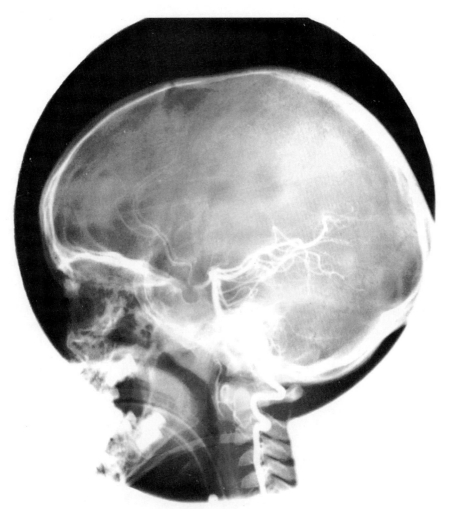

Figure 17–12 Lateral vertebral arteriogram. Male aged 20 years.

17. A 55-year-old man with a history of hypertension collapsed in the street while walking to work. He complained of a sudden severe headache. After 5 minutes, his face began to sag on the right side and his speech became slurred. On admission to the hospital, his right arm and leg were found to be weaker than the left, and the muscles were hypotonic. The eyes were deviated to the left. Later, the right arm and leg showed complete paralysis and were insensitive to pinprick. A positive Babinski sign was present on the right side. Two hours later, the patient relapsed into a deep coma with bilateral dilated fixed pupils. Later, the respirations became deep and irregular, and the patient died 6 hours later. Using your knowledge of neuroanatomy, make the diagnosis.

18. What is the blood supply to the spinal cord? Which areas of the spinal cord are supplied by the anterior spinal artery? Which regions of the spinal cord are most susceptible to ischemia?

Answers to Clinical Problem Solving

1. Once the terminal branches of the cerebral arteries enter the brain substance, no further anastomoses occur. Blockage of such end arteries by disease is quickly followed by neuronal death and necrosis. The surrounding neuroglia then usually proliferates and invades the area, producing a neuroglial scar or forming a cystic cavity. The following important anastomoses exist between the cerebral arteries: (a) the circle of Willis; (b) anastomoses between the branches of the cerebral arteries on the surface of the cerebral hemi-

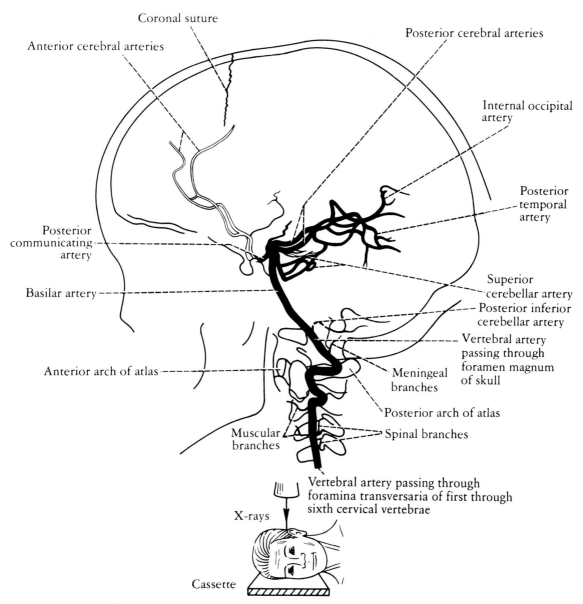

Figure 17–13 Main features shown in the radiograph in Figure 17-12.

spheres and the cerebellar hemispheres; and (c) anastomoses between the branches of the internal and external carotid arteries: (i) at their origin at the common carotid artery, (ii) at the anastomosis between the branches of the ophthalmic artery within the orbit and the facial and maxillary arteries, and (iii) between the meningeal branches of the internal carotid artery and the middle meningeal artery.

2. The work of McDonald and Potter in 1951 showed that the posterior communicating artery is the site at which the streams of blood from the internal carotid and vertebral arteries on the same side come together, and since their pressures at this point are equal, they do not mix. Nevertheless, in clinical practice, good filling of the posterior cerebral artery with radiopaque material

as shown by carotid angiography occurs in about 25 percent of patients. Slight filling also may be seen in other normal individuals. The variable results can be explained on the basis that the size of the arteries making up the arterial circle is subject to considerable variation and consequently the blood flow in different individuals may vary.

3. Occlusion of the cortical branches of the left posterior cerebral artery will give rise to right-sided homonymous hemianopia because of ischemia of the primary visual area in the calcarine fissure. The escape of the macular region could be accounted for by the overlapping of the arterial supply of this area of the occipital lobe by the left posterior and left middle cerebral arteries. The right-sided hemianesthesia and the severe burning pain in

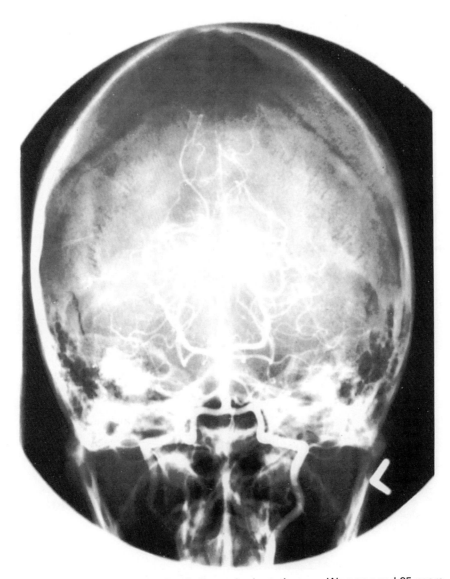

Figure 17–14 Anteroposterior (angled) vertebral arteriogram. Woman aged 35 years.

the right leg are referred to clinically as the thalamic syndrome and are due to occlusion of one of the central branches of the left posterior cerebral artery that supplies the sensory nuclei of the left thalamus. The presence of a mild fleeting right-sided hemiparesis could be explained by a temporary occlusion of a branch of the left posterior cerebral artery to the left cerebral peduncle.

4. Atheromatous plaques tend to occur at the following sites: (a) carotid sinus of the internal carotid artery at or just beyond the bifurcation of the common carotid artery, (b) the first main bifurcation of the middle cerebral artery, (c) where the vertebral arteries join to form the basilar artery, (d) where the anterior cerebral artery curves superiorly and posteriorly over the genu of the corpus callosum, and (e) where the posterior cerebral

artery passes around the lateral side of the cerebral peduncle.

5. A stroke may be defined as a sudden development of a neurological defect, usually associated with the development of some degree of hemiplegia and sometimes accompanied by unconsciousness; it is usually caused by a cerebrovascular accident. The symptoms and signs will depend on the cause of the interruption of cerebral blood flow and the size of the artery involved. For example, cerebral embolism or cerebral hemorrhage is a sudden event, whereas the development of atherosclerosis in a patient with hypertension is a slow process that suddenly may become worse when thrombosis occurs at the site of the atheromatous plaque. Hemiplegia is the most common sign, but many additional sensory defects may develop, depending on the artery blocked.

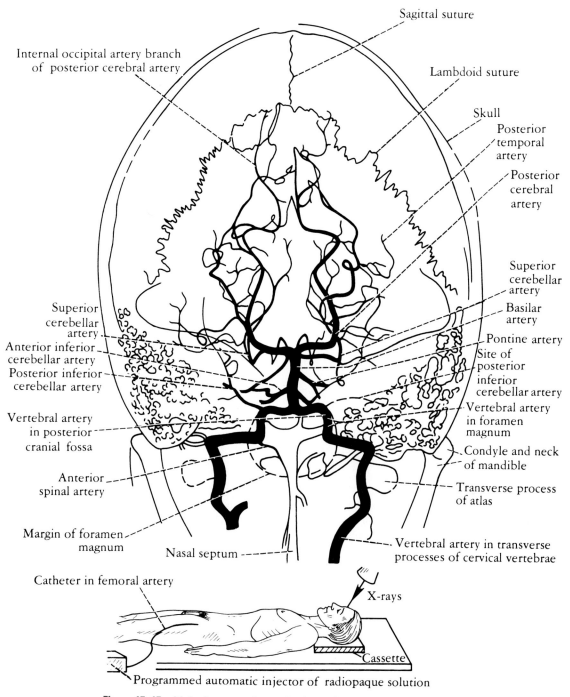

Figure 17–15 Main features shown in the radiograph in Figure 17-14.

Examples are hemianesthesia, hemianopia, dysphasia, and dysarthria.

6. Occlusion of the middle cerebral artery or its branches can produce, in addition to paralysis of the muscles of the opposite side of the body, contralateral hemianesthesia owing to ischemia of the postcentral gyrus and homonymous hemianopia owing to ischemia of the optic radiation.

Occlusion of the anterior cerebral artery or its branches may produce contralateral sensory loss in the leg, foot, and toes owing to ischemia of the leg area of the cerebral cortex. Occlusion of the posterior cerebral artery or its branches may produce contralateral homonymous hemianopia owing to ischemia of the primary visual area in the region of the calcarine fissure. If the branches to the thalamus also are blocked, there

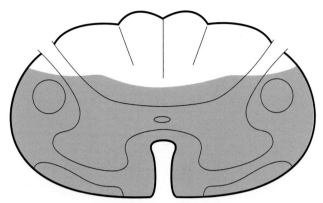

Figure 17–16 Anterior spinal artery occlusion. Red area denotes region of spinal cord affected.

will also be contralateral hemianesthesia and possibly the development of severe pain in the same areas.

The above sensory deficits are the main ones seen. The degree of sensory involvement will depend on the size and number of branches of the artery occluded.

7. The internal carotid and the basilar arteries are equally affected by disease. The internal carotid artery supplies predominantly one cerebral hemisphere through the anterior cerebral and middle cerebral branches and, therefore, occlusion of the internal carotid artery will produce contralateral hemiplegia, hemianesthesia, hemianopia, and aphasia and agnosia, depending on whether the dominant hemisphere is involved. On the other hand, the basilar artery contributes to the blood supply of both sides of the brain through the two posterior cerebral arteries and the many branches to both sides of the brainstem. Consequently, occlusion of the basilar artery will result in bilateral motor and sensory losses and involvement of the cranial nerves and cerebellum on both sides of the body.

8. The dominant hemisphere possesses the language function. In right-handed individuals (and in some left-handed persons) language is a function of the left hemisphere. A cerebrovascular accident involving the middle cerebral artery on the left side will therefore be more serious than one on the right side, since it will involve the cortical speech area and cause a total sensory motor aphasia. In persons who have a dominant right hemisphere, the reverse occurs.

9. The middle cerebral artery, in addition to giving off cortical branches, gives off central branches that supply part of the posterior limb of the internal capsule and the optic radiation. Occlusion of these branches will cause contralateral homonymous hemianopia.

10. Since so many important ascending and descending tracts travel in the internal capsule, an occlusion of its blood supply would produce a widespread neurological deficit. The internal capsule is supplied by the medial and lateral striate central branches of the middle cerebral artery and by the central branches of the anterior cerebral artery.

11. This patient has the symptoms of the carotid sinus syndrome. For a full description of this syndrome, see page 483.

12. It has been estimated that irreversible changes start to occur in the cerebral nervous tissue about 4 minutes following the complete arrest of cerebral blood flow. (This figure may be higher if the patient's body has been cooled.)

13. The impairment of vision of the right eye with motor symptoms in the left leg strongly suggests partial occlusion of the right internal carotid artery. When these are coupled with impairment of memory and a systolic bruit over the right internal carotid artery, the diagnosis is almost certain. The right-sided headaches are also common symptoms in this condition. A right-sided carotid angiogram can confirm the presence of extreme narrowing of the internal carotid artery at its origin. Ophthalmodynamometric measurements can show diminished retinal arterial pressure on the right side owing to diminished pressure in the right ophthalmic artery.

14. This patient had a congenital aneurysm of the anterior communicating artery. The sudden onset of a severe headache, which is often so dramatic that the patient feels as though he or she has been hit on the head, is characteristic of rupture of a congenital aneurysm into the subarachnoid space. The stiff or rigid neck is due to meningeal irritation caused by the presence of blood in the subarachnoid space. This patient had no evidence of previous pressure on the optic nerve leading to unilateral visual defect, which sometimes occurs when the aneurysm is situated on the anterior part of the circle of Willis. The loss of tone in the left leg muscles is difficult to explain, although it may be due to the sudden hemorrhage into the subarachnoid space causing damage to the right cerebral hemisphere.

15. This patient had a right-sided extradural hemorrhage due to a fracture of the anterior part of the parietal bone, which tore the anterior division of the right middle meningeal artery. The history of the patient being found unconscious, then recovering consciousness for a period only to relapse into unconsciousness, is a characteristic finding. The initial trauma usually is responsible for the initial loss of consciousness. The relapse into an unconscious state is due to the accumulation of a large blood clot under arterial pressure outside the meningeal layer of dura. This is responsible for the dilated pupil on the right side due to indirect pressure on the right oculomotor nerve. The pressure on the right precentral gyrus causes the hemiplegia and weakness of the left leg; it also causes the positive Babinski sign on the left side. The presence of a large blood clot in the intracranial cavity was easily recognized on a CT scan. The presence of the clot was also responsible for the raised cerebrospinal fluid pressure. The slight blood staining of the fluid obtained from a spinal tap was due to a small leakage of blood from the extradural space into the subarachnoid space at the fracture site.

16. This patient had a chronic subdural hematoma following trauma to the head 3 weeks previously. This resulted from one of the superior cerebral veins tearing at its point of entrance into the superior sagittal sinus. The blood accumulated under low pressure between the dura and the arachnoid. The headaches, drowsiness, and mental confusion were due to the raised intracranial pressure. The blood clot could be seen easily on the CT scan. The blood clot was successfully removed through a burr hole in the skull and the patient had no further symptoms.

17. The history of hypertension, sudden onset of severe headache, slurring of speech, right lower facial weakness, right-sided hemiplegia, right positive Babinski sign, right-sided hemianesthesia, and deviation of the eyes to the left side are all diagnostic of a cerebrovascular accident involving the left cerebral hemisphere. The perforating central branches of the left middle cerebral artery were found at autopsy to be extensively affected by atherosclerosis. One of these arteries had ruptured, resulting in a large hemorrhage into the left lentiform nucleus and left internal capsule. The combination of hypertension and atherosclerotic degeneration of the artery was responsible for the fatal hemorrhage. The dilated fixed pupils, the irregularity in breathing, and, finally, death were due to the raised pressure within the hemisphere causing downward pressure effects within the brainstem.

18. The blood supply to the spinal cord is fully described on page 481. The anterior spinal artery supplies the anterior two-thirds of the spinal cord. The upper and lower thoracic segments of the spinal cord have a relatively poor supply of blood because the anterior spinal artery in this region may be extremely small, and therefore are more susceptible to ischemia.

Review Questions

Directions: Each of the numbered items in this section is followed by answers that are positively phrased. Select the ONE lettered answer that is an EXCEPTION.

1. The following statements concerning the blood supply to the brain are correct **except:**
   (a) The brain receives its blood supply directly and indirectly from the two internal carotid and the two vertebral arteries that lie within the subarachnoid space.
   (b) The circle of Willis is formed by the anterior cerebral, the internal carotid, the posterior cerebral, the basilar, and the anterior and posterior communicating arteries.
   (c) The cerebral arteries anastomose on the surface of the brain.
   (d) There are no anastomoses between the branches of the cerebral arteries once they have entered the substance of the brain.
   (e) The main blood supply to the internal capsule is from the central branches of the anterior cerebral artery.

2. The areas of the cerebral cortex listed below receive their arterial supply as indicated **except:**
   (a) The precentral gyrus (face area) is supplied by the middle cerebral artery.
   (b) The postcentral gyrus (foot area) is supplied by the anterior cerebral artery.
   (c) The cuneus is supplied by the posterior cerebral artery.
   (d) The inferior temporal gyrus is supplied by the middle cerebra artery.
   (e) Wernicke's area is supplied by the middle cerebral artery.

3. The arteries listed below arise from the main stem arteries as indicated **except:**
   (a) The ophthalmic artery is a branch of the middle cerebral artery.
   (b) The pontine arteries are branches of the basilar artery.
   (c) The posterior communicating artery is a branch of the internal carotid artery.
   (d) The posterior spinal artery arises from the vertebral artery.
   (e) The posterior inferior cerebella artery is a branch of the vertebral artery.

4. The veins listed below drain into the venous sinuses indicated **except:**
   (a) The superior cerebral veins drain into the superior sagittal sinus.
   (b) The great cerebral vein drains into the straight sinus.
   (c) The superior cerebellar veins drain into the straight sinus.
   (d) The spinal veins drain into the internal vertebral venous plexus.
   (e) The great cerebral vein drains into the straight sinus.

5. The following statements concerning the cerebral blood flow are correct **except:**
   (a) The sympathetic postganglionic fibers exert very little control over the diameter of the cerebral blood vessels.
   (b) The cerebral blood flow varies only slightly with changes in the general blood pressure.
   (c) High oxygen tension in the cerebral blood causes vasodilation of the cerebral blood vessels.

(d) One of the most powerful vasodilators of cerebral blood vessels is carbon dioxide.

(e) The blood flow for a particular area of nervous tissue following occlusion of a cerebral artery depends on the adequacy of the collateral circulation.

6. The following statements concerning cerebral ischemia are correct **except:**

(a) Atheromatous degeneration of a cerebral artery may cause degeneration of the nerve cells in the avascular area and proliferation of the microglial cells in the surrounding area.

(b) Neuronal function ceases after the blood flow has stopped for about 1 minute.

(c) Irreversible cerebral damage starts to occur after the blood flow has ceased for about 4 minutes.

(d) Shock occurring as the result of severe physical trauma can result in cerebral ischemia.

(e) Cooling of the patient's body following a cerebrovascular accident speeds up cerebral degeneration.

Directions: Matching Questions
In Figure 17-17, match the numbered arteries listed below with the appropriate lettered arteries. Each lettered option may be selected once, more than once, or not at all.

7. Number 1
8. Number 2

9. Number 3
10. Number 4
11. Number 5
12. Number 6

(a) Middle cerebral artery
(b) Anterior communicating artery
(c) Posterior cerebral artery
(d) Basilar artery
(e) None of the above

Directions: In the next item the possible answers are positively phrased. Select the ONE lettered answer that is an EXCEPTION.

13. The following statements concerning the blood supply to the spinal cord are correct **except:**

(a) The posterior spinal arteries supply the posterior third of the spinal cord.

(b) The veins communicate with the veins of the brain and the venous sinuses.

(c) The arteria radicularis magna (artery of Adamkiewicz) arises in the upper thoracic region from the arch of the aorta.

(d) The anterior spinal artery is single but usually arises from both vertebral arteries.

(e) The spinal arteries are reinforced by radicular arteries, which are branches of local arteries.

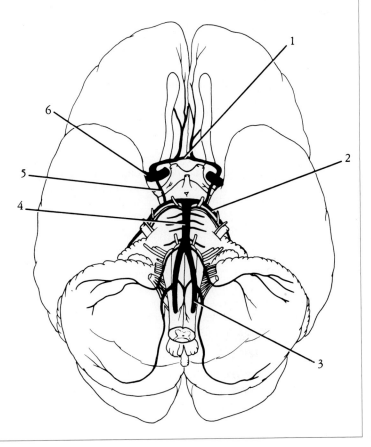

Figure 17–17   The arteries of the inferior surface of the brain.

Directions: Read the case histories then answer the questions. You will be required to select ONE BEST lettered answer.

A 58-year-old man, while eating his evening meal, suddenly complained of a severe headache. Moments later, he slumped forward and lost consciousness.

14. On being admitted to the hospital the examining physician could have found the following physical signs **except:**
    (a) He was in a deep coma and his breathing was deep and slow.
    (b) The patient's head was turned to the left.
    (c) The right side of his face was flattened and saliva was drooling out of the right corner of his mouth.
    (d) The muscle tone of the limbs was less on the right side than on the left.
    (e) The right abdominal reflexes were absent and there was a positive Babinski response on the left side.

15. Three days later the patient regained consciousness and the following additional signs could have become apparent **except:**
    (a) The right arm and, to a lesser extent, the right leg were paralyzed.
    (b) Movements of the left arm and leg and the left side of the face were normal.
    (c) The upper and lower parts of the right side of his face were paralyzed.
    (d) The patient had difficulty in swallowing.
    (e) The patient was unable to speak.

16. During the next two weeks the following signs could have developed **except:**
    (a) The muscles of the limbs on the right side became hypertonic.
    (b) The tendon reflexes on the right side became hyperactive.
    (c) The patient had some sensory loss on the right side.
    (d) The patient was suffering from urinary incontinence.
    (e) The muscles on the left side exhibited hypotonia.

17. The neurologist in charge of this patient interpreted the findings as follows. All his interpretations were likely to be correct **except:**
    (a) The sudden onset of a severe headache followed by loss of consciousness is a common finding in patients with a blockage of a cerebral artery.
    (b) The depth of coma is unrelated to the extent of the arterial blockage.
    (c) Paralysis of the face on the right side indicated the presence of a lesion on the left side of the brain.
    (d) The patient's head and eyes were turned to the left, i.e., to the side of the lesion.
    (e) The loss of right sided abdominal reflexes indicated the presence of a lesion on the left side of the brain.

18. The following physical signs and known anatomical data strongly suggested the involvement of the left middle cerebral artery **except:**
    (a) Paralysis of the right side of the face and the right arm was more severe than that of the right leg.
    (b) The presence of Aphasia.
    (c) The central branches of the middle cerebral artery do not supply the lentiform nucleus, the caudate nucleus and the internal capsule.
    (d) The left middle cerebral artery supplies the entire lateral surface of the cerebral hemisphere, except for the narrow strip supplied by the anterior cerebral artery.
    (e) The left posterior cerebral artery supplies the occipital pole and the inferolateral surface of the cerebral hemisphere.

A 60-year-old man was admitted to the emergency department, complaining of the sudden onset of excruciating, sharp, tearing pain localized to the back of the chest and the back. After a thorough physical and radiological examination, a diagnosis of dissection of the descending thoracic aorta was made. Within a few hours the patient started to experience "girdle" pain involving the fourth thoracic dermatome on both sides. Later, he was found to have bilateral thermoanesthesia and analgesia below the level of the fourth thoracic dermatome. Position sense, vibration, and light touch remained normal. Complete spastic paralysis of both legs quickly developed.

19. The sudden onset of "girdle" pain in this patient was **most likely caused by:**
    (a) Pressure on the fourth thoracic spinal nerves.
    (b) Blockage of the origins of the posterior intercostal arteries that give rise to the segmental spinal arteries by the aortic dissection.
    (c) Discomfort caused by the expanding aneurysm.
    (d) Osteoarthritis of the vertebral column.

20. The development of bilateral thermoanesthesia and analgesia below the level of the fourth thoracic segment of the cord and the later development of paraplegia **could be caused by:**
    (a) Absent circulation in the posterior spinal arteries.
    (b) Cerebral hemorrhage.
    (c) Absent circulation in the anterior spinal artery.
    (d) Collapse of the fourth thoracic vertebral body.

Answers to Review Questions

1. E
2. D
3. A
4. C
5. C
6. E
7. B
8. C
9. E
10. D
11. E
12. A
13. C
14. E. A positive Babinski sign was present on the right side.
15. C. The muscles of the upper part of the face on the right side are not affected by a lesion involving the upper motor neurons on the left side of the brain. This is due to the fact that the part of the facial nucleus of the seventh cranial nerve that controls the muscles of the upper part of the face receives corticonuclear fibers from both cerebral hemispheres (see p. 345).
16. E. The cerebral lesion was on the left side of the brain and the muscles of the left leg were completely unaffected by the vascular accident.
17. B. The depth of coma is related to the extent of the arterial blockage.
18. C. The central branches of the right middle cerebral artery do supply the right lentiform and caudate nuclei and the right internal capsule.

19. B. In the thoracic region, the posterior intercostal arteries arise directly from the thoracic aorta and can be blocked by a blood clot as the aortic dissection progresses. The segmental spinal arteries, which are branches of the posterior intercostal arteries, give origin to the radicular arteries that supply the spinal nerves and their roots. If these arteries are compromised, severe pain is experienced in the distribution of the spinal nerves involved, hence, the "girdle" pain.
20. C. The blood supply to the spinal cord is meager and if the segmental arteries that reinforce the anterior and posterior spinal arteries are compromised, ischemia of the spinal cord could follow. In this patient, the circulation in the anterior spinal artery ceased and the blood supply to the anterior two-thirds of the spinal cord was cut off. This would explain the sudden development of bilateral thermoanesthesia and analgesia (spinothalamic tracts in both lateral white columns) and the paraplegia (corticospinal tracts in both lateral white columns). The sparing of the sensations of position, vibration, and light touch, which travel in the fasciculus gracilis and fasciculus cuneatus, can be explained by the fact that the posterior white columns are supplied by the posterior spinal arteries, in which the circulation was adequate.

ADDITIONAL READING

Angerson, W.J., et al. (eds). *Blood Flow in the Brain.* New York, Oxford University Press, 1989.

Ascher, G. F., Ganti, S. R., Hilal, S. K. Cerebral Angiography. In R. N. Rosenberg (ed.). *The Science and Practice of Clinical Medicine. Vol. 5, Neurology.* New York: Grune & Stratton, 1980.

Bannister, R. *Brain's Clinical Neurology* (6th ed.). London and New York: Oxford University Press, 1985.

Bes, A. (ed.). *Proceedings of the Eleventh International Symposium on Cerebral Blood Flow and Metabolism.* New York: Raven, 1983.

Brazis, P. W., Masden, J. C., Biller, J. *Localization in Clinical Neurology* (2nd ed.). Boston: Little, Brown, 1990.

Brust, J.C.M. Cerebral Infarction. In: L.P. Rowland (ed.). *Merritt's Textbook of Neurology,* 9th ed., pp. 246-256. Philadelphia, PA: Lea & Febiger, 1995.

Capra, N. F. Anatomy of the Cerebral Venous System. In J. P. Kapp and H. H. Schmidek (eds.), *Cerebral Venous System and Its Disorders.* New York: Grune & Stratton, 1984. P. 1.

Duvernoy, H. M. *The Superficial Veins of the Human Brain.* Berlin: Springer-Verlag, 1975.

Duvernoy, H. M., Delon, S., Vanson, J. L. Cortical blood vessels of the human brain. *Brain Res. Bull.* 7:519, 1981.

Edvinsson, L., et al. *Cerebral Blood Flow and Metabolism.* New York, Raven Press, 1993.

Pulsinelli, W.A. Cerebrovascular Diseases. In: J.C. Bennett, F. Plum (eds). *Cecil Textbook of Medicine,* 20th ed., pp. 2057-2080, Philadelphia, PA: Saunders, 1996.

Reed, G., Devous, M. Cerebral blood flow autoregulation and hypertension. *Am. J. Med. Sci.* 289:37, 1985.

Snell, R. S. *Clinical Anatomy for Medical Students* (6th ed.). Philadelphia: Lippincott, Williams & Wilkins, 2000.

Snell, R. S., Wyman, A. C. *An Atlas of Normal Radiographic Anatomy.* Boston: Little, Brown, 1976.

Williams, P. L., et al. (eds.). *Gray's Anatomy* (38th Br. ed.). New York, Edinburgh: Churchill Livingstone, 1995.

Weisberg, L. A., Strub, R. L., Garcia, C. A. Stroke. In *Essentials of Clinical Neurology.* Baltimore: University Park Press, 1983. p. 147.

CHAPTER 18

The Development of the Nervous System

A pediatrician examined a newborn baby boy after a difficult delivery, and found a soft, fluctuant swelling over the vertebral column in the lumbosacral region. The swelling measured about 3 inches (7.5 cm) in diameter and was covered with a thin layer of intact skin. Transillumination of the sac revealed what appeared to be solid nervous tissue. Any neurological deficit was then carefully looked for and it was noted that the baby moved both legs normally and appeared to respond normally to painful stimulation of the leg skin. Examination of the anal sphincter showed normal tone. Careful examination for other congenital anomalies, especially hydrocephalus, was then made, but nothing abnormal was detected.

A diagnosis of meningomyelocele was made. In this condition there is a failure in the development of the vertebral arches with herniation of the meninges and nervous tissue through the defect. Later, the child was operated upon and the lower end of the spinal cord and the cauda equina were returned to the vertebral canal and the vertebral defect repaired. The child made an uneventful recovery.

CHAPTER OUTLINE

CHAPTER OBJECTIVES

This chapter is a brief overview of the development of the nervous system. It has been included to assist the students who have difficulty visualizing the relationship of different parts of the nervous system to one another; it also serves to explain in many instances how the different nerve tracts insinuate themselves between the central masses of gray matter.

 EARLY DEVELOPMENT

Before the formation of the nervous system in the embryo, three main cell layers become differentiated. The innermost layer, the **entoderm,** gives rise to the gastrointestinal tract, the lungs, and the liver. The **mesoderm** gives rise to the muscle, connective tissues, and the vascular system. The third and outermost layer, the **ectoderm,** formed of columnar epithelium, gives rise to the entire nervous system.

During the third week of development, the ectoderm on the dorsal surface of the embryo between the primitive knot and the buccopharyngeal membrane becomes thickened to form the **neural plate.** The plate, which is pear-shaped and wider cranially, develops a longitudinal **neural groove.** The groove now deepens so that it is bounded on either side by **neural folds** (Fig. 18-1). With further development, the neural folds fuse, converting the neural groove into a **neural tube.** Fusion starts at about the midpoint along the groove and extends cranially and caudally so that in the earliest stage the cavity of the tube remains in communication with the amniotic cavity through the **anterior** and **posterior neuropores** (Fig. 18-1). The anterior neuropore closes first, and 2 days later the posterior neuropore closes. Thus, normally the neural tube closure is complete within 28 days. Meanwhile, the neural tube has sunk beneath the surface ectoderm.

During the invagination of the neural plate to form the neural groove, the cells forming the lateral margin of the plate do not become incorporated in the neural tube but form a strip of ectodermal cells that lie between the neural tube and the covering ectoderm. This strip of ectoderm is called the **neural crest** (Fig. 18-1), and subsequently this group of cells will migrate ventrolaterally on each side around the neural tube. Ultimately, the neural crest cells will differentiate into the cells of the **posterior root ganglia, the sensory ganglia of the cranial nerves, autonomic ganglia, the cells of the suprarenal medulla,** and the **melanocytes.** It is also believed that these cells give rise to mesenchymal cells in the head and neck.

Meanwhile, the proliferation of cells at the cephalic end of the neural tube causes it to dilate and form **three primary brain vesicles:** the **forebrain vesicle,** the **midbrain vesicle,** and the **hindbrain vesicle** (Fig. 18-2, Table 18-1). The rest of the tube elongates and remains smaller in diameter; it will form the **spinal cord.**

The subsequent differentiation of cells in the neural tube is brought about by the inductive interactions of one group of cells with another. The inducing factors influence the control of the gene expression in the target cells. Ultimately, the simplest progenitor cell will differentiate into neurons and neuroglial cells. It is interesting to note that excessive numbers of neurons and neuroglial cells are developed and many (nearly half of the developing neurons) will be programmed to die by a process known as **programmed cell death.** Research into the identification of neurotrophic factors that promote the development and survival of neurons

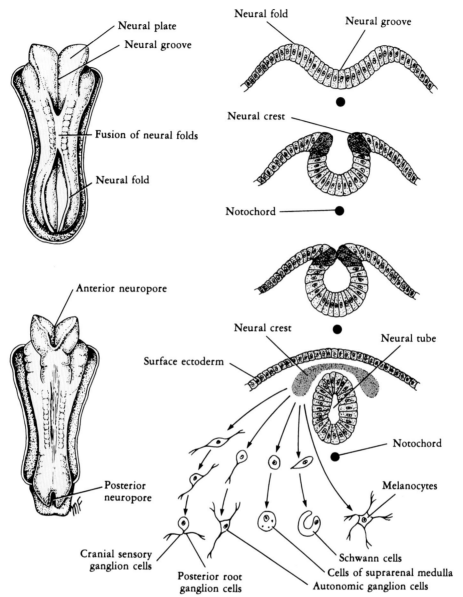

Figure 18–1 Formation of the neural plate, neural groove, and neural tube. The cells of the neural crest differentiate into the cells of the posterior root ganglia, the sensory ganglia of cranial nerves, autonomic ganglia, neurilemmal cells (Schwann cells), the cells of the suprarenal medulla, and melanocytes.

Table 18–1 The Primary Divisions of the Developing Brain

Primary Vesicle	Primary Division	Subdivision	Adult Structures
Forebrain vesicle	Prosencephalon (forebrain)	Telencephalon	Cerebral hemisphere, basal ganglia, hippocampus
		Diencephalon	Thalamus, hypothalamus, pineal body, infundibulum
Midbrain vesicle	Mesencephalon (midbrain)	Mesencephalon (midbrain)	Tectum, tegmentum, crus cerebri
Hindbrain vesicle	Rhombencephalon (hindbrain)	Metencephalon	Pons, cerebellum
		Myelencephalon	Medulla oblongata

is of great importance, since the results could possibly be applied to the problem of regeneration of the spinal cord neurons following trauma, or the inhibition of degenerative diseases, such as Alzheimer disease.

 SPINAL CORD

The wall of the neural tube consists of a single layer of pseudostratified columnar epithelial cells, called the **matrix cells** (Fig. 18-2). This thick zone of epithelium, which extends from the cavity of the tube to the exterior, is referred to as the **ventricular zone.** The nuclei of these cells move in toward the cavity of the tube to divide, and out toward the periphery during the intermitotic phases of the cell cycle (Fig. 18-2C). Repeated division of the matrix cells results in an increase in length and diameter of the neural tube. Eventually the early **neuroblasts** are formed, and are incapable of further division. These cells migrate peripherally to form the **intermediate zone** (Fig. 18-2). The intermediate zone will form the **gray matter** of the spinal cord.

The neuroblasts now give rise to nerve fibers that grow peripherally and form a layer external to the intermediate zone called the **marginal zone.** The nerve fibers in the marginal zone become myelinated and form the **white matter** of the spinal cord.

While the neuroblasts are being formed, the matrix cells also give rise to the **astrocytes** and the **oligodendrocytes** of the neuroglia. Later the **microglial cells,** which are derived from the surrounding mesenchyme, migrate into the developing spinal cord along with blood vessels. The **ependymal cells** are formed from the matrix cells that line the neural tube.

The cavity of the neural tube now becomes narrowed to form a dorsiventral cleft with thick lateral walls and thin **floor** and **roof plates** (Fig. 18-3). The intermediate zone of the lateral wall of the tube forms a large anterior thickening known as the **basal plate** and a smaller posterior thickening known as the **alar plate** (Fig. 18-3). The neuroblasts in the basal plate will form the motor cells of the anterior column (horn), while the neuroblasts in the alar plate will become the sensory cells of the posterior column. The motor

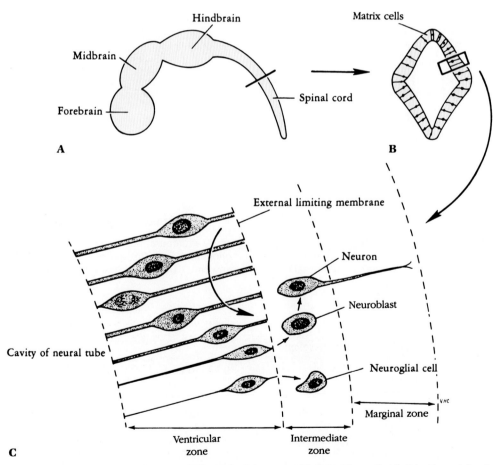

Figure 18–2   A. Expansion of the cephalic end of the neural tube to form the forebrain, midbrain, and hindbrain vesicles. **B** and **C.** Cross section of the developing neural tube in the region of the spinal cord. The cells of the neuroepithelial layer have been widely separated for clarity.

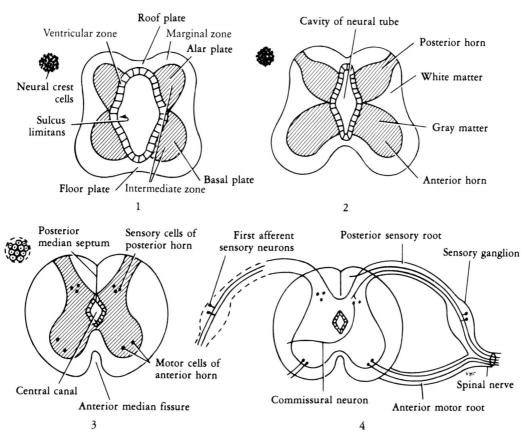

Figure 18–3 Different stages in the development of the spinal cord, showing the neural crest cells, which will form the first afferent neurons in the sensory pathway.

basal plate and the sensory alar plate are separated on each side by the **sulcus limitans.** The roof and floor plates remain thin and the cells contribute to the ependyma.

Continued growth of the basal plates on each side of the midline forms a deep longitudinal groove called the **anterior median fissure** (Fig. 18-3). The alar plates also increase in size and extend medially, compressing the posterior part of the lumen of the neural tube. Ultimately, the walls of the posterior portion of the tube fuse, forming the **posterior median septum.** The lumen of the neural tube becomes the **central canal** (Fig. 18-3).

Further Development of the Motor Neurons

The medial group of motor neurons form large multipolar cells whose axons will leave the anterior surface of the spinal cord to supply the musculature of the body. How the axons from a developing neuron are guided from their points of origin to a specific target is now occupying the minds of researchers. It is believed that the growing end of the axon possesses numerous receptors that respond to chemical cues along the way.

The lateral group of neurons gives rise to axons that will leave the anterior surface of the spinal cord as autonomic preganglionic fibers. Between the first thoracic and second or third lumbar segments of the mature spinal cord, the lateral group of neurons will form the **lateral gray column (horn)**, that is, the **sympathetic outflow.** Collectively, the axons leaving the anterior surface of the spinal cord will form the **anterior roots of the spinal nerves** (Fig. 18-3).

Development of the First Afferent Neurons in the Sensory Pathway

The first neurons in this pathway have their cell bodies situated outside the spinal cord and are derived from the neural crest (Figs. 18-1 and 18-3). The neural crest cells migrate to a posterolateral position on either side of the developing spinal cord and become segmented into cell clusters. Some of the cells in each cluster now differentiate into neuroblasts. Each neuroblast develops two processes, a peripheral process and a central process. The peripheral processes grow out laterally to become typical axons of sensory nerve fibers. The central processes, also axons, grow into the posterior part of the developing spinal cord and either end in the posterior gray column or ascend through the marginal zone (white matter) to one of the higher brain centers. These central processes are referred to collectively as the **posterior root of the spinal nerve** (Fig. 18-3). The peripheral processes join the anterior root to form the **spinal nerve.**

Some of the neural crest cells form the **capsular** or **satellite cells,** which surround the unipolar nerve cell bodies in a ganglion. Each **posterior root ganglion** is thus formed of the unipolar neurons and the capsular cells.

Further Development of the Sensory Neurons in the Posterior Gray Column

The neuroblasts that have entered the alar plates now develop processes that enter the marginal zone (white matter) of the cord on the same side and either ascend or descend to a higher or lower level. Other nerve cells send processes to the opposite side of the cord through the floor plate, where they ascend or descend for variable distances (Fig. 18-3).

Development of the Meninges and the Relation of the Spinal Cord to the Vertebral Column

The **pia mater, arachnoid mater,** and **dura mater** are formed from the mesenchyme (sclerotome) that surrounds the neural tube. The **subarachnoid space** develops as a cavity in the mesenchyme, which becomes filled with **cerebrospinal fluid.** The **ligamentum denticulatum** is formed from areas of condensation of the mesenchyme.

During the first 2 months of intrauterine life, the spinal cord is the same length as the vertebral column. Thereafter the developing vertebral column grows more rapidly than the spinal cord, so that at birth the coccygeal end of the cord lies at the level of the third lumbar vertebra. In the adult, the lower end of the spinal cord lies at the level of the lower border of the body of the first lumbar vertebra. As a result of this disproportion in the rate of growth of the vertebral column and spinal cord, the anterior and posterior roots of the spinal nerves below the first lumbar segment of the spinal cord descend within the vertebral canal until they reach their appropriate exits through the intervertebral foramina. Moreover the pia mater, which attached the coccygeal end of the spinal cord to the coccyx, now extends down as a slender fibrous strand from the lower end of the cord to the coccyx and forms the **filum terminale.** The obliquely coursing anterior and posterior roots of the spinal nerves and the filum terminale, which now occupy the lower end of the vertebral canal, form collectively the **cauda equina.**

It is now understood how the cauda equina is enclosed within the subarachnoid space down as far as the level of the second sacral vertebra. It is in this region, below the level of the lower end of the spinal cord, that a **spinal tap** can be performed (see p.18).

As the result of the development of the limb buds during the fourth month and the additional sensory and motor neurons, the spinal cord becomes swollen in the cervical and lumbar regions to form the **cervical** and **lumbar enlargements.**

 BRAIN

Once the neural tube has closed, the **three primary vesicles**—the **forebrain vesicle,** the **midbrain vesicle,** and the **hindbrain vesicle**—complete their development (Fig. 18-4). The forebrain vesicle will become the forebrain (**prosencephalon**), the midbrain vesicle will become the midbrain (**mesencephalon**), and the hindbrain vesicle will become the hindbrain (**rhombencephalon**).

By the fifth week the forebrain and hindbrain vesicles divide into two secondary vesicles (Fig. 18-4). The forebrain vesicle forms (1) the **telencephalon,** with its primitive cerebral hemispheres, and (2) the **diencephalon,** which develops optic vesicles. The hindbrain vesicle forms (1) the **metencephalon,** the future pons and cerebellum, and (2) the **myelencephalon,** or medulla oblongata (see Table 18-1).

The basic pattern of the ventricular system now is established. The cavity in each cerebral hemisphere is known as the **lateral ventricle.** The cavity of the diencephalon is known as the **third ventricle.** With continued growth, the cavity of the midbrain vesicle becomes small and forms the **cerebral aqueduct** or **aqueduct of Sylvius.** The cavity of the hindbrain vesicle forms the **fourth ventricle,** which is continuous with the central canal of the spinal cord. The lateral ventricles communicate with the third ventricle through the **interventricular foramina (foramina of Monro).** The ventricular system and the central canal of the spinal cord are lined with ependyma and are filled with cerebrospinal fluid. In the earliest stages, the cerebrospinal fluid within the ventricular system is not continuous with that of the subarachnoid space.

Early in development, the embryo is a flat disc and the neural tube is straight. Later, with the development of the head fold and tail fold, the neural tube becomes curved.

Medulla Oblongata (Myelencephalon)

The walls of the hindbrain vesicle initially show the typical organization seen in the neural tube, with the anterior thickenings, the **basal plates,** and the posterior thickenings, the **alar plates,** the two being separated by the **sulcus limitans** (Fig. 18-5). As development proceeds, the lateral walls are moved laterally (like an opening clamshell) at higher levels by the expanding fourth ventricle. As a result, the alar plates come to lie lateral to the basal plates. The neurons of the basal plate form the motor nuclei of cranial nerves IX, X, XI, and XII and are situated in the floor of the fourth ventricle medial to the sulcus limitans. The neurons of the alar plate form the sensory nuclei of cranial nerves V, VIII, IX, and X and the **gracile** and **cuneate nuclei.** Other cells of the alar plate migrate ventrolaterally and form the **olivary nuclei.**

The roof plate becomes stretched into a thin layer of ependymal tissue. The vascular mesenchyme lying in contact with the outer surface of the roof plate forms the pia mater, and the two layers together form the **tela choroidea.** Vascular tufts of tela choroidea project into the cavity of the fourth ventricle to form the **choroid plexus** (Fig. 18-5). Between the fourth and fifth months, local resorptions of

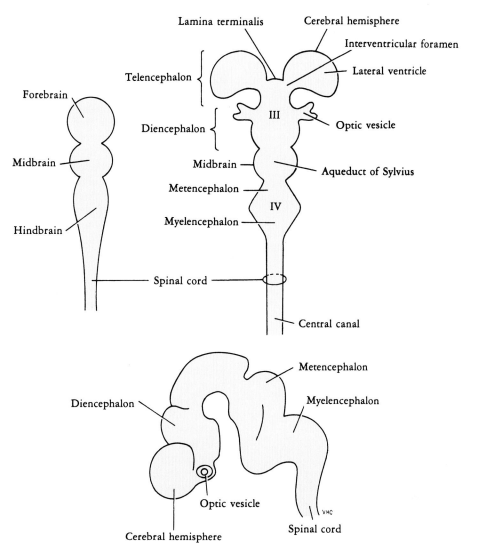

Figure 18–4 Division of the forebrain vesicle into the telencephalon and the diencephalon, and the hindbrain vesicle into the metencephalon and myelencephalon. Also shown is the way in which the cerebral hemisphere on each side develops as a diverticulum from the telencephalon.

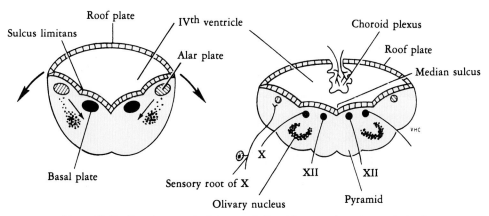

Figure 18–5 Development of the medulla oblongata (myelencephalon).

the roof plate occur, forming paired lateral foramina, the **foramina of Luschka,** and a median foramen, the **foramen of Magendie.** These important foramina allow the escape of the cerebrospinal fluid, which is produced in the ventricles, into the subarachnoid space (see p. 452).

The floor plate remains narrow and forms the region of the median sulcus. In the marginal layer on the anterior aspect of the medulla, descending axons from the neurons in the motor areas of the cerebral cortex (precentral gyrus) produce prominent swellings called the **pyramids.**

Pons (Ventral Part of the Metencephalon)

The pons arises from the anterior part of the metencephalon (Fig. 18-6), but it also receives a cellular contribution from the alar part of the myelencephalon.

The neurons of the basal plates form the motor nuclei of cranial nerves V, VI, and VII. The neurons of the ventromedial part of each alar plate form the main sensory nucleus of cranial nerve V, a sensory nucleus of cranial nerve VII, and the vestibular and cochlear nuclei of cranial nerve VIII; they also form the **pontine nuclei.** The axons of the pontine nuclei grow transversely to enter the developing cerebellum of the opposite side, thus forming the **transverse pontine fibers** and the **middle cerebellar peduncle.**

Cerebellum (Posterior Part of the Metencephalon)

The cerebellum is formed from the posterior part of the alar plates of the metencephalon. On each side, the alar plates bend medially to form the **rhombic lips** (Fig. 18-7). As they enlarge, the lips project caudally over the roof plate of the fourth ventricle and unite with each other in the midline to form the cerebellum (Figs. 18-7 and 18-8). At the twelfth week, a small midline portion, the **vermis,** and two lateral portions, the **cerebellar hemispheres,** may be recog-

nized. At about the end of the fourth month, fissures develop on the surface of the cerebellum and the characteristic folia of the adult cerebellum gradually develop.

The neuroblasts derived from the matrix cells in the ventricular zone migrate toward the surface of the cerebellum and eventually give rise to the neurons forming the **cerebellar cortex.** Other neuroblasts remain close to the ventricular surface and differentiate into the **dentate** and other deep cerebellar nuclei. With further development, the axons of neurons forming these nuclei grow out into the mesencephalon (midbrain) to reach the forebrain and these fibers will form the greater part of the superior cerebellar peduncle. Later, the growth of the axons of the pontocerebellar fibers and the corticopontine fibers will connect the cerebral cortex with the cerebellum, and so the middle cerebellar peduncle will be formed. The inferior cerebellar peduncle will be formed largely by the growth of sensory axons from the spinal cord, the vestibular nuclei, and olivary nuclei.

Midbrain (Mesencephalon)

The midbrain develops from the midbrain vesicle, the cavity of which becomes much reduced to form the **cerebral aqueduct** or **aqueduct of Sylvius** (Fig. 18-9). The sulcus limitans separates the alar plate from the basal plate on each side, as seen in the developing spinal cord. The neuroblasts in the basal plates will differentiate into the neurons forming the nuclei of the **third** and **fourth cranial nerves** and possibly the **red nuclei,** the **substantia nigra,** and the **reticular formation.** The marginal zone of each basal plate enlarges considerably, thus forming the **basis pedunculi** by the descent of nerve fibers from the cerebral cortex to the lower motor centers in the pons and spinal cord, that is, the **corticopontine, corticobulbar,** and **corticospinal tracts.**

The two alar plates and the original roof plate form the **tectum.** The neuroblasts in the alar plates differentiate into the sensory neurons of the **superior** and **inferior colliculi** (Fig. 18-9). Four swellings representing the four colliculi ap-

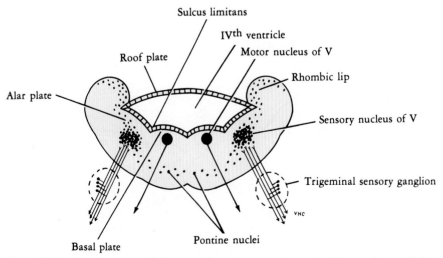

Figure 18–6 Development of the pons from the anterior part of the metencephalon.

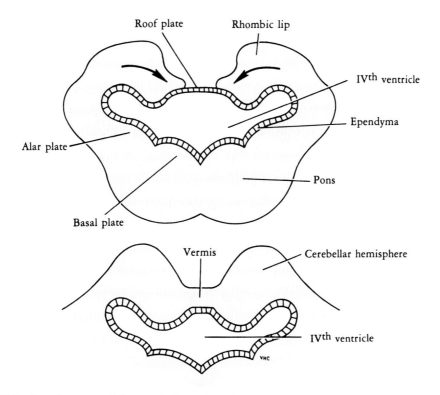

Figure 18–7 Development of the cerebellum. Also shown is the fusion of the rhombic lips in the midline to form the dumbbell-shaped cerebellum.

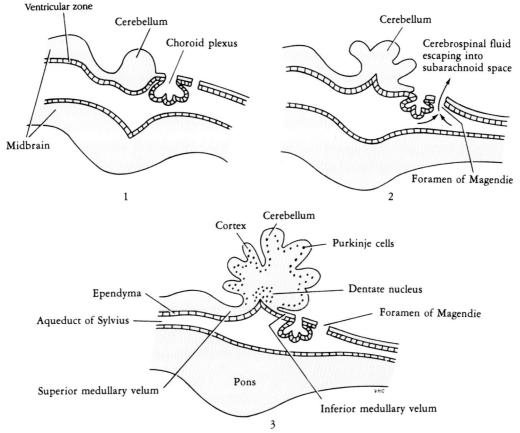

Figure 18–8 Sagittal sections of the developing cerebellum.

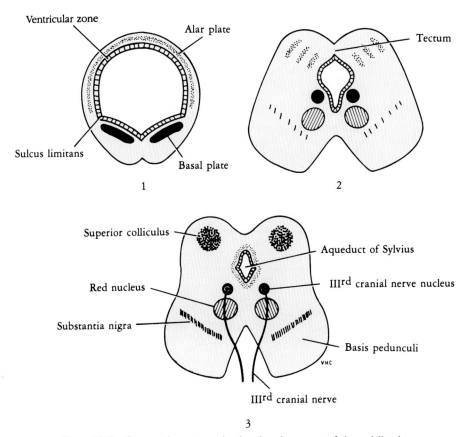

Figure 18–9 Successive stages in the development of the midbrain.

pear on the posterior surface of the midbrain. The superior colliculi are associated with visual reflexes and the inferior colliculi are associated with auditory reflexes.

With further development, the fibers of the fourth cranial nerve emerge on the posterior surface of the midbrain and decussate completely in the superior medullary velum. The fibers of the third cranial nerve emerge on the anterior surface between the cerebral peduncles.

Forebrain (Prosencephalon)

The forebrain develops from the forebrain vesicle. The roof and floor plates remain thin, whereas the lateral walls become thick, as in the developing spinal cord. At an early stage, a lateral diverticulum called the **optic vesicle** appears on each side of the forebrain. That part of the forebrain that lies rostral to the optic vesicle is the telencephalon, and the remainder is the diencephalon (Fig. 18-10). The optic vesicle and stalk ultimately will form the retina and optic nerve.

The telencephalon now develops a lateral diverticulum on each side of the cerebral hemisphere, and its cavity is known as the **lateral ventricle.** The anterior part of the third ventricle therefore is formed by the medial part of the telencephalon and ends at the **lamina terminalis,** which

represents the rostral end of the neural tube. The opening into each lateral ventricle is the future **interventricular foramen.**

Fate of the Diencephalon

The cavity of the diencephalon forms the greater part of the third ventricle (Fig. 18-10). Its roof shows a small diverticulum immediately anterior to the midbrain, which will form the **pineal body.** The remainder of the roof forms the **choroid plexus of the third ventricle** (Fig. 18-11). In the lateral wall of the third ventricle the **thalamus** arises as a thickening of the alar plate on each side. Posterior to the thalamus, the **medial** and **lateral geniculate bodies** develop as solid buds. With the continued growth of the two thalami, the ventricular cavity becomes narrowed, and in some individuals the two thalami may meet and fuse in the midline to form the **interthalamic connection** of gray matter that crosses the third ventricle (Fig. 18-12).

The lower part of the alar plate on each side will differentiate into a large number of **hypothalamic nuclei.** One of these becomes conspicuous on the inferior surface of the hypothalamus and forms a rounded swelling on each side of the midline called the **mammillary body.**

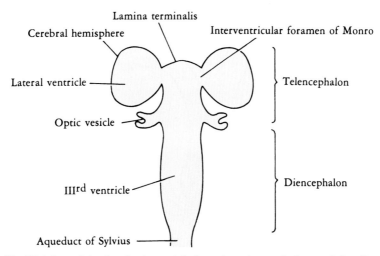

Figure 18–10   Division of the forebrain vesicle into the telencephalon and the diencephalon.

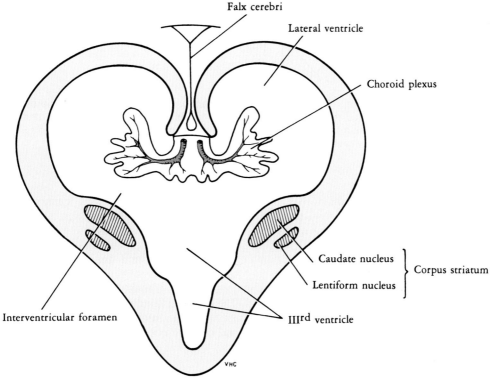

Figure 18–11   Diagrammatic representation of a coronal section of the cerebral hemispheres showing the developing choroid plexuses in the third and lateral ventricles.

The **infundibulum** develops as a diverticulum from the floor of the diencephalon and from it will originate the **stalk** and **pars nervosa of the hypophysis.**

Fate of the Telencephalon

The telencephalon forms the anterior end of the third ventricle, which is closed by the lamina terminalis, while the diverticulum on either side forms the cerebral hemisphere.

Cerebral Hemispheres

Each cerebral hemisphere arises at the beginning of the fifth week of development. As it expands superiorly, its walls thicken and the interventricular foramen becomes reduced in size (see Figs. 18-10, 18-11, and 18-12). The mesenchyme between each cerebral hemisphere condenses to form the **falx cerebri.** As development proceeds, the cerebral hemispheres grow and expand rapidly, first anteriorly to form the **frontal lobes,** then laterally and superiorly to form the

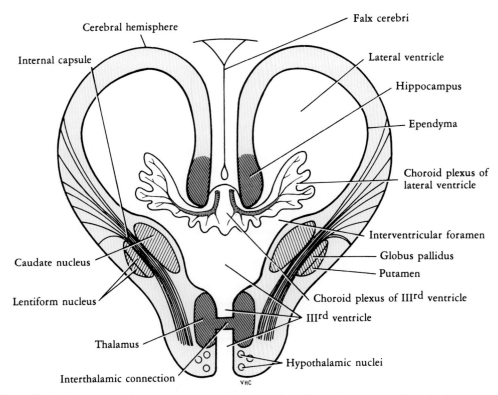

Figure 18–12 Diagrammatic representation of a coronal section of the cerebral hemispheres showing the choroid plexuses in the third and lateral ventricles. Also shown are the caudate and lentiform nuclei and the thalami. The ascending and descending nerve tracts can be seen passing between the masses of gray matter to form the internal capsule.

parietal lobes, and finally posteriorly and inferiorly to produce the **occipital** and **temporal lobes.** As the result of this great expansion, the hemispheres cover the midbrain and hindbrain (Fig. 18-13).

The medial wall of the cerebral hemisphere remains thin and is formed by the ependymal cells. This area becomes invaginated by vascular mesoderm, which forms the **choroid plexus of the lateral ventricle** (Fig. 18-12). The occipital lobe of the cerebral hemisphere is separated from the cerebellum by mesenchyme, which condenses to form the **tentorium cerebelli.**

Meanwhile, the matrix cells lining the floor of the forebrain vesicle proliferate, producing large numbers of neuroblasts. These collectively form a projection that encroaches on the cavity of the lateral ventricle and is known as the **corpus striatum** (Fig. 18-11). Later this differentiates into two parts: the dorsomedial portion, the **caudate nucleus,** and a ventrolateral part, the **lentiform nucleus.** The latter becomes subdivided into a lateral part, the **putamen,** and a medial part, the **globus pallidus** (Fig. 18-12). As each hemisphere expands, its medial surface approaches the lateral surface of the diencephalon so that the caudate nucleus and thalamus come in close contact.

A further longitudinal thickening occurs in the wall of the forebrain vesicle and the thickening protrudes into the lateral ventricle and forms the **hippocampus** (Fig. 18-12).

While these various masses of gray matter are developing within each cerebral hemisphere, maturing neurons in different parts of the nervous system are sending axons either to or from the differentiating cortex. These axons form the large **ascending** and **descending tracts** which, as they develop, are forced to pass between the thalamus and caudate nucleus medially and the lentiform nucleus laterally. The compact bundle of ascending and descending tracts is known as the **internal capsule** (see Fig. 18-12). The **external capsule** consists of a few cortical projection fibers that pass lateral to the lentiform nucleus.

Cerebral Cortex

As each cerebral hemisphere rapidly expands, the **convolutions** or **gyri** separated by **fissures** or **sulci** become evident on its surface. The cortex covering the lentiform nucleus remains as a fixed area called the **insula** (Fig. 18-13). Later this region becomes buried in the **lateral sulcus** as the result of overgrowth of the adjacent temporal, parietal, and frontal lobes.

The matrix cells lining the cavity of the cerebral hemisphere produce large numbers of neuroblasts and **neuroglial cells** that migrate out into the marginal zone. The remaining matrix cells ultimately will form the **ependyma,** which lines the lateral ventricle. In the twelfth week, the cor-

Brain **511**

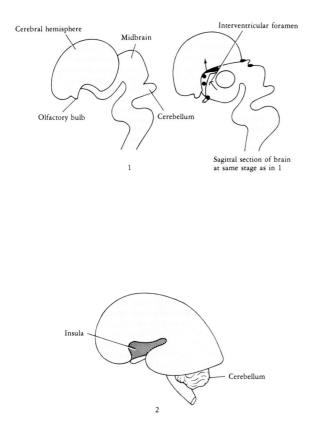

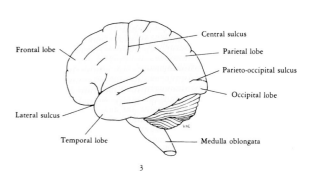

Figure 18–13   Successive stages in the development of the cerebral cortex.

tex becomes very cellular because of the migration of large numbers of neuroblasts. At term, the neuroblasts have become differentiated and have assumed a stratified appearance as the result of the presence of incoming and outgoing fibers. Different areas of the cortex soon show specific cell types; thus the motor cortex contains a large number of **pyramidal cells,** whereas the sensory areas are characterized mainly by **granular cells.**

Commissures

The **lamina terminalis,** which is the cephalic end of the neural tube, forms a bridge between the two cerebral hemispheres and enables nerve fibers to pass from one cerebral hemisphere to the other (Fig. 18-10).

The **anterior commissure** is the first commissure to develop. It runs in the lamina terminalis and connects the olfactory bulb and the temporal lobe of the cortex on one side with the same structures of the opposite hemisphere.

The **fornix** is the second commissure to develop and connects the cortex of the hippocampus in each hemisphere.

The **corpus callosum,** the largest and most important commissure, is the third commissure to develop. Its first fibers connect the frontal lobes of both sides and later the parietal lobes. As the corpus callosum increases in size because of increased numbers of fibers, it arches back over the

roof of the developing third ventricle. The remains of the lamina terminalis, which lie between the corpus callosum and the fornix, become stretched out to form a thin septum, the **septum pellucidum.** The **optic chiasma** is formed in the inferior part of the lamina terminalis; it contains fibers from the medial halves of the retinae, which cross the midline to join the optic tract of the opposite side and so pass to the **lateral geniculate body** and the **superior colliculus.**

Myelination in the Central Nervous System

The myelin sheath in the central nervous system is formed and maintained by the oligodendrocytes of the neuroglia (see p. 75).

Myelination in the spinal cord begins first in the cervical region, and from here the process extends caudally. The process of myelination begins within the cord at about the fourth month, and the sensory fibers are affected first. The last affected are the descending motor fibers.

Myelination in the brain begins at about the sixth month of fetal life but is restricted to the fibers of the basal ganglia. Later the sensory fibers passing up from the spinal cord myelinate, but the progress is slow so that at birth the brain still is largely unmyelinated. In the newborn there is very little cerebral function; motor reactions such as respiration, sucking, and swallowing are essentially reflex. After birth, the corticobulbar, corticospinal, tectospinal, and corticopontocerebellar fibers begin to myelinate. This process of myelination is not haphazard but systematic, occurring in different nerve fibers at specific times. The corticospinal fibers, for example, start to myelinate at about 6 months after birth, and the process is largely complete by the end of the second year. It is believed that some nerve fibers in the brain and spinal cord do not complete myelination until puberty.

CLINICAL NOTES

CONGENITAL ANOMALIES

Practically any part of the nervous system can show defects of development, and these produce a wide variety of clinical signs and symptoms. Only the common defects of the central nervous system are considered here. Spina bifida, hydrocephalus, and anencephaly each occur about 6 times per 1000 births and are therefore the more common congenital anomalies.

Spina Bifida

In spina bifida, the spines and arches of one or more adjacent vertebrae fail to develop. The condition occurs most frequently in the lower thoracic, lumbar, and sacral regions. Beneath this defect the meninges and spinal cord may or may not be involved to varying degrees. The condition is a result of failure of the mesenchyme, which grows in between the neural tube and the surface ectoderm, to form the vertebral arches in the affected region. The types of spina bifida are as follows:

1. **Spina bifida occulta.** The spines and arches of one or more vertebrae, usually in the lumbar region, are absent, and the vertebral canal remains open posteriorly (Fig. 18-14). The spinal cord and nerve roots usually are normal. The defect is covered by the postvertebral muscles and cannot be seen from the surface. A small tuft of hair or a fatty tumor may be present over the defect. Most cases are symptomless and are diagnosed by chance when the vertebral column is x-rayed.
2. **Meningocele.** The meninges project through the defect in the vertebral arches, forming a cystic swelling beneath the skin and containing cerebrospinal fluid, which communicates with the subarachnoid space (Fig. 18-14). The spinal cord and nerves usually are normal.
3. **Meningomyelocele.** The normal spinal cord, or cauda equina, lies within the meningeal sac, which projects through the vertebral arch defect (Fig. 18-14). The spinal cord or nerve roots are adherent to the inner wall of the sac.
4. **Myelocele.** The neural tube fails to close in the region of the defect (Fig. 18-14). An oval raw area is found on the surface; this represents the neural groove whose lips are fused. The central canal discharges clear cerebrospinal fluid onto the surface.
5. **Syringomyelocele.** This condition is rare. A meningomyelocele is present, and in addition the central canal of the spinal cord at the level of the bony defect is grossly dilated (Fig. 18-14).

Spina bifida occulta is the commonest defect. The next most common defect is myelocele, and many afflicted infants are born dead. If the child is born alive, death from infection of the spinal cord may occur within a few days.

Most cases of spina bifida occulta require no treatment. A meningocele should be removed surgically within a few days of birth. Infants with meningomyelocele should also be treated surgically. The sac is opened and the spinal cord or nerves are freed and carefully replaced in the vertebral canal. The meninges are sutured over the cord and the postvertebral muscles are approximated.

As the result of advances in medical and surgical care, many infants with the severe forms of spina bifida now survive. Unfortunately, these children are likely to have life long disabilities and psychosocial problems. The neurologic deficits alone may result in deformation of the limbs and spine, and bladder, bowel and sexual dysfunction.

Hydrocephalus

Hydrocephalus is an abnormal increase in the volume of cerebrospinal fluid within the skull. The condition may be associated with spina bifida and meningocele. Hydrocephalus alone may be caused by stenosis of the cerebral aqueduct or, more commonly, by the normal single channel being represented by many inadequate minute tubules. Another cause, which is progressive, is the overgrowth of neuroglia around the aqueduct. Inadequate development or failure of development of the interventricular foramen, or the foramina of Magendie and Luschka, may also be responsible.

In cases of hydrocephalus with spina bifida, the **Arnold-Chiari phenomenon** may occur. During development, the cephalic end of the spinal cord is fixed by virtue of the brain's residing in the skull, and in the presence of spina bifida the caudal end of the cord may also be fixed. The longitudinal growth of the vertebral column is more rapid and greater than that of the spinal cord, and this results in traction pulling the medulla and part of the cerebellum through the foramen magnum. This displacement of the hindbrain downward obstructs the flow of cerebrospinal fluid through the foramina in the roof of the fourth ventricle.

Hydrocephalus may occur before birth, and if it is advanced, it could obstruct labor. It usually is noticed during

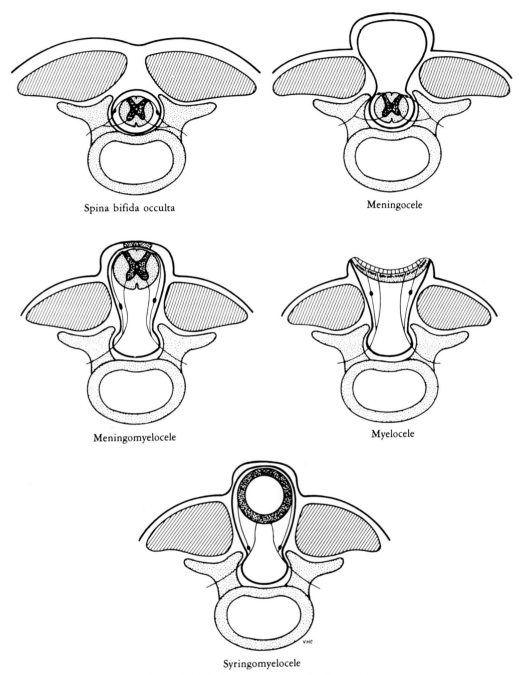

Spina bifida occulta

Meningocele

Meningomyelocele

Myelocele

Syringomyelocele

Figure 18–14   Different types of spina bifida.

the first few months of life because of the enlarging head, which may attain a huge size, sometimes measuring more than 30 inches in diameter (Fig. 18-15). The cranial sutures are widely separated and the anterior fontanelle is much enlarged. The veins of the scalp are distended and the eyes look downward. Cranial nerve paralyses are common. The ventricles of the brain become markedly dilated. This ventricular expansion occurs largely at the expense of the white matter, and the neurons of the cerebral cortex are mostly spared. This results in the preservation of cerebral function, but the destruction of the tracts, especially the corticobulbar and corticospinal tracts, produces a progressive loss of motor function.

If the condition is diagnosed by sonography while the fetus is in utero, it is possible to perform prenatal surgery with the introduction of a catheter into the ventricles of the brain and the drainage of the cerebrospinal fluid into the amniotic cavity. Should the diagnosis be delayed until after birth, a drainage tube fitted with a nonreturn valve can connect the ventricles to the internal jugular vein in the neck.

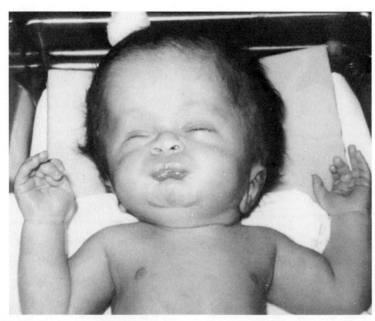

Figure 18–15   Hydrocephalus. Note the large size of the head. (Courtesy Dr. G. Avery.)

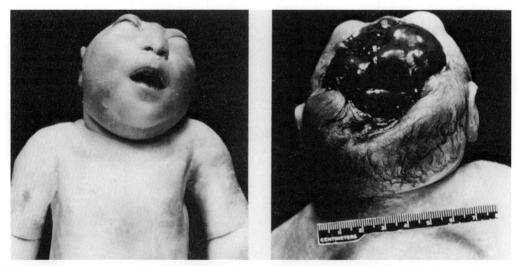

Figure 18–16   Example of anencephaly. Note that the greater part of the brain and the vault of the skull are absent. In the posterior view, the remainder of the brain is exposed. (Courtesy Dr. M. Platt.)

Anencephaly

In anencephaly the greater part of the brain and the vault of the skull are absent (Fig. 18-16). The anomaly is caused by the failure of the rostral end of the neural tube to develop and as a consequence its cavity remains open. In place of the normal neural tissue are thin-walled vascular channels resembling the choroid plexus and masses of neural tissue. Although the eyes are present, the optic nerves are absent. The condition commonly involves the spinal cord, and the neural tube remains open in the cervical region. The condition is commonly diagnosed before birth with sonography or x-ray studies. Most anencephalic infants are stillborn or die shortly after birth.

Prevention of Neural Defects with Folic Acid

The development and closure of the neural tube are normally completed within 28 days. In practical terms, this means that neural tube defects have occurred before many women are aware that they are pregnant.

Extensive clinical research has demonstrated that environmental and genetic factors have a joint role in the causation of neural tube defects. The increased risk of neural defects in the lower socioeconomic groups suggested that poor nutrition may also be an important factor. More recent clinical research has demonstrated that the risk of recurrent neural defects is significantly reduced among women who took 4000 Ug of **folic acid** daily than those that did not. Further studies have shown that a daily dose that is ten times lower is effective in preventing the defect. These findings have stimulated much new research to identify the genetic and biochemical bases of neural tube defects.

Because as many as 50% of pregnancies in the United States are unplanned, and since the neural tube closes before most women know that they are pregnant, physicians should strongly urge women capable of becoming pregnant to consume at least 400 Ug of folic acid per day, preferably in a multivitamin supplement.

Clinical Problem Solving

1. A 10-year-old boy fell off his bicycle and hurt his back. Following a complete physical examination in the emergency department, nothing abnormal was found. An x-ray examination, however, revealed the complete absence of the spine and laminae of the fifth lumbar vertebra. How would you explain the presence of the bony defect?

2. A male child was delivered normally to a 20-year-old woman. A pediatrician examined the infant and found a large swelling in the lower part of his back over the fourth and fifth lumbar vertebrae. On closer examination, the summit of the swelling had an oval raw area from which a clear fluid was discharging. The legs showed hyperextension of the knees, and the feet were held in the position of talipes calcaneus. What is the diagnosis? How would you explain the congenital defect on the back?

3. A 2-month-old girl was taken to a pediatrician because her mother was concerned about the size of her head. "She looks top-heavy," she said. Examination showed the head to be large and globular in shape. The anterior fontanelle was greatly enlarged and extended posteriorly to the enlarged posterior fontanelle. The enlarged head contrasted markedly with the small face. Neurological examination revealed some evidence of optic atrophy on both sides and there was increased tone in the muscles of both lower limbs. What is the diagnosis? How can you explain this congenital anomaly? What is the prognosis if the patient is left untreated?

Answers to Clinical Problem Solving

1. This patient has spina bifida occulta involving the fifth lumbar vertebra. The condition is a result of failure of the mesenchyme to grow between the neural tube and the surface ectoderm and form the vertebral arch; the vertebral canal remains open posteriorly. The defect therefore has existed since before birth and could not be seen or felt on physical examination because it was covered by the postvertebral muscles. The spinal cord and spinal nerve roots usually are normal. No treatment is required.

2. This child has a myelocele. In addition to the failure of the formation of the vertebral arches of the fourth and fifth lumbar vertebrae, the neural tube failed to close in this region. The oval raw area seen in this patient is the neural groove whose lips have not united. The central canal is discharging clear cerebrospinal fluid onto the skin surface. The deformities of the knee joints and feet are the result of the maldevelopment of the spinal cord in the lumbar region, with consequent interference with the innervation of certain muscle groups in the legs.

3. This child has hydrocephalus. A postmortem examination performed 1 year later showed that the cerebral aqueduct was not normally developed and consisted of a number of small tubules. This had resulted in the excessive accumulation of cerebrospinal fluid within the lateral and third ventricles of the brain. The distention of the ventricles, with the consequent enlargement of the brain and increased intracranial pressure, forced apart the bones of the cranial vault so that the head became greatly enlarged. The optic atrophy probably was caused by the stretching of the optic nerve on each side. The increased muscle tone of the lower limbs was almost certainly the result of destruction of the corticospinal and other descending tracts by the expanding lateral ventricles. Although in some cases the head ceases to enlarge spontaneously, in most patients the hydrocephalus is progressive and death ultimately occurs. Surgical treatment of hydrocephalus may be attempted (see p. 513).

Review Questions

Directions: Each of the numbered items in this section is followed by answers that are positively phrased. Select the ONE lettered answer that is an EXCEPTION.

1. The following statements concerning the neural tube are correct **except:**
   (a) It is lined by stratified squamous cells.
   (b) The neuroblasts migrate peripherally to form the intermediate zone.
   (c) The repeated division of the matrix cells results in an increase in the length and diameter of the tube.
   (d) The intermediate zone will form the gray matter of the spinal cord.
   (e) The nerve fibers in the marginal zone become myelinated and form the white matter of the spinal cord.

2. The following statements concerning the neural crest cells are correct **except:**
   (a) They are formed from the lateral margin of the neural plate.
   (b) They give rise to the posterior root ganglia.
   (c) They form the neurons of the autonomic ganglia.
   (d) The Schwann cells of peripheral nerves are formed from neural crest cells.
   (e) They form the cells of the suprarenal cortex.

3. The following statements concerning the developing spinal cord are correct **except:**
   (a) The alar plates form the neurons in the posterior gray columns.
   (b) The nerve cells of the sympathetic outflow are formed from the basal plates.
   (c) In the adult the lower end of the spinal cord lies at the level of the lower border of the first lumbar vertebra.
   (d) At birth the lower end of the spinal cord lies at the level of the third sacral vertebra.
   (e) The meninges surrounding the spinal cord are developed from the mesenchyme.

4. The following statements concerning the development of the brainstem are correct **except:**
   (a) The cerebellum is formed from the dorsal part of the alar plates of the metencephalon.
   (b) The neurons of the deep cerebellar nuclei are derived from the matrix cells lining the cavity of the hindbrain vesicle.
   (c) The neuroblasts in the basal plates will form the nuclei of the trochlear and oculomotor nerves.
   (d) The neuroblasts of the superior and inferior colliculi are also formed from the neurocytes in the basal plates.
   (e) The pons arises from the anterior part of the metencephalon with cellular contributions from the alar part of the myelencephalon.

5. The following statements concerning the fate of the forebrain vesicle are correct **except:**
   (a) The optic vesicle grows out of the forebrain vesicle.
   (b) The thalamus is formed from the alar plates in the lateral walls of the diencephalon.
   (c) The lamina terminalis is formed from the rostral end of the telencephalon.
   (d) The pars nervosa of the hypophysis is formed from the floor of the diencephalon.
   (e) The hypothalamic nuclei are formed from the basal plates of the diencephalon.

6. The following statements concerning the development of the cerebral hemispheres are correct **except:**
   (a) The corpus striatum is formed from the proliferation of the matrix cells lining the floor of the forebrain vesicle.
   (b) The interventricular foramen is formed by the cavity of the telencephalon.
   (c) The choroid plexus of the lateral ventricle is formed by vascular mesenchyme covered by ependymal cells.
   (d) The internal capsule is formed by the developing ascending and descending tracts growing between the developing thalamus and caudate nucleus medially and the lentiform nucleus laterally.
   (e) The cortical neurons develop in situ and do not migrate out laterally from the matrix cells lining the cavity of the cerebral hemisphere.

7. The following statements concerning the development of myelination in the brain are correct **except:**
   (a) Myelination begins at birth.
   (b) The sensory fibers are myelinated first.
   (c) The process of myelination is not haphazard.
   (d) Myelination of the nerve tracts is largely complete by the second year of life.
   (e) Myelination is carried out by oligodendrocytes and not by neurons.

8. The following statements concerning the condition of spina bifida are correct **except:**
   (a) It is one of the more common congenital anomalies of the central nervous system.
   (b) The commonest form of spina bifida is syringomyelocele.
   (c) The condition occurs most often in the lower thoracic, lumbar, and sacral regions.
   (d) In a myelocele, the neural tube fails to close in the region of the defect.
   (e) Most cases of spina bifida occulta require no treatment.

Directions: Read the following case history then answer the questions. You will be required to select ONE BEST lettered answer.

A 6-month-old girl was seen by a plastic surgeon because of the presence of a swelling at the root of the nose. The mother said that she had noticed the swelling when the child was born and that since then it had gradually increased in size.

9. The surgeon examined the child and found the following likely signs **except:**
    (a) The swelling was situated at the root of the nose in the midline.
    (b) The swelling was located between the frontal and nasal bones.
    (c) The swelling was fluctuant and on gentle pressure could be reduced in size.
    (d) The swelling was pulsatile and the pulse coincided with the heart rate.
    (e) The pulse did not coincide with the pulse felt over the anterior fontanelle of the skull.

10. A neurosurgeon was consulted and the following possible additional findings were ascertained **except:**
    (a) A lateral radiograph of the skull revealed a defect in the membranous bones involving the nasal process of the frontal bone.
    (b) The defect in the membranous bones is known as cranioschisis.
    (c) The condition was associated with a cephalic meningocele.
    (d) There was a herniation of the meninges through the defect in the skull
    (e) Brain tissue is never found within the hernia.

Answers to Review Questions

1. A
2. E
3. D
4. D
5. E
6. E
7. A
8. B
9. E. In a cephalic meningocele, the cerebrospinal fluid within the swelling is in direct communication with that in the subarachnoid space. The pulsation of the swelling is produced by the pulse wave of the cerebral arteries through the cerebrospinal fluid. This pulse wave will coincide with the pulse felt over the anterior fontanelle of the skull.

10. E. Cranioschisis is characterized by a defect in the membranous bones of the skull through which meninges or meninges and neural tissue may protrude. The defect usually occurs in the midline in the occipital region or between the frontal and nasal bones. The condition probably is the result of anomalous formation and separation of the neural tube from the surface ectoderm of the embryo.

 ADDITIONAL READING

Anderson, D.J. Cellular and Molecular Biology of Neural Crest Cell Lineage Determination. *Trends Genet.* 13:276-280,1997.

Anderson, S. A., Eisenstat, D.D., Shi, L., Rubenstein, J.L. Interneuron Migration from Basal Forebrain to Neocortex: Dependence on D1x genes. *Science* 278: 474-476,1997.

Berry, R.J. et al. Prevention of Neural Tube Defects with Folic Acid in China. *N. Engl. J. Med.* 341:1485-1490,1999.

Botto, L.D., Moore, C.A., Khoury, M.J., Erickson, J.D. Medical Progress: Neural Tube Defects. *N. Engl. J. Med.* 341:1509-1519,1999.

Crossley, P.H., Martinez, S., Martin, G.R. Midbrain Development Induced by FGF8 in the Chick Embryo. *Nature* 380:66-68,1996.

Ericson, J., Briscoe, J., Rashbass, P., van Heyningen, V., Jessell, T.M. Graded Sonic Hedgehog Signaling and the Specification of Cell Fate in the Ventral Neural Tube, Cold Spring Harb. *Symp. Quant. Biol.* 62:451-466,1997.

Francis, N.J., Landis, S.C. Cellular and Molecular Determinants of Sympathetic Neuron Development. *Annu. Rev. Neurosci.* 22:541-566, 1999.

Hatten, M.E. Central Nervous System Neuronal Migration. *Annu. Rev. Neurosci.* 22:261-294,1999.

Henderson, C.E. Programmed Cell Death in the Developing Nervous System. *Neuron* 17:579-585,1996.

Lee, K.J., Jessell, T.M. The Specification of Dorsal Cell Fates in the Vertebrate Central Nervous System. *Annu. Rev. Neurosci.* 22:261-294,1999.

Liem, J.F. Jr, Tremml, G., Roelink, H., Jessell, T.M. Dorsal Differentiation of Neural Plate Cells Induced by BMP-mediated Signals from Epidermal Ectoderm. *Cell* 82:969-979,1995.

Lumsden, A., Gulisano, M. Neocortical Neurons: Where Do They Come From? *Science* 278:402-403,1997.

Marigo, V., Davey, R.A., Zuo, Y., Cunningham, J.M., Tabin, C.J. Biochemical Evidence that Patched is the Hedgehog Receptor. *Nature* 384:176-179,1996.

Mueller, B.K. Growth Cone Guidance:First Steps Towards a Deeper Understanding. *Annu. Rev. Neurosci.* 22:351-388, 1999.

O'Leary, D.D., Wilkinson, D.G. Eph Receptors and Ephrins in Neural Development. *Curr. Opin. Neurobiol.* 9:65-73, 1999.

Song, H.J. Poo, M.M. Signal Transduction Underlying Growth Cone Guidance by Diffusible Factors. *Curr. Opin. Neurobiol.* 9:355-363, 1999.

Tanabe, Y. Jessell, T.M. Diversity and Pattern in the Developing Spinal Cord. *Science* 274:1115-1123,1997.

Tessier-Lavigne, M., Goodman, C.S. The Molecular Biology of Axon Guidance. *Science* 274:1123-1133, 1996.

Williams, P. L., et al.(eds.). *Gray's Anatomy* (38th Br. Ed.). New York Edinburgh: Churchill Livingstone, 1995.

Wolpert, L., Beddington, R. Brockes, J. Jessell, T.M., Lawrence, P.A., Meyerowitz, E. *Principles of Development.* New York: Oxford Univ. Press, 1998.

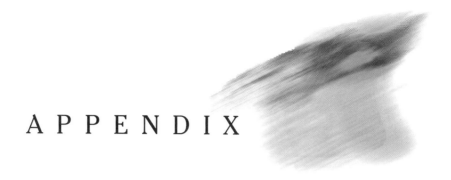

APPENDIX

IMPORTANT NEUROANATOMICAL DATA OF CLINICAL SIGNIFICANCE

Baseline of the Skull

This baseline extends from the lower margin of the orbit backward through the upper margin of the external auditory meatus. The **cerebrum** lies entirely above the line, and the **cerebellum** lies in the posterior cranial fossa below the posterior third of the line (Fig. A-1).

Falx Cerebri, Superior Sagittal Sinus, and the Longitudinal Cerebral Fissure Between the Cerebral Hemispheres

The position of these structures can be indicated by passing a line over the vertex of the skull in the sagittal plane that joins the root of the nose to the external occipital protuberance.

Parietal Eminence

This is a raised area on the lateral surface of the parietal bone and can be felt about 2 in. (5 cm) above the auricle. It lies close to the lower end of the **central cerebral sulcus of the brain** (Fig. A-1).

Pterion

This is the point where the greater wing of the sphenoid bone meets the anteroinferior angle of the parietal bone. Lying 11/2 in. (4 cm) above the midpoint of the zygomatic arch (Fig. A-1), it is not marked by an eminence or a depression, but it is important since the **anterior branches of the middle meningeal artery and vein lie beneath it.**

Clinical Neuroanatomy of Techniques for Treating Intracranial Hematomas
BURR HOLES

Indications for Burr Holes. Cranial decompression is performed in a patient with a history of progressive neurologic deterioration and signs of brain herniation, in spite of adequate medical treatment. The presence of a hematoma should be confirmed by a CT scan if possible.

Anatomy of the Technique for a Temporal Burr Hole

1. The patient is placed in a supine position with the head rotated so that the side for the burr hole is uppermost. For example, in a patient with a right-sided fixed dilated pupil, indicating herniation of the right uncus with pressure on the right oculomotor nerve, a hematoma on the right side must be presumed, and a burr hole is placed on the right side.
2. The temporal skin is shaved and prepared for surgery in the usual way.
3. A 3-cm vertical skin incision is made two fingerbreadths anterior to the tragus of the ear and three fingerbreadths above this level (Fig. A-2).
4. The following structures are then incised:
   a. Skin
   b. Superficial fascia containing small branches of the superficial temporal artery.
   c. Deep fascia covering the outer surface of the temporalis muscle.
   d. The temporalis muscle is then incised vertically down to the periosteum of the squamous part of the temporal bone (Fig. A-2).
   e. The temporalis muscle is elevated from its attachment to the skull and a retractor is positioned (some muscular bleeding will be encountered).

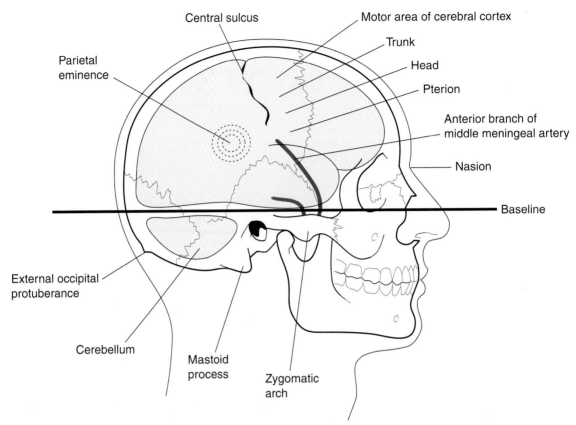

Figure A–1 Surface landmarks on the right side of the head. The relations of the middle meningeal artery and the brain to the surface of the skull are shown.

f. A small hole is then drilled through the outer and inner tables of the skull at right angles to the skull surface, and the hole is enlarged with a burr (unless a blood clot is present between the inner table and the endosteal layer of dura).

g. The white meningeal layer of dura is flexible and gives slightly on gentle pressure.

h. The hole may be enlarged with a curette, and bleeding from the diploe may be controlled with bone wax.

The surgical wound is closed in layers with interrupted sutures placed in the temporalis muscle, the deep fascia covering the temporalis muscle, and the scalp.

Burr Hole for Epidural Hematoma. Once the inner table of the squamous part of the temporal bone (or the anterior inferior angle of the parietal bone) is pierced with a small bit and enlarged with a burr, the dark red clotted blood beneath the endosteal layer of dura is usually easily recognized. However, bright red liquid blood means that the middle meningeal artery or one of its branches is bleeding. The meningeal artery is located deep to the clot and between the endosteal layer of dura and the meningeal layer of dura or in the substance the endosteal layer of dura; or it may lie in a tunnel of bone.

Burr Hole for Subdural Hematoma. When the squamous part of the temporal bone is penetrated, as described above, the endosteal layer of dura will be exposed. In this case there is no blood clot between the endosteal layer of dura and the meningeal layer of dura, but both fused layers of dura will be dark bluish. The dura (endosteal and meningeal layers) is gently incised to enter the space between the meningeal layer of dura and the arachnoid mater. The subdural blood usually gushes out, leaving the unprotected brain covered only by arachnoid and pia mater in the depths of the hole.

Clinical Neuroanatomy of the Technique of Ventriculostomy
INDICATIONS FOR VENTRICULOSTOMY

Ventriculostomy is indicated in acute hydrocephalus, in which there is a sudden obstruction to the flow of cerebrospinal fluid.

Anatomy of the Technique of Ventriculostomy

The needle is inserted into the lateral ventricle through either a frontal or parietal burr hole. The anatomy of these

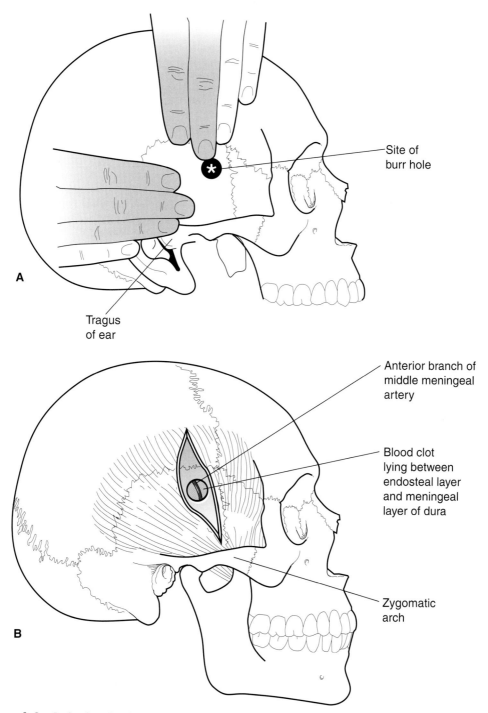

Figure A–2 **A**. Surface landmarks for a temporal burr hole. **B**. The vertical incision passes through the temporalis muscle down to bone. The middle meningeal artery lies between the endosteal and meningeal layers of dura and is embedded in the endosteal layer of dura or lies in a bony tunnel.

burr holes has been described previously. The needle is inserted through the burr hole using the following anatomical landmarks.

1. **Frontal Approach.** The needle is inserted through the frontal burr hole and is directed downward and forward in the direction of the inner canthus of the ipsilateral eye (Fig. A-3).
2. **Parietal Approach.** The needle is inserted through the parietal burr hole and is directed downward and forward in the direction of the pupil of the ipsilateral eye (Fig. A-3).

The needle is inserted to a depth of about 5.5 cm from the skull opening; in cases of chronic hydrocephalus with gross dilatation of the ventricles, the depth of penetration to the ventricular cavity may be much less.

Vertebral Numbers and Spinal Cord Segments

Table A-1 relates which vertebral body is related to a particular spinal cord segment.

Segmental Innervation of Muscles

It is possible to test for the integrity of the segmental innervation of muscles by performing the following simple muscle reflexes on the patient.

Table A–1

Vertebrae	Spinal Segment
Cervical vertebrae	Add 1
Upper thoracic vertebrae	Add 2
Lower thoracic vertebrae (7–9)	Add 3
Tenth thoracic vertebra	L1 and 2 cord segments
Eleventh thoracic vertebra	L3 and 4 cord segments
Twelfth thoracic vertebra	L5 cord segment
First lumbar vertebra	Sacral and coccygeal cord segments

Biceps brachii tendon reflex C5-**6** (flexion of the elbow joint by tapping the biceps tendon).

Triceps tendon reflex C6-7, and **8** (extension of the elbow joint by tapping the triceps tendon).

Brachioradialis tendon reflex C5-**6,** and 7 (supination of the radioulnar joints by tapping the insertion of the brachioradialis tendon).

Abdominal superficial reflexes (contraction of underlying abdominal muscles by stroking the skin). Upper abdominal skin T6-7; middle abdominal skin T8-9; lower abdominal skin T10-12.

Patellar tendon reflex (knee jerk) L2, **3,** and **4** (extension of knee joint on tapping the patellar tendon).

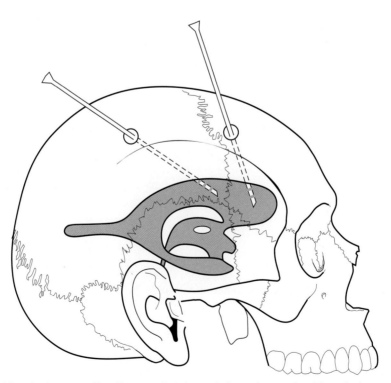

Figure A–3   Ventriculostomy. Needles passing through frontal or parietal burr holes to enter the lateral ventricle are shown. The needle is inserted to a depth of about 5.5 cm from the skull opening in order to enter the lateral ventricle.

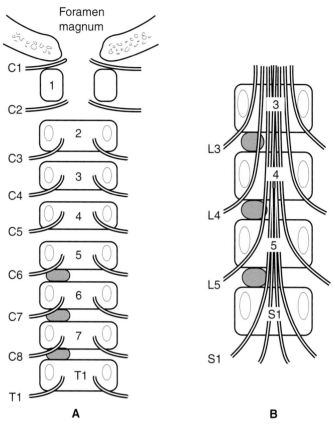

Figure A–4   A and B. Posterior views of vertebral bodies in the cervical and lumbar regions showing the relationship that might exist between herniated nucleus pulposus (red) and spinal nerve roots. Note there are eight cervical nerves and only seven cervical vertebrae. In the lumbar region, for example, the emerging L4 nerve roots pass out laterally close to the pedicles of the fourth lumbar vertebra and are not related to the intervertebral disc between the fourth and fifth lumbar vertebrae. Pressure on the L5 motor nerve root produces weakness of dorsiflexion of ankle; pressure on the S1 motor nerve root produces weakness of plantar flexion of the ankle joint.

Achilles tendon reflex (ankle jerk) S1 and 2 (plantar flexion of ankle joint on tapping the Achilles tendon-tendo calcaneus.

Relationship Between Possible Intervertebral Disc Herniations and Spinal Nerve Roots

It is useful to be able to relate possible nucleus pulposus herniations with spinal nerve roots. These are shown for the cervical and lumbar regions in Figure A-4.

A correlation between the nerve roots involved, the pain dermatome, the muscle weakness, and the missing or diminished reflex is shown in Table A-2.

Surface Landmarks for Performing a Spinal Tap

The patient is placed in the lateral prone position or in the upright sitting position. The trunk is then bent well forward, to open up to the maximum the space between adjoining laminae in the lumbar region. A groove runs down the middle of the back over the tips of the spines of the thoracic and the upper four lumbar vertebrae. The spines are made more prominent when the vertebral column is flexed. An imaginary line joining the highest points on the iliac crests passes over the fourth lumbar spine. With a careful aseptic technique and under local anesthesia, the spinal tap needle, fitted with a stylet, is passed into the vertebral canal above or below the fourth lumbar spine.

STRUCTURES PIERCED BY SPINAL TAP NEEDLE

The following structures are pierced by the needle before it enters the subarachnoid space (Fig. A-5):

1. Skin
2. Superficial fascia
3. Supraspinous ligament
4. Interspinous ligament
5. Ligamentum flavum

Table A–2 Correlation Between Nerve Roots Involved, the Pain Dermatome, the Muscle Weakness, and the Missing or Diminished Reflex

Root Injury	Dermatome Pain	Muscles Supplied	Movement Weakness	Reflex Involved
C5	Lower lateral aspect of upper arm	Deltoid and biceps	Shoulder abduction, elbow flexion	Biceps
C6	Lateral aspect of forearm	Extensor carpi radialis longus and brevis	Wrist extensors	Brachioradialis
C7	Middle finger	Triceps and flexor carpi radialis	Extension of elbow and flexion of wrist	Triceps
C8	Medial aspect of forearm	Flexor digitorum superficialis and profundus	Finger flexion	None
L1	Groin	Iliopsoas	Hip flexion	Cremaster
L2	Anterior aspect of thigh	Iliopsoas, sartorius, hip adductors	Hip flexion, hip adduction	Cremaster
L3	Medial aspect of knee	Iliopsoas, sartorius, quadriceps, hip adductors	Hip flexion, knee extension, hip adduction	Patellar
L4	Medial aspect of calf	Tibialis anterior, quadriceps	Foot inversion, knee extension	Patellar
L5	Lateral part of lower leg and dorsum of foot	Extensor hallucis longus, extensor digitorum longus	Toe extension, ankle dorsiflexion	None
S1	Lateral edge of foot	Gastrocnemius, soleus	Ankle plantar flexion	Ankle jerk
S2	Posterior part of thigh	Flexor digitorum longus, flexor hallucis longus	Ankle plantar flexion, toe flexion	None

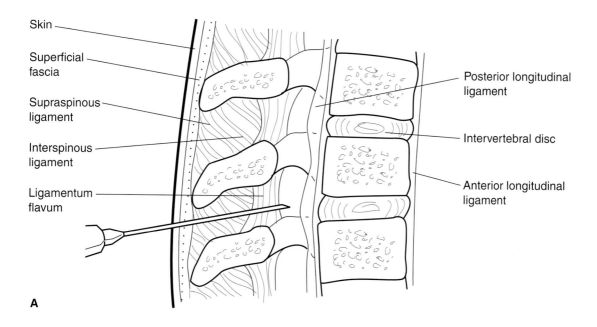

Skin
Superficial fascia
Supraspinous ligament
Interspinous ligament
Ligamentum flavum

Posterior longitudinal ligament
Intervertebral disc
Anterior longitudinal ligament

A

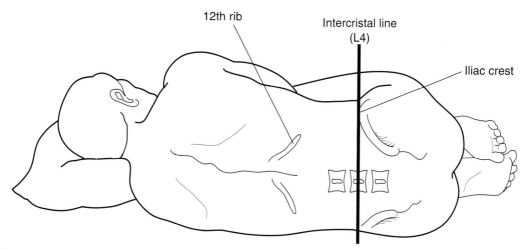

12th rib
Intercristal line (L4)
Iliac crest

B

Figure A–5   **A**. Structures penetrated by the spinal tap needle before it reaches the dura mater. **B**. Important anatomic landmarks when performing a spinal tap. Although this is usually performed in a lateral recumbent position with the vertebral column well flexed, the patient may be placed in the sitting position and bent well forward.

6. Areolar tissue containing the internal vertebral venous plexus in the epidural space
7. Dura mater
8. Arachnoid mater

The **depth** to which the needle will have to pass will vary from an inch or less in children to as much as 4 in. (10 cm) in obese adults.

The **pressure** of the cerebrospinal fluid in the lateral recumbent position is normally about 60–150 mm of water.

See Table A-3 for physical characteristics and composition of the cerebrospinal fluid.

Table A–3   The Physical Characteristics and Composition of the Cerebrospinal Fluid

Appearance	Clear and colorless
Volume	130 ml
Rate of production	0.5 ml/min
Pressure (lumbar puncture with patient in lateral recumbent position)	60–150 mm of water
Composition	
Protein	15–45 mg/100 ml
Glucose	50–85 mg/100 ml
Chloride	720–750 mg/100 ml
No. of cells	0–3 lymphocytes/cu mm

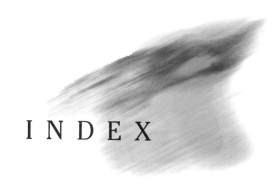

INDEX